New Frontiers in Clinical Pathology

New Frontiers in Clinical Pathology

Edited by Cecilia Bryant

hayle
medical

New York

Hayle Medical,
750 Third Avenue, 9th Floor,
New York, NY 10017, USA

Visit us on the World Wide Web at:
www.haylemedical.com

ISBN: 978-1-63241-730-5

Cataloging-in-Publication Data

New frontiers in clinical pathology / edited by Cecilia Bryant.
    p. cm.
Includes bibliographical references and index.
ISBN 978-1-63241-730-5
1. Diagnosis, Laboratory. 2. Diagnosis. 3. Pathology. I. Bryant, Cecilia.
RB37 .N49 2019
616.075--dc23

Table of Contents

Permissions

List of Contributors

Index

Preface

Every book is a source of knowledge and this one is no exception. The idea that led to the conceptualization of this book was the fact that the world is advancing rapidly; which makes it crucial to document the progress in every field. I am aware that a lot of data is already available, yet, there is a lot more to learn. Hence, I accepted the responsibility of editing this book and contributing my knowledge to the community.

The diagnosis of diseases based on a laboratory analysis of bodily fluids, such as urine, blood, etc. and tissue homogenates or extracts, is under the scope of clinical pathology. Such investigations are guided by an understanding of chemistry, hematology, microbiology and molecular pathology. It is aided by tools such as microscopes, analyzers, centrifugal machines and strips, etc. A diagnosis is made by performing a macroscopic examination, a microscopic examination, automated analysis and a culture. The visual examination of a sample is part of the macroscopic analysis, while the microscopic analysis allows a pathologist to determine whether the liquid is normal, infectious, inflammatory or tumoral. The latter stage also allows the determination of the causal infectious agent, if any, such as a mould, yeast, bacterium, parasite or a virus. Automated analyzers measure different chemicals and other parameters with minimal human assistance. Clinical pathology, primarily for medical purposes use a culture media for various examinations. It is a field of medical science that has undergone rapid development over the past few decades. This book explores all the important aspects of clinical pathology, in the present day scenario. In this book, using case studies and examples, constant effort has been made to make the understanding of the difficult concepts of clinical pathology as easy and informative as possible, for the readers.

While editing this book, I had multiple visions for it. Then I finally narrowed down to make every chapter a sole standing text explaining a particular topic, so that they can be used independently. However, the umbrella subject sinews them into a common theme. This makes the book a unique platform of knowledge.

I would like to give the major credit of this book to the experts from every corner of the world, who took the time to share their expertise with us. Also, I owe the completion of this book to the never-ending support of my family, who supported me throughout the project.

Editor

Clinical chemistry profiles in injection heroin users from Coastal Region, Kenya

Tom Were[1*], Jesca O Wesongah[2], Elly Munde[3], Collins Ouma[3], Titus M Kahiga[4], Francisca Ongecha-Owuor[5], James N Kiarie[6], Aabid A Ahmed[7], Ernest P Makokha[8] and Valentine Budambula[9]

Abstract

Background: Although the co-burden of injection drug use and HIV is increasing in Africa, little is known about the laboratory markers of injection drug use and anti-retroviral treatment (ART) in Kenyan injection drug users. This study, therefore, aimed at determining the clinical chemistry profiles and identifying the key laboratory markers of HIV infection during ART in injection heroin users (IHUs).

Methods: Clinical chemistry measurements were performed on serum samples collected from HIV-1 infected ART-experienced (n = 22), naive (n = 16) and HIV-1 negative (n = 23) IHUs, and healthy controls (n = 15) from Mombasa, coastal Kenya.

Results: HIV uninfected IHUs had lower alanine aminotransferase (ALT) levels ($P = 0.023$) as ART-exposed IHUs exhibited lower albumin ($P = 0.014$) and higher AST to platelet index (APRI) ($P < 0.0001$). All IHUs presented with lower aspartate aminotransferase to ALT values ($P = 0.001$) and higher C-reactive protein (CRP) levels ($P = 0.002$). ART-naive IHUs had higher globulin levels ($P = 0.013$) while ART-experienced and naive IHUs had higher albumin to total protein ($P < 0.0001$) and albumin to globulin ($P < 0.0001$) values. In addition, CD4+ T cells correlated with ALT ($\rho = -0.522$, $P = 0.011$) and CRP (rho, $\rho = 0.529$, $P = 0.011$) in HIV negative and ART-experienced IHUs, respectively. HIV-1 viral load correlated with albumin to globulin index in ART-experienced ($\rho = -0.468$, $P = 0.037$) and naive ($\rho = -0.554$, $P = 0.040$) IHUs; and with albumin to total protein index ($\rho = -0.554$, $P = 0.040$) and globulin ($\rho = 0.570$, $P = 0.033$) in ART-naive IHUs.

Conclusion: Absolute ALT, albumin, globulin, and CRP measurements in combination with APRI, AST to ALT, albumin to total protein and albumin to globulin indices may be useful laboratory markers for screening IHUs for initiating and monitoring treatment.

Keywords: Injection heroin user, Clinical chemistry markers, HIV-1 infection, Anti-retroviral treatment

Background

Of the 14 million people who inject drugs worldwide, 1.64 million are HIV infected [1]. In addition, more than 40% of new HIV infections in the world are attributed to injection drug use [2]. HIV sero-prevalence rates among injection drug users (IDUs) in Kenya are exceedingly high at 18%, and at least, 17% of new HIV infections in the country are linked to injection drug use [3]. Moreover, the rates of HIV transmission in injection drug users in the country are higher relative to the spread in the general population [4],

suggesting that injection drugs and substance use are important in promoting the spread of HIV in Kenya.

Although CD4+ T cell measurements are commonly used in initiating and monitoring disease progression and treatment in HIV-1 infected individuals [5], other biomarkers may not be specific to HIV infection due to concomitant illicit drug and poly-substance use among injection drug users. Since, addictive drugs such as opioids largely cause persistent immune stimulation inducing chronic inflammation [6], while anti-retroviral therapy cumulatively cause hepatotoxic injury [7], it is likely that HIV-1 infected injection drug users progressively develop intense inflammation and hepatotoxicity

---

* Correspondence: mugogwe@yahoo.com
[1]Department of Clinical Medicine, University of Kabianga, P. O. Box 2030–20200, Kericho, Kenya
Full list of author information is available at the end of the article

that can be indirectly assessed through determining hepatic functionality.

Injection drugs usually cause chronic liver degeneration and marked derangements in hepatic synthetic functions [6,8,9]. Elevated alanine aminotransferase (ALT), aspartate aminotransferase (AST), globulin, aspartate aminotransferase to platelet index (APRI), and C-reactive protein (CRP) levels are linked to injection drug use in both HIV infected and uninfected individuals [10-14]. In contrast, addictive heroin doses promote reductions in hepatic albumin synthesis [15]. Taken together, these studies suggest increased inflammatory-mediated hepatic derangements in both HIV infected and uninfected injection drug users.

However, no studies to date have investigated clinical chemistry profiles in injection heroin users, resident at coastal Mombasa, Kenya. The identification of clinical chemistry laboratory markers in this sub-population is of great importance, since it can assist in the clinical management of HIV in injection drug users. The current study, therefore, examined clinical chemistry laboratory markers in HIV-1 infected ART-experienced, naïve and HIV-1 non-infected injection heroin users, and healthy controls.

Methods
Study site and population
This cross-sectional clinical laboratory study was conducted as part of a larger study investigating the microbiological and immunological determinants of HIV infection among adult injection drug users. The study was undertaken at Bomu Hospital, a social enterprise facility in Mombasa, a coastal region of Kenya. Mombasa has a large injection drug using population of about 26,000, with heroin being the predominant injection drug [3]. Injection drug users were recruited via respondent driven sampling, snowball and makeshift outreach methods. Only individuals (age ≥18 yrs.) exhibiting needle scars, reporting injection heroin use at least once in the previous month and providing written informed consent were recruited into the study. Healthy controls were recruited from among HIV negative individuals presenting no evidence of illness and history of drug use.

Sample collection
From each injection drug user and healthy control, 10 ml of venous blood was collected. Of this, 5 ml was placed into both the EDTA and plain BD vacutainer® tubes (BD, Franklin Lakes, USA). The EDTA blood samples were used immediately after collection for hematological measurements and the enumeration of CD4+ T cells. Serum was obtained from clotted blood after clot retraction and centrifugation at 15,000 r.p.m for 10 minutes. The serum samples were used for the determinations of clinical chemistry analytes, HIV and hepatitis virus sero-testing, and viral loads.

HIV-1 diagnosis
HIV-1 testing was performed using rapid immunochromatographic tests, Determine™ (Abbott Laboratories, Tokyo, Japan) and Unigold™ (Trinity Biotech Plc, Bray, Ireland). Study participants with positive results for both Determine and Unigold were considered HIV infected based on the Kenyan national HIV testing algorithm [16].

HBV and HCV testing
Sero-diagnosis for the presence of hepatitis B virus (HBV) and hepatitis C virus (HCV) infections was performed using the one-step HBV-5 panel, and anti-HCV rapid diagnostic tests, respectively (Healthaw Medical limited, Hangzhou, China). Serum samples were tested for sero-reactivity against the HBV panel markers and anti-HCV. HBsAg and anti-HCV reactive individuals were considered sero-positive for HBV and/or HCV infection.

Clinical chemistry measurements
Direct clinical chemistry determinations were performed for ALT, AST, gamma-glutamyl transpeptidase (GGT), total protein, albumin, creatinine, urea, total cholesterol, high density lipoprotein (HDL), CRP, phosphocreatine kinase isoenzymes (CK-MB), and vitamin D using the automated clinical chemistry analyzer (Roche COBAS® 6000, Lausanne, Switzerland). Globulin was calculated by subtracting albumin concentrations from the total protein levels and the albumin to globulin ratio >1 was considered normal [17]. The reference values were based on our laboratory established reference ranges. APRI was determined as previously described [18], with AST upper limit values from laboratory established reference values (<37 U/L).

CD4+ T cell enumerations
Baseline CD4+ T cell counts were determined in an automated fashion using the BD FACSCalibur flow cytometer (Becton-Dickinson™, Franklin Lakes, USA). Briefly, 5.0 µl of EDTA blood samples were placed in a tube and RBC lysis buffer added. After 5 minute incubation, the cells were washed and fluorescent-tagged antibodies (anti-CD3, anti-CD4, and anti-CD45) were added. The cells were incubated for 30 minutes after which the samples were washed and the CD4+ T cells enumerated on the flow cytometer.

HIV-1 viral load
HIV-1 viral loads were determined using the automated Abbott m2000 System according to the manufacturer's instructions (Abbott Molecular Inc., Illinois, USA). Briefly, RNA was extracted from 0.2 ml serum samples and reverse-transcribed into cDNA. The cDNA was amplified using HIV-1-specific and internal control primers. Fluorescence intensity of the HIV-1 probe was converted into viral loads by the analyzer.

Ethical considerations

Ethical approval for the study was obtained from Kenyatta University Ethical Review Committee. Each participant gave written informed consent prior to enrolment into the study. Confidentiality of the study participant's information was ensured throughout the study by coding and limiting accessibility of the study information. The study participants benefited from free health education on HIV, tuberculosis (TB), hepatitis B and C, sexually transmitted infections, hygiene and nutrition. HIV-positive, TB-positive and HIV-TB co-infected individuals were referred to the comprehensive care centers at Bomu Hospital or the Coast General Provincial Hospital for treatment, support and care.

Statistical analysis

Statistical analysis was conducted using IBM® SPSS Statistics 19.0 (SPSS Inc. Chicago, USA). Continuous data (age, and laboratory measures) summarized as medians (IQR) and categorical data (gender, duration of injection, and non-injection drugs) presented as proportions were tabulated. Differences in the proportions were determined using the chi-square tests. Statistical comparisons of the continuous data across the study groups were performed using non-parametric ANOVA (Kruskal Wallis) tests followed by Bonferroni post-hoc corrections for multiple comparisons. Spearman's rank correlation tests were used to determine the associations of clinical chemistry measures with CD4+ T cells and viral loads within the study groups. A two-sided probability value <0.05 was considered statistically significant. Bonferroni correction for multiple comparisons were determined by dividing the criterion $P < 0.05$ by the total number of the study groups ($P < 0.05/4 = P < 0.0125$). The $P < 0.0125$ was then used for statistical inferences following between-group Mann Whitney U comparisons.

Results

Demographic and laboratory characteristics of the study participants

The study population comprised both male (n = 39) and female (n = 37) adult participants. These comprised of HIV-1 infected ART-experienced (n = 22), naive (n = 16) and HIV-1 non-infected (n = 23) injection heroin users, and healthy controls (HC, n = 15). Table 1 summarizes the clinical, laboratory and demographic characteristics of the study participants. The ages of the study participants were significantly different ($P = 0.008$). Additionally, between-group analysis showed that the anti-retroviral treatment-exposed injection heroin users were relatively older than the healthy controls ($P = 0.003$). The proportions of male and female participants were comparable across the study groups ($P = 0.351$). Use of heroin as an injection drug was common in all the injection heroin users ($P = 0.999$). As

non-injection drugs; the use of *bhang*, rohypnol, cigarettes, cocktail and alcohol were not significantly different among the injection heroin users ($P = 0.584$, $P = 0.338$, $P = 0.972$, $P = 0.351$ and $P = 0.076$, respectively). Across group analysis revealed a statistically significant difference in the CD4+ T cell counts/μL ($P < 0.0001$) with the anti-retroviral treatment-exposed (median, 301; IQR, 426) and treatment-naive (median, 448; IQR, 337) groups presenting with lower counts in comparison to HIV uninfected injection heroin users (median, 986; IQR, 474) and healthy controls (median, 755; IQR 463) ($P < 0.0001$ for all between-group comparisons). The lower limit of HIV-1 viral load quantification was 150 (2.18 $\log_{10}$) copies/ml of serum sample, and median viral loads were comparable between both anti-retroviral treatment-naive and anti-retroviral treatment-exposed individuals ($P = 0.163$) (Table 1).

Clinical chemistry measurements

While across group analysis did not show significant differences in the levels of phosphocreatine kinase iso-enzymes (CK-MB) ($P = 0.964$), the levels of CRP differed significantly across the study groups ($P = 0.002$). Subsequent post-hoc corrections revealed significantly higher levels of CRP in anti-retroviral treatment-exposed (median, 4.0 mg/L; IQR, 7.8; $P = 0.001$), anti-retroviral treatment-naive (median, 3.8 mg/L; IQR, 14.2; $P < 0.0001$) and in HIV-1 uninfected injection heroin users (median, 6.1 mg/L; IQR, 8.4; $P = 0.001$) in comparison to healthy controls (median, 0.7 mg/L; IQR, 0.9) signifying the importance of CRP as an inflammation marker of injection heroin use.

Additional analyses revealed statistical differences in the activity of ALT among the study groups ($P = 0.023$). Between-group tests showed lower ALT levels (U/L) in HIV uninfected injection heroin users (median, 11.0; IQR, 5.5) compared to healthy controls (median, 13.7; IQR, 12.7; $P = 0.005$). However, across group analysis did not reveal any differences in the activity of AST and GGT among the study groups ($P = 0.341$ and $P = 0.504$, respectively). Furthermore, no statistical differences were found in the levels of total cholesterol, HDL cholesterol and the ratio of total cholesterol to HDL cholesterol across the study groups ($P = 0.176$, $P = 0.828$ and $P = 0.117$, respectively). The levels of total protein, creatinine, urea and vitamin D were also comparable across the study groups ($P = 0.147$, $P = 0.840$, $P = 0.135$ and $P = 0.064$, respectively). Across group comparison of albumin levels (g/L) further revealed that there were significant differences ($P = 0.014$), with a further between-group analyses indicating that in anti-retroviral treatment-exposed injection heroin users, albumin levels (median, 41.1; IQR, 10.5) were significantly lower compared to the healthy controls (median, 48.0; IQR, 3.7; $P < 0.0001$). Further analysis indicated that the levels of globulin (g/L) in the anti-retroviral

Table 1 Demographic, clinical and laboratory characteristics of the study participants

Characteristic	HIV-1 uninfected		HIV-1 infected		P
	HC, n = 15	IHUs, n = 23	ART-naive IHUs, n = 16	ART-exposed IHUs, n = 22	
Age, yrs.	25.6 (8.7)	29.2 (7.1)	31.2 (5.9)	33.1 (8.5)[a]	**0.008**
Female/male, (%)	40.0/60.0	39.1/60.9	50.0/50.0	63.6/36.4	0.351
Injection drugs, n (%)					
Heroin	-	23 (100.0)	16 (100.0)	22 (100.0)	0.999
Diazepam	-	0 (0.0)	3 (18.8)	2 (9.1)	-
Duration of injection, n (%)					
<1 yr.	-	12 (52.2)	2 (12.5)	4 (18.2)	
1-3 yrs.	-	7 (30.4)	9 (56.2)	5 (22.7)	-
>3 yrs.	-	4 (17.4)	5 (31.3)	13 (59.1)	
Non-injection drugs, n (%)					
Bhang	-	8 (34.8)	7 (43.8)	11 (50.0)	0.584
Brown sugar	-	3 (13.1)	2 (12.5)	5 (22.7)	-
Rohypnol	-	12 (52.2)	9 (56.2)	16 (72.7)	0.338
Cigarettes	-	18 (78.3)	12 (75.0)	17 (77.3)	0.972
Khat	-	5 (21.7)	3 (18.8)	8 (36.4)	-
Cocktail	-	5 (21.7)	6 (37.5)	9 (40.9)	0.351
Alcohol	-	8 (34.8)	9 (56.2)	15 (68.2)	0.076
CD4+ T cell count/µl	755 (463)	986 (474)	448 (337)[a,b]	301 (426)[a,b]	**<0.0001**
Viral loads, copies/µl	-	-	13,470 (81,176)	150 (17,761)	0.163
Hepatitis B	-	1 (4.3)	2 (12.5)	1 (4.5)	-
Hepatitis C	-	1 (4.3)	3 (18.8)	5 (22.7)	-

Data shown are medians (IQR) unless indicated. HC, healthy controls. ART, anti-retroviral treatment. HIV-1, human immunodeficiency virus-1. IHUs, injection heroin users. Brown sugar, crude heroin. Cocktail, cigarette and bhang mixture. Data analysis was conducted using chi-square for proportions; and Kruskal Wallis tests for continuous data. Following the Kruskal Wallis tests, post-hoc Bonferroni corrections for multiple comparisons were performed based on the Mann Whitney between-group tests (significant at P < 0.0125). [a]ART-exposed and ART-naive IHUs vs. HC, P < 0.01. [b]ART-exposed and ART-naive IHUs vs. HIV-1 uninfected IHUs, P < 0.0001. Values in bold are statistically significant at P-values indicated.

treatment-naive injection heroin users (median, 51.2; IQR, 17.5) were higher compared to the healthy controls (median, 35.1; IQR, 11.1; $P < 0.0001$) and the HIV uninfected injection heroin users (median, 36.6; IQR 10.4; $P < 0.0001$) (Table 2).

AST, ALT, albumin, globulin and platelet ratios

Values for the AST to ALT ratio varied across the groups ($P = 0.001$) and were higher in the anti-retroviral treatment-exposed injection heroin users (median, 1.6; IQR, 0.8; $P < 0.01$), anti-retroviral treatment-naive injection heroin users (median, 2.1; IQR, 0.9; $P < 0.01$) and HIV negative injection heroin users (median, 1.8; IQR, 1.0; $P < 0.01$) relative to healthy controls (median, 1.1; IQR, 0.7). In addition, at least a quarter of the anti-retroviral treatment-exposed (27.3%), treatment-naive (62.5%) and HIV negative injection heroin users (43.5%) had AST to ALT ratio ≥2.0, indicating increased liver damage in both HIV infected and uninfected injection heroin users.

Albumin to total protein ratio differed in the groups ($P < 0.0001$) and were significantly lower in the anti-retroviral treatment-exposed (median, 0.5; IQR, 0.1) and treatment-naive (median, 0.4; IQR, 0.2) groups compared to HIV negative injection heroin users (median, 0.6; IQR, 0.1) and healthy controls (median, 0.6; IQR, 0.1; $P < 0.01$ and $P < 0.0001$, respectively). Likewise, albumin to globulin ratio varied in the study groups ($P < 0.0001$) such that the anti-retroviral treatment-experienced (median, 1.0; IQR, 0.5) and naive (median, 0.8; IQR, 0.6) individuals had lower values in comparison to HIV negative group (median, 1.5; IQR, 0.4; $P = 0.002$) and healthy controls (median, 1.4; IQR, 0.3; $P < 0.0001$).

APRI differed significantly across the study groups ($P = 0.005$) with the anti-retroviral treatment-exposed group (median, 0.25; IQR, 0.20) having higher values compared to the healthy controls (median, 0.14; IQR, 0.10; $P = 0.001$). Moreover, the frequency of moderate-to-severe forms (i.e., APRI ≥ 0.5) of liver damage was only noted in anti-retroviral treatment-exposed (18.2%)

Table 2 Clinical chemistry measurements of the study participants

Marker	HIV-1 uninfected		HIV-1 infected		P
	HC, n = 15	IHUs, n = 23	ART-naive IHUs, n = 16	ART-exposed IHUs, n = 22	
CK-MB, U/L	18.0 (15.0)	17.0 (12.0)	17.5 (16.3)	18.0 (26.8)	0.946
CRP, mg/L	0.7 (0.9)	6.1 (8.4)[a]	3.8 (14.2)[a]	4.0 (7.8)[a]	**0.002**
CRP > 5.0 mg/L, n (%)	1 (6.7)	14 (60.9)	7 (43.8)	9 (40.9)	-
ALT, U/L	13.7 (12.7)	11.0 (5.5)[a]	10.7 (5.4)	15.2 (11.0)	**0.023**
M > 40; F > 31, n (%)	2 (13.3)	0 (0.0)	1 (6.3)	2 (9.1)	-
AST, U/L	19.5 (9.4)	21.7 (13.0)	22.4 (10.8)	24.9 (14.1)	0.341
AST/ALT	1.1 (0.7)	1.8 (1.0)[a]	2.1 (0.9)[a]	1.6 (0.8)[a]	**0.001**
AST/ALT ≥2.0, n (%)	0 (0.0)	10 (43.5)	10 (62.5)	6 (27.3)	-
APRI	0.14 (0.10)	0.23 (0.20)	0.19 (0.10)	0.25 (0.20)[a]	**0.005**
APRI ≥0.5, n (%)	0 (0.0)	0 (0.0)	1 (6.3)	4 (18.2)	-
GGT, U/L	23.0 (28.1)	27.0 (20.1)	27.5 (39.0)	41.5 (45.0)	0.504
TC, mmol/L	5.0 (1.5)	4.1 (2.0)	4.3 (1.9)	4.2 (1.6)	0.176
HDL, mmol/L	1.3 (0.5)	1.3 (0.7)	1.1 (0.7)	1.1 (0.8)	0.828
TC/HDL	3.5 (1.0)	3.3 (1.7)	3.9 (1.0)	4.0 (1.5)	0.117
ALB, g/L	48.0 (3.7)	45.3 (17.8)	41.5 (14.3)	41.1 (10.5)[a]	**0.014**
ALB <32.0 g/L, n (%)	0 (0.0)	1 (4.3)	2 (12.5)	2 (9.1)	-
Total PROT, g/L	82.3 (15.9)	84.4 (22.8)	90.2 (27.7)	82.0 (27.8)	0.147
ALB/PROT	0.6 (0.1)	0.6 (0.1)	0.4 (0.2)[a,b]	0.5 (0.1)[a,b]	**<0.0001**
GLB, g/L	35.1 (11.1)	36.6 (10.4)	51.2 (17.5)[a,b]	41.5 (32.9)	**0.013**
ALB/GLB	1.4 (0.3)	1.5 (0.4)	0.8 (0.6)[a,b]	1.0 (0.5)[a,b]	**<0.0001**
ALB/GLB ≤1, n (%)	0 (0.0)	3 (13.0)	10 (62.5)	11 (50.0)	-
Creatinine, µmol/L	80.0 (23.0)	72.0 (30.0)	75.0 (30.0)	81.0 (29.0)	0.840
Urea, mmol/L	3.5 (1.2)	2.9 (2.5)	2.8 (0.6)	3.0 (1.4)	0.135
Vitamin D, ng/ml	30.7 (8.2)	32.0 (15.0)	35.3 (23.3)	38.3 (13.3)	0.064

Data presented are medians (IQR) unless indicated. HC, healthy controls. ART, anti-retroviral treatment. HIV-1, human immunodeficiency virus-1. IHUs, injection heroin users. CK-MB, phosphocreatine kinase isoenzymes. CRP, C-reactive protein. AST, aspartate aminotransferase. ALT, alanine aminotransferase. APRI, aspartate to platelet index. GGT, gamma-glutamyl transpeptidase. TC, total cholesterol. HDL, high density lipoprotein cholesterol. PROT, protein. ALB, albumin. GLB, globulin. Vitamin D3, 1,25-dihydroxyvitamin D. Data analysis was conducted using chi-square for proportions; and Kruskal Wallis tests for continuous data. Following the Kruskal Wallis tests, post-hoc Bonferroni corrections for multiple comparisons were performed based on the Mann Whitney between-group tests (significant at $P < 0.0125$). [a]ART-exposed, ART-naive or HIV uninfected IHUs vs. HC, $P < 0.01$. [b]ART-exposed and ART-naive IHUs vs. HIV-1 uninfected IHUs, $P < 0.01$. Values in bold are statistically significant at P-values indicated.

and -naive (6.3%) individuals (Table 2), suggesting increased liver derangements in HIV infected injection heroin users.

Correlation of the clinical chemistry markers with CD4+ T cells and HIV viral loads

CD4+ T cells inversely correlated with ALT levels ($\rho = -0.522$; $P = 0.011$; Figure 1A) in HIV uninfected injection heroin users and positively with the CRP levels ($\rho = 0.529$; $P = 0.011$; Figure 1B) in HIV infected anti-retroviral treatment-experienced injection heroin users.

HIV-1 viral loads inversely correlated with albumin to globulin ($\rho = -0.468$, $P = 0.037$; Figure 2A) ratio in HIV infected anti-retroviral treatment-exposed injection heroin users. In addition, the HIV-1 viral loads inversely

correlated with albumin to globulin ($\rho = -0.554$; $P = 0.040$; Figure 2B) and the albumin to total protein ($\rho = -0.554$; $P = 0.040$; Figure 2C) values, and positively with globulin ($\rho = 0.570$; $P = 0.033$; Figure 2D) in HIV infected anti-retroviral treatment-naive injection heroin users.

Discussion

Clinical chemistry laboratory analysis constitutes a key step in patient assessment for initiating and monitoring response to anti-retroviral treatment [5]. The reliability and accuracy of clinical chemistry analytes, however, is confounded by complex interaction between injection drug use and anti-retroviral drugs. Therefore, this cross-sectional clinical laboratory study determined the clinical chemistry markers in

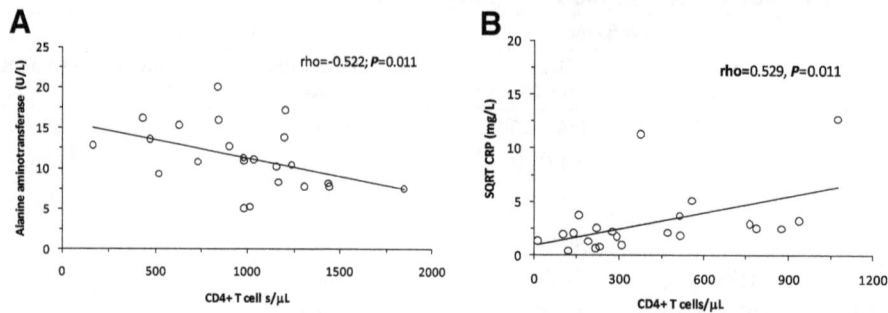

Figure 1 Correlations of CD4+ T cell counts with alanine aminotransferase and C-reactive protein. Correlations of the CD4+ T cells with alanine aminotransferase and C-reactive protein levels were determined using the Spearman's rank correlation test. **(A)** Correlation between CD4+ T cells and alanine aminotransferase in HIV uninfected injection heroin users (n = 23). **(B)** Correlation between CD4+ T cells and square root of the C-reactive protein (SQRT CRP) in HIV infected ART-exposed injection heroin users (n = 22).

HIV infected and uninfected injection heroin users from coastal Kenya.

Absolute albumin levels and albumin to total protein ratio reductions observed in the HIV-1 infected injection drug users are indications of derangements in protein metabolism. The decreases in the albumin levels can be attributed to low dietary intake of proteins that is linked to low synthesis of albumin [19], a feature of malnutrition that is frequently observed among injection drug users presenting with and without HIV infection [20]. It is also possible that suppression of albumin results from inhibition of hepatic synthesis at abusive doses of heroin

[15]. In addition, opioid-induced hepatotoxicities and inflammatory-mediated hepatic damage cause reduced hepatic synthetic functions [15,21]. Thus, findings presented here suggest that injection heroin use among HIV-infected individuals promote increased reductions in the albumin levels and marked alterations in the albumin to total protein ratio.

The inverse associations of HIV viral load and albumin to total protein and albumin to globulin indices in the anti-retroviral-naive injection heroin users signify disease progression but during treatment the albumin to globulin ratio is inverted indicating reductions in the

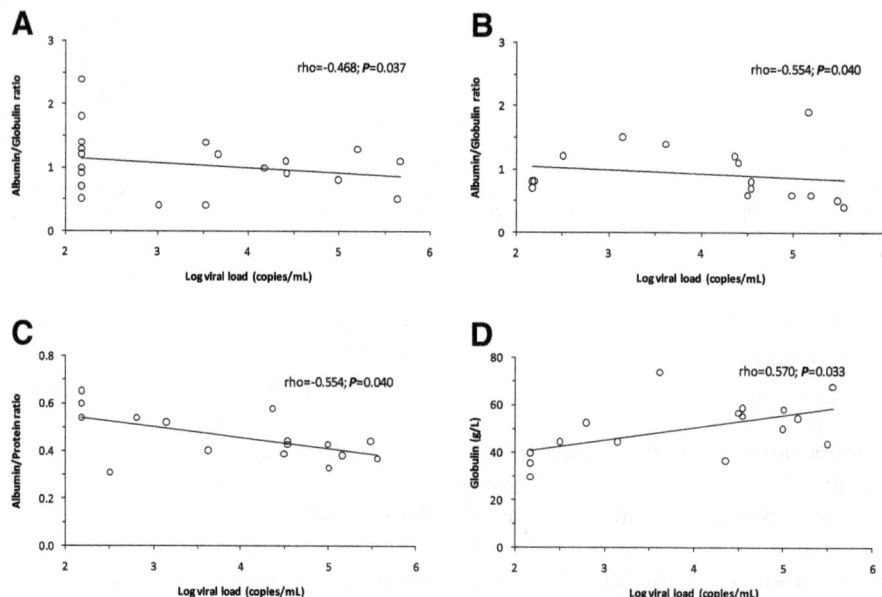

Figure 2 Correlations of HIV-1 viral load with albumin to globulin, albumin to total protein and globulin. Correlations of the HIV-1 viral loads with albumin to globulin, albumin to total protein and globulin levels were determined using the Spearman's rank correlation test. **(A)** Correlation between HIV-1 viral load and albumin to globulin index in anti-retroviral treatment-exposed injection heroin users (n = 22). **(B)** Correlation between HIV-1 viral load and albumin to globulin index in anti-retroviral treatment-naive injection heroin users (n = 16). **(C)** Correlation between HIV-1 viral load and albumin to total protein index in anti-retroviral treatment-naive injection heroin users (n = 16). **(D)** Correlation between HIV-1 viral load and calculated globulin in anti-retroviral treatment-naive injection heroin users (n = 16).

viral loads and immune reconstitution. This premise is, in part, consistent with clinical studies in HIV infected patients commencing highly active anti-retroviral therapy showing that hypoalbuminaemia is associated with morbidity and mortality [22,23]. Therefore, reduced albumin and low albumin to total protein ratio are important laboratory measures in injection heroin users that can be utilized as important surrogates for screening and for initiating and monitoring of anti-retroviral treatment in HIV infected injection heroin users.

In contrast to previous studies, a higher globulin level was found in the HIV infected injection heroin users naive for anti-retroviral treatment [17]. This finding suggests that hyperglobulinaemia is an important laboratory marker of HIV infected patients injecting illicit drugs. Hyperglobulinaemia characterizes B cell dysfunction during primary HIV infections and persisting into chronic infections [24]. The lower median albumin to globulin values in the presence of higher proportions of ratios ≤1.0, and the correlations of HIV viral loads with globulin in the anti-retroviral treatment-naive individuals, further corroborate increased derangements in B cell functions in both HIV infected and uninfected injection heroin users. The findings of the current study also parallel studies showing elevated globulin and the albumin to globulin ratio in Australian drug addicts [12]. In addition, elevations in total IgM and IgG, specific anti-morphine IgM, and cross-reactive IgM auto-antibodies were recorded in HIV infected and uninfected opioid users [25-27]. Hence, it appears heroin-induced antibodies promote inflammation leading to liver damage in injection users. Elevated globulin with concomitant lower albumin to globulin ratio may thus be a useful biomarker for clinical laboratory assessment of HIV infected and uninfected injection heroin users.

Reduced absolute ALT levels found in the HIV sero-negative injection heroin users, indicate reduced hepatic functionality. However, the higher AST to ALT ratio and proportions of AST to ALT ratio ≥2.0 in the HIV sero-negative and infected injection heroin users naive or on anti-retroviral treatment, suggest synergistic heroin and anti-retroviral drug-induced hepatic inflammation. These results are similar to observations showing that the AST to ALT ratio is a better measure of liver enzyme activity [28]. In addition, the results are, in part, supported by the elevated AST, AST to ALT ratios, and higher proportions of ALT observed in patients on anti-retroviral treatment [10-12]. Since a large number of the injection heroin users in the present study were concomitantly consuming alcohol and *khat*, it is possible that these non-injection substances synergistically promote the alterations in the ALT levels [10,29]. Importantly, the inverse correlations of absolute ALT levels and the CD4+ T cell counts in the HIV sero-negative

injection heroin users, suggests that the CD4+ T cell count can also be utilized as a surrogate marker of liver function in the management of HIV negative heroin users.

The greater magnitude APRI median values and proportions ≥0.5 in the HIV infected injection heroin users on anti-retroviral treatment, suggests, that APRI is a better screening indicator of heroin and anti-retroviral treatment in this population. This observation is, in part, parallel to the time-dependent increases and prognostic value of APRI among HIV and hepatitis C co-infected patients undergoing anti-retroviral treatment [7], and studies in injection drug users showing the utility of APRI in predicting hepatic fibrosis [30]. It is, therefore, likely that increased hepatotoxicity in HIV patients on anti-retroviral treatment results from the synergistic effect of anti-retroviral drugs, heroin and poly-substance consumption. Hence, APRI and proportions of APRI ≥0.5 are important measures for evaluating the degree of hepatoxicity in HIV infected injection heroin users undergoing anti-retroviral treatment.

Elevations of the C-reactive protein in all the study groups of injection heroin users is similar to previous studies showing elevated C-reactive protein in Australian drug addicts [12], and higher C-reactive protein levels in buprenorphine injection users in Singapore [31]. Higher levels and proportions of individuals of this acute phase protein in both HIV infected and uninfected injection heroin users in the present study are indicative of increased liver synthesis following consumption of the illicit drugs, infection and cytokine release [32]. In addition, the increases indicate heightened liver damage through illicit drug- and anti-retroviral treatment-mediated necrosis, apoptosis, and immune mechanisms. Of significance are analyses showing positive correlations between the C-reactive protein levels and the CD4+ T cell count in injection heroin users on anti-retroviral treatment. This result may reflect development of immune reconstitution inflammatory syndrome (IRIS) in the injection heroin users on anti-retroviral treatment resulting from poor adherence and illicit drug use. Consistent with this hypothesis, previous studies illustrated a link between IRIS and low adherence to anti-retroviral therapy, alcohol use, and low suppression of viral load among South African adults initiating anti-retroviral therapy [33]. Implications of this observation include utilization of the C-reactive protein in assessing immune reconstitution following initiation of anti-retroviral treatment in injection heroin users.

Our results clearly show high rates of poly-drug use among injection heroin users in Mombasa. It is highly likely that the complex interactions of opioids and/or active compounds in bhang (Δ9-tetrahydrocannabinol), cigarettes (nicotine), rohypnol (benzodiazepines), alcohol, khat (cathinone), and anti-retroviral drugs promote the occurrence of drug dependence and adverse events. With regards to clinical chemistry profiles, such complex interactions induce hepatic metabolic derangements leading to toxicity and altered profiles of clinical chemistry markers. Consistent with these propositions, previous studies among drug users showed that interactions between opioids and benzodiazepines or alcohol increase occurrence of adverse events, overdose and death [34], as nicotine increase rates of opioid consumption [35]. In addition, drugs of abuse (alcohol, opioids, benzodiazepines, marijuana, and nicotine) reduce the efficacy of anti-retroviral drugs leading to toxicity, treatment failure and high viral loads [36]. Taken together, poly-drug use appears to promote toxicity leading to altered clinical chemistry profiles in both HIV-1 infected and uninfected injection drug users.

While a prospective design would have been important in examining the utility of clinical chemistry markers, in response to drug rehabilitation and HIV treatment, this cross-sectional study provides the first baseline information for screening of injection drug users for initiating and monitoring anti-retroviral treatments in Kenya. Although recruitment into this study was based on self-reported injection heroin use, it is possible that the study participants were also using other opioids, hence the need to carry out toxicological analyses to provide additional insights into the complex interactions between injection drugs and anti-retroviral treatment. These collectively can be linked to clinical laboratory markers and patient prognosis in a prospective approach.

Conclusions

This study provides further evidence that chronic inflammation in HIV infected and uninfected injection heroin users is characterized by derangements in hepatic synthetic functions. Our data suggest that injection heroin, HIV infection and anti-retroviral treatment differentially alter ALT; albumin; APRI and AST to ALT, albumin to total protein and albumin to globulin indices; C-reactive protein; and globulin in injection drug users.

Competing interests

None of the authors have a commercial relationship or financial conflict of interest as part of this study.

Authors' contributions

TW and VB conceived and designed the study, and performed the experiments, and along with AA, JW, CO, TMK, FO, and JNK designed the study. TW performed statistical analyses and interpretation of data, and co-drafted the manuscript with EM and VB. EPM and CO critically revised the manuscript. All authors have read and approved the manuscript.

Acknowledgements

We thank the study participants for making this study possible. We are grateful to the management and staff of the Bomu Hospital for their support during the study. This study was supported, in part, by the Kenya National Commission for Science, Technology and Innovation [NCST/5/003/065], and Partnership for Innovative Medical Education in Kenya (NIH 1R24TW008889) grants to TW and VB.

Author details

[1]Department of Clinical Medicine, University of Kabianga, P. O. Box 2030-20200, Kericho, Kenya. [2]Department of Medical Laboratory Sciences, Jomo Kenyatta University of Agriculture and Technology, Juja, Kenya. [3]Department of Biomedical Sciences and Technology, Maseno University, Maseno, Kenya. [4]Department of Pharmacy and Complementary Medicine, Kenyatta University, Nairobi, Kenya. [5]Department of Medicine, Therapeutics, Dermatology and Psychiatry, Kenyatta University, Nairobi, Kenya. [6]Department of Obstetrics and Gynaecology, University of Nairobi, Nairobi, Kenya. [7]Bomu Hospital, Mombasa, Kenya. [8]Centre for Virus Research, Kenya Medical Research Institute, Nairobi, Kenya. [9]Department of Environment and Health Sciences, Technical University of Mombasa, Mombasa, Kenya.

References

1. UNODC: World Drug Report 2013. New York: The United Nations Office on Drugs and Crime; 2013.
2. UNAIDS: Global Report: UNAIDS Report on the Global AIDS Epidemic 2013. New York: Joint United Nations Programme on HIV/AIDS; 2013.
3. NASCOP: Rapid Situational Assessment of HIV Prevalence and Related Risky Behaviours Among Injecting Drug Users in Nairobi and Coast Provinces of Kenya. Kenya. National AIDS and STI Control Programme, Ministry of Health; 2012.
4. NASCOP: Kenya AIDS Indicator Survey 2012 Report. Kenya: National AIDS and STI Control Programme, Ministry of Health; 2013.
5. NASCOP: Guidelines for Antiretroviral Therapy in Kenya 2011. Kenya: National AIDS and STI Control Programme, Ministry of Health; 2012.
6. Reece AS: Chronic immune stimulation as a contributing cause of chronic disease in opiate addiction including multi-system ageing. Med Hypotheses 2010, 75(6):613–619.
7. Moodie EE, Pant Pai N, Klein MB: Is antiretroviral therapy causing long-term liver damage? A comparative analysis of HIV-mono-infected and HIV/hepatitis C co-infected cohorts. PLoS One 2009, 4(2):e4517.
8. Chen CK, Su LW, Lin SK: Characteristics of hospitalized heroin smokers and heroin injectors in Taiwan. Changgeng Yi Xue Za Zhi 1999, 22(2):197–203.
9. Weller IV, Cohn D, Sierralta A, Mitcheson M, Ross MG, Montano L, Scheuer P, Thomas HC: Clinical, biochemical, serological, histological and ultrastructural features of liver disease in drug abusers. Gut 1984, 25(4):417–423.
10. Drumright LN, Hagan H, Thomas DL, Latka MH, Golub ET, Garfein RS, Clapp JD, Campbell JV, Bonner S, Kapadia F, Thiel TK, Strathdee SA: Predictors and effects of alcohol use on liver function among young HCV-infected injection drug users in a behavioral intervention. J Hepatol 2011, 55(1):45–52.
11. Langohr K, Sanvisens A, Fuster D, Tor J, Serra I, Rey-Joly C, Rivas I, Muga R: Liver enzyme alterations in HCV-monoinfected and HCV/HIV-coinfected patients. Open AIDS J 2008, 2:82–88.
12. Reece AS: Evidence of accelerated ageing in clinical drug addiction from immune, hepatic and metabolic biomarkers. Immun Ageing 2007, 4:6.
13. Mehta SH, Vogt SL, Srikrishnan AK, Vasudevan CK, Murugavel KG, Saravanan S, Anand S, Kumar MS, Ray SC, Celentano DD, Solomon S, Solomon SS: Epidemiology of hepatitis C virus infection & liver disease among injection drug users (IDUs) in Chennai, India. Indian J Med Res 2011, 132:706–714.
14. Samikkannu T, Rao KV, Arias AY, Kalaichezian A, Sagar V, Yoo C, Nair MP: HIV infection and drugs of abuse: role of acute phase proteins. J Neuroinflammation 2013, 10:113.
15. Gomez-Lechon MJ, Ponsoda X, Jover R, Fabra R, Trullenque R, Castell JV: Hepatotoxicity of the opioids morphine, heroin, meperidine, and methadone to cultured human hepatocytes. Mol Toxicol 1987, 1(4):453–463.
16. NASCOP: Guidelines for HIV Testing and Counselling and Kenya. Kenya: National AIDS and STI Control Programme, Ministry of Health; 2010.
17. Serpa J, Haque D, Valayam J, Breaux K, Rodriguez-Barradas MC: Effect of combination antiretroviral treatment on total protein and calculated

globulin levels among HIV-infected patients. *Int J Infect Dis* 2010, **14**(Suppl 3):e41–e44.

18. Wai CT, Greenson JK, Fontana RJ, Kalbfleisch JD, Marrero JA, Conjeevaram HS, Lok AS: **A simple noninvasive index can predict both significant fibrosis and cirrhosis in patients with chronic hepatitis C.** *Hepatology* 2003, **38**(2):518–526.

19. Kaysen GA, Yeun J, Depner T: **Albumin synthesis, catabolism and distribution in dialysis patients.** *Miner Electrolyte Metab* 1997, **23**(3–6):218–224.

20. Forrester JE: **Nutritional alterations in drug abusers with and without HIV.** *Am J Infect Dis* 2006, **2**(3):173–179.

21. Valente MJ, Carvalho F, Bastos M, de Pinho PG, Carvalho M: **Contribution of oxidative metabolism to cocaine-induced liver and kidney damage.** *Curr Med Chem* 2012, **19**(33):5601–5606.

22. Dao CN, Peters PJ, Kiarie JN, Zulu I, Muiruri P, Ong'ech J, Mutsotso W, Potter D, Njobvu L, Stringer JS, Borkowf CB, Bolu O, Weidle PJ: **Hyponatremia, hypochloremia, and hypoalbuminemia predict an increased risk of mortality during the first year of antiretroviral therapy among HIV-infected Zambian and Kenyan women.** *AIDS Res Hum Retroviruses* 2011, **27**(11):1149–1155.

23. Sudfeld CR, Isanaka S, Aboud S, Mugusi FM, Wang M, Chalamilla GE, Fawzi WW: **Association of serum albumin concentration with mortality, morbidity, CD4 T-cell reconstitution among Tanzanians initiating antiretroviral therapy.** *J Infect Dis* 2013, **207**(9):1370–1378.

24. Titanji K, Chiodi F, Bellocco R, Schepis D, Osorio L, Tassandin C, Tambussi G, Grutzmeier S, Lopalco L, De Milito A: **Primary HIV-1 infection sets the stage for important B lymphocyte dysfunctions.** *AIDS* 2005, **19**(17):1947–1955.

25. Blanck RR, Ream N, Deegan MJ: **Immunoglobulins in heroin users.** *Am J Epidemiol* 1980, **111**(1):81–86.

26. Gamaleya N, Tagliaro F, Parshin A, Vrublevskii A, Bugari G, Dorizzi R, Ghielmi S, Marigo M: **Immune response to opiates: new findings in heroin addicts investigated by means of an original enzyme immunoassay and morphine determination in hair.** *Life Sci* 1993, **53**(2):99–105.

27. McGowan JP, Shah SS, Small CB, Klein RS, Schnipper SM, Chang CJ, Rosenstreich DL: **Relationship of serum immunoglobulin and IgG subclass levels to race, ethnicity and behavioral characteristics in HIV infection.** *Med Sci Monit* 2006, **12**(1):CR11–CR16.

28. Sorbi D, Boynton J, Lindor KD: **The ratio of aspartate aminotransferase to alanine aminotransferase: potential value in differentiating nonalcoholic steatohepatitis from alcoholic liver disease.** *Am J Gastroenterol* 1999, **94**(4):1018–1022.

29. Roelandt P, George C, D'Heygere F, Aerts R, Monbaliu D, Laleman W, Cassiman D, Verslype C, Van Steenbergen W, Pirenne J, Wilmer A, Nevens F: **Acute liver failure secondary to khat (Catha edulis)-induced necrotic hepatitis requiring liver transplantation: case report.** *Transplant Proc* 2011, **43**(9):3493–3495.

30. Wilson LE, Torbenson M, Astemborski J, Faruki H, Spoler C, Rai R, Mehta S, Kirk GD, Nelson K, Afdhal N, Thomas DL: **Progression of liver fibrosis among injection drug users with chronic hepatitis C.** *Hepatology* 2006, **43**(4):788–795.

31. Ho RC, Ho EC, Mak A: **Cutaneous complications among i.v. buprenorphine users.** *J Dermatol* 2009, **36**(1):22–29.

32. Lobo SM: **Sequential C-reactive protein measurements in patients with serious infections: does it help?** *Crit Care* 2012, **16**(3):130.

33. Nachega JB, Morroni C, Chaisson RE, Goliath R, Efron A, Ram M, Maartens G: **Impact of immune reconstitution inflammatory syndrome on antiretroviral therapy adherence.** *Patient Prefer Adherence* 2012, **6**:887–891.

34. Gudin JA, Mogali S, Jones JD, Comer SD: **Risks, management, and monitoring of combination opioid, benzodiazepines, and/or alcohol use.** *Postgrad Med* 2013, **125**(4):115–130.

35. Spiga R, Schmitz J, Day J II: **Effects of nicotine on methadone self-administration in humans.** *Drug Alcohol Dep* 1998, **50**(2):157–165.

36. Pal D, Kwatra D, Minocha M, Paturi DK, Budda B, Mitra AK: **Efflux transporters- and cytochrome P-450-mediated interactions between drugs of abuse and antiretrovirals.** *Life Sci* 2011, **88**(21–22):959–971.

2

Enrichment of the embryonic stem cell reprogramming factors Oct4, Nanog, Myc, and Sox2 in benign and malignant vascular tumors

Clarissa N. Amaya and Brad A. Bryan[*]

Abstract

Background: The "stem cell theory of cancer" states that a subpopulation of cells with stem cell-like properties plays a central role in the formation, sustainment, spread, and drug resistant characteristics of malignant tumors. Recent studies have isolated distinct cell populations from infantile hemangiomas that display properties equivalent to aberrant progenitor cells, suggesting that, in addition to malignant tumors, benign tumors may also contain a stem cell-like component.

Methods: In this study, the expression levels of the embryonic stem cell reprogramming factors Oct4, Nanog, Myc, Sox2, and Klf4 were examined via immunohistochemistry in a panel of 71 benign, borderline, and malignant vascular tumors including capillary hemangioma, cavernous hemangioma, granulomatous hemangioma, venous hemangioma, hemangioendothelioma, hemangiopericytoma, and angiosarcoma. Antigenicity for each protein was quantified based on staining intensity and percentage of tissue positive for each antigen, and subsequently compared to data obtained from two control tissue sets: 10 vascular tissues and a panel of 58 various malignant sarcomas.

Results and discussion: With the exception of Myc (which was only present in a subset of benign, borderline, and malignant tumors), Oct4, Nanog, Sox2, and Klf4 were detectable at variable levels across both normal and diseased tissues. Semi-quantitative evaluation of our immunohistochemical staining revealed that protein expression of Oct4, Nanog, Myc, and Sox2, but not Klf4, was significantly increased in benign, borderline, and malignant vascular tumors relative to non-diseased vascular tissue controls. Interestingly, the enhanced levels of Oct4, Nanog, Myc, and Sox2 protein were approximately equivalent between benign, borderline, and malignant vascular tumors.

Conclusions: These findings provide supporting evidence that enrichment for proteins involved in pluripotency is not restricted solely to malignant tumors as is suggested by the "stem cell theory of cancer", but additionally extends to common benign vascular tumors such as hemangiomas.

Background

The origin of cancer remains unclear, however the "cancer stem cell theory" postulates that a subpopulation of cancer cells with stem cell-like properties is responsible for sustaining long term tumor growth [1]. In addition, cancer stem cells give rise to metastases and can act as a reservoir that potentially leads to relapse after treatment has eliminated all observable signs of the cancer. These cancer stem cells are believed to be genotypically and/or phenotypically related to normal stem cells and share many of the features of normal stem cells such as self-renewal, drug resistance, and a proliferative potential to generate a multi-potent cellular lineage [2, 3]. The core transcription factors that control "stemness" in embryonic stem cells include Oct4, Sox2, Nanog, Myc, and Klf4, and the combination of these factors has been shown to successfully reprogram differentiated somatic cells into pluripotent stem cells [4]. There is substantial evidence that cancer stem cells express these specific markers and their activity contributes to the oncogenic properties inherent in this disease [5].

[*] Correspondence: brad.bryan@ttuhsc.edu
Department of Biomedical Sciences, Paul L. Foster School of Medicine, Texas Tech University Health Sciences Center, El Paso, TX, USA

In addition to malignant tumors, benign prostate, breast, and angiomyolipoma tumors express various stem cell markers, suggesting the expression of these markers is not limited exclusively to malignant tumors [6–9]. It was recently reported that benign infantile hemangiomas, which are the most common tumors of infancy, express higher levels of neural crest and stem cell markers at the mRNA level than dermal microvascular endothelial cells [10], and within this tumor type resides multiple cellular subpopulations expressing Oct4 and Nanog proteins [11]. Moreover, it was recently revealed that a clonogenic subpopulation of cells isolated from cutaneous infantile hemangiomas was capable of differentiating into endothelial cells, smooth muscle, or adipocytes [12], suggesting that a stem cell-like component may drive the etiology of this benign vascular tumor. These fascinating findings suggest that the "stem cell theory of cancer" may serve as a more generalized theory than is currently accepted, and extend to benign vascular tumors.

Thus, in this study we used immunohistochemical analysis to examine the expression of the stem cell reprogramming factors Oct4, Sox2, Nanog, Myc, and Klf4 in 71 diverse benign and malignant vascular tumors. Our findings surprisingly revealed that, relative to normal endothelial tissues, staining of benign and malignant vascular tumors demonstrated significantly higher expression of these stem cell reprogramming factors.

Methods

Immunohistochemistry (IHC)

Blood vessel disease spectrum tissue arrays containing various vascular tumors and non-diseased controls were purchased from US Biomax, Inc. (#SO8010). The sarcoma tissue arrays were purchased from Novus Biologicals (#NBP2 = 30332). For detection of protein expression, tissue arrays were labeled with anti-Myc (Cat# ab32072; Abcam), anti-Oct4 (Cat# ab18976; Abcam), anti-Sox2 (Cat# ab97959; Abcam), anti-Klf4 (Cat# ab118961; Abcam), and anti-Nanog (Cat# ab80892; Abcam) antibodies. Antigenicity was detected using Alkaline Phosphatase reactivity (CellMarque). Positive (primary antibody included) and negative (primary antibody excluded) controls from human intestine (Klf4), human testicle (Oct4 and Nanog), rat brain (Sox2), or human colon cancer (Myc) which have been reported by the Human Protein Atlas (HPA) (www.proteinatlas.org) were subjected to immunohistochemistry to validate the specificity of each antibody tested (Additional file 1: Figure S1). In addition, immunohistochemistry for each antigen was performed on adipose tissue as a negative control, given the HPA revealed no to very low expression of each protein in this tissue type (Additional file 1: Figure S1). Immunopositivity was quantified by two metrics: the percentage of tissue with positive staining (<25 %, 25–50 %, 50–75 %, or >75 %) and the

staining intensity (0 = no staining, + = weak staining, ++ = moderate staining, +++ = high staining). IHC scores were determined by multiplying the staining intensity (0 = 0, + = 1, ++ = 2, +++ = 3) by the percent of tissue stained (<25 % = 1, 25–50 % = 2, 50–75 % = 3, >75 % = 4) based on previously described methods [13]. For statistical analysis, the Mann-Whitney rank sum test was used. Statistical significance was determined if the two-sided P value of the test was < 0.05. Use of human tissues for research was approved by TTUHSC board review #11027.

Results

Included in this study were 71 diseased vascular tissue samples originally collected from human patients, representing malignant (seven angiosarcomas, two hemangiopericytomas), borderline (six hemangioendothelioma), and benign (five infantile hemangioma, one capillary hemangioma, 45 cavernous hemangiomas, three granulomatous hemangiomas, one venous hemangioma) vascular tumors and one thrombophlebitis. Known characteristics of patients grouped according to biopsy classification are reported in Table 1. As controls, we included two tissue sets in this analysis: 1) ten non-diseased blood vessel tissues and 2) a diverse panel of 58 human sarcoma tumors. The non-diseased blood vessel tissues were chosen to evaluate the expression of stem cell reprogramming factors in normal vasculature, while the various sarcomas were selected to compare the levels of stem cell reprogramming factors in borderline and malignant vascular sarcomas to that of other malignant mesenchymal tumors.

IHC staining for the stem cell reprogramming factors Oct4, Nanog, Myc, Klf4, and Sox2 was performed in the vascular tumor samples as well as the two control tissue sets. Representative images of each staining are depicted in Figs. 1, 2, 3, 4 and 5. With the exception of Myc, each of these proteins was detectable at variable levels across non-diseased vascular tissues, ranging from 50 % of normal tissues displaying Nanog and Klf4 immunoreactivity to 90 % of normal tissues displaying Oct4 immunoreactivity (Table 2). Expression of these "stem cell regulators" in non-diseased adult tissue is not surprising given that the HPA reports detection of Oct4, Nanog, Klf4, and Sox2 in approximately 70, 11, 29, and 51 % of normal human tissues, respectively. Though HPA reports Myc expression in

Table 1 Vascular tumor and control patient characteristics

Variable	Overall	Malignant	Borderline	Benign	Normal
# patient samples	81	9	6	56	10
Age [mean years (s.d.)]	41 ± 17	53 ± 19	36 ± 15	40 ± 17	34 ± 14
Age [median years (range)]	42 (80)	53 (64)	35 (44)	42 (71)	32 (44)
Sex	42 F, 39 M	4 F, 5 M	6 F, 0 M	27 F, 29 M	5 F, 5 M

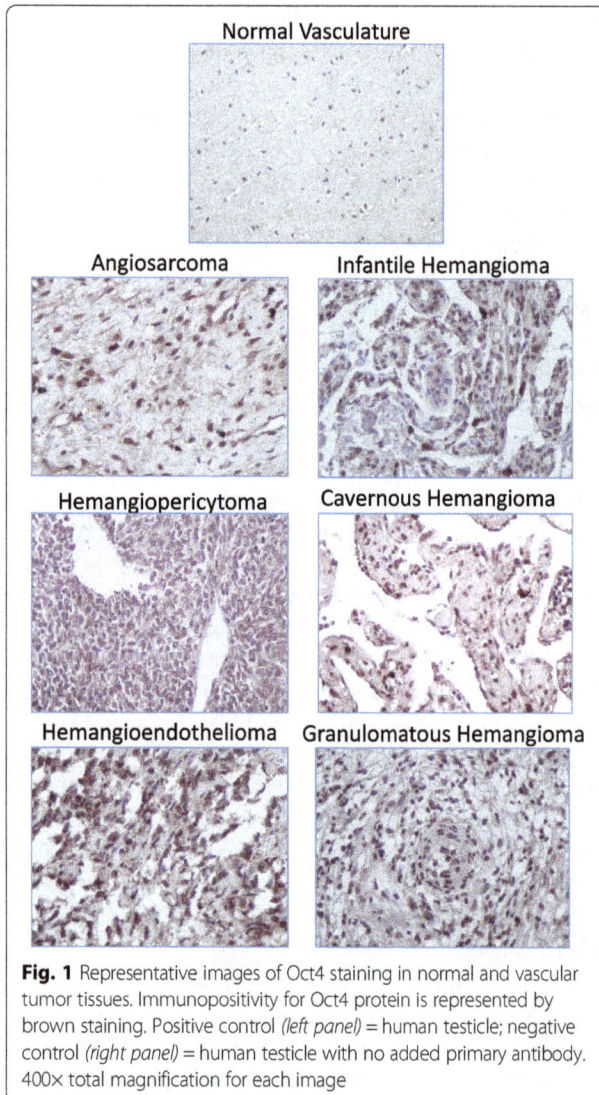

Fig. 1 Representative images of Oct4 staining in normal and vascular tumor tissues. Immunopositivity for Oct4 protein is represented by brown staining. Positive control *(left panel)* = human testicle; negative control *(right panel)* = human testicle with no added primary antibody. 400× total magnification for each image

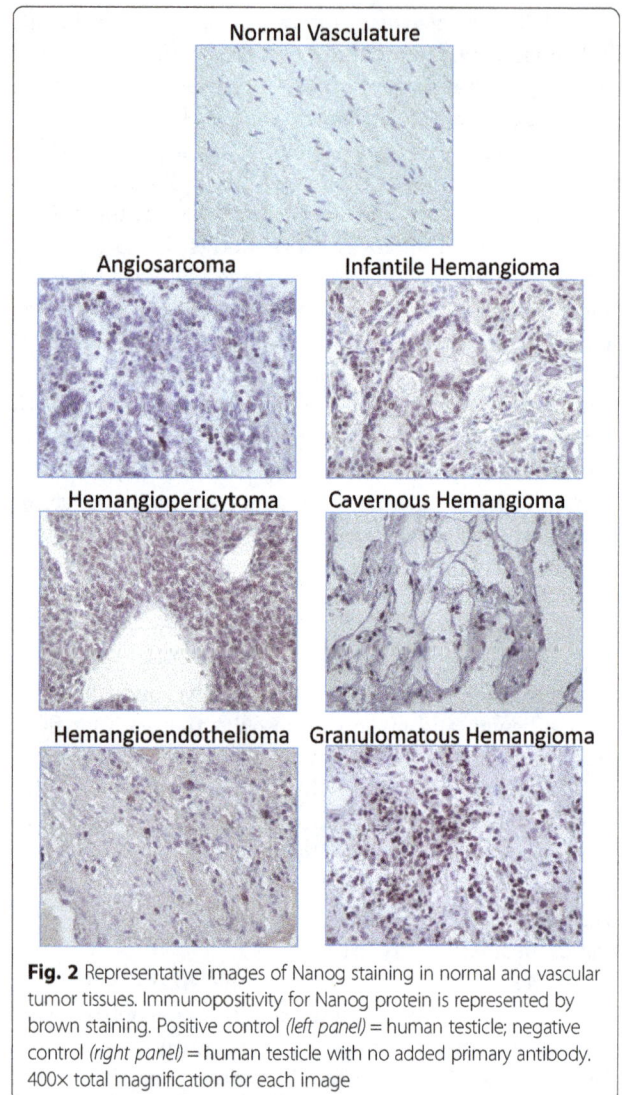

Fig. 2 Representative images of Nanog staining in normal and vascular tumor tissues. Immunopositivity for Nanog protein is represented by brown staining. Positive control *(left panel)* = human testicle; negative control *(right panel)* = human testicle with no added primary antibody. 400× total magnification for each image

56 % of normal human tissues, we did not detect this protein in any non-diseased vascular tissues tested in this analysis. While immunostaining for these stem cell regulators was observed in non-diseased vasculature, the IHC score for these tissues was relatively low given that staining intensity for each stem cell marker was weak to moderate and often occurred in a very small fraction (<25 %) of the cells comprising the tissue (Fig. 6, Additional file 2: Table S1).

In contrast to the non-diseased vascular rich tissue controls, benign vascular tumors and the single thrombophlebitis sample exhibited significantly increased staining (in both intensity and percentage of positive tissue) for Oct4, Nanog, Myc, and Sox2, with no statistically significant increase in antigenicity for Klf4 (Fig. 6, Additional file 2: Table S1). It is worth noting that unlike the absence of Myc expression in normal vasculature, 46 % of the benign tumors tested were positive for Myc protein. The data obtained from malignant and borderline vascular tumors were remarkably similar to that demonstrated from the benign vascular tumors. Malignant and borderline vascular sarcomas displayed 100 % immunoreactivity for Oct4, Nanog, and Sox2, while Myc protein was present in 50 % of malignant and borderline vascular tumors (Table 2). The IHC scores for all proteins tested except Klf4 were significantly increased in the malignant and borderline vascular tumors relative to the non-diseased controls, and were surprisingly very similar to the levels observed in benign vascular tumors. The elevated IHC scores observed for malignant and borderline vascular tumors correlated to the results obtained in a diverse panel of malignant sarcoma cells, revealing immunoreactivity for Oct4, Nanog, and Sox2 in 100 % of various sarcoma tissues and 72 % for Myc and Kfl4 (Additional file 2: Table S2). While Klf4 protein expression was not significantly different between any of the vascular tumors or vascular tissue controls, this protein did show a significantly increased mean IHC score

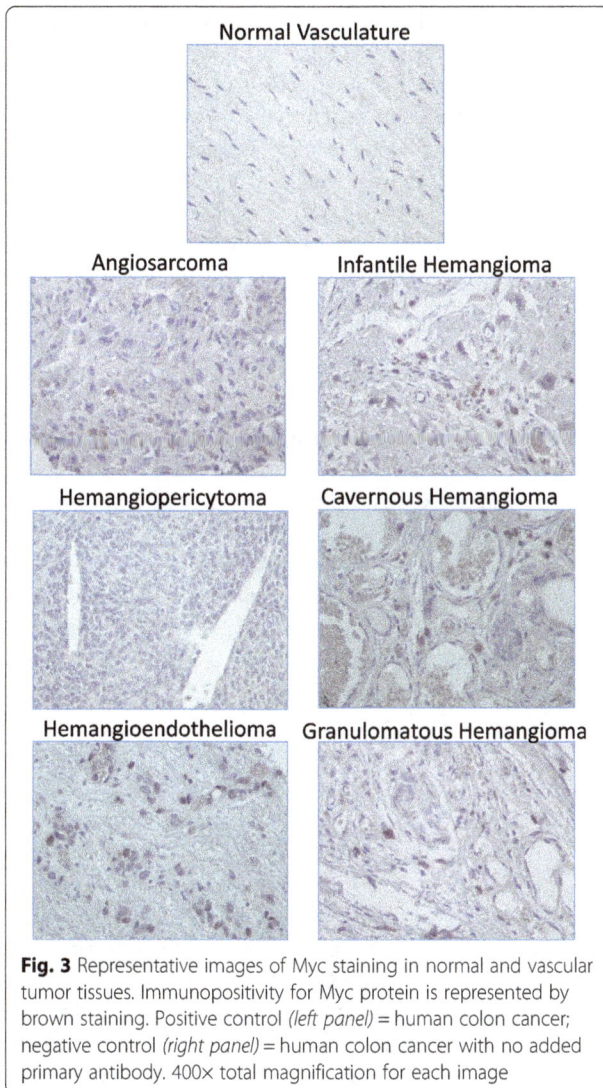

Fig. 3 Representative images of Myc staining in normal and vascular tumor tissues. Immunopositivity for Myc protein is represented by brown staining. Positive control *(left panel)* = human colon cancer; negative control *(right panel)* = human colon cancer with no added primary antibody. 400× total magnification for each image

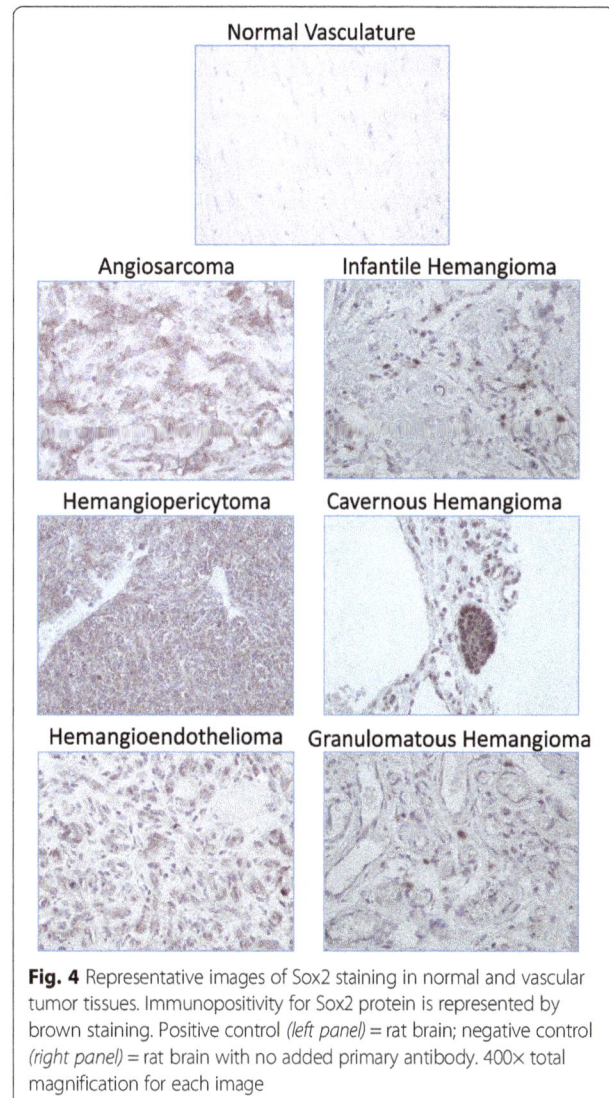

Fig. 4 Representative images of Sox2 staining in normal and vascular tumor tissues. Immunopositivity for Sox2 protein is represented by brown staining. Positive control *(left panel)* = rat brain; negative control *(right panel)* = rat brain with no added primary antibody. 400× total magnification for each image

in the sarcoma tissue control set (Fig. 6, Additional file 2: Table S2). The expression of Oct4, Nanog, Myc, Sox2, and Klf4 in the current study correlated well with data reported in the HPA which reveals expression of Oct4 in 88 % of cancers, Sox2 in 88 % of cancers, Myc in 78 % of cancers, Klf4 in 28 % of cancers, and Nanog in 7 % of cancers.

Discussion

This study directly stems from the results of a handful of recent publications which suggest that the benign vascular tumor, infantile hemangioma, harbors a subpopulation of stem cell-like progenitor cells. mRNA and protein expression of neural crest and stem cell markers was previously confirmed in a panel of hemangioma samples, revealing variable expression levels for Oct4, Myc, Sox2, and Nanog [10, 11]. These publications suggest that infantile hemangiomas may contain cells that are capable of differentiating into all three embryonic germ layers and

additionally point to a possible mechanism of clonality in these tumors. Indeed, implantation of isolated CD133+ stem cell populations from infantile hemangiomas produce hemangioma-like tumors in xenograft animal models [14], however Oct4 and Nanog positive subpopulations from infantile hemangiomas failed to form teratomas in SCID/NOD mice [11], a hallmark of embryonic stem cell-derived tumors [15], suggesting they do not function like true embryonic stem cells. Substantial lines of evidence controversially suggest that congenital and infantile hemangiomas originate from metastatic spread of placental chorangiomas [16–20], creating a possibility in which the etiology of some childhood hemangiomas (at least in their earliest stages) may be more similar to metastatic tumors than benign tumors. Thus, our observations that both infantile hemangiomas and malignant vascular tumors such as angiosarcomas and hemangiopericytomas expressed stem cell reprogramming factors at significantly increased

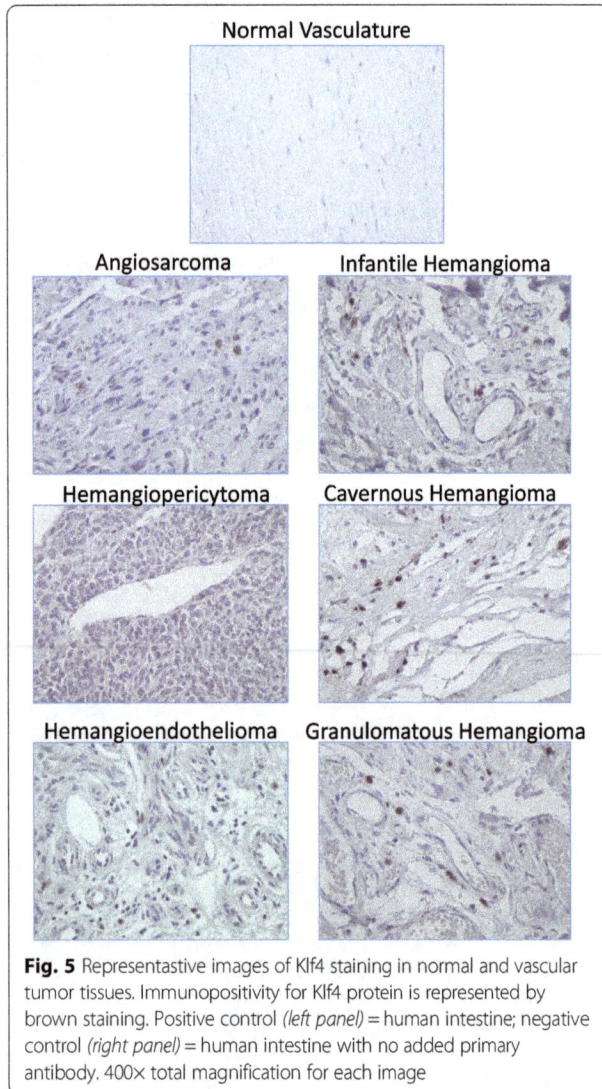

Normal Vasculature

Angiosarcoma | Infantile Hemangioma

Hemangiopericytoma | Cavernous Hemangioma

Hemangioendothelioma | Granulomatous Hemangioma

Fig. 5 Representastive images of Klf4 staining in normal and vascular tumor tissues. Immunopositivity for Klf4 protein is represented by brown staining. Positive control *(left panel)* = human intestine; negative control *(right panel)* = human intestine with no added primary antibody. 400× total magnification for each image

quite surprising. These benign tumors often occur in the third to fourth decade of life, thus their origin cannot be attributed easily to distal neoplasms as arguably may occur in infantile hemangiomas. These expression patterns in diverse benign vascular tumors are intriguing given that the presence of "stemness" proteins in malignant tumors is well established in the literature and forms the basis for the "stem cell theory of cancer"; however our data provide strong evidence that these proteins could potentially contribute to the formation and/or properties associated with a diverse array of benign vascular tumors. Though more studies must be performed for definitive arguments either way, it is possible that the "stem cell theory of cancer" is too narrowly defined in its current state and may need to be broadened to include benign neoplasms. This subject should be treaded lightly and with careful future evaluation as, while Oct4 has been shown to maintain pluripotency during early embryogenesis, its role as a pure stem cell marker has been questioned given that it is also expressed in differentiated cells [21, 22]. Nanog expression has been reported in E18 stage rat myocardial tissues, and is detectable in post-natal stages up to 30 days after birth and after acute myocardial infarction [23, 24].

Compared to the abundance of research performed in carcinomas and hematopoietic cancers, relatively minimal work has been reported evaluating the presence of stem cells as driving components in malignant mesenchymal tumors, and much of these efforts have focused exclusively on pediatric bone and musculoskeletal sarcomas [25–27]. For instance, osteosarcomas and Ewing's sarcomas express Oct4 and Nanog [25, 28, 29] and rhabdomyosarcomas express Oct4, Nanog, and Sox2 [30]. Moreover, the EWS-FLI1 fusion gene, present in nearly 85 % of Ewing's sarcomas, induces the expression of Oct4, Nanog, and Sox2 in human pediatric mesenchymal stem cells but not their adult counterparts [31]. Though drug resistant progenitor-like cell populations have been reported for angiosarcomas [32, 33], only expression of Myc as an embryonic stem cell marker has been thoroughly examined in malignant vascular tumors [34]. It has been reported that Myc gene amplification and overexpression occurs in post-irradiation induced angiosarcomas, but not in primary cutaneous angiosarcomas or in other radiation-associated vascular proliferations [35, 36]; however several other studies provide evidence that Myc amplification and overexpression is not a definitive marker of radiation-induced tumorigenesis in angiosarcomas [37–39]. Our data additionally demonstrates that Oct4, Nanog, Sox2, Klf4, and Myc are widely expressed at high levels across a wide variety of sarcomas and benign vascular tumors at elevated levels. While the data reported in this study in no way indicate that the cells expressing these markers are cancer stem cells (which generally make up single digit or less percentages of the total cancer cell population in a tumor), the

and relatively similar levels compared to non-diseased vascular tissue, is not entirely surprising.

In contrast, our highly novel observations that other benign vascular tumors such as adult capillary, cavernous, granulomatous, and venous hemangiomas as well as the single thrombophlebitis sample displayed expression of Oct4, Nanog, Myc, and Sox2 in similarly elevated rates and intensities as seen in malignant sarcomas was

Table 2 Percentage of tumors with positive antigenicity for embryonic stem cell reprogramming factors

Protein	Normal	Benign	Borderline	Malignant	Various Sarcomas
Oct4	90 %	100 %	100 %	100 %	100 %
Nanog	50 %	98 %	100 %	100 %	100 %
Myc	0 %	46 %	50 %	50 %	72 %
Sox2	60 %	98 %	100 %	100 %	100 %
Klf4	50 %	59 %	67 %	63 %	72 %

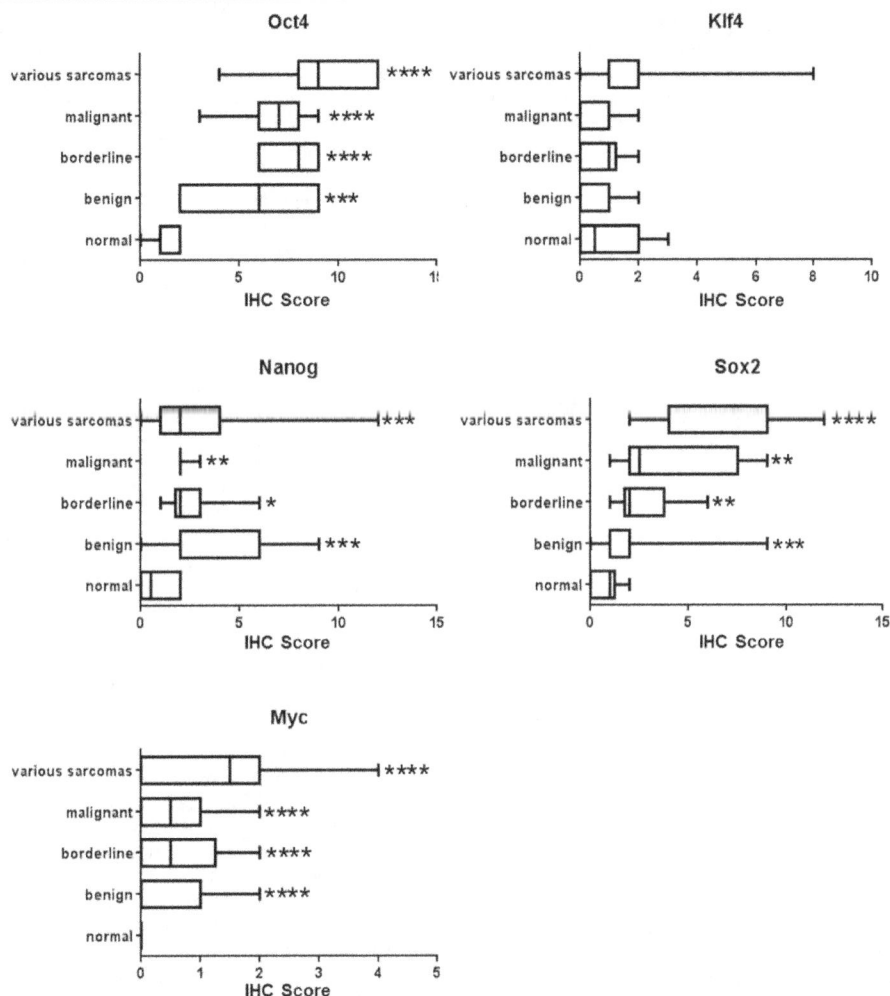

Fig. 6 Antigenicity for embryonic stem cell reprogramming factors in normal tissue and vascular tumors. Box and whisker plots depicting the IHC scores for Oct4, Nanog, Myc, Sox2, and Klf4 in normal vasculature, benign, borderline or malignant vascular tumors, or across a panel of various sarcomas. The Mann-Whitney rank sum test was used to determine statistical significance. Significance was determined if the two-sided P value of the test was < 0.05. Asterisks indicate level of significance relative to normal vasculature (* $p < 0.05$, ** $p < 0.05$, *** $p < 0.005$, **** $p < 0.0005$)

statistically significant increases in Oct4, Nanog, Sox2, and Myc expression in benign and malignant tumors relative to normal tissues provides correlative support that overexpression of these proteins could contribute to their overall tumorigenic properties.

Conclusion

In conclusion, the data presented in this study demonstrate that the protein expression of embryonic stem cell reprogramming factors is enriched in benign, borderline, and malignant vascular tumors. This finding could translate to future therapeutic targeting of tumor cell populations that express embryonic stem cell reprogramming factors to disrupt tumor cell clonality, long term growth, and drug resistance.

Additional files

Additional file 1: Figure S1. Positive and negative staining controls. For each indicated antigen detected by immunohistochemistry, three controls were performed. The Negative Control column represents images acquired following immunohistochemistry against the indicated antigen on adipocyte tissue, which has been shown by the HPA to express no to low levels of each protein. The No Primary Antibody column represents images acquired following immunohistochemistry using no primary antibody on tissues as indicated in the Materials and Methods section to demonstrate that the detection system was no causing background staining on the samples. The Positive Control column represents images acquired from immunohistochemistry using the indicated antibody on tissues as indicated in the Materials and Methods section that are known to strongly express each antigen.

Additional file 2: Table S1. Immunopositivity for stem cell reprogramming factors in malignant and benign vascular tumors. Table S2. Immunopositivity for stem cell reprogramming factors in a panel of diverse sarcomas.

Abbreviations

CD133: Cluster of differentiation 133 protein; EWS-FLI1: Ewings sarcoma oncogene-friend leukemia virus integration 1; HPA: Human protein atlas; IHC: Immunohistochemistry; Klf4: Kruppel-like factor 4; Myc: Myelocytomatosis viral oncogene homolog; Nanog: Homeobox protein Nanog; Oct4: Octamer-binding transcription factor 3/4; SCID/NOD: Severe combined immunodeficiency disease/non-obese diabetic; SOX2: Sex determining region Y box 2 protein; TTUHSC: Texas Tech University Health Sciences Center.

Competing interests

The authors declare that they have no competing interests.

Authors' contributions

AM carried out all IHC analysis and statistical analysis. BB designed the study, drafted the manuscript. Both authors read and approved the final manuscript.

Authors' information

Not applicable.

Acknowledgements

We would like to thank Dolores Diaz of the TTUHSC Histology Core for assistance with IHC methodology.

Funding

This analysis was funded through a Liddy Shriver Sarcoma Initiative Grant and TTUHSC seed funding to BB.

References

1. Bjerkvig R, Tysnes BB, Aboody KS, Najbauer J, Terzis AJ. Opinion: the origin of the cancer stem cell: current controversies and new insights. Nat Rev Cancer. 2005;5(11):899–904.
2. Dean M, Fojo T, Bates S. Tumour stem cells and drug resistance. Nat Rev Cancer. 2005;5(4):275–84.
3. Kreso A, Dick JE. Evolution of the cancer stem cell model. Cell Stem Cell. 2014;14(3):275–91.
4. Patel M, Yang S. Advances in reprogramming somatic cells to induced pluripotent stem cells. Stem Cell Rev. 2010;6(3):367–80.
5. Ben-Porath I, Thomson MW, Carey VJ, Ge R, Bell GW, Regev A, et al. An embryonic stem cell-like gene expression signature in poorly differentiated aggressive human tumors. Nat Genet. 2008;40(5):499–507.
6. da Arnaud Cruz P, Marques O, Rosa AM, de Fatima Faria M, Rema A, Lopes C. Co-expression of stem cell markers ALDH1 and CD44 in non-malignant and neoplastic lesions of the breast. Anticancer Res. 2014;34(3):1427–34.
7. Lim SD, Stallcup W, Lefkove B, Govindarajan B, Au KS, Northrup H, et al. Expression of the neural stem cell markers NG2 and L1 in human angiomyolipoma: are angiomyolipomas neoplasms of stem cells? Mol Med. 2007;13(3–4):160–5.
8. Prajapati A, Gupta S, Mistry B, Gupta S. Prostate stem cells in the development of benign prostate hyperplasia and prostate cancer: emerging role and concepts. BioMed Res Intl. 2013;2013:107954.
9. Ugolkov AV, Eisengart LJ, Luan C, Yang XJ. Expression analysis of putative stem cell markers in human benign and malignant prostate. Prostate. 2011;71(1):18–25.
10. Spock CL, Tom LK, Canadas K, Sue GR, Sawh-Martinez R, Maier CL, et al. Infantile hemangiomas exhibit neural crest and pericyte markers. Ann Plast Surg. 2015;74(2):230–6.
11. Itinteang T, Tan ST, Brasch HD, Steel R, Best HA, Vishvanath A, et al. Infantile haemangioma expresses embryonic stem cell markers. J Clin Pathol. 2012;65(5):394–8.
12. Huang L, Nakayama H, Klagsbrun M, Mulliken JB, Bischoff J. Glucose transporter 1-positive endothelial cells in infantile hemangioma exhibit features of facultative stem cells. Stem Cells. 2015;33(1):133–45.
13. Krajewska M, Smith LH, Rong J, Huang X, Hyer ML, Zeps N, et al. Image analysis algorithms for immunohistochemical assessment of cell death events and fibrosis in tissue sections. J Histochem Cytochem : Off J Histochemistry Soc. 2009;57(7):649–63.
14. Khan ZA, Boscolo E, Picard A, Psutka S, Melero-Martin JM, Bartch TC, et al. Multipotential stem cells recapitulate human infantile hemangioma in immunodeficient mice. J Clin Investig. 2008;118(7):2592–9.
15. Xu C, Inokuma MS, Denham J, Golds K, Kundu P, Gold JD, et al. Feeder-free growth of undifferentiated human embryonic stem cells. Nat Biotechnol. 2001;19(10):971–4.
16. Bakaris S, Karabiber H, Yuksel M, Parmaksiz G, Kiran H. Case of large placental chorioangioma associated with diffuse neonatal hemangiomatosis. Pediatr Dev Pathol: Off J Soc Pediatr Pathol Paediatr Pathol Soc. 2004;7(3):258–61.
17. Baruteau J, Joomye R, Muller JB, Vinceslas C, Baraton L, Joubert M, et al. Chorioangiomatosis: a rare etiology of nonimmune hydrops fetalis. Obstetric and pediatric implications for patient care. Arch Pediatr: Organe Off de la Soc Francaise de Pediatrie. 2009;16(10):1341 5.
18. Maymon R, Hermann G, Reish O, Herman A, Strauss S, Sherman D, et al. Chorioangioma and its severe infantile sequelae: case report. Prenat Diagn. 2003;23(12):976–80.
19. Miliaras D, Conroy J, Pervana S, Meditskou S, McQuaid D, Nowak N. Karyotypic changes detected by comparative genomic hybridization in a stillborn infant with chorioangioma and liver hemangioma. Birth Defects Res A Clin Mol Teratol. 2007;79(3):236–41.
20. Selmin A, Foltran F, Chiarelli S, Ciullo R, Gregori D. An epidemiological study investigating the relationship between chorangioma and infantile hemangioma. Pathol Res Pract. 2014;210(9):548–53.
21. Tai MH, Chang CC, Kiupel M, Webster JD, Olson LK, Trosko JE. Oct4 expression in adult human stem cells: evidence in support of the stem cell theory of carcinogenesis. Carcinogenesis. 2005;26(2):495–502.
22. Zangrossi S, Marabese M, Broggini M, Giordano R, D'Erasmo M, Montelatici E, et al. Oct-4 expression in adult human differentiated cells challenges its role as a pure stem cell marker. Stem Cells. 2007;25(7):1675–80.
23. Guo ZK, Guo K, Luo H, Mu LM, Li Q, Chang YQ. The expression analysis of nanog in the developing rat myocardial tissues. Cellular Physiology Biochemistry : Interl J Experimental Cellular Physiology, Biochemistry, Pharmacology. 2015;35(3):866–74.
24. Luo H, Li Q, Pramanik J, Luo J, Guo Z. Nanog expression in heart tissues induced by acute myocardial infarction. Histol Histopathol. 2014;29(10):1287–93.
25. Gibbs CP, Kukekov VG, Reith JD, Tchigrinova O, Suslov ON, Scott EW, et al. Stem-like cells in bone sarcomas: implications for tumorigenesis. Neoplasia. 2005;7(11):967–76.
26. Levings PP, McGarry SV, Currie TP, Nickerson DM, McClellan S, Ghivizzani SC, et al. Expression of an exogenous human Oct-4 promoter identifies tumor-initiating cells in osteosarcoma. Cancer Res. 2009;69(14):5648–55.
27. Wu C, Wei Q, Utomo V, Nadesan P, Whetstone H, Kandel R, et al. Side population cells isolated from mesenchymal neoplasms have tumor initiating potential. Cancer Res. 2007;67(17):8216–22.
28. Martins-Neves SR, Lopes AO, do Carmo A, Paiva AA, Simoes PC, Abrunhosa AJ, et al. Therapeutic implications of an enriched cancer stem-like cell population in a human osteosarcoma cell line. BMC Cancer. 2012;12:139.
29. Suva ML, Riggi N, Stehle JC, Baumer K, Tercier S, Joseph JM, et al. Identification of cancer stem cells in Ewing's sarcoma. Cancer Res. 2009;69(5):1776–81.
30. Salerno M, Avnet S, Bonuccelli G, Hosogi S, Granchi D, Baldini N. Impairment of lysosomal activity as a therapeutic modality targeting cancer stem cells of embryonal rhabdomyosarcoma cell line RD. PLoS One. 2014;9(10), e110340.
31. Riggi N, Suva ML, De Vito C, Provero P, Stehle JC, Baumer K, et al. EWS-FLI-1 modulates miRNA145 and SOX2 expression to initiate mesenchymal stem cell reprogramming toward Ewing sarcoma cancer stem cells. Genes Dev. 2010;24(9):916–32.
32. Gorden BH, Saha J, Khammanivong A, Schwartz GK, Dickerson EB. Lysosomal drug sequestration as a mechanism of drug resistance in vascular sarcoma cells marked by high CSF-1R expression. Vascular Cell. 2014;6:20.
33. Khammanivong A, Gorden BH, Frantz AM, Graef AJ, Dickerson EB. Identification of drug-resistant subpopulations in canine hemangiosarcoma. Vet Comp Oncol. 2014. doi:10.1111/vco.12114.
34. Kurisetty V, Bryan BA. Aberrations in Angiogenic Signaling and MYC Amplifications are Distinguishing Features of Angiosarcoma. Angiology: Open access. 2013;1.

35. Guo T, Zhang L, Chang NE, Singer S, Maki RG, Antonescu CR. Consistent MYC and FLT4 gene amplification in radiation-induced angiosarcoma but not in other radiation-associated atypical vascular lesions. Genes Chromosomes Cancer. 2011;50(1):25–33.

36. Mentzel T, Schildhaus HU, Palmedo G, Buttner R, Kutzner H. Postradiation cutaneous angiosarcoma after treatment of breast carcinoma is characterized by MYC amplification in contrast to atypical vascular lesions after radiotherapy and control cases: clinicopathological, immunohistochemical and molecular analysis of 66 cases. Modern Pathol : Off J US Canadian Acad Pathol, Inc. 2012;25(1):75–85.

37. Hadj-Hamou NS, Lae M, Almeida A, de la Grange P, Kirova Y, Sastre-Garau X, et al. A transcriptome signature of endothelial lymphatic cells coexists with the chronic oxidative stress signature in radiation-induced post-radiotherapy breast angiosarcomas. Carcinogenesis. 2012;33(7):1399–405.

38. Italiano A, Chen CL, Thomas R, Breen M, Bonnet F, Sevenet N, et al. Alterations of the p53 and PIK3CA/AKT/mTOR pathways in angiosarcomas: a pattern distinct from other sarcomas with complex genomics. Cancer. 2012;118(23):5878–87.

39. Tran D, Verma K, Ward K, Diaz D, Kataria E, Torabi A, et al. Functional genomics analysis reveals a MYC signature associated with a poor clinical prognosis in liposarcomas. Am J Pathol. 2015;185(3):717–28.

3

Practice of percutaneous needle autopsy; a descriptive study reporting experiences from Uganda

Janneke A Cox[1,2]*, Robert L Lukande[3], Sam Kalungi[3,4], Koen Van de Vijver[5], Eric Van Marck[6], Ann M Nelson[7], Asafu Munema[3], Yukari C Manabe[2,8] and Robert Colebunders[1,9]

Abstract

Background: Percutaneous needle autopsy can overcome a number of barriers that limit the use of complete autopsies. We performed blind-and ultrasound guided needle autopsies in HIV-infected adults in Uganda. In this study we describe in detail the methods we used, the ability of both procedures to obtain sufficient tissue for further examination and the learning curve of the operators over time.

Methods: If written informed consent was granted from the next of kin, we first performed a blind needle autopsy, puncturing brain, heart, lungs, liver, spleen and kidneys using predefined surface marking points. We then performed an ultrasound guided needle autopsy puncturing heart, liver, spleen and kidneys. The number of attempts, expected success and duration of the procedure were noted. A pathologist read the slides and indicated if the target tissue was present and of sufficient quality for pathological review. We report the predicted and true success rates, compare the yield of blind to ultrasound guided needle biopsies and evaluate the failure rate over time.

Results: Two operators performed 96 blind needle autopsies and 95 ultrasound guided needle autopsies. For blind needle biopsies true success rates varied from 56-99% and predicted success rates from 89-99%. For ultrasound guided needle biopsies true success rates varied from 72-100% and predicted success rates from 84-98%. Ultrasound guidance led to a significantly higher success rate in heart and left kidney. A learning curve was observed over time with decreasing failure rates with increasing experience and a shorter duration of the needle autopsy.

Conclusion: Needle autopsy can successfully obtain tissue for further pathological review in the vast majority of cases, with a decrease in failure rate with increasing experience of the operator. The benefit of ultrasound guidance will depend on the population, the disease and organ of interest and the local circumstances. Our results justify further evaluation of needle autopsies as a method to establish a cause of death.

Keywords: Needle autopsy, Partial autopsy, Minimal invasive autopsy, Needle biopsy, Ultra-sound guided biopsy, Tru-cut biopsy, Post mortem, Uganda, Sub Saharan Africa

* Correspondence: jannekecox@xs4all.nl
[1]Department of Clinical Sciences, Institute of Tropical Medicine, Nationalestraat 155, 2000 Antwerpen, Belgium
[2]Infectious Diseases Institute, Makerere University College of Health Sciences, Kampala, Uganda
Full list of author information is available at the end of the article

Background

Needle autopsy was first described in 1955 when in 24 corpses tissue was obtained by percutaneous biopsies. Its use was motivated by low acceptance rates and limited accessibility of complete autopsy outside the hospital [1]. Since then, needle autopsy has been used in various settings and for various reasons including increased acceptability, simplicity and decreased risk of disease transmission when compared to complete autopsies [2,3].

However, an important disadvantage of needle autopsy is the lack of direct visual judgment. This may lead to sampling error of both the target organ and the target lesion. Reported success rates to obtain tissue vary widely depending on the organ involved. The largest postmortem needle biopsy study retrospectively evaluated 394 biopsies that were performed between 1948 and 1968 by 32 different pathology residents in the United States. The success rates ranged from 34% for the kidneys to 92% for the liver [2]. Smaller studies in various adult populations have shown successful biopsy rates of 98-100% for the liver, 76-94% for the lungs, 50-100% for the heart and 10-80% for the kidneys [3-6].

The addition of ultrasound guidance could compensate for the loss of visual judgment. For clinical biopsies in living patients ultrasound guidance is well established and used to increase tissue yield and to prevent complications [7-9]. For needle autopsies, the use of ultrasound guidance was reported in one study [10]. However, since postmortem there is no apparent limit to the number of biopsies and complications no longer need to be prevented, its benefit may be less obvious.

We conducted a study in Uganda in which we subsequently performed blind needle autopsy, ultrasound guided needle autopsy and complete autopsy in deceased HIV-infected hospitalized adults. Our results on the concordance in cause of death between needle and complete autopsy have been published elsewhere [11]. Herein, we report in detail the methods we used, the success rates for the individual organs and the observed learning curve over time. Moreover, we compare the success rates per organ of blind and ultrasound guided needle autopsies.

Methods

Setting and population

The study was conducted in Mulago hospital, a tertiary teaching hospital in Kampala, Uganda from February until June 2013. Written informed consent for study participation was obtained from the next of kin of HIV-infected adults (>18 years old) that died during hospitalization. Postpartum deaths and deaths after trauma were excluded.

General information

The needle autopsy took place within 4 hours after consent was granted. Two medical doctors (JAC, RLL), without previous experience in needle biopsies or ultrasound use performed all needle autopsies in the hospital mortuary. Prior to study initiation, an experienced radiologist instructed the two medical doctors on the performance of ultrasound guided needle biopsies. One automated biopsy needle 14G*16cm (Bard® Max-Core® disposable core biopsy instrument) was used per patient. For each procedure the start and end-time were recorded. The operator assessed nutritional status on gross examination of the corpse (emaciated, thin, well nourished or obese). After completing all study procedures the body was embalmed free of charge and any needle-entry sites leaking bodily fluids were sutured.

The operator was free to perform as many punctures as needed, however a minimum of 3 attempts and a reasonable maximum of approximately 10 attempts was set. The operator noted the number of attempts and the number of expected successful core biopsies per organ.

The core biopsies (brain, heart, liver, spleen, right and left kidney, right and left lung) were collected in 3 separate specimen containers filled with formalin 10%. For the blind biopsies container 1 collected brain, heart, liver and spleen, container 2 left kidney and left lung and container 3 right kidney and right lung. For the ultrasound guided biopsies container 1 collected heart, liver and spleen, container 2 left kidney and container 3 right kidney.

Autopsy procedures

For the blind needle autopsy, surface marking points and palpation were used to estimate the location of each individual target organ. The following surface marking points for needle entry were used: the brain through the nose and the cribriform plate, the spleen along the mid-clavicular line under the rib arch pointing the needle in dorso-lateral direction or from the 11th intercostal space mid-axillary in case of a sample error (i.e. no tissue in the biopsy needle), the liver along the mid-clavicular line under the rib arch, both lungs at the level of the 3rd intercostal space below the deltoid tubercle or in case of a sample error from the 6-7th intercostal space mid-axillary, the heart 5th intercostal space lateral from the sternum and both kidneys dorsal below the 12th rib just lateral from the spine. The operator was allowed to change the needle position during the procedure if the macroscopic appearance of the core biopsy would imply so.

Ultrasound guided needle biopsies were taken from the heart, liver, spleen and both kidneys using a pocket-size, portable ultrasound scan (Vscan® V1.2, GE Healthcare, USA). The ultrasound scan was used for real-time guidance of the needle to the target organ. However, if the ultrasound scan identified any specific lesion(s) in the target-organ, an attempt was made to also puncture this lesion.

Histological assessment

For the needle autopsy, one paraffin-embedded tissue block was made per specimen container. Therefore, 6 tissue blocks per patient were made with 4/6 tissue blocks containing core biopsies of more than one organ. An effort was made by the lab-technicians to embed all tissue-cores on the same level, so that when cutting the block all tissue-cores would be present.

From each block, a hematoxylin and eosin (H&E) stained slide was made. A pathologist read each slide and noted per slide if the target tissue was present and of sufficient quality for histological review. If a slide did not contain all the expected tissues, the block was reviewed and when needed re-embedded to ensure all tissue-cores were at one level on the cut-surface. A new H&E stained slide would be made and reread by the pathologist in the same manner as before.

Definition of outcomes

A successful biopsy was defined as at least one representative core biopsy of a specific organ on the slide where it should be present. This definition was used because within a patient target tissue could be obtained unintentionally when trying to puncture another organ but missed when intending to puncture that organ, e.g. heart tissue could be present on the slide that should contain left lung but not present on the slide that should contain heart tissue. In that case, the heart biopsy was classified as unsuccessful. We report the true success rate, i.e. the proportion of successful biopsies after histological review and the predicted success rate, i.e. the proportion of successful biopsies predicted by the operators during the procedure.

Statistical methods

Proportions are reported with 95% confidence intervals (CI) and medians with inter-quartile ranges (IQR). When comparing proportions a McNemar test, a Chi square test or a Fisher's exact test were performed when appropriate. When evaluating the relation between number of attempts and success rates, logistic regression was used. A p-value <0.05 was considered statistically significant. Data were analyzed using STATA version 11.0 (Stata Corp., College Station, TX, Texas, USA).

Ethics statement

The study received ethical approval from the Joint Clinical Research Center Research and Ethics Committee (Uganda), the Mulago Internal Review Board (Uganda) and the Institute of Tropical Medicine Institutional Review Board (Belgium). The study received final approval and registration by the Uganda National Council of Science and Technology (HS1300).

Results

We conducted 96 blind needle autopsies and 95 ultrasound guided autopsies; in one patient the ultrasound-guided biopsy was not performed due to generalized cutaneous lesions with extreme desquamation. After processing, 4 kidney-containing ultrasound guided tissue blocks were missing. Therefore we were able to analyze 768 blind biopsies (8 target organs in 96 patients) and 471 ultrasound-guided biopsies (5 target organs in 95 patients, minus 4).

Fifty-seven percent of patients were female, the median age was 35 years (IQR 29–40), 31% were classified emaciated, 38% thin, 27% well nourished and 4% obese. Nine percent of all tissue blocks were re-embedded after initial pathological review. No leakage of fluid from entry-sites was observed and no suturing was performed.

Blind needle autopsy

The true success rates for the different organs varied from 56-99% (Table 1). The heart had the lowest true success rate, 56% (95%CI 46-66%), followed by the right and left lung, respectively 71% (95%CI 62-80%) and 66% (95%CI 56-75%) and the right and left kidney, respectively 73% (95%CI 64-82%) and 71% (95%CI 62-80%). When combining the biopsies of the left and right lung and the left and right kidney for each patient, the true success rates for the lung increased to 82% (95% CI 75–90) and for the kidney to 83% (95% CI 76-91%).

The true success rates were significantly lower than the predicted success rates for all organs, except brain and liver. The predicted success rates varied from 89-99% (Table 1).

Because a variable number of attempts were allowed to obtain a biopsy, we calculated the true success rate per attempt (Table 1). For this analysis we selected 80 patients for whom the number of attempts was noted for all 8 target-organs. The true success rates in these 80 patients were not significantly different than the true success rates of the whole cohort. We found no significant correlation between an increasing number of attempts and true success rate in any organ. For the spleen, an increasing number of attempts lead to a lower true success rate (p = 0.003).

There were 188 (24%) unsuccessful biopsies in 68 (71%) patients (Table 2). Thirty-five (19%) of these were predicted by the operator. This could be because of several reasons: the operator could have failed to pierce the cribriform plate in case of a brain biopsy or the macroscopic appearance of the core biopsy made the operator doubt if he/she had punctured the target organ. In 16 (9%) unsuccessful biopsies, the target tissue was present but of insufficient quality for histological review. Patients classified as "thin" had more unsuccessful biopsies compared to all others (p = 0.01).

Table 1 Success rates per organ for blind and ultra-sound guided needle biopsies

	Blind				Ultrasound			
	Predicted success rate (%, 95% CI)	True success rate (%, 95% CI)	Median# of attempts (IQR)	True success rate/ total# of attempts[§] (95% CI)	Predicted success rate (%, 95% CI)	True success rate (%, 95% CI)	Median# of attempts (IQR)	True success rate/ total# of attempts[§] (95% CI)
Brain	92 (87–98)	93 (87–98)	3 (3–4)	0.27 (0.26-0.29)	-	-	-	-
Lung right	99 (97–100)	71 (62–80)*	5 (4–7)	0.15 (0.12-0.17)	-	-	-	-
Lung left	99 (97–100)	66 (56–75)*	5 (4–6)	0.13 (0.11-0.15)	-	-	-	-
Both lungs	99 (97–100)	82 (75–90)*	10 (8–12)	0.08 (0.07-0.09)	-	-	-	-
Heart	97 (93–100)	56 (46–66)*	4 (3–5)	0.14 (0.11-0.16)	91 (85–97)	72 (62–81)*/**	3 (3–5)	0.20 (0.17-0.23)***
Liver	99 (97–100)	99 (97–100)	3 (3–4)	0.27 (0.26-0.29)	98 (95–100)	100	3 (3–4)	0.29 (0.28-0.30)
Spleen	89 (83–96)	76 (67–85)*	5 (3–7)	0.14 (0.12-0.17)	84 (77–92)	72 (62–81)*	5 (3–6)	0.15 (0.12-0.17)
Kidney right	91 (86–97)	73 (64–82)*	5 (4–6)	0.15 (0.13-0.17)	91 (85–97)	83 (75–91)	4 (3–5)	0.20 (0.18-0.23)***
Kidney left	90 (84–96)	71 (62–80)*	5 (4–6)	0.16 (0.13-0.18)	91 (85–97)	86 (79–93)**	4 (3–6)	0.20 (0.17-0.22)***
Both kidneys	97 (97–100)	83 (76–91)*	10 (8–11)	0.09 (0.08-0.10)	96 (92–100)	91 (86–97)	9 (7–11)	0.11 (0.10-0.11)

CI: Confidence interval; #: Number IQR: Inter quartile range.
[§]: Selection of 80 patients for which the number of attempts were noted for each organ. True success rates were not significantly different in these 80 patients when compared to the whole cohort both for blind and ultrasound guided needle biopsies. The minimum number of attempts was 3, therefore the maximum rate is 0.33.
*: Predicted and true success rate significantly different.
**: True success rate significantly different between blind and ultrasound guided needle biopsy.
***: True success rate/total# of attempts significantly different between blind and ultrasound guided biopsy.

Ultrasound guided needle autopsy

For the ultrasound-guided biopsies the true success rate varied from 72-100% (Table 1). The predicted success rates varied from 84-98% and were significantly higher than the true success rate for the heart and the spleen. When considering the same 80-patient subset mentioned before, we found a significant correlation with an increasing number of attempts leading to lower true success rates for the heart, the spleen and right kidney (respectively p = 0.002, p = 0.02 and p = 0.01). Ultrasound imaging detected no specific lesions within the target organs and only once a large abdominal lesion outside a target organ was seen and successfully punctured.

The use of ultrasound guidance led to a significantly higher true success rate for the heart (72% versus 56%, p = 0.03) and the left kidney (86% versus 71%, p = 0.01) when compared to blind biopsy. The true success rate for kidney tissue irrespective of the side was not significantly different between ultrasound guided and blind needle autopsy (91% versus 83%, p = 0.09). Moreover, the true success rate per number of attempts was significantly higher with ultrasound guidance for the heart (0.2 versus 0.13, p = 0.0001) and the right kidney (0.2 versus 0.15, p = 0.002). Ultrasound guided needle autopsy had fewer unsuccessful biopsies (18% versus 24%, p = 0.01) and more expected unsuccessful biopsies (22% versus

Table 2 Unsuccessful biopsies for each organ

	Blind			Ultrasound		
	Total	Predicted n (%)	QNS n (%)	Total	Predicted n (%)	QNS n (%)
Brain	7	6 (86)	-	-	-	-
Right lung	28	1 (4)	5 (18)	-	-	-
Left lung	33	1 (3)	3 (9)	-	-	-
Heart	42	3 (7)	2 (5)	27	8 (30)	2 (7)
Liver	1	1 (100)	-	-	-	-
Spleen	23	7 (30)	-	27	13 (48)	1 (4)
Right kidney	26	8 (31)	4 (15)	16	6 (38)	-
Left kidney	28	8 (29)	2 (7)	13	5 (38)	-
Total	188	34 (18)	16 (9)	83	32 (39)*	3 (4)

n: Absolute number; QNS = Quality not sufficient.
*Significantly different when compared to the proportion of predicted unsuccessful biopsies in the blind needle autopsy.

39%, p = 0.01), when taking only into account the 5 organs that were punctured in both procedures.

Experience over time

Operator 1 performed 13 (14%) blind and 12 (13%) ultrasound guided biopsies and operator 2 performed the remaining 83 blind and 83 ultrasound-guided biopsies. The mean number of unsuccessful biopsies per patient was similar for both operators when comparing the blind biopsies from operator 1 (4.3, 95% CI 3.6-5.0) to the first 13 blind biopsies from operator 2 (3.8, 95% CI 3.1-4.6) and when comparing the ultrasound guided biopsies from operator 1 (2, 95% CI 1,2-2,8) to the first 12 ultrasound-guided biopsies of operator 2 (1.7, 95% CI 1.1-2.2) (Figure 1). For operator 2, over time the cumulative number of unsuccessful biopsies leveled off; when considering the last 13 blind and last 12 ultrasound guided biopsies, the mean number of unsuccessful biopsies per patient was 0.7 (0.1-1.3) and 0.2 (95% CI 0–0.4) respectively, implying a learning curve over time for both procedures.

For operator 1 and 2, the mean duration of the first 13 blind needle biopsies was 25 min (95% CI 19–31) and 20 minutes (95% CI 18–22) respectively. The last 13 blind needle biopsies took performer 2 on average 16 min (95% CI 15–18). For operator 1 and 2 the mean duration of the first 12 ultrasound-guided biopsies was 24 min (95% CI 18–31) and 23 minutes (95% CI 21–26) respectively. The last 12 blind needle biopsies took performer 2 on average 14 min (95% CI 12–15).

Discussion

We found postmortem needle biopsies using surface marking-points to be a successful method for obtaining adequate tissue for further pathological review in the majority of cases. Operators tended to overestimate the success of the needle biopsy. The addition of ultrasound guidance lead to higher true success rates and success rates per attempt in the heart and the individual kidneys. A learning curve was observed in the performance of needle autopsy.

The success rates of blind needle biopsies for the different organs are very comparable to the results of others that performed needle autopsy in adults; the heart, the lungs and the kidneys were most difficult to successfully biopsy [2-4,6]. These organs cannot be easily palpated, which partly explains why they have the lowest biopsy success rates. Any benefit of ultrasound guidance would be expected mainly in those organs and was indeed found for the heart and the individual kidneys. Another study that used ultrasound guidance for postmortem biopsies of spleen (n = 39), kidneys (n = 39) and heart (n = 3) reported a yield of respectively 87%, 100% and 100% [10]. So the tissue yield for certain organs can be increased by the addition of ultrasound guidance. However, ultrasound guidance also has disadvantages; it requires the availability of an ultrasound machine and it decreases the simplicity of the procedure. Moreover, ultrasound guidance is unsuitable for some organs (brain and lungs). Therefore, whether ultrasound guidance should be recommended depends on the setting and the organs of interest. In our population of severely

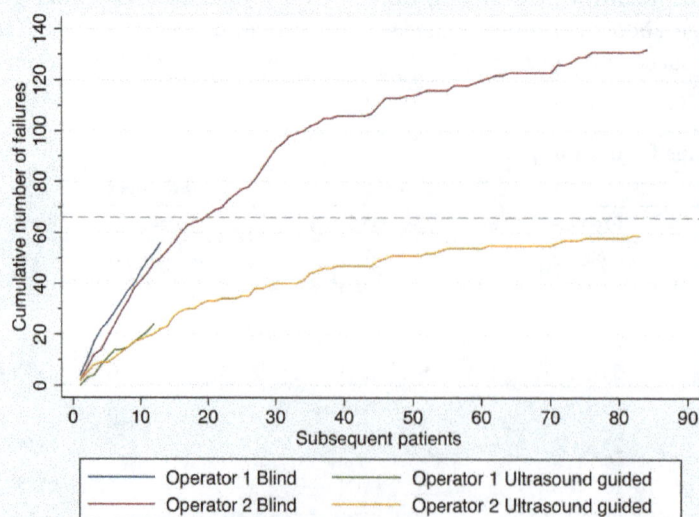

Figure 1 Cumulative number of unsuccessful biopsies per operator in each subsequent procedure performed. The dashed line indicates 50% of cumulative unsuccessful biopsies for operator 2 in the blind needle biopsies.

immune-compromised HIV-infected adults the addition of ultrasound guidance did not lead to the identification of more causes of death, however, for other populations e.g. where renal or cardiac diseases are more prevalent, this might be different [11].

The entry points we used rely on normative general anatomy. Alternative entry points have been reported, although their descriptions are vague: a 'bonesaw tract' to biopsy the brain and a 'lateral position' to biopsy the kidneys [4,6]. For organs with a relative low yield alternative entry points should be further explored, e.g. below the xyphoid pointing the needle towards the left axilla for the heart or the 9th or 10th intercostal space behind the mid axillary line for the spleen. Moreover, to evaluate and compare needle autopsy it is important to know what exact methods are being used. Detailed methodological descriptions, e.g. what needle entry points are used, how many punctures are performed per organ, how tissue collection and processing takes place, should therefore be reported in needle autopsy studies.

We had set a reasonable maximum of 10 biopsy-attempts per organ and often far fewer attempts were made. A way to increase the yield could be to increase the number of attempts. However, we found for some organs a decrease in success rate with an increasing number of attempts, implying more punctures were done on 'difficult' organs without increasing the number of successful punctures. Therefore, merely increasing the number of attempts will unlikely increase the number of successful biopsies. Changing the entry point and/or position during the procedure may increase the success rate. This information was not collected during our study. Moreover, we found that predicted success rates did not correspond well to the true success rates. Therefore, the judgment of the operator should not be used to guide the sampling. A possible way forward to increase tissue yield would be to biopsy organs that are notoriously difficult more often and use different entry point and/or needle positions for each subsequent attempt.

Others showed the degree of experience and motivation of the person performing the biopsies influenced the yield [2]. We also observed a clear learning curve over time. Moreover, the procedure was fast, the visible marks after the needle autopsy were limited and no suturing of needle entry points was needed. Although medically trained people performed the needle autopsies, they were laymen in the field of needle biopsies. This offers perspectives for needle autopsies to be performed on a broader scale. Potential possibilities include practice outside a hospital setting by trained lower level healthcare workers.

This study has several limitations. The reported learning curve over time is based on the performance of 1 operator. Moreover, the subsequent performance of the blind, ultrasound guided and complete autopsy may have influenced the learning curve, for example the macroscopic assessment of the organs during the complete autopsy gave the operator feedback on the successfulness of the needle autopsy. Also, the increased failure rate in thin but not in emaciated patients was significant but difficult to interpret. The assessment of the nutritional status might have been inaccurate and also the numbers of patients in the categories "well nourished" and "obese" were small. These results should therefore be interpreted with caution. Finally, we assumed the absence of target tissue was the result of a failed biopsy. However, some small, fragile tissue cores may have also got lost during tissue processing.

Conclusion

We found that the use of surface marking points led to adequate tissue cores for further pathological review in the vast majority of organs assessed. Whether these will be adequate to diagnose the actual underlying causes of death depends on the population and the diseases and organs involved. However, the ability to obtain adequate tissue biopsies justifies further evaluation of this technique that overcomes many of the barriers of complete autopsy practices.

Competing interests
The authors declare that they have no competing interests.

Authors' contributions
Conception and design: JAC, RLL, AMN, YM, RC. Acquisition of data: JAC, RLL, SK, KVdV, EVM, AMN, AM. Analysis and interpretation of data: JAC, RLL, YM, RC. Drafting and/or revising the article: JAC, RLL, SK, KVdV, EVM, AMN, AM, YM, RC. All authors have approved the manuscript.

Acknowledgements
The authors want to thank all relatives that provided consent for study participation. Moreover, we want to thank Moses Kamya, Head of the Department of Medicine, Makerere University and the staff of the medicine wards of Mulago Hospital. We also particularly thank Dr. Male-Mutumba and Dr. Eva Mbwilo, the staff of the Mulago Hospital mortuary, particularly Mr. Edrisa Katende and the staff of the Makerere University Pathology lab, particularly Miss Betty Namwase. We want to thank the staff of the Infectious Diseases Institute, particularly Andrew Kambugu head of the research department for his scientific input and Mr. Michael Enyakoit and Mrs. Allen Mukhwana for their logistic support.

Author details
[1]Department of Clinical Sciences, Institute of Tropical Medicine, Nationalestraat 155, 2000 Antwerpen, Belgium. [2]Infectious Diseases Institute, Makerere University College of Health Sciences, Kampala, Uganda. [3]Department of Pathology, College of Health Sciences, Makerere University, Kampala, Uganda. [4]Department of Pathology, Mulago Hospital Complex, Kampala, Uganda. [5]Department of Diagnostic Oncology & Molecular Pathology, Netherlands Cancer Institute - Antoni van Leeuwenhoek Hospital, Amsterdam, The Netherlands. [6]Department of Pathology, University Hospital Antwerp, University of Antwerp, Antwerp, Belgium. [7]Joint Pathology Center, Silver Spring, USA. [8]Division of Infectious Diseases, Department of Medicine, Johns Hopkins University School of Medicine, Baltimore, Maryland. [9]Faculty of Medicine, University of Antwerp, Antwerp, Belgium.

References

1. Terry R: **Needle necropsy.** *J Clin Pathol* 1955, **8**(1):38–41.
2. Wellmann K: **The needle autopsy: a retrospective evaluation of 394 consecutive cases.** *Am J Clin Pathol* 1969, **52**(4):441–444.
3. Guerra I, Ortiz E, Portu J, Atares B, Aldamiz-Etxebarria M, De Pablos M: **Value of limited necropsy in HIV-positive patients.** *Pathol Res Pract* 2001, **197**(3):165–168.
4. Foroudi F, Cheung K, Duflou J: **A comparison of the needle biopsy post mortem with the conventional autopsy.** *Pathology* 1995, **27**(1):79–82.
5. Baumgart KW, Cook M, Quin J, Painter D, Gatenby PA, Garsia RJ: **The limited (needle biopsy) autopsy and the acquired immunodeficiency syndrome.** *Pathology* 1994, **26**(2):141–143.
6. Huston BM, Malouf NN, Azar HA: **Percutaneous needle autopsy sampling.** *Mod Pathol* 1996, **9**(12):1101–1107.
7. Flemming JA, Hurlbut DJ, Mussari B, Hookey LC: **Liver biopsies for chronic hepatitis C: should nonultrasound-guided biopsies be abandoned?** *Can J Gastroenterol* 2009, **23**(6):425–430.
8. Maya ID, Maddela P, Barker J, Allon M: **Percutaneous renal biopsy: comparison of blind and real-time ultrasound-guided technique.** *Semin Dial* 2007, **20**(4):355–358.
9. Sperandeo M, Rotondo A, Guglielmi G, Catalano D, Feragalli B, Trovato GM: **Transthoracic ultrasound in the assessment of pleural and pulmonary diseases: use and limitations.** *Radiol Med* 2014, **119**(10):729–740.
10. Wong EB, Omar T, Setlhako GJ, Osih R, Feldman C, Murdoch DM, Martinson NA, Bangsberg DR, Venter WD: **Causes of death on antiretroviral therapy: a post-mortem study from South Africa.** *PLoS One* 2012, **7**(10):e47542.
11. Cox JA, Lukande RL, Kalungi S, Van Marck E, Van de Vijver K, Kambugu A, Nelson AM, Manabe YC, Colebunders R: **Needle autopsy to establish the cause of death in HIV-infected hospitalized adults in Uganda: a comparison to complete autopsy.** *J Acquir Immune Defic Syndr* 2014, **67**(2):169–176.

4

Prognostic and predictive significance of podocalyxin-like protein expression in pancreatic and periampullary adenocarcinoma

Margareta Heby, Jakob Elebro, Björn Nodin, Karin Jirström and Jakob Eberhard[*]

Abstract

Background: Adenocarcinoma of the periampullary region is associated with poor prognosis and new prognostic and treatment predictive biomarkers are needed for improved treatment. Membranous expression of podocalyxin-like 1(PODXL), which is a cell-adhesion glycoprotein and stem cell marker, has been found to correlate with an aggressive tumour phenotype and adverse outcome in several cancer types. The aim of the present study was to examine the clinicopathological correlates, prognostic and predictive significance of tumour-specific PODXL expression in a retrospective cohort of pancreatic and periampullary carcinoma, morphologically divided into intestinal type (I-type) and pancreatobiliary type (PB-type) tumours.

Methods: Immunohistochemical expression of PODXL was analysed in tissue microarrays with primary tumours and a subset of paired lymph node metastases from 175 patients operated with pancreaticoduodenectomy for periampullary adenocarcinoma. Chi square test was applied to analyse the relationship between PODXL expression and clinicopathological parameters. Kaplan Meier analysis and Cox regression models were applied to estimate differences in 5-year overall survival (OS) and recurrence-free survival (RFS) in strata according to membranous and non-membranous PODXL expression.

Results: Membranous PODXL expression was significantly higher in primary PB-type (49.5 %) as compared with I-type (17.5 %) tumours. In PB-type tumours, PODXL expression was significantly associated with female sex ($p = 0.005$), location to the pancreas ($p = 0.005$), and poor differentiation grade ($p = 0.044$). Membranous PODXL expression was significantly associated with a reduced RFS (HR = 2.44, 95 % CI 1.10–5.44) and OS (HR = 2.32, 95 % CI 1.05–5.12) in I-type tumours and with a reduced RFS (HR = 1.63, 95 % CI 1.07–2.49) but not OS in PB-type tumours. PODXL remained a significant independent prognostic factor only in I-type tumours (HR = 5.12, 95 % CI 1.43–18.31 for RFS and HR = 7.31, 95 % CI 2.12–25.16 for OS). Patients with I-type tumours displaying membranous PODXL expression had a significant beneficial effect of adjuvant chemotherapy regarding 5-year OS.

Conclusion: Membranous expression of PODXL is significantly higher in PB-type than in I-type periampullary adenocarcinomas and an independent factor of poor prognosis in the latter. The results further indicate a beneficial effect of adjuvant chemotherapy on I-type tumours with membranous PODXL expression, suggesting the potential utility of PODXL as a biomarker for improved treatment stratification of these patients.

Keywords: Periampullary adenocarcinoma, Pancreatic cancer, Podocalyxin-like 1, Immunohistochemistry, Biomarkers, Prognosis, Response prediction

* Correspondence: jakob.eberhard@med.lu.se
Department of Clinical Sciences Lund, Division of Oncology and Pathology,
Lund University, Skåne University Hospital, 221 85 Lund, Sweden

Background

Adenocarcinoma of the periampullary region, including tumours originating in the distal bile duct, pancreas, ampulla of Vater and the periampullary duodenum, are a heterogeneous group of neoplasms and despite advances in surgery, radiotherapy, chemotherapy and targeted agents, patients still suffer from a poor prognosis. The incidence of these tumours has markedly increased over the past decades and in 2012 pancreatic cancers of all types were the seventh most common cause of cancer deaths, resulting in 330.000 deaths globally [1]. The overall 5-year survival is 5 %, all stages of the disease combined, and the median survival has been reported to be 5–8 months [2–4]. There are no early detection tests and most patients with localized disease have no recognizable symptoms or signs, resulting in late diagnosis in the majority of cases. Only 15-20 % of the tumours are resectable at presentation [5], resectability often being limited by early local invasion of the surrounding anatomical structures, such as mesenteric arteries, or distant metastasis. There are two major morphological types of periampullary adenocarcinomas, i.e. pancreatobiliary (PB-type) adenocarcinomas (including pancreatic cancer, distal bile duct cancer, and some of the ampullary carcinomas) and intestinal type (I-type) periampullary adenocarcinomas (including duodenal carcinoma and some of the ampullary carcinomas). Morphological type seems to provide more important prognostic information in resected periampullary carcinoma than the tumour origin, with PB-type tumours being associated with significantly shorter survival rates than I-type tumours [6, 7]. The present diagnostic and prognostic information provided by histopathological parameters is far from sufficient, strongly implicating the need for additional molecular-based biomarkers to better define clinically relevant subgroups of these tumours for improved treatment stratification.

Podocalyxin-like protein (PODXL) is a member of the CD34 family of transmembrane sialomucins. PODXL is expressed on the apical surface of glomerular epithelial cells and podocytes [8], where it plays an integral role in maintaining adequate filtration [9], and it is also expressed on vascular endothelia [10] and hematopoietic stem cells [11, 12]. PODXL is upregulated in several types of cancer, and strong expression, in particular in the cell membrane, has been demonstrated to signify more aggressive tumours and poor prognosis in e.g. breast cancer [13], colorectal cancer [14-17] ovarian cancer [18], urinary bladder cancer [19], and glioblastoma [20].

PODXL has been found to be more frequently expressed (44 %) in pancreatic ductal adenocarcinoma as compared with other types of adenocarcinomas of the gastrointestinal and biliary tracts [21]. In another study, sialofucosylated PODXL was demonstrated to be a functional E- and L-selectin ligand expressed by metastatic pancreatic cancer

cells *in vitro*, and was also found to be overexpressed, with membranous localization, in 69 % of 105 pancreatic ductal adenocarcinomas [22]. To our knowledge, the prognostic or predictive impact of PODXL expression in pancreatic or periampullary adenocarcinoma has not yet been described. The aim of the present study was therefore to examine the clinicopathological correlates, prognostic and predictive significance of tumour-specific PODXL expression in a retrospective cohort of pancreatic and periampullary adenocarcinoma, with particular reference to morphological subtypes thereof.

Methods

Patients

The study consists of a retrospective consecutive cohort of 175 patients with primary periampullary adenocarcinomas, surgically treated with pancreaticoduodenectomy at the University hospitals of Lund and Malmö, Sweden, from January 1 2001 until December 31 2011 [23–25]. Out of 175 cases in the entire cohort, there were 110 pancreatobiliary-type and 65 intestinal-type adenocarcinomas. Survival data were collected from the Swedish National Civil Register. Follow-up started at the date of surgery and ended at death, at 5 years after surgery or at December 31, 2013, whichever came first. Information on neoadjuvant and adjuvant treatment and recurrence was obtained from patient records.

All haematoxylin & eosin stained slides from all cases were re-evaluated by one pathologist (JEL), blinded to the original report and outcome. The decision on tumour origin and morphological type was based on several criteria, as previously described [23].

The study has been approved by the Ethics Committee of Lund University (ref nr 445/07).

Tissue microarray construction

Tissue microarrays (TMAs) were constructed using a semi-automated arraying device (TMArrayer, Pathology Devices, Westminister, MD, USA). A standard set of three tissue cores (1 mm) were obtained from each of the 175 primary tumours and from lymph node metastases from 105 of the cases, whereby one to three lymph node metastases were sampled in each case. Paired samples with non-malignant pancreatic tissue from the resection specimens were also obtained from 50 of the cases, using a standard set of two 1 mm tissue cores.

Immunohistochemistry and staining evaluation

For immunohistochemical analysis of PODXL expression, 4 μm TMA-sections were automatically pre-treated using the PT Link system and then stained in an Autostainer Plus (DAKO; Glostrup, Copenhagen, Denmark) with the affinity-purified polyclonal, monospecific PODXL antibody (HPA002110; Atlas Antibodies AB, Stockholm,

Sweden) diluted 1: 250. This antibody, originally generated within the Human Protein Atlas (HPA) project, has also been used in and validated in several previous biomarker studies on e.g. colorectal, bladder, pancreatic and testicular cancer [14, 19, 22, 26]. The expression of PODXL was recorded as negative (0), weak cytoplasmic positivity in any proportion of cells (1), moderate cytoplasmic positivity in any proportion of cells (2), distinct membranous positivity in < = 50 % of cells (3) and distinct membranous positivity in >50 % of cells (4) as previously described [14-16, 19]. Staining of PODXL was evaluated by two independent observers (MH and KJ) who were blinded to clinical and outcome data. Scoring differences were discussed in order to reach consensus.

Statistical analysis

Chi square test was applied to analyse the relationship between PODXL expression and clinicopathological parameters. Two patients with PB-type adenocarcinomas who had received neoadjuvant chemotherapy were excluded from the correlation and survival analyses. Three additional patients were excluded from the survival analyses; two with I-type adenocarcinomas who died within one month from surgery due to complications and one with PB-type adenocarcinoma who emigrated 5 months after surgery.

Kaplan Meier analysis and log rank test were applied to estimate differences in 5-year overall survival (OS) and recurrence-free survival (RFS) in strata according to membranous and non-membranous PODXL expression. Hazard ratios (HR) for death and recurrence within 5 years were calculated by Cox regression proportional hazard´s modelling in unadjusted analysis and in a multivariable model adjusted for age, sex, T-stage, N-stage, differentiation grade, lymphatic invasion, vascular invasion, perineural invasion, infiltration in peripancreatic fat, resection margins, tumour origin, and adjuvant chemotherapy. A backward conditional method was used for variable selection in the adjusted model. To estimate the interaction effect between adjuvant treatment and PODXL expression in order to measure any possible difference in treatment effect based on PODXL expression, the following interaction variable was constructed; any adjuvant treatment $(+/-) \times$ PODXL $(+/-)$.

All tests were two sided. *P-values* <0.05 were considered significant. All statistical analyses were performed using IBM SPSS Statistics version 20.0 (SPSS Inc., Chicago, IL, USA).

Results

PODXL expression in non-malignant pancreas, primary tumours and lymph node metastases

Sample immunohistochemical images of PODXL expression are shown in Fig. 1. PODXL expression could be assessed in in 63/65 (96.9 %) primary I-type carcinomas and 24/30 (80.0 %) lymph node metastases, and in 107/108 (99.1 %) primary PB-type carcinomas and 63/75 (84.0 %) corresponding lymph node metastases. PODXL expression could be assessed in 49/50 (98 %) paired non-malignant samples, all displaying negative or very weak PODXL expression in acini and ducts. The distribution of PODXL expression in primary tumours and metastases, which did not differ significantly, by histological subtype, is shown in Fig. 2. Membranous PODXL expression was denoted in 11/63 (17.5 %) primary and 2/24 (8.3 %) metastatic I-type carcinomas, and in 53/107 (49.5 %) primary and 23/63 (36.5 %) metastatic PB-type carcinomas. In I-type tumours, membranous PODXL in the metastasis was seen in 1/21 (4.8 %) cases denoted as having non-membranous expression in the primary tumour, and non-membranous PODXL expression in the metastasis was denoted in 2/3 (66.7 %) cases with primary tumours displaying membranous PODXL expression. In PB-type tumours, the number of cases with non-membranous to membranous conversion was 2/32 (6.2 %) and with membranous to non-membranous conversion 10/31 (32.3 %). In all further statistical analyses, a dichotomized variable of non-membranous (score 0, 1, 2) versus membranous (score 3, 4) PODXL expression in the primary and/or metastatic component is applied. According to this combined variable, 12/63 (19.0 %) I-type cases and 55/107 (51.4 %) PB-type cases displayed membranous PODXL expression in any component.

Associations of PODXL expression with clinicopathological factors

The associations between PODXL expression and clinicopathological factors in I-type and PB-type tumours, respectively, are shown in Table 1. In I-type tumours, there were no significant associations between PODXL expression and clinicopathological factors. In PB-type tumours, membranous PODXL expression was significantly associated with female sex ($p = 0.005$), with location to the pancreas ($p = 0.005$), and with poor differentiation grade ($p = 0.044$). There was no statistically significant association between PODXL expression and other clinicopathological factors including age at diagnosis, tumour size, T-stage, N-stage, resection margins, presence of vascular- lymphatic and neural invasion and growth in peripancreatic fat.

Prognostic and potential predictive value of PODXL expression

As demonstrated in Fig. 3, Kaplan-Meier analysis revealed significant associations of membranous PODXL expression with a reduced RFS (logrank $p = 0.024$) and OS (logrank $p = 0.032$) in I-type tumours and with a reduced RFS (logrank $p = 0.022$) but not OS in PB-type tumours. These associations were confirmed in univariable Cox regression

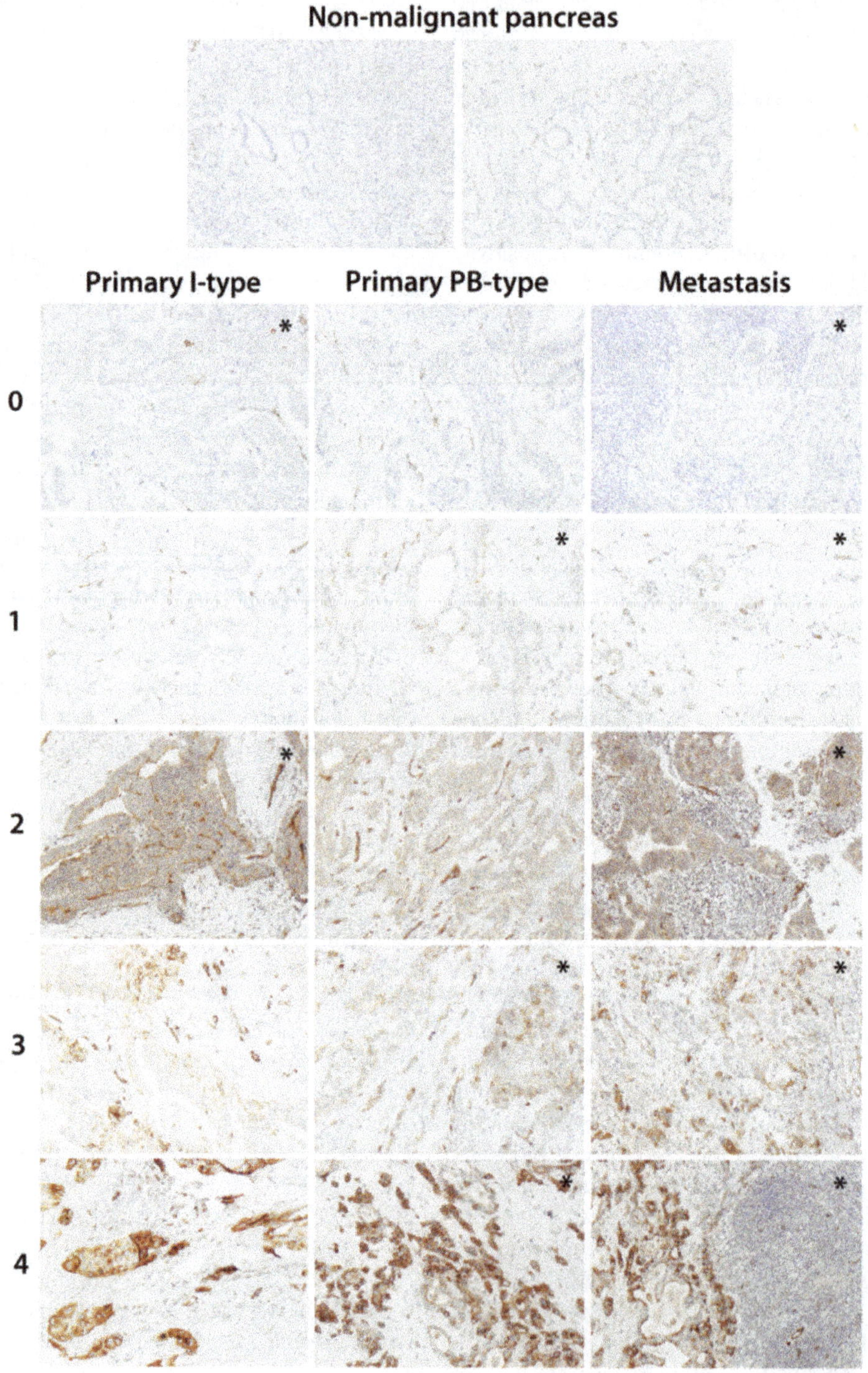

Fig. 1 Sample immunohistochemical images. Immunohistochemical images of PODXL- negative non-malignant pancreatic tissue from two cases (*top row*), primary intestinal-type (*I-type*) tumours (*left column*), primary pancreatobiliary-type (*PB-type*) tumours (*mid-column*) and metastases (*right column*) with different PODXL staining scores (*0–4*). Asterisks indicate paired samples; i.e. from the same case/resection specimen. Score 0 = negative staining, score 1 = weak cytoplasmic positivity in any proportion of cells, score 2: moderate-strong cytoplasmic positivity in any proportion of cells, score 3: distinct membranous positivity in < = 50 % of cells and score 4 = distinct membranous positivity in >50 % of cells. All images with 10X original magnification

analysis for both RFS (Table 2) and OS (Table 3) in I-type tumours (HR = 2.44, 95 % CI 1.10–5.44, and HR = 2.32, 95 % CI 1.05–5.12, respectively) and for RFS (Table 2), but not OS (Table 3) in PB-type tumours (HR = 1.63, 95 % CI 1.07–2.49, logrank $p = 0.022$). In multivariable analysis, PODXL remained a significant prognostic factor only in

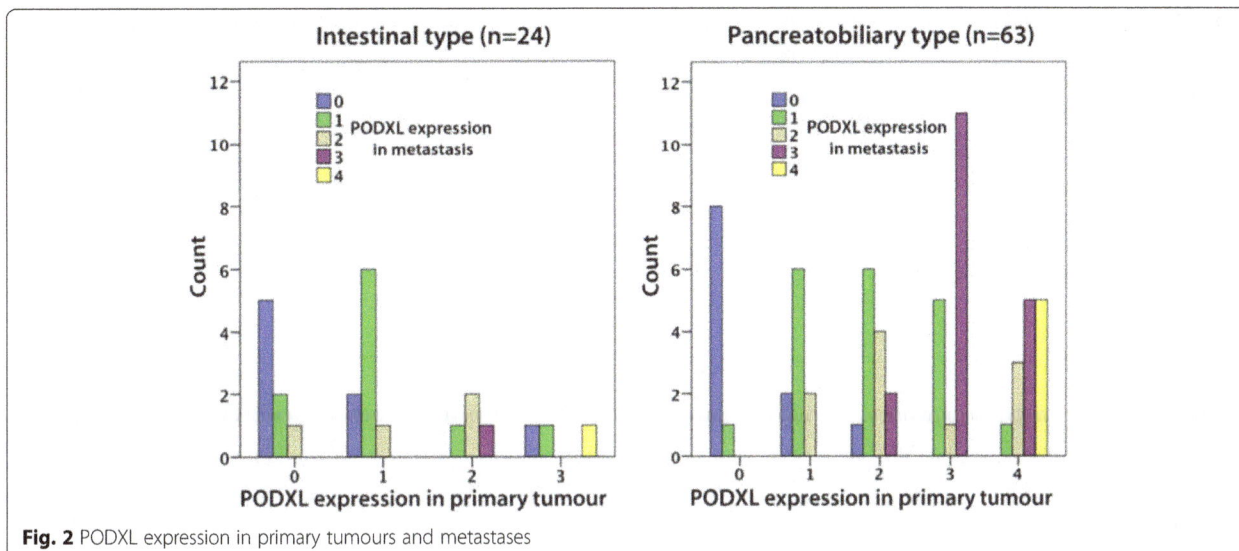

Fig. 2 PODXL expression in primary tumours and metastases

I-type tumours (HR = 5.12, 95 % CI 1.43–18.31 for RFS, Table 2, and HR = 7.31, 95 % CI 2.12–25.16 for OS, Table 3).

Next, we examined the potential predictive impact of PODXL expression on survival in strata according to adjuvant treatment. As demonstrated in Fig. 4, patients with I-type tumours displaying membranous PODXL expression had a significant beneficial effect of adjuvant chemotherapy regarding 5-year OS. When ampullary PB-type tumours, expressing membranous PODXL in a similar proportion to I-type tumours, were included in the analysis, the beneficial value of adjuvant chemotherapy was even more pronounced (Fig. 4). Hazard ratios for 5-year OS according to adjuvant treatment and PODXL expression are shown in Additional file 1. The results demonstrate that survival did not differ significantly by membranous PODXL-expression in patients with I-type tumours or the extended group of I-type + ampullary PB-type tumours having received adjuvant chemotherapy. In contrast, the adverse prognostic impact of membranous PODXL expression was even more evident in patients not receiving adjuvant chemotherapy compared to the entire group (unadjusted HR = 4.38, 95 % CI 1.57–12.18 in I-type tumours, and unadjusted HR = 7.13; 95 % CI 2.64–19.26 in I-type + ampullary PB-type tumours). These associations remained significant in multivariable analysis, but there was no significant treatment interaction (Additional file 1). These associations were not significant in relation to RFS (data not shown) or in PB-type tumours (data not shown). The prognostic and predictive impact of membranous PODXL expression was similar when only its expression in the primary tumour was considered (data not shown). The prognostic value of the full range of PODXL scores (0–4) in relation to RFS and OS, in the entire cohort and by morphological subtype, is shown in Additional file 2. All survival analyses were also performed using a dichotomized

variable of score 0–1 vs 2–4, with allover less significant results (data not shown).

Discussion

Pancreatic cancer is an extremely lethal type of cancer. On average, patients die from the disease within 6 months from diagnosis. Therefore it is of uttermost importance to find both predictive and prognostic factors so as to improve treatment. The results from this study provide a first demonstration of the prognostic and potential predictive value of PODXL in pancreatic, distal bile duct, ampullary and duodenal adenocarcinoma. PODXL-expression was found to be significantly higher in PB-type as compared with I-type tumours, with the exception for ampullary PB-type tumours. These findings are in line with the expected and provide further evidence of PODXL being associated with a more aggressive tumour phenotype and a biomarker of poor prognosis in human cancer.

The study cohort encompasses a retrospective cohort of 110 pancreatobiliary-type and 65 intestinal-type adenocarcinomas, including paired normal tissue and lymph node metastases from a subset of cases, thus providing a thorough characterization of PODXL expression in a wide range of periampullary adenocarcinomas. In the present study, membranous PODXL expression was denoted in 49.5 % of primary PB-type carcinomas, which is somewhat lower than in the previous study by Dallas et al., including tumours from 105 cases assembled in TMAs, wherein membranous PODXL expression was found in 69 % of the cases [22]. In primary I-type carcinomas, membranous PODXL expression was denoted in 17.5 %, which is well in line with previous TMA-based studies on colorectal cancer wherein membranous expression was found in 13.4 % and 9.6 % respectively [14, 15]. This observation further supports the theory that I-type carcinomas of the

Table 1 Associations between membranous and non-membranous PODXL expression with clinciopathological parameters in intestinal type and pancreatobiliary type tumours, respectively

	Intestinal type			Pancreatobiliary type		
	PODXL NM	PODXL M	P	PODXL NM	PODXL M	P
	(*n* = 51)	(*n* = 12)		(*n* = 52)	(*n* = 55)	
Age						
(median, range)	66.0 (38.0–83.0)	67.5 (44.0–74.0)	0.972	66.0 (44.0–81.0)	68.0 (44.0–81.0)	0.613
Sex						
Women	28 (82.4)	6 (17.6)	0.761	17 (34.0)	33 (66.0)	0.005
Men	23 (79.3)	6 (20.7)		35 (61.4)	22 (38.6)	
Tumour origin						
Duodenum	12 (85.7)	2 (14.3)	0.610			
Ampulla intestinal type	39 (79.6)	10 (20.4)				
Ampulla pancreatobiliary type				14 (73.7)	5 (26.3)	0.005
Distal bile duct				23 (51.1)	22 (48.9)	
Pancreas				15 (34.9)	28 (65.1)	
Tumour size mm						
(median, range)	30.0 (5.0–90.0)	26.5 (12.0–40.0)	0.923	30.0 (5.0 70.0)	30.0 (15.0–70.0)	0.313
Differentiation grade						
Well-moderate	26 (83.9)	5 (16.1)	0.565	24 (61.5)	15 (38.5)	0.044
Poor	25 (78.1)	7 (21.9)		28 (41.2)	40 (58.8)	
T-stage						
T1	4 (100.0)	0 (0.0)	0.246	2 (100.0)	0 (0.0)	0.392
T2	9 (81.8)	2 (18.2)		4 (40.0)	6 (60.0)	
T3	21 (84.0)	4 (16.0)		34 (43.6)	44 (56.4)	
T4	17 (73.9)	6 (26.1)		12 (70.6)	5 (29.4)	
N-stage						
N0	28 (84.8)	5 (5.2)	0.936	17 (56.7)	13 (43.3)	0.315
N1	13 (68.4)	6 (31.6)		21 (46.7)	24 (53.3)	
N2	10 (90.9)	1 (9.1)		14 (43.8)	18 (56.2)	
Margins						
R0	15 (88.2)	2 (11.8)	0.375	3 (50.0)	3 (50.0)	0.944
R1-Rx	36 (78.3)	10 (21.7)		49 (48.5)	52 (51.5)	
Perineural growth						
No	38 (86.4)	6 (13.6)	0.099	14 (63.6)	8 (36.4)	0.115
Yes	13 (68.4)	6 (31.6)		38 (44.7)	47 (55.3)	
Invasion of lymphatic vessels						
No	26 (89.7)	3 (10.3)	0.107	16 (50.0)	16 (50.0)	0.850
Yes	25 (73.5)	9 (26.5)		36 (48.0)	39 (52.0)	
Invasion of blood vessels						
No	48 (82.8)	10 (17.2)	0.217	35 (50.0)	35 (50.0)	0.691
Yes	3 (60.0)	2 (40.0)		17 (45.9)	20 (54.1)	
Growth in peripancreatic fat						
No	35 (85.4)	6 (14.6)	0.227	13 (59.1)	9 (40.9)	0.271
Yes	16 (72.7)	6 (27.3)		39 (45.9)	46 (54.1)	

Table 1 Associations between membranous and non-membranous PODXL expression with clinciopathological parameters in intestinal type and pancreatobiliary type tumours, respectively (Continued)

Adjuvant chemotherapy						
None	40 (88.9)	5 (11.1)	0.145	23 (46.0)	27 (54.0)	0.348
5-FU-analogue	2 (40.0)	3 (60.0)		5 (62.5)	3 (37.5)	
Gemcitabine	4 (57.1)	3 (42.9)		20 (45.5)	24 (54.5)	
Gemcitabine + capecitabine	1 (100.0)	0 (0.0)		1 (50.0)	1 (50.0)	
Oxaliplatin + 5-FU analogue	4 (100.0)	0 (0.0)		1 (100.0)	0 (0.0)	
Gemcitabine + oxaliplatin	0 (0.0)	1 (100.0)		2 (100.0)	0 (0.0)	

M membranous PODXL expression, *NM* non-membranous PODXL expression
R0 radical resection, *R1* non-radical resection, *RX* uncertain resection margins

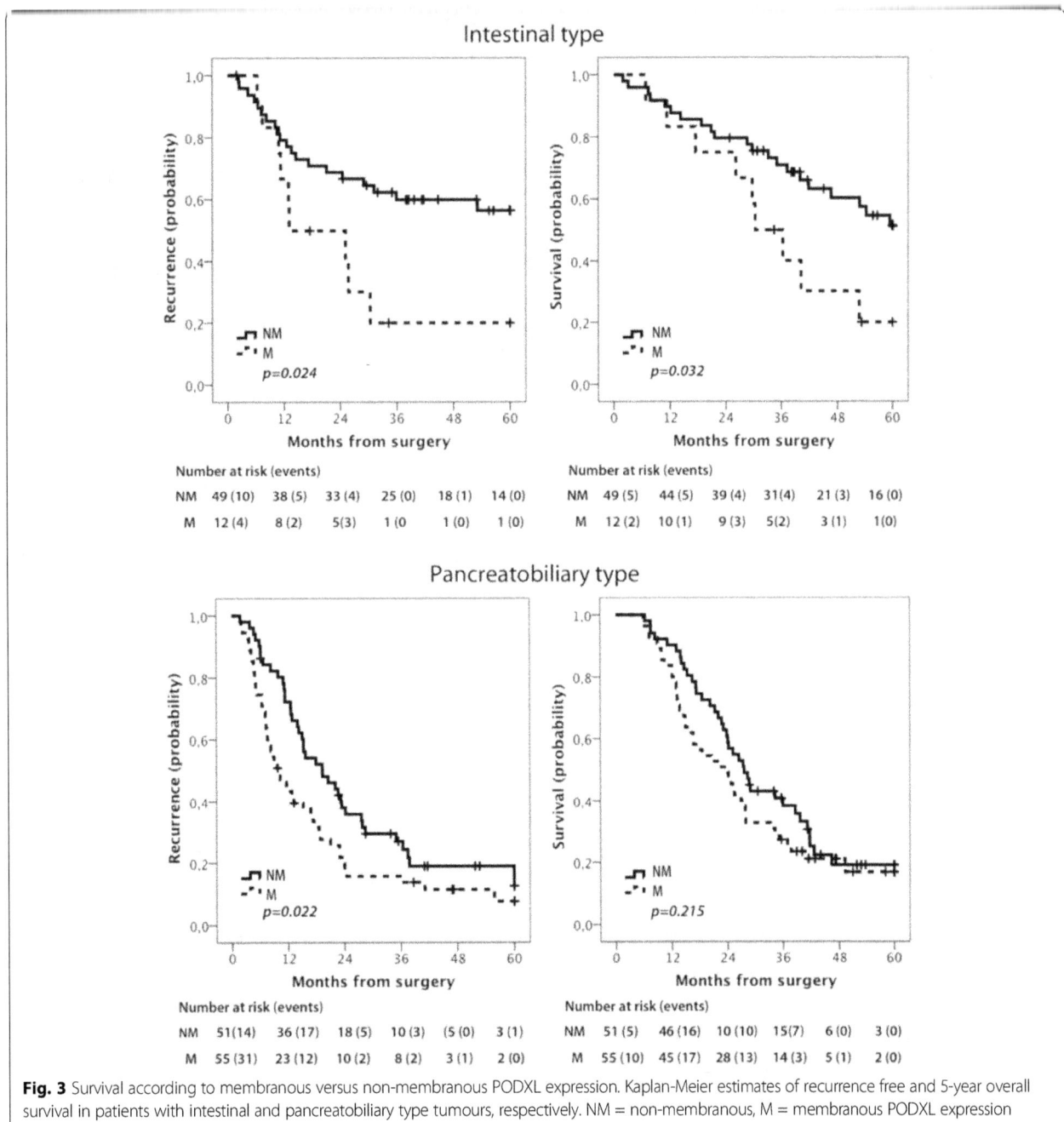

Fig. 3 Survival according to membranous versus non-membranous PODXL expression. Kaplan-Meier estimates of recurrence free and 5-year overall survival in patients with intestinal and pancreatobiliary type tumours, respectively. NM = non-membranous, M = membranous PODXL expression

Table 2 Unadjusted and adjusted hazard ratios for recurrence within five years in intestinal and pancreatobiliary type tumours

	Intestinal type			Pancreatobiliary type		
	n(events)	Unadjusted HR(95 % CI)	Adjusted HR(95 % CI)	n(events)	Unadjusted HR(95 % CI)	Adjusted HR(95 % CI)
Age						
Continuous	61 (29)	1.00 (0.96–1.03)	1.07 (1.02–1.13)	106 (88)	0.98 (0.96–1.01)	1.00 (0.96–1.03)
Gender						
Female	34 (11)	1.00	1.00	50 (42)	1.00	1.00
Male	27 (18)	2.31 (1.08–4.94)	2.40 (0.94–6.14)	56 (46)	1.06 (0.70–1.61)	0.88 (0.53–1.49)
Tumour origin						
Duodenum	13 (4)	1.00	1.00	–	–	
Ampulla-Intestinal type	48 (25)	2.18 (0.76–6.27)	6.82 (1.32–35.12)	–	–	
Ampulla-Pancreatobiliary type		–	–	19 (16)	1.00	1.00
Distal Bile duct		–	–	44 (38)	1.10 (0.61–1.98)	1.52 (0.78–2.94)
Pancreas		–	–	43 (34)	1.06 (0.58–1.93)	0.93 (0.49–1.77)
Tumour size						
Continuous	61 (30)	1.00 (0.98–1.02)	1.04 (1.00–1.09)	106 (88)	1.03 (1.02–1.05)	1.02 (0.99–1.04)
T-stage						
T1	4 (1)	1.00	1.00	2 (1)	1.00	1.00
T2	10(3)	1.28 (0.13–12.30)	3.71 (0.34–40.64)	10 (6)	1.61 (0.19–13.36)	0.66 (0.07–6.08)
T3	25 (9)	1.86 (0.24–14.71)	5.72 (0.50–65.06)	77 (66)	4.67 (0.64–33.96)	1.21 (0.15–9.92)
T4	22 (16)	5.44 (0.72–41.21)	6.36 (0.21–195.20)	17 (15)	4.31 (0.56–33.10)	1.83 (0.08–40.27)
N-stage						
N0	33 (11)	1.00	1.00	29 (21)	1.00	1.00
N1 (metastasis in 1–3 lgl)	19 (11)	2.07 (0.90–4.78)	1.00 (0.37–2.70)	45 (37)	2.17 (1.25–3.78)	2.04 (1.13–3.67)
N2 (metastasis in 4 or more lgl)	9 (7)	4.06 (1.55–10.59)	6.88 (1.81–26.15)	32 (30)	3.11 (1.72–5.61)	2.61 (1.42–4.83)
Differentiation grade						
Well-moderate	30 (11)	1.00	1.00	39 (29)	1.00	1.00
Poor	31 (18)	2.16 (1.02–4.57)	1.38 (0.40–4.79)	67 (59)	2.32 (1.45–3.71)	2.02 (1.20–3.39)
Involved margins, status						
R0	17 (3)	1.00	1.00	6 (4)	1.00	1.00
R1 & Rx	44 (26)	4.51 (1.36–14.94)	2.23 (0.62–8.03)	100 (84)	2.31 (0.84–6.36)	2.39 (0.84–6.76)
Lymphatic growth						
Absent	28 (5)	1.00	1.00	32 (23)	1.00	1.00
Present	33 (24)	6.16 (2.34–16.19)	6.19 (1.76–21.82)	74 (65)	1.77 (1.09–2.88)	1.05 (0.59–1.85)
Vascular growth						
Absent	56 (24)	1.00	1.00	70 (55)	1.00	1.00
Present	5 (5)	8.16 (2.86–23.30)	1.62 (0.39–6.65)	36 (33)	2.30 (1.47–3.61)	2.08 (1.28–3.36)
Perineural growth						
Absent	42 (15)	1.00	1.00	22 (14)	1.00	1.00
Present	19 (14)	2.72 (1.31–5.66)	1.01 (0.27–3.81)	84 (74)	2.93 (1.57–5.46)	2.04 (1.06–3.90)
Growth in peripancreatic fat						
Absent	40 (12)	1.00	1.00	22 (13)	1.00	1.00
Present	21 (17)	4.74 (2.23–10.10)	3.60 (1.43–9.07)	84 (75)	2.60 (1.42–4.75)	1.45 (0.76–2.77)

Table 2 Unadjusted and adjusted hazard ratios for recurrence within five years in intestinal and pancreatobiliary type tumours (Continued)

Adjuvant treatment						
No	43 (21)	1.00	1.00	49 (40)	1.00	1.00
Yes	18 (8)	0.87 (0.38–1.96)	0.12 (0.04–0.44)	57 (48)	1.08 (0.70–1.65)	0.89 (0.54–1.49)
PODXL expression						
Non-membranous	49 (20)	1.00	1.00	51 (40)	1.00	1.00
Membranous	12 (9)	2.44 (1.10–5.44)	5.12 (1.43–18.31)	55 (88)	1.63 (1.07–2.49)	1.53 (0.99–2.38)

R0 radical resection, *R1* non-radical resection, *RX* uncertain resection margins

pancreatic region resemble tumours with colorectal origin in a stronger way than PB-types. In line with the study by Ney et al., PODXL was negative or only weakly expressed in normal pancreatic parenchyma from the resection specimens [21].

In a previous study on colorectal cancer, wherein a PODXL expression was compared in full-face sections from 31 primary tumours and all available lymph node metastases ($n = 140$), there was an excellent concordance in that all primary tumours with non-membranous PODXL expression had metastases with non-membranous expression, whereas a few primary tumours with membranous PODXL expression had a varying proportion of metastatic lymph nodes with membranous and non-membranous PODXL expression [16]. These findings led to the conclusion that for prognostic or predictive purposes, analysis of the primary tumour would be sufficient [16]. In the present study, although negative conversion of membranous PODXL expression from primary tumour to lymph node metastasis was far more common than positive conversion, a few cases displayed the latter phenomenon. Of note, all analyses were based on TMA-samples, and therefore, future studies based on full-face sections are warranted to further examine the rate of positive conversion of membranous PODXL expression in pancreatic and periampullary cancers, so as to determine whether biomarker analysis of the primary tumour will be sufficient in the clinical setting.

In the present study membranous PODXL expression was an independent predictor of reduced 5-year overall and recurrence-free survival in I-type but not in PB-type tumours, although there was a significant association between membranous PODXL expression and a reduced RFS in the latter in unadjusted analysis. These findings are well in line with previous publications regarding the prognostic significance of PODXL expression in several other major types of cancer [13–15, 18–20]. In addition, and importantly, we found that patients with I-type tumours displaying membranous PODXL had a beneficial effect of adjuvant chemotherapy. When ampullary PB-type tumours, expressing membranous PODXL in a similar proportion to I-type tumours, were included in the analysis, the effect by adjuvant chemotherapy was even

more pronounced. This supports earlier data that patients with PODXL positive tumours benefit from adjuvant chemotherapy, irrespective of treatment regime, as seen in colorectal cancer [14, 15]. Moreover, these findings indicate that I-type tumours with high expression of PODXL are more likely to benefit from adjuvant therapy than PB-type tumours. Today, all patients with pancreatic and periampullary adenocarcinoma are recommended adjuvant treatment. Since adjuvant treatment often is associated with toxicity and adverse side effects, it is important to identify novel predictive and prognostic factors, such as PODXL, to support and improve clinical decisions. Therefore, the results from the present study indicate that PODXL could be used as a predictive marker for adjuvant treatment of periampullary cancer with intestinal morphology, and possibly also ampullary PB-type tumours. Of note, given the retrospective nature of the present study, the term "predictive" should be applied with caution. It must however be pointed out that the study cohort encompasses a consecutive series of clinically and histopathologically well-annotated pancreatoduodenectomy cases, of which only approximately half have been given adjuvant chemotherapy, which should allow for a fairly good assessment of both prognostic and predictive biomarkers even in the retrospective setting. Thus, the herein observed prognostic and potential predictive value of PODXL, in particular in I-type tumours, is of potential clinical relevance and merits further study in additional retrospective cohorts as well as in a controlled, prospective trial. Targeting PODXL with monoclonal antibodies may also be a future treatment option [27].

Membranous PODXL expression was considerably higher in PB-type as compared with I-type tumours, which is in line with the former being clinically more aggressive. In PB-type tumours, the prognostic value of PODXL was only significant for RFS, and not after adjustment for other clinicopathological factors, and there was no evident predictive value. The choice of prognostic cutoff, i.e. membranous vs non-membranous PODXL expression, can be considered appropriate for the herein used antibody, since the same antibody and cutoff has been used in the previous study on pancreatic cancer by Dallas et al. [22] and since this dichotomization yielded the strongest prognostic and predictive

Table 3 Unadjusted and adjusted hazard ratios for death within five years in intestinal and pancreatobiliary type tumours

	Intestinal type			Pancreatobiliary type		
	n(events)	Unadjusted HR(95 % CI)	Adjusted HR(95 % CI)	n(events)	Unadjusted HR(95 % CI)	Adjusted HR(95 % CI)
Age						
Continuous	61 (30)	1.02 (0.98–1.06)	1.07 (1.02–1.13)	106 (82)	0.99 (0.96–1.02)	1.01 (0.98–1.05)
Gender						
Female	34 (13)	1.00	1.00	50 (36)	1.00	1.00
Male	27 (17)	1.85 (0.89–3.84)	2.12 (0.86–5.22)	56 (46)	1.20 (0.78–1.87)	1.22 (0.76–1.95)
Tumour origin						
Duodenum	13 (5)	1.00	1.00			
Ampulla-Intestinal type	48 (25)	1.49 (0.57–3.88)	7.77 (1.86–32.39)		–	–
Ampulla-Pancreatobiliary type		–	–	19 (16)	1.00	1.00
Distal Bile duct		–	–	44 (32)	0.74 (0.40–1.34)	1.03 (0.50–2.15)
Pancreas		–	–	43 (34)	0.91 (0.50–1.65)	1.06 (0.52–2.19)
Tumour size						
Continuous	61 (30)	1.00 (0.98–1.03)	1.05 (1.01–1.10)	106 (82)	1.03 (1.01–1.05)	1.01 (0.99–1.04)
T-stage						
T1	4 (2)	1.00	1.00	2 (1)	1.00	1.00
T2	10(3)	0.65 (0.11–3.88)	0.55 (0.07–4.50)	10 (6)	1.43 (0.17–11.85)	0.77 (0.08–7.56)
T3	25 (9)	0.94 (0.20–4.37)	1.49 (0.19–11.34)	77 (60)	2.95 (0.41–21.34)	0.84 (0.10–7.08)
T4	22 (16)	2.55 (0.58–11.15)	1.88 (0.19–18.25)	17 (15)	3.77 (0.50–28.71)	2.12 (0.09–48.78)
N-stage						
N0	33 (15)	1.00	1.00	29 (18)	1.00	1.00
N1 (metastasis in 1–3 lgl)	19 (9)	1.17 (0.51–2.68)	0.55 (0.20–1.50)	45 (37)	2.41 (1.35–4.29)	2.85 (1.57–5.17)
N2 (metastasis in 4 or more lgl)	9 (6)	2.08 (0.80–5.37)	8.96 (2.47–32.51)	32 (27)	2.59 (1.40–4.78)	2.45 (1.30–4.63)
Differentiation grade						
Well-moderate	30 (12)	1.00	1.00	39 (24)	1.00	1.00
Poor	31 (18)	1.98 (0.95–4.11)	2.16 (0.77–6.03)	67 (58)	2.44 (1.50–3.95)	2.13 (1.28–3.54)
Involved margins, status						
R0	17 (4)	1.00	1.00	6 (2)	1.00	1.00
R1 & Rx	44 (26)	2.56 (0.89–7.36)	0.46 (0.12–1.69)	100 (80)	3.49 (0.86–14.25)	2.57 (0.62–10.60)
Lymphatic growth						
Absent	28 (7)	1.00	1.00	32 (22)	1.00	1.00
Present	33 (23)	3.61 (1.55–8.44)	5.85 (1.93–17.77)	74 (60)	1.51 (0.92–2.48)	0.96 (0.55–1.70)
Vascular growth						
Absent	56 (25)	1.00	1.00	70 (47)	1.00	1.00
Present	5 (5)	7.78 (2.74–22.11)	1.70 (0.40–7.31)	36 (35)	2.39 (1.54–3.72)	2.45 (1.54–3.87)
Perineural growth						
Absent	42 (17)	1.00	1.00	22 (14)	1.00	1.00
Present	19 (13)	2.15 (1.04–4.44)	3.81 (1.55–9.37)	84 (68)	1.88 (1.05–3.38)	0.92 (0.48–1.76)
Growth in peripancreatic fat						
Absent	40 (14)	1.00	1.00	22 (14)	1.00	1.00
Present	21 (16)	3.49 (1.68–7.25)	0.75 (0.06–9.94)	84 (68)	1.80 (1.00–3.25)	1.25 (0.64–2.43)
Adjuvant treatment						
No	43 (24)	1.00	1.00	49 (39)	1.00	1.00

Table 3 Unadjusted and adjusted hazard ratios for death within five years in intestinal and pancreatobiliary type tumours (Continued)

Yes	18 (6)	0.60 (0.25–1.47)	0.03 (0.01–0.16)	57 (43)	0.90 (0.58–1.39)	0.67 (0.43–1.04)
PODXL expression						
Non-membranous	49 (21)	1.00	1.00	51 (38)	1.00	1.00
Membranous	12 (9)	2.32 (1.05–5.12)	7.31 (2.12–25.16)	55 (44)	1.32 (0.85–2.03)	1.10 (0.67–1.81)

R0 radical resection, *R1* non-radical resection, *RX* uncertain resection margins

value. It is however noteworthy that the category of tumours with moderate-strong cytoplasmic staining (score 2) is a somewhat ambiguous group with an intermediate prognosis, undoubtedly harbouring some cases with a prognosis equally poor to cases with membranous PODXL expression. While it is possible that in some of these cases, the presence of membranous expression may be masked by a strong cytoplasmic expression, this category of tumours may also constitute a different biological entity, possibly constituting an "intermediate" between tumours with negative/weak and membranous PODXL expression. In a comparative study on colorectal cancer, membranous expression of the herein used antibody and cytoplasmic expression of an in-house generated antibody were both found to be independent predictors of poor prognosis, and combined use of the antibodies was found to detect a group with an even worse prognosis [28].

Previous studies have demonstrated PODXL to be a functional ligand of E- and L- selectins in pancreatic cancer suggesting that its expression may promote haemotogenic spread of metastases by facilitating binding of circulating tumour cells to selectin-expressing host cells [22]. These findings further support the theory of PODXL overexpression being associated with more aggressive tumours [22]. Moreover, similar to the situation in colorectal [14, 15, 16] and urinary bladder [19] cancer, PODXL expression was observed predominantly on the invasive tumour front, also suggesting its importance in the metastatic spread of the disease. Of note, in the study on bladder cancer, the herein used polyclonal antibody was compared with two other monoclonal antibodies, all showing 100 % concordance regarding the detection of membranous PODXL expression, whereas the degree of cytoplasmic expression detected by the monoclonal antibodies was substantially weaker [19].

Our results are derived from TMA-based analyses on retrospectively collected tumour samples. Of note, the TMA-technique was also used in the study by Dallas et al. [22]. For characterization of key molecular alterations and expression of investigative biomarkers in tumours from large patient cohorts, whether retrospectively or prospectively defined, the TMA-technology is essential [29].

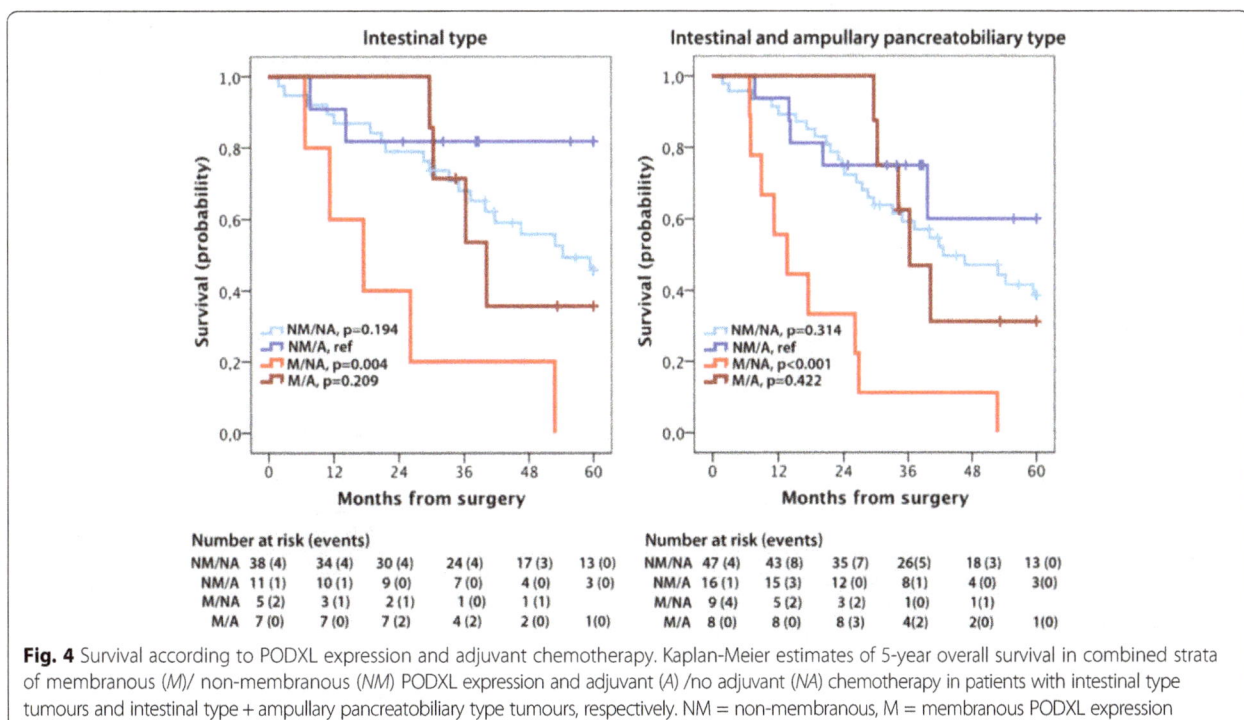

Fig. 4 Survival according to PODXL expression and adjuvant chemotherapy. Kaplan-Meier estimates of 5-year overall survival in combined strata of membranous (*M*)/ non-membranous (*NM*) PODXL expression and adjuvant (*A*) /no adjuvant (*NA*) chemotherapy in patients with intestinal type tumours and intestinal type + ampullary pancreatobiliary type tumours, respectively. NM = non-membranous, M = membranous PODXL expression

However, some limitations related to the TMA-technique must be considered, most importantly its ability to accurately reflect the expression of heterogeneously expressed markers. To compensate for this one needs to ensure that tumour cores are sampled from different regions of the tumour. In the present study, the cores from the primary tumour were, whenever possible, obtained from different donor blocks, and different lymph nodes were sampled in cases with more than one metastatic node.

Conclusions

Membranous expression of PODXL is significantly higher in pancreatobiliary type as compared with intestinal type periampullary adenocarcinomas and an independent factor of poor prognosis in the latter. The herein presented results also indicate a beneficial effect of adjuvant chemotherapy on intestinal type tumours with membranous PODXL expression, suggesting the potential utility of PODXL as a biomarker for improved treatment stratification of these patients.

Additional files

Additional file 1: Cox proportional hazards analysis of the impact of PODXL expression on overall survival according to adjuvant treatment intestinal-type and intestinal-type + ampullary pancreatobiliary-type adenocarcinomas.

Additional file 2: Survival according to PODXL score. Kaplan-Meier estimates of recurrence free survival and 5-year overall survival, respectively, in (A,B) the entire cohort, (C, D) patients with intestinal type tumours and (E, F) patients with pancreatobiliary type tumours. Score 0 = negative staining, score 1 = weak cytoplasmic positivity in any proportion of cells, score 2: moderate-strong cytoplasmic positivity in any proportion of cells, score 3: distinct membranous positivity in < = 50 % of cells and score 4 = distinct membranous positivity in >50 % of cells.

Abbreviations

PODXL: Podocalyxin-like protein 1; PB-type: Pancreatobiliary type adenocarcinoma; I-type: Intestinal type adenocarcinoma; TMA: Tissue microarray; OS: Overall survival; RFS: Recurrence free survival; HR: Hazard ratio; CI: Confidence interval.

Competing interests

The authors declare that they have no competing interests.

Authors' contributions

MH collected clinical data, annotated the immunohistochemical staining, performed the statistical analyses and drafted the manuscript. JEL collected clinicopathological data, assisted with TMA construction and helped draft the manuscript. BN constructed the tissue microarray and performed the IHC stainings. KJ conceived the study, evaluated the immunohistochemical staining and helped draft the manuscript. JEB collected clinical data, conceived the study and helped draft the manuscript. All authors read and approved the final manuscript.

Acknowledgments

This study was supported by grants from the Knut and Alice Wallenberg Foundation, the Swedish Cancer Society, the Gunnar Nilsson Cancer Foundation, the Swedish Government Grant for Clinical Research, Lund University Faculty of Medicine and University Hospital Research Grants.

References

1. C.P, SBWW. World Cancer Report 2014. In: Bernard W, editor. World Cancer Report 2014. Stewart CPW: IARC; 2014.
2. Heinemann V, Boeck S, Hinke A, Labianca R, Louvet C. Meta-analysis of randomized trials: evaluation of benefit from gemcitabine-based combination chemotherapy applied in advanced pancreatic cancer. BMC Cancer. 2008;8:82.
3. Jemal A, Siegel R, Ward E, Hao Y, Xu J, Thun MJ. Cancer statistics, 2009. CA Cancer J Clin. 2009;59(4):225–49.
4. Sultana A, Tudur Smith C, Cunningham D, Starling N, Neoptolemos JP, Ghaneh P. Meta-analyses of chemotherapy for locally advanced and metastatic pancreatic cancer: results of secondary end points analyses. Br J Cancer. 2008;99(1):6–13.
5. Herreros-Villanueva M, Hijona E, Cosme A, Bujanda L. Adjuvant and neoadjuvant treatment in pancreatic cancer. World J Gastroenterol. 2012;18(14):1565–72.
6. Westgaard A, Tafjord S, Farstad IN, Cvancarova M, Eide TJ, Mathisen O, et al. Pancreatobiliary versus intestinal histologic type of differentiation is an independent prognostic factor in resected periampullary adenocarcinoma. BMC Cancer. 2008;8:170.
7. Bronsert P, Kohler I, Werner M, Makowiec F, Kuesters S, Hoeppner J, et al. Intestinal-type of differentiation predicts favourable overall survival: confirmatory clinicopathological analysis of 198 periampullary adenocarcinomas of pancreatic, biliary, ampullary and duodenal origin. BMC Cancer. 2013;13:428.
8. Kerjaschki D, Sharkey DJ, Farquhar MG. Identification and characterization of podocalyxin–the major sialoprotein of the renal glomerular epithelial cell. J Cell Biol. 1984;98(4):1591–6.
9. Doyonnas R, Kershaw DB, Duhme C, Merkens H, Chelliah S, Graf T, et al. Anuria, omphalocele, and perinatal lethality in mice lacking the CD34-related protein podocalyxin. J Exp Med. 2001;194(1):13–27.
10. Horvat R, Hovorka A, Dekan G, Poczewski H, Kerjaschki D. Endothelial cell membranes contain podocalyxin–the major sialoprotein of visceral glomerular epithelial cells. J Cell Biol. 1986;102(2):484–91.
11. Doyonnas R, Nielsen JS, Chelliah S, Drew E, Hara T, Miyajima A, et al. Podocalyxin is a CD34-related marker of murine hematopoietic stem cells and embryonic erythroid cells. Blood. 2005;105(11):4170–8.
12. McNagny KM, Pettersson I, Rossi F, Flamme I, Shevchenko A, Mann M, et al. Thrombomucin, a novel cell surface protein that defines thrombocytes and multipotent hematopoietic progenitors. J Cell Biol. 1997;138(6):1395–407.
13. Somasiri A, Nielsen JS, Makretsov N, McCoy ML, Prentice L, Gilks CB, et al. Overexpression of the anti-adhesin podocalyxin is an independent predictor of breast cancer progression. Cancer Res. 2004;64(15):5068–73.
14. Larsson A, Johansson ME, Wangefjord S, Gaber A, Nodin B, Kucharzewska P, et al. Overexpression of podocalyxin-like protein is an independent factor of poor prognosis in colorectal cancer. Br J Cancer. 2011;105(5):666–72.
15. Larsson AH, Fridberg M, Gaber A, Nodin B, Leveen P, Jonsson GB, et al. Validation of podocalyxin-like protein as a biomarker of poor prognosis in colorectal cancer. BMC Cancer. 2012;12(1):282.
16. Larsson AH, Nodin B, Syk I, Palmquist I, Uhlen M, Eberhard J, et al. Podocalyxin-like protein expression in primary colorectal cancer and synchronous lymph node metastases. Diagn Pathol. 2013;8:109.
17. Kaprio T, Fermer C, Hagstrom J, Mustonen H, Bockelman C, Nilsson O, et al. Podocalyxin is a marker of poor prognosis in colorectal cancer. BMC Cancer. 2014;14:493.
18. Cipollone JA, Graves ML, Kobel M, Kalloger SE, Poon T, Gilks CB, et al. The anti-adhesive mucin podocalyxin may help initiate the transperitoneal metastasis of high grade serous ovarian carcinoma. Clin Exp Metastasis. 2012;29(3):239–52.
19. Boman K, Larsson AH, Segersten U, Kuteeva E, Johannesson H, Nodin B, et al. Membranous expression of podocalyxin-like protein is an independent factor of poor prognosis in urothelial bladder cancer. Br J Cancer. 2013;108(11):2321–8.
20. Binder ZA, Siu IM, Eberhart CG, Ap Rhys C, Bai RY, Staedtke V, et al. Podocalyxin-like protein is expressed in glioblastoma multiforme stem cells and is associated with poor outcome. PLoS One. 2013;8(10):e75945.
21. Ney JT, Zhou H, Sipos B, Buttner R, Chen X, Kloppel G, et al. Podocalyxin-like protein 1 expression is useful to differentiate pancreatic ductal adenocarcinomas from adenocarcinomas of the biliary and gastrointestinal tracts. Hum Pathol. 2007;38(2):359–64.
22. Dallas MR, Chen SH, Streppel MM, Sharma S, Maitra A, Konstantopoulos K. Sialofucosylated podocalyxin is a functional E- and L-selectin ligand expressed by metastatic pancreatic cancer cells. Am J Physiol Cell Physiol. 2012;303(6):C616–24.
23. Elebro J, Jirstrom K. Use of a standardized diagnostic approach improves the prognostic information of histopathologic factors in pancreatic and periampullary adenocarcinoma. Diagn Pathol. 2014;9(1):80.

24. Fristedt R, Elebro J, Gaber A, Jonsson L, Heby M, Yudina Y, et al. Reduced expression of the polymeric immunoglobulin receptor in pancreatic and periampullary adenocarcinoma signifies tumour progression and poor prognosis. PLoS One. 2014;9(11):e112728.

25. Elebro J, Heby M, Gaber A, Nodin B, Jonsson L, Fristedt R, et al. Prognostic and treatment predictive significance of SATB1 and SATB2 expression in pancreatic and periampullary adenocarcinoma. J Transl Med. 2014;12(1):289.

26. Cheung HH, Davis AJ, Lee TL, Pang AL, Nagrani S, Rennert OM, et al. Methylation of an intronic region regulates miR-199a in testicular tumor malignancy. Oncogene. 2011;30(31):3404–15.

27. Snyder KA, Hughes MR, Hedberg B, Brandon J, Hernaez DC, Bergqvist P, et al. Podocalyxin enhances breast tumor growth and metastasis and is a target for monoclonal antibody therapy. Breast Cancer Res. 2015;17(1):46.

28. Kaprio T, Hagstrom J, Fermer C, Mustonen H, Bockelman C, Nilsson O, et al. A comparative study of two PODXL antibodies in 840 colorectal cancer patients. BMC Cancer. 2014;14:494.

29. Torhorst J, Bucher C, Kononen J, Haas P, Zuber M, Kochli OR, et al. Tissue microarrays for rapid linking of molecular changes to clinical endpoints. Am J Pathol. 2001;159(6):2249–56.

5

The use of dried blood spot sampling for the measurement of HbA1c: a cross-sectional study

Claudio A. Mastronardi[1†], Belinda Whittle[2†], Robert Tunningley[2], Teresa Neeman[3] and Gilberto Paz-Filho[1*]

Abstract

Background: The use of dried blood spot (DBS) sampling is an alternative to traditional venous blood collection, and particularly useful for people living in rural and remote areas, and for those who are infirm, house-bound or time-poor. The objective of this study was to assess whether the measurement of glycated haemoglobin A1c (HbA1c) in DBS samples provided comparative and acceptably precise results.

Methods: Venous and capillary blood samples were collected from 115 adult participants. After proper instruction, each participant punctured his/her own finger and collected capillary blood samples on pieces of a proprietary cellulose filter paper. Each filter paper was subsequently placed inside a breathable envelope, stored at room temperature, and processed on the same day (D0), four (D4), seven (D7) and fourteen (D14) days after collection. HbA1c was measured in duplicates/triplicates in whole venous blood (WB), capillary blood (capDBS) and venous blood placed on the matrix paper (venDBS), by turbidimetric inhibition immunoassay. Intra-assay coefficients of variation (CV) were calculated. DBS values were compared to WB results using linear regression, Bland-Altman plots and cross-validation models.

Results: Eleven and 56 patients had type 1 and type 2 diabetes mellitus, respectively. Mean HbA1c levels were 6.22 ± 1.11 % for WB samples (n = 115). The median intra-assay CV was lower than 3 % for WB and capDBS on all days. Results from capDBS and venDBS showed high correlation and agreement to WB results, with narrow 95 % limits of agreement (except for results from D14 samples), as observed in Bland-Altman plots. When capDBS values were applied to equations derived from regression analyses, results approached those of WB values. A cross-validation model showed that capDBS results on D0, D4 and D7 were close to the WB results, with prediction intervals that were narrow enough to be clinically acceptable.

Conclusions: The measurement of HbA1c from DBS samples provided results that were comparable to results from WB samples, if measured up to seven days after collection. Intra-assay coefficients of variation were low, results were in agreement with the gold-standard, and prediction intervals were clinically acceptable. The measurement of HbA1c through DBS sampling may be considered in situations where traditional venipuncture is not available.

Keywords: Diabetes, Dried blood spot testing, HbA1c, Hemoglobin A1c, Turbidimetry

* Correspondence: Gilberto.Pazfilho@anu.edu.au
†Equal contributors
[1]Department of Genome Sciences, The John Curtin School of Medical Research, The Australian National University, 131 Garran Rd, Canberra, Acton ACT 2601, Australia
Full list of author information is available at the end of the article

Background

Glycated haemoglobin (HbA1c) is a biomarker that is fundamental for the diagnosis of diabetes and for monitoring glycaemic control [1]. Traditionally, its measurement depends on venipuncture, and on processing, transportation and storage of whole blood (WB) samples, which can be logistically challenging [2]. These challenges can sometimes compromise proper diagnosis and treatment of patients with diabetes mellitus.

An alternative blood sampling method, based on the use of a dry matrix, was first described in the literature over a century ago [3], and subsequently applied in the clinics to detect metabolic defects through the collection of heel capillary blood samples from newborns [4]. This method is centred on collecting blood samples obtained from finger or heel puncturing on a matrix paper, which is subsequently dried. These dried blood spots (DBS) can then be used for the measurement of diverse substances, including HbA1c, and requires minimal training of staff, is cheaper and safer, eliminates the need for special transportation logistics, and is more acceptable to study participants [5–7].

DBS sampling has been routinely and successfully used for the screening of congenital metabolic and endocrine diseases, such as phenylketonuria and hypothyroidism [8]. More recently, studies have shown that measurements of inflammatory markers, cytokines, serum antibodies, human immunodeficiency virus (HIV) loads and blood hormone levels provide results that are comparable to those obtained from standard venous samples [5, 9–11].

Dried blood spot sampling is also useful for the measurement of HbA1c in individuals with and without diabetes. A recent meta-analysis of seventeen heterogeneous studies demonstrated that HbA1c results from DBS were correlated to those obtained through venipuncture [12]. However, there is still a need for standardisation of sample collection, transportation, storage and analysis. In this study, we evaluated HbA1c levels collected on a novel matrix paper and measured through immunoturbidity, up to 14 days after DBS collection. Subsequently, to demonstrate whether DBS provide results comparable to WB samples, DBS results were compared against those obtained from standard methods.

Methods

This study was approved by the Australian National University Human Research Ethics Committee, and all participants provided informed consent. We recruited participants from the general population living within the Australian Capital Territory region, Australia. Inclusion criteria allowed all adults over 18 years-old from all genders and ethnicities that had no restrictions to having their blood drawn (i.e. due to religious matters, or blood donation in the previous 4 weeks, or difficulty in providing venous blood samples). Participants were advised not to consume food, alcohol or caffeine for 12 h prior to the collection.

Venous blood was collected from an arm vein following standard sterile techniques, into EDTA-coated plastic tubes, providing WB samples. For the collection of capillary DBS (capDBS) samples, we used a 2 x 3 inch dry matrix cellulose paper with nine 10-mm outer diameter circles printed on the surface (ITL Healthcare Pty Ltd). Each printed circle has the capacity to hold 30 to 40 microlitres of blood. Participants were instructed to collect their capillary blood through finger pricking and placing one drop of blood onto each of the pre-defined circles of the dry matrix paper, at room temperature (23 ° C). The matrix paper was then placed into a breathable envelope (ITL Healthcare Pty Ltd) for transportation to the testing laboratory, and blood spots were allowed to dry at room temperature for >2 h before transportation. Forty-microlitre drops of venous blood were also pipetted from collection tubes with no anticoagulant and immediately placed on another dry matrix card, providing venous DBS (venDBS) samples.

All blood samples were transported to the pathology laboratory for analysis. HbA1c levels were determined by a direct turbidimetric inhibition immunoassay that determines HbA1c as a percentage of total haemoglobin (%HbA1c) (Thermo Fisher Scientific). Assays were performed on an Indiko Plus (Thermo Fisher Scientific) automated biochemistry analyser, and results were reported as %HbA1c NGSP values.

Processing of DBS samples (capDBS and venDBS): For each participant sample, two punches were taken from one DBS near the outer edge of the spot. Each punch had 3.2 mm in diameter and contains approximately 1.4 μL of serum. Punches were placed in haemolysing reagent (Thermo Fisher Scientific), in duplicate or triplicate, and incubated at room temperature with shaking. For each duplicate, one milliliter of haemolysate was processed in the Indiko analyser as per the standard protocol for whole blood. capDBS and venDBS samples were processed and analysed on the same day (D0), and on D4, D7 and D14, in duplicates or triplicates for the calculation of intra-assay coefficients of variation (CV).

Processing of WB samples: WB samples were prepared and processed as per standard protocol (Thermo Fisher Scientific). WB samples were processed and analysed on the same day (D0), in duplicates.

Results were presented as mean ± SD or median and range. Linear regression models for predicting WB from DBS were fit and goodness-of-fit measures [mean standard error (MSE) and R-squared] were estimated using cross-validation (R program developed for the cross-validation available upon request). From these models, we predicted WB from DBS values of 4 %, 7 %, 7.5 %

Table 1 Characteristics of the studied population

	All	No diabetes	Type 1 diabetes	Type 2 diabetes
Gender (Males:Females)	51 M:64 F	20 M:28 F	2 M:9 F	28 M:28 F
Age (years; mean ± SD)	55.9 ± 15.3	46.2 ± 14.4	45.0 ± 12.8	64.8 ± 10.0
WB HbA1c (%; mean ± SD)	6.22 ± 1.11 %	5.41 ± 0.35 %	7.80 ± 0.81 %	6.61 ± 1.11 %

Note: WB = whole blood; SD = standard deviation

and 10 % and in addition, obtained 95 % prediction intervals for all days. DBS values were applied to equations derived from linear regression analyses from D0, D4, D7 and D14 data, in order to obtain corrected DBS values (*i.e.*, to bring uncorrected DBS values closer to the line of equality). Bland-Altman plots were constructed with corrected D0, D4, D7 and D14 results.

Results

A total of 115 participants (n = 51 males, n = 64 females) were recruited. Mean age was 55.9 ± 15.3 years-old; 11 participants (9.6 %) had been previously diagnosed with type 1 diabetes, and 56 individuals (48.7 %) had type 2 diabetes. Overall mean whole blood HbA1c levels were 6.22 ± 1.11 % (5.41 ± 0.35 % for participants without diabetes, 7.80 ± 0.81 % for volunteers with type 1 diabetes, and 6.61 ± 1.11 % among individuals with type 2 diabetes). Characteristics of the studied participants are summarised in Table 1.

Whole blood and dried blood spot samples (capillary and venous) were measured in duplicates or triplicates, allowing the determination of intra-assay CV. The median intra-assay CVs were 1.19 % for WB (range 0–4.1 %), and lower than 3 % for all other samples (Table 2).

Mean ± SD capillary DBS (capDBS) levels of HbA1c were 6.62 ± 1.16 % when measured on D0 (n = 77), 6.92 ± 1.32 % on D4 (n = 96), 6.85 ± 1.29 % on D7 (n = 81), and 6.62 ± 1.44 % on D14 (n = 79). Venous DBS (venDBS) samples ranged from 6.72 ± 1.20 % on D0 to 7.36 ± 1.47 % on D7. Mean capDBS and venDBS values were applied to correction formulas obtained from linear regression analyses for each day. Corrected DBS values were closer to WB results (except for D14). Table 2 summarizes the results from WB and DBS samples (corrected and uncorrected).

Bland-Altman plots of difference in HbA1c values in WB and corrected capDBS (Fig. 1), and in WB and corrected venDBS (Fig. 2) showed good correlation and agreement between the two methods, with few samples falling outside the 95 % limits of agreement for each comparison (average difference ± 1.96 standard deviation of the difference). However, limits of agreement were broader on D14 (Table 3).

From any given capDBS result, the linear regression models predicted WB values that were generally lower than the measured capDBS values. For example, for capDBS HbA1c results of 4 %, the predicted WB values were 3.84 % on Day 0, 3.86 % on Day 4, 3.97 % on Day 7, and 4.48 % on Day 14. For capDBS HbA1c results of 7 %, the predicted WB values were 6.76 % on Day 0, 6.33 % on Day 4, 6.37 % on Day 7, and 6.33 % on Day 14. For capDBS HbA1c results of 7.5 %, the predicted WB values were 7.25 % on Day 0, 6.73 % on Day 4, 6.77 % on Day 7, and 6.64 % on Day 14. For capDBS HbA1c results of 10 %, the predicted WB values were 9.69 % on Day 0, 8.79 % on Day 4, 8.78 % on Day 7, and 8.19 % on Day 14. The width of the 95 % prediction intervals (a measure of how precisely WB can be estimated) varied more broadly on D14. The estimated mean squared error (MSE) was lower on Days 0 and 4 when using the linear regression model, which also determined further decreases in R^2 values on D7 and D14 (Table 4).

Table 2 Summary of HbA1c results from WB, capillary DBS and venous DBS samples

Day	Sample	HbA1c (%, Mean ± SD)	Intra-assay CV % (median, range)
D0	WB	6.22 ± 1.11 (N = 115)	1.19, 0–4.10
	Uncorrected capDBS	6.62 ± 1.16 (N = 77)	2.28, 0–10.10
	Corrected capDBS	6.39 ± 1.17 (N = 77)	N/A
	Uncorrected venDBS	6.72 ± 1.20 (N = 81)	1.68, 0–6.86
	Corrected venDBS	6.42 ± 1.18 (N = 81)	N/A
D4	Uncorrected capDBS	6.92 ± 1.32 (N = 96)	2.28, 0–9.87
	Corrected capDBS	6.26 ± 1.18 (N = 96)	N/A
	Uncorrected venDBS	7.15 ± 1.39 (N = 81)	2.14, 0–11.79
	Corrected venDBS	6.42 ± 1.21 (N = 81)	N/A
D7	Uncorrected capDBS	6.85 ± 1.29 (N = 81)	1.98, 0–16.04
	Corrected capDBS	6.25 ± 1.15 (N = 81)	N/A
	Uncorrected venDBS	7.36 ± 1.47 (N = 75)	2.81, 0–26.42
	Corrected venDBS	6.51 ± 1.23 (N = 75)	N/A
D14	Uncorrected capDBS	6.62 ± 1.44 (N = 79)	2.62, 0–17.68
	Corrected capDBS	6.10 ± 1.33 (N = 79)	N/A
	Uncorrected venDBS	7.30 ± 1.65 (N = 79)	2.54, 0–26.52
	Corrected venDBS	6.44 ± 1.29 (N = 79)	N/A

Note: WB = whole blood; ven = venous; cap = capillary; DBS = dried blood spot; SD = standard deviation; CV = coefficient of variation; N/A = not applicable

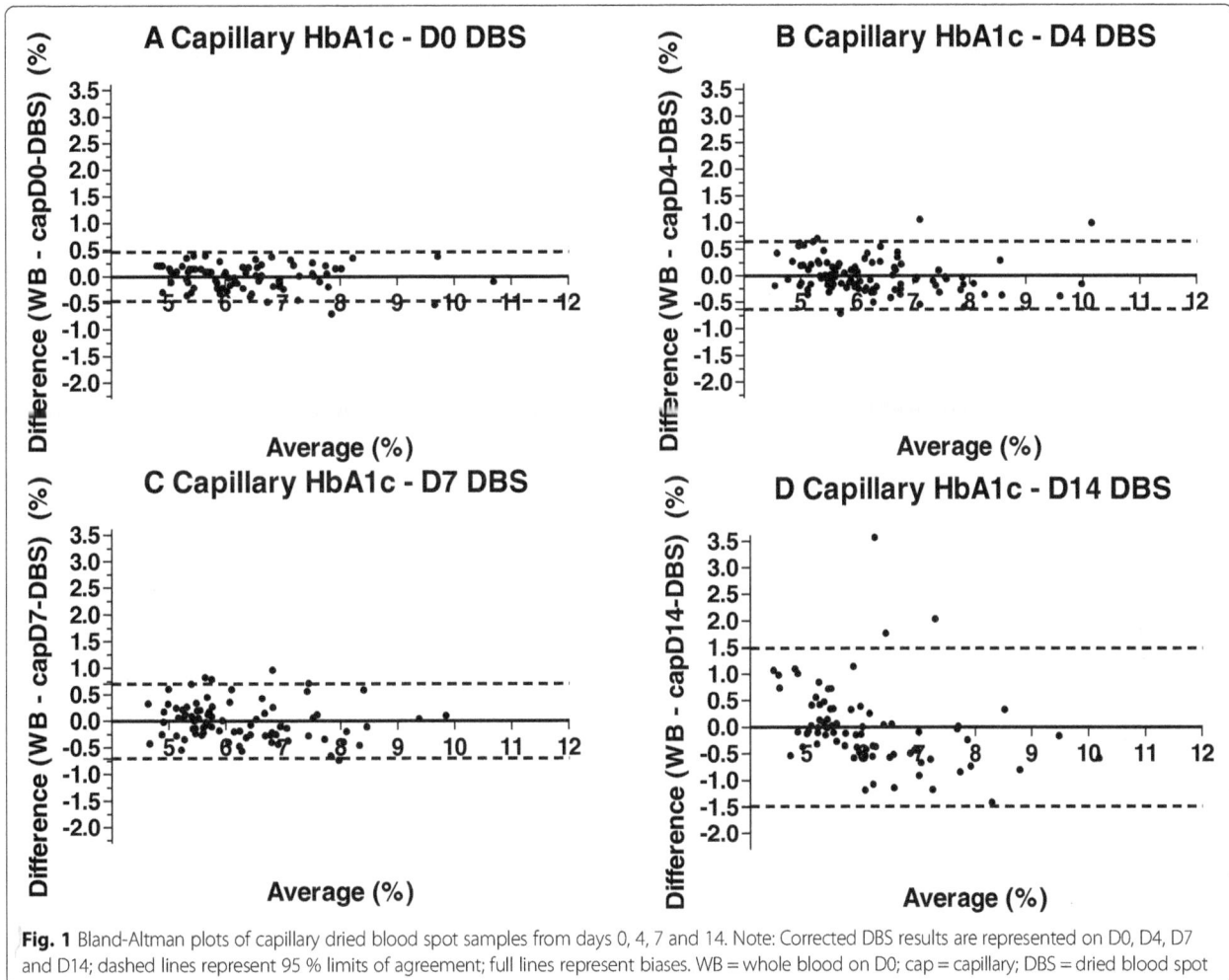

Fig. 1 Bland-Altman plots of capillary dried blood spot samples from days 0, 4, 7 and 14. Note: Corrected DBS results are represented on D0, D4, D7 and D14; dashed lines represent 95 % limits of agreement; full lines represent biases. WB = whole blood on D0; cap = capillary; DBS = dried blood spot

Discussion

There is growing demand for human pathology test services in Australia and around the world, driven by the ageing global population and increasing incidence of chronic diseases [13]. Dried blood spot sampling is an alternative to traditional blood sampling, and has been used in clinical and epidemiological studies for several decades [6, 8, 14]. This method provides results that are comparable to those obtained through traditional venipucture [2, 12], without its logistical obstacles regarding sample collection, processing, transportation and storage. For the measurement of HbA1c, DBS has also been shown to produce results that are comparable to those obtained through venous sampling [15–25]. In our study, we showed that HbA1c levels from DBS samples collected via finger pricking from volunteers with and without diabetes were comparable to those measured from venous samples, when measured up to seven days after collection.

In our study, DBS samples collected from finger pricking (capDBS) were analysed on the same day (D0),

four (D4), seven (D7) and fourteen (D14) days after collection. High correlation and agreement between capDBS results on D0 and venous blood HbA1c values showed that the analysis of samples collected on matrix paper and analysed immediately provides results that are similar to those obtained and processed by traditional methods.

In a real-life scenario, DBS samples are mailed or shipped to the pathology laboratory that performs the assays. Therefore, DBS samples are not analysed immediately. To assess whether this gap between collection and analysis may interfere with the results, we performed analyses also four, seven and fourteen days after collection. We observed that, over time, the correlation between DBS and venous blood results becomes weaker, and the 95 % limits of agreement become wider, especially for D14 results, which may be clinically unacceptable. It is noteworthy that WB samples also degrade over time when not analysed immediately, particularly if not kept refrigerated. Haemoglobin degradation products may show up in

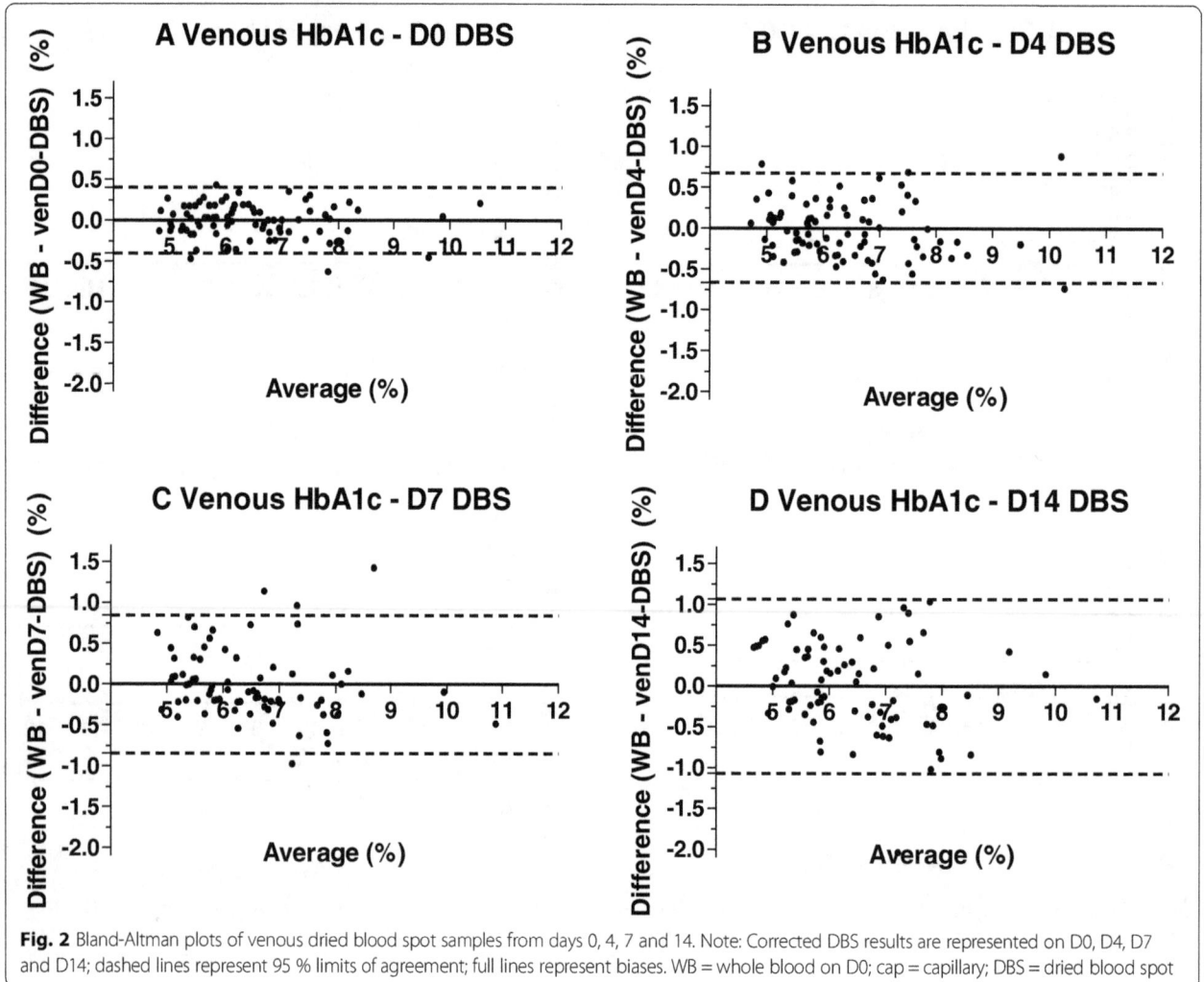

Fig. 2 Bland-Altman plots of venous dried blood spot samples from days 0, 4, 7 and 14. Note: Corrected DBS results are represented on D0, D4, D7 and D14; dashed lines represent 95 % limits of agreement; full lines represent biases. WB = whole blood on D0; cap = capillary; DBS = dried blood spot

Table 3 95% limits of agreement for capillary and venous DBS results, uncorrected and corrected

		Upper limit		Lower limit	
		Uncorrected	Corrected	Uncorrected	Corrected
D0	Capillary	0.2308	0.462	−0.6828	−0.463
	Venous	0.1174	0.404	−0.7051	−0.402
D4	Capillary	0.1117	0.638	−1.428	−0.636
	Venous	0.1203	0.671	−1.567	−0.666
D7	Capillary	0.2383	0.668	−1.436	−0.668
	Venous	0.2345	0.845	−1.943	−0.845
D14	Capillary	1.111	1.484	−2.151	−1.485
	Venous	0.6642	1.065	−2.373	−1.069

samples that have coagulated and aged. These products may co-elute with, or be incompletely separated from, HbA1c. In these cases, the HbA1c value obtained may be reported as higher than it actually is [26]. This effect is particularly evident for venDBS samples, which were collected without anticoagulant.

We used a linear regression model for cross-validation, to ensure unbiased measures of goodness-of-fit and prediction intervals for WB. In that model, capD0-DBS results were closer to the predicted WB values for all evaluated HbA1c steps (4 %, 7 %, 7.5 %, and 10 %), and the prediction intervals were narrower. On the remaining days, capDBS results were further away from the predicted WB values, and the prediction intervals broadened over time. In the clinics, capD0-DBS samples would provide the most accurate HbA1c results, closer to the predicted WB results and with a narrower prediction interval. However, the difference between predicted WB and both capD4- and capD7-DBS results

Table 4 Prediction intervals for WB from capillary DBS values of 4 %, 7 %, 7.5 % and 10 %, obtained through linear regression models

	capDBS 4 %			capDBS 7 %			capDBS 7.5 %			capDBS 10 %			MSE	Adjusted R²
	pWB	Lower 95 % CI	Upper 95 % CI	pWB	Lower 95 % CI	Upper 95 % CI	pWB	Lower 95 % CI	Upper 95 % CI	pWB	Lower 95 % CI	Upper 95 % CI		
D0	3.84	3.36	4.32	6.76	6.30	7.23	7.25	6.78	7.72	9.69	9.20	10.18	0.0554	0.9463
D4	3.86	3.22	4.51	6.33	5.70	6.95	6.74	6.11	7.36	8.79	8.14	9.43	0.0992	0.9064
D7	3.97	3.26	4.67	6.37	5.68	7.06	6.77	6.08	7.46	8.77	8.06	9.49	0.1247	0.8267
D14	4.48	3.20	5.76	6.33	5.08	7.59	6.64	5.38	7.90	8.19	6.89	9.48	0.3905	0.5268

Note: pWB = predicted whole blood; capDBS = capillary dried blood spot; MSE: mean standard error; CI: confidence interval

may be clinically acceptable, as well as their prediction intervals. In the case of capD14-DBS results, their prediction intervals may be too wide to be clinically acceptable. We applied four different capDBS values to the model, but any result can be applied to it (R program available upon request), providing similar behaviour.

In some cases, patients may have difficulty in collecting sufficient amount of blood samples from finger pricking on the matrix paper. That difficulty was evidenced by the fact that the sample size for each day was not equal to the total number of recruited participants. Therefore, we assessed whether venous blood collected through standard methods and spotted on the matrix paper would produce similar results. In those analyses, venous DBS samples were correlated to traditionally-processed venous blood samples in a similar way as capillary DBS. Also, there was high correlation and agreement between capDBS and venDBS results.

In our study, we recruited 67 diabetic patients. Most of them had type 2 diabetes, and had HbA1c levels that are considered adequate (particularly among participants with type 2 diabetes). Only three participants had HbA1c levels higher than 9 %. Therefore, results might have been different should more participants with decompensated diabetes had been recruited. Samples were measured at least in duplicates, and the median intra-assay coefficients of variation were clinically acceptable, lower than 3 % at all times. However, some participants had heterogeneous results. It is unclear why results using the same sample and assay method may vary in some participants.

One of the key issues to be considered for the employment of DBS sampling is the standardization of the analysis of the DBS measurements. It is essential to predict, with the highest possible level of accuracy, the concentration of HbA1c in WB from the values measured in the DBS tests. In a recent study, a meta-analysis of seventeen heterogeneous studies (employing different methods for measuring HbA1c) was performed by Affan et al., and a correction formula to approximate the DBS results to the WB values was

published (12). We employed their correction formula in our current studies (results not presented), but the outcomes of the corrected DBS values resulted in a poorer approximation to the WB values. It appears that the time elapsed between sample collection and processing is a key component of the variability observed in the DBS sampling. Indeed, we found that there are significant differences among the Bland-Altman plots constructed from data on each particular day (e.g. D0, D4, D7 and D14) between DBS vs. WB. Thus, in our current analytical method, we analysed the data of each processed day independently by proposing mean values and prediction intervals for each particular processing day. Additionally, we corrected capillary DBS results by applying a correction formula that derived from regression analyses for each particular day, to approximate the regression line to the equality line. Thus, we obtained a different formula for each day, and observed that corrected capillary DBS results were closer to the predicted WB ones on all days except D14, when MSE was higher (i.e., WB results were less precisely predicted).

We acknowledge that our study is limited by the fact that participants were evaluated in a controlled research setting, and results may be different when capillary HbA1c is evaluated in a real-life scenario. Future studies need to evaluate samples from participants who collect their capillary DBS samples on their own, and mail them to the testing laboratory via standard postal services (subjected to confounding factors such as delays and temperature variations). Furthermore, future studies should evaluate the prediction intervals for other elapsed times such as D1, D2, and D3, and also determine how these prediction intervals can be applied in the management of diabetes. To answer those questions, future studies should evaluate healthy individuals and those with diabetes who are treatment-naïve, and compare their DBS values and their prediction intervals with their WB HbA1c outcomes. By considering their WB values as the gold-standard, a more accurate clinical interpretation of the prediction intervals, as proposed here, could be established.

Conclusion

In conclusion, HbA1c measured from DBS samples collected via finger pricking provided results that were comparable to those obtained from venous samples and measured by standard procedures. When results from DBS samples (processed up to 7 days after their collection) were applied to correction equations, HbA1c results with the most accuracy and the least clinically-acceptable variability were obtained, with high correlation and agreement to HbA1c results from whole venous blood, and with narrow 95 % limits of agreement. Those findings were further confirmed by a cross-validation model, which provided prediction intervals that were narrow enough to be clinically acceptable. In order for the measurement of HbA1c through DBS sampling to be considered in situations where traditional venipuncture is not available, further studies need to evaluate the effects of external factors, in a broader population.

Competing interests

This study was funded by MyHealthTest Pty. MyHealthTest Pty funded the article-processing charge; MyHealthTest Pty staff instructed participants how to collect their capillary blood samples. MyHealthTest Pty had no role in study design, data analysis and interpretation of data, writing of the manuscript, and decision to submit the manuscript for publication. All authors had and have full access to the study data.

Authors' contributions

BW performed samples collection, developed the DBS elution protocol, performed samples assays, performed data analysis, wrote the manuscript; CAM designed the study, performed data analysis, wrote the manuscript. RT performed samples collection, developed the DBS elution protocol, performed samples assays. TN designed the study, performed data analysis, wrote the manuscript. GP-F designed the study, performed samples collection, performed data analysis, wrote the manuscript. All authors read and approved the final manuscript.

Authors' information

Claudio A. Mastronardi and Belinda Whittle considered co-first authors.

Acknowledgements

We thank MyHealthTest Pty staff, Dr. Marianne Gould (for logistical assistance), and Ms. Jennifer Orr (for her assistance with capillary blood samples collection). We also thank DiabetesACT for their assistance with the recruitment of volunteers. This study was funded by MyHealthTest Pty, including the article-processing charge.

Author details

[1]Department of Genome Sciences, The John Curtin School of Medical Research, The Australian National University, 131 Garran Rd, Canberra, Acton ACT 2601, Australia. [2]Australian Phenomics Facility, The Australian National University, 117 Garran Rd, Canberra, Acton ACT 2601, Australia. [3]Statistical Consulting Unit, The Australian National University, 27 Union Lane, Canberra, Acton ACT 2601, Australia.

References

1. American Diabetes A. Standards of medical care in diabetes–2014. Diabetes Care. 2014;37 Suppl 1:S14–80.
2. McDade TW. Development and validation of assay protocols for use with dried blood spot samples. Am J Hum Biol. 2014;26(1):1–9.
3. Bang I. Ein verfahren zur mikrobestimmung von blutbestandteilen. Biochem Ztschr. 1913;49:19–39.
4. Guthrie R, Susi A. A Simple Phenylalanine Method for Detecting Phenylketonuria in Large Populations of Newborn Infants. Pediatrics. 1963;32:338–43.
5. Mei JV, Alexander JR, Adam BW, Hannon WH. Use of filter paper for the collection and analysis of human whole blood specimens. J Nutr. 2001;131(5):1631S–6.
6. Parker SP, Cubitt WD. The use of the dried blood spot sample in epidemiological studies. J Clin Pathol. 1999;52(9):633–9.
7. Bhatti P, Kampa D, Alexander BH, McClure C, Ringer D, Doody MM, et al. Blood spots as an alternative to whole blood collection and the effect of a small monetary incentive to increase participation in genetic association studies. BMC Med Res Methodol. 2009;9:76.
8. Wilcken B, Wiley V. Newborn screening. Pathology. 2008;40(2):104–15.
9. Corran PH, Cook J, Lynch C, Leendertse H, Manjurano A, Griffin J, et al. Dried blood spots as a source of anti-malarial antibodies for epidemiological studies. Malar J. 2008;7:195.
10. Sherman GG, Stevens G, Jones SA, Horsfield P, Stevens WS. Dried blood spots improve access to HIV diagnosis and care for infants in low-resource settings. J Acquir Immune Defic Syndr. 2005;38(5):615–7.
11. Xu YY, Pettersson K, Blomberg K, Hemmila I, Mikola H, Lovgren T. Simultaneous quadruple-label fluorometric immunoassay of thyroid-stimulating hormone, 17 alpha-hydroxyprogesterone, immunoreactive trypsin, and creatine kinase MM isoenzyme in dried blood spots. Clin Chem. 1992;38(10):2038–43.
12. Affan ET, Praveen D, Chow CK, Neal BC. Comparability of HbA1c and lipids measured with dried blood spot versus venous samples: a systematic review and meta-analysis. BMC Clin Pathol. 2014;14:21.
13. Britt H. An analysis of pathology test use in Australia. Australian Association of Pathology Practices Inc. 2008. Available from http://pathologyaustralia. com.au/wp-content/uploads/2013/03/DOD-paper-+-append.pdf. Accessed 7 May 2015.
14. Williams SR, McDade TW. The use of dried blood spot sampling in the national social life, health, and aging project. J Gerontol B Psychol Sci Soc Sci. 2009;64 Suppl 1:i131–6.
15. Anjali, Geethanjali FS, Kumar RS, Seshadri MS. Accuracy of filter paper method for measuring glycated hemoglobin. J Assoc Physicians India. 2007;55:115–9.
16. Egier DA, Keys JL, Hall SK, McQueen MJ. Measurement of hemoglobin A1c from filter papers for population-based studies. Clin Chem. 2011;57(4):577–85.
17. Fokkema MR, Bakker AJ, de Boer F, Kooistra J, de Vries S, Wolthuis A. HbA1c measurements from dried blood spots: validation and patient satisfaction. Clin Chem Lab Med. 2009;47(10):1259–64.
18. Gay EC, Cruickshanks KJ, Chase HP, Klingensmith G, Hamman RF. Accuracy of a filter paper method for measuring glycosylated hemoglobin. Diabetes Care. 1992;15(1):108–10.
19. Jeppsson JO, Jerntorp P, Almer LO, Persson R, Ekberg G, Sundkvist G. Capillary blood on filter paper for determination of HbA1c by ion exchange chromatography. Diabetes Care. 1996;19(2):142–5.
20. Jones TG, Warber KD, Roberts BD. Analysis of hemoglobin A1c from dried blood spot samples with the Tina-quantR II immunoturbidimetric method. J Diabetes Sci Technol. 2010;4(2):244–9.
21. Lacher DA, Berman LE, Chen TC, Porter KS. Comparison of dried blood spot to venous methods for hemoglobin A1c, glucose, total cholesterol, high-density lipoprotein cholesterol, and C-reactive protein. Clin Chim Acta. 2013;422:54–8.
22. Lakshmy R, Gupta R. Measurement of glycated hemoglobin A1c from dried blood by turbidimetric immunoassay. J Diabetes Sci Technol. 2009;3(5):1203–6.
23. Little RR, McKenzie EM, Wiedmeyer HM, England JD, Goldstein DE. Collection of blood on filter paper for measurement of glycated hemoglobin by affinity chromatography. Clin Chem. 1986;32(5):869–71.
24. Lomeo A, Bolner A, Scattolo N, Guzzo P, Amadori F, Sartori S, et al. HPLC analysis of HbA1c in dried blood spot samples (DBS): a reliable future for diabetes monitoring. Clin Lab. 2008;54(5–6):161–7.
25. Wikblad K, Smide B, Bergstrom A, Wahren L, Mugusi F, Jeppsson JO. Immediate assessment of HbA1c under field conditions in Tanzania. Diabetes Res Clin Pract. 1998;40(2):123–8.
26. Selvin E, Coresh J, Jordahl J, Boland L, Steffes MW. Stability of haemoglobin A1c (HbA1c) measurements from frozen whole blood samples stored for over a decade. Diabet Med. 2005;22(12):1726–30.

6

P53 nuclear stabilization is associated with *FHIT* loss and younger age of onset in squamous cell carcinoma of oral tongue

Raju SR Adduri[1], Viswakalyan Kotapalli[1], Neha A Gupta[1,6], Swarnalata Gowrishankar[2], Mukta Srinivasulu[3], Mohammed Mujtaba Ali[3], Subramanyeshwar Rao[3,7], Shantveer G Uppin[4], Umanath K Nayak[2], Snehalatha Dhagam[5], Mohana Vamsy Chigurupati[5] and Murali Dharan Bashyam[1*]

Abstract

Background: Squamous cell carcinoma of tongue (SCCT) is expected to harbor unique clinico-pathological and molecular genetic features since a significant proportion of patients are young and exhibit no association with tobacco or alcohol.

Methods: We determined P53, epidermal growth factor receptor, microsatellite instability, human papilloma virus infection and loss of heterozygosity status at several tumor suppressor loci in one hundred and twenty one oral SCCT (SSCOT) samples and analyzed their association with clinico-pathological features and patient survival.

Results: Our results revealed a significantly higher incidence of p53 nuclear stabilization in early (as against late) onset SCCOT. *FHIT* loss was significantly associated with p53 nuclear stabilization and the association was stronger in patients with no history of tobacco use. Samples harboring mutation in p53 DNA binding domain or exhibiting p53 nuclear stabilization, were significantly associated with poor survival.

Conclusion: Our study has therefore identified distinct features in SCCOT tumorigenesis with respect to age and tobacco exposure and revealed possible prognostic utility of p53.

Keywords: Oral tongue cancer, TP53, *FHIT*, EGFR, Disease specific survival

Background

Squamous cell carcinoma of tongue (SCCT) is believed to be associated with late onset and tobacco use similar to other Head and neck squamous cell carcinoma (HNSCC) subtypes. An increased incidence in the young [1] and in individuals with no history of smoking and alcohol consumption [2] is reported for squamous cell carcinoma of oral tongue (SCCOT). SCCOT has the highest burden of young patients among all HNSCC subtypes and a significant proportion of patients belonging to this age group appear to include non-smokers [3]. In addition, young patients with SCCOT have frequent loco-regional recurrence [4] and poor prognosis [3]. Despite advances in cancer therapy, SCCOT five year survival rate has not improved in the last few decades [5]. All these factors make SCCOT a unique HNSCC subtype and yet molecular genetic studies designed specifically for this important cancer have been rare; most studies have been restricted to a single prognostic marker and/or a small cohort of patients [6].

We have conducted a retrospective study involving comprehensive molecular genetic and clinico-pathological analyses of one hundred and twenty one SCCOT samples; results revealed significant association of p53 nuclear stabilization with age of onset, *FHIT* loss and survival.

Methods
Patient samples
Previously untreated, surgically resected primary SCCOT specimens were collected from three hospitals in Hyderabad, India following informed consent and approval from respective hospital ethics committees (Institutional Ethics

* Correspondence: bashyam@cdfd.org.in
[1]Laboratory of Molecular Oncology, Centre for DNA Fingerprinting and Diagnostics, Nampally, Hyderabad 500001, India
Full list of author information is available at the end of the article

Committee of MNJ Institute of Oncology & Regional Cancer Centre, Institutional Ethics Committee of Apollo Hospitals and Ethics Committee of Omega Hospitals), as per modified Helsinki declaration of 2008 (http://www.wma.net/en/30publications/10policies/b3/). The study included a total of 121 tumor/normal sample pairs (all oral tongue; 106 freshly resected and 15 archived); all samples were from patients not associated with family history for any cancer. Median age of patients was 50 years with a male to female ratio of 2.0. Patients aged ≤45 years were considered as 'young' where as those aged ≥46 were considered as 'old'. Surgically resected fresh tumor and matched normal tissues were collected in liquid nitrogen and preserved at −70°C after collecting representative pieces in buffered formalin for embedding in paraffin. 4 μM sections from tumor and matched normal formalin fixed and paraffin embedded (FFPE) blocks for each sample were stained with hematoxylin and eosin (H&E) to evaluate grade and absence of tumor infiltration, respectively. Clinical data and information pertaining to use of tobacco, alcohol and family history were obtained via personal interview in the form of questionnaire or from hospital medical records. Majority of tumors were well differentiated (86/121; 71.07%). Clinicopathological details of the patient samples are given in Additional file 1: Table S1.

Immunohistochemistry (IHC)

IHC was performed as per standard protocols [7] on tissues embedded into FFPE blocks mentioned above, as per standard practice though we are aware that this slice of tissue may not represent the whole tumor. 4 μM tumor sections were deparafinized and rehydrated in graded series of alcohol followed by heat induced epitope retrieval in citrate buffer at pH 6.0 (for p53) or proteinase K pretreatment (for epidermal growth factor receptor (EGFR)) and subjected to peroxidase quenching using 0.6% hydrogen peroxide in methanol. Sections were incubated with 1 μg/ml anti-p53 (DO-1, EMD Millipore Calbiochem, Darmstadt, Germany) or 0.15 μg/ml anti-EGFR (Clone: 31G7, Zymed laboratories, Carlsbad, CA, USA) antibodies separately for one hour followed by incubation with HRP-conjugated anti-mouse secondary antibody (Dako REAL Envision Detection System, Dako, Glostrup, Denmark) for 30 minutes and subsequently with DAB chromogen (Dako REAL Envision Detection System, Dako, Glostrup, Denmark) for 3 and 7 minutes for p53 and EGFR, respectively. Sections were counter stained with hematoxylin. The slides were scored by two experienced pathologists blinded for clinical and molecular data. Samples exhibiting nuclear stain in more than 20% tumor epithelium were considered as positive for p53. For EGFR, staining intensity (negative, weak, moderate and strong) and fractional epithelium positivity (≤25%, 25 ≤ 50%, 50 ≤ 75% and 75 ≤ 100%) were scored as 0–3. A summated score greater than 3 was considered as positive.

DNA isolation
From FFPE blocks
8 μM FFPE tissue sections from tumor and matched normal blocks were stained with hematoxylin after deparaffinization. Tumor rich areas identified by the pathologist were scraped off and DNA was isolated using SDS-proteinase K lysis and subsequent phenol-chloroform extraction followed by alcohol precipitation.

From frozen tissues
DNA was isolated from fresh resected tumor tissues using the DNeasy Kit (Qiagen, Hamburg, Germany) as per manufacturer's protocol after confirming ≥70% neoplastic cellularity.

TP53 mutation and human papilloma virus (HPV) screening
Bidirectional sequencing of *TP53* exons 5–8 was carried out on a 3100 Genetic analyzer (ABI inc., Foster city, CA, USA) after PCR amplification using FFPE tumor DNA as template. Primer sequences are given in supplementary Additional file 2: Table S2. Suspected in-dels were confirmed using TA cloning vector (Invitrogen, Carlsbad, CA, USA) as per standard procedure. PCR based screening of HPV was carried out as per standard protocol [7] with GP5+ and GP6+ primers using DNA isolated from frozen tumor tissue as template. Primer sequences are given in supplementary Additional file 2: Table S2.

Microsatellite instability (MSI) screening and loss of heterozygosity (LOH) analysis
MSI analysis was performed for the 106 fresh samples using the standard NCI panel of five microsatellites (two mononucleotide repeats *viz.* BAT25 and BAT26 and three dinucleotide repeats *viz.* D2S123, D5S346 and D17S250) using FFPE DNA as template as described earlier [8]. Primer sequences are listed in supplementary Additional file 2: Table S2. Samples were classified as MSI if two or more microsatellites exhibited instability and as microsatellite stable (MSS) if one or none exhibited instability.

LOH analysis was performed (only for fresh samples) based on polymorphic microsatellites located close to putative tongue cancer tumor suppressor genes including tp53CA (*TP53*-17pl3.1), D3S1300 (*FHIT*-3p14.2) and D9S1748 (*CDKN2A*-9p21). LOH status was also assessed for all three dinucleotide microsatellites of the NCI panel namely D2S123 (*hMSH2*-2p15-16), D5S346 (*APC*-5q21) and D17S250 (*BRCA1*-17q11.2). Primer sequences are listed in supplementary Additional file 2: Table S2. Experimental procedure was identical to that of MSI

Table 1 Correlation of p53 nuclear stabilization with patient age

Age	n	NS+	NS-	p-value
Young (≤45 years)	46	36	10	0.0184
Old (≥46 years)	75	42	33	
Total	121	78	43	

n, Number of samples; NS+, Nuclear stabilization; NS-, Absence of nuclear stabilization;
p value corresponds to Fisher's exact test.

analysis and LOH status was determined as described earlier [7].

Statistical analysis

Association between clinico-pathological and molecular variables was examined using Fisher's exact test. Disease specific survival time was calculated as the duration between tumor resection and death. For patients who were lost to follow up or died of reasons other than SCCOT, survival times were censored to the last date on which patients were known to be alive. Kaplan-Meier method was used to estimate survival probability. Log rank test was used to estimate significant differences in survival rates between different groups. Cox proportional hazards model was used to assess the effect of covariates in multivariate analysis.

Results

Among 121 samples analyzed, 78 (64.46%) exhibited p53 nuclear stabilization (Table 1 and Figure 1A and B).

Surprisingly, we observed a significant difference (p = 0.0184) in p53 nuclear staining between young (36/46; 78.26%), and old (42/75; 56%) patients (Table 1). There was no significant association however between p53 stabilization and tobacco use (data not shown). We next screened mutations in exons 5–8 of *TP53* that encode the DNA binding domain and are known to harbor majority of mutations [9]. Mutations (listed in Additional file 3: Table S3), were detected in fifteen of thirty five tumor samples that exhibited p53 nuclear stabilization and in three of twenty six that did not. We did not observe differences in frequency of mutation in young and old patients stratified by p53 nuclear stabilization (5/16, 31.25% in young and 10/19, 52.63% in old among p53 positive tumors; and 0/5, 0% in young and 3/21, 14.28% in older patients among p53 negative tumors). Proportion of transitions, transversions and indels were similar to previous reports for SCCT as per the International Agency for Research on Cancer TP53 database (Additional file 4: Figure S1) and were not significantly different between the two age groups (data not shown). We identified a novel 33 bp deletion, c.616-648del33 (Additional file 5: Figure S2), located in exon 5 in a p53 positive tumor sample obtained from a chronic tobacco chewer that is expected to result in loss of eleven amino acids (143–153). The deleted amino acids include four (143–146) that form part of β-sheet S3 which is important in stabilizing the loop- β sheet- α helix motif, a key domain in formation of p53 DNA binding surface [10]. Majority of p53 positive tumors harboring mutation (12/15) exhibited p53 positivity

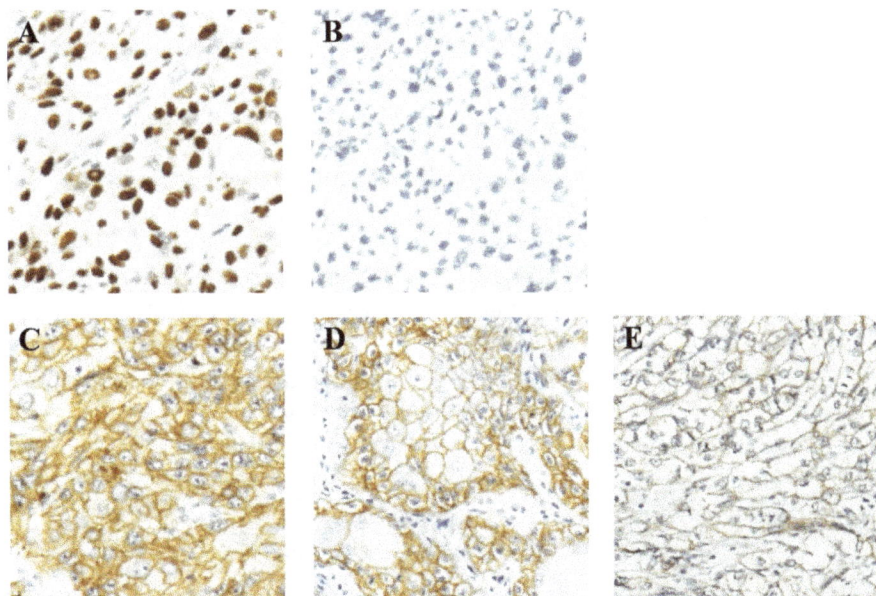

Figure 1 Immunohistochemistry based detection of p53 and EGFR in primary SCCOT samples. Representative results of nuclear stabilization (**A**) and negative staining (**B**) of p53 are shown. Panels **C**, **D** and **E** show representative results for strong, moderate and weak EGFR staining, respectively. Original magnification 100x.

Table 2 LOH frequency at different loci

Microsatellite	D2S123/*hMSH2*	D5S345/*APC*	D17S143/*BRCA2*	TP53CA/*TP53*	D3S1300/*FHIT*	D9S1748/*CDKN2A*
Informative cases	94	95	90	98	91	89
Frequency of LOH*	2.12 (02)	6.31 (06)	6.67 (06)	11.22 (11)	26.37 (24)	28.09 (25)

LOH, loss of heterozygosity.
*In percentage; Number of samples exhibiting LOH is shown in parenthesis.

in greater than 50% tumor cells (Additional file 3: Table S3). In contrast, frequency of mutation was significantly lower (3/14; 21.42%) (Additional file 3: Table S3) in p53 positive tumors exhibiting stabilization in less than 50% cells. In addition, of the three p53 negative tumors that harbored p53 mutation, two exhibited complete absence of staining. Interestingly, missense/inframe mutations were predominantly identified in tumors exhibiting p53 stabilization whereas frameshift mutations resulting in protein truncation were identified exclusively in p53 negative tumors (Additional file 3: Table S3).

A significant proportion of HNSCC has been found to express EGFR at high levels [11] and the same was observed in the current study as well (97/121; 80.17%) (Additional file 6: Table S4) (Figure 1C-E). There was no significant difference in EGFR staining in tumors from young and old patients (data not shown). We also analyzed EGFR expression status in matched normal samples for 25 tumors; staining was weak to moderate and was limited to the basal and suprabasal layers (non-keratinized cells). In the corresponding tumors however, strong staining was observed throughout the tumor (data not shown). In addition, in normal epithelium, staining was observed predominantly in cell membrane whereas in tumor cells, cytoplasmic staining was also observed (data not shown).

PCR based screening revealed low proportion of HPV infection (14/106; 13.2%) (Additional file 6: Table S4) and MSI 14/106 (13.2%) (Additional file 7: Figure S3A-E) in our sample cohort. Dinucleotide microsatellites exhibited frequent instability (40/318; 12.58%) compared to mononucleotide microsatellites (13/212; 6.13%) (data not shown). LOH was more frequently observed in *CDKN2A* (28.09%) and *FHIT* (26.37%) than other loci tested (Table 2) (Additional file 7: Figure S3F-G). Nineteen of fifty six samples (33.92%) positive for p53 staining in contrast to only five of thirty five (14.29%) p53 negative samples, exhibited

LOH at *FHIT* indicating *FHIT* loss could be a more frequent event in tumors exhibiting p53 nuclear stabilization (p = 0.0508) (Table 3). In addition, this association was stronger (p = 0.0094) in patients with no history of tobacco use (Table 4).

Survival data was collected for a total of seventy nine patients; median survival was 30.5 months. Though we did not detect correlation of disease specific survival with pathological stage or grade, there is a significant difference in survival rate between patients with p53 positive and negative tumors (p = 0.0003) (Figure 2A and Table 5). As expected, patients with tumors harboring p53 DNA binding domain mutation were significantly associated with poor survival (p = 0.0117) (Figure 2B and Table 5). *FHIT* loss also exhibited significant effect on disease specific survival (p = 0.0302) (Figure 2C and Table 5) but it was not an independent predictor of worse prognosis, as determined by Cox proportional hazard model.

Discussion

Abrogation of p53 tumor suppressor activity is a frequent event in many cancers, including HNSCC [12]. The frequency of p53 nuclear stabilization identified in SCCOT in the present cohort (64.46%) is in accordance with previous reports from India [13] as well as from the West [14]. Interestingly, frequency of p53 nuclear stabilization was high in young patients (Table 1), suggesting possible role of genetic factors. An earlier study conducted on 724 HNSCC cases reported a similar difference of p53 stabilization between young and older patients [15]. Of interest, a study conducted on aging mice showed a two-fold decline in p53 activity with advancing age, when exposed to radiation [16]. It can perhaps be postulated that age related decline in p53 transcriptional

Table 3 Correlation of p53 stabilization with *FHIT* LOH

FHIT status	n	p53 status		p-value
		NS+	NS-	
FHIT LOH+	24	19	05	0.0508
FHIT LOH-	67	37	30	

FHIT LOH+, *FHIT* LOH present; *FHIT* LOH-, *FHIT* LOH absent; NS+, p53 Nuclear stabilization; NS-, absence of p53 nuclear stabilization; n, Number of samples; LOH, loss of heterozygosity.
p value corresponds to Fisher's exact test.

Table 4 Correlation of *FHIT* LOH with p53 stabilization and tobacco use

P53 status	n	Tobacco users (50)		Tobacco never users (23)	
		FHIT LOH+	*FHIT* LOH-	*FHIT* LOH+	*FHIT* LOH-
NS+	45	09	24	08	4
NS-	28	04	13	01	10
				p value = 0.0094	

FHIT LOH+, *FHIT* LOH present; *FHIT* LOH-, *FHIT* LOH absent; NS+, p53 nuclear stabilization; NS-, absence of p53 nuclear stabilization; n, Number of samples; LOH, loss of heterozygosity.
p value corresponds to Fisher's exact test.

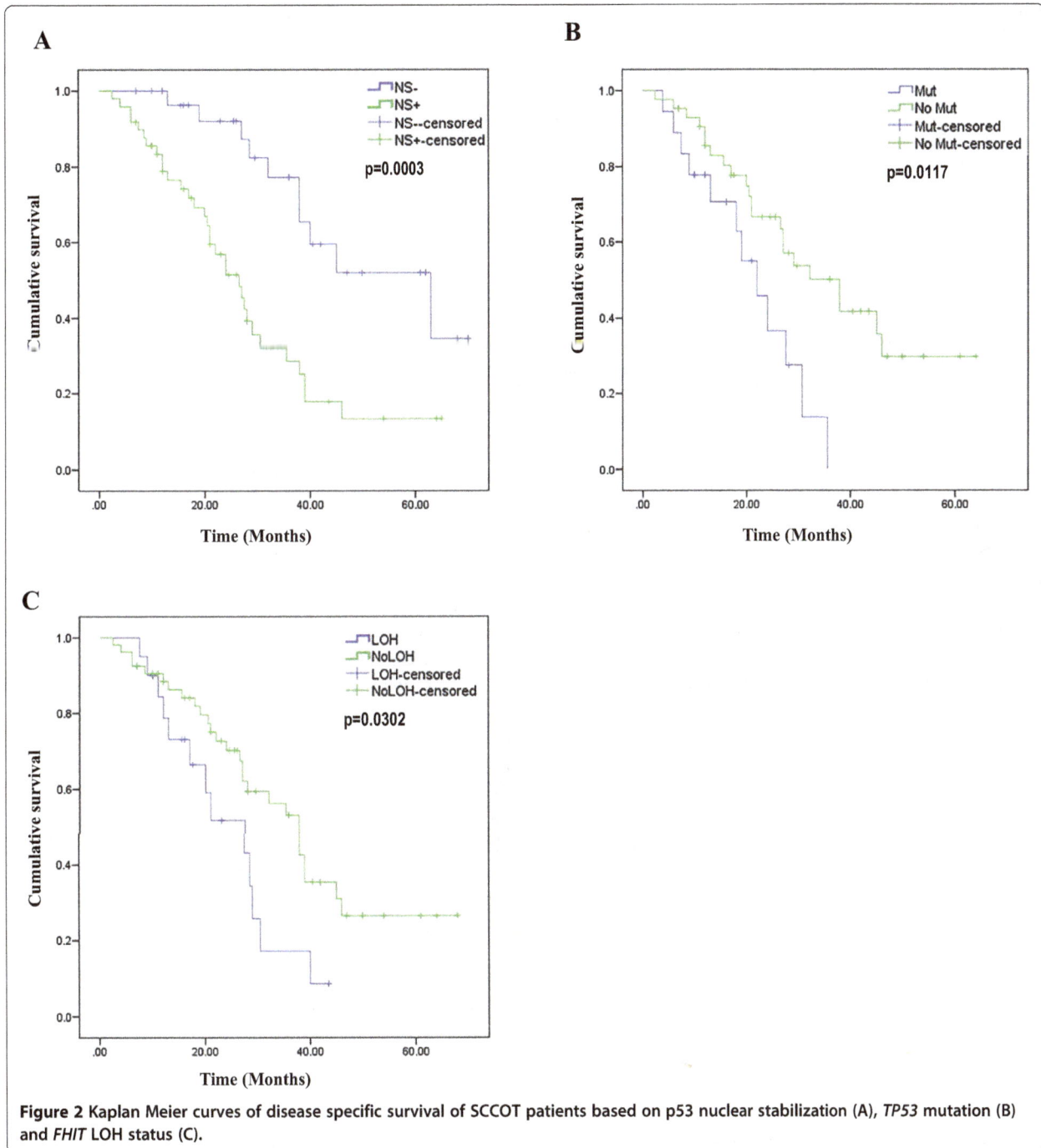

Figure 2 Kaplan Meier curves of disease specific survival of SCCOT patients based on p53 nuclear stabilization (A), *TP53* mutation (B) and *FHIT* LOH status (C).

activity may independently contribute to tumorigenesis in old patients perhaps by mimicking mutational inactivation. The distinct occurrence of *TP53* mutation exclusively in samples exhibiting strong or absent p53 immunostain has been observed earlier in ovarian cancer [17]. However, we cannot rule out the possibility of dilution of mutant allele by the wild type allele in samples exhibiting p53 staining in less than 50% cells. Since p53 mutations were also identified in samples not exhibiting nuclear stabilization, using immunostaining alone to identify p53 status may not

be an ideal approach. Interestingly, we observed that young patients with p53 nuclear stabilization also exhibited DNA binding domain mutation similar to older SCCOT patients. This is in contrast to a study conducted on SCCOT patients in USA where none of the young patients who exhibited p53 nuclear stabilization harbored mutation [18,19]. There is no previous report of HPV screening performed specifically on SCCOT from India, though few studies on oral squamous cell carcinoma (OSCC) revealed a higher frequency of HPV infection [20], probably due to inclusion

Table 5 Association of p53 nuclear stabilization and *FHIT* loss with disease specific survival of SCCOT patients

	Total (n)	Dead (n)	% Dead	Median survival (months)	Hazard ratio[a]	95% CI	Significance[b]
Total	79	42	53.16				
P53 nuclear stabilization							
NS-	30	10	33.3	63	-	-	0.0003
NS+	49	32	65.31	26.5	3.35.1	1.8293-6.1350	
P53 mutation							
Mutation	18	12	66.67	22			0.0117
No mutation	43	22	51.16	38	0.4274	0.1811 to 1.0084	
***FHIT* LOH**							
LOH	20	13	65	21	-	-	0.0302
No LOH	53	27	50.94	38	0.4967	0.2265-1.0893	

[a]Hazard ratio was calculated to the first variable in a subgroup (indicated by empty cells).
[b]Corresponds to Log Rank test (Mantel-Cox).

of other oral cancer subtypes. Base of tongue squamous cell carcinoma is known to exhibit higher frequency of HPV infection [21].

Previous studies undertaken on HNSCC showed significant variation in MSI (ranging from 1- 65%) across populations, though number of markers analyzed varied significantly [22-24]. Our results suggest the presence of a higher frequency of MSI in SCCOT compared to other HNSCC subtypes, as also reported previously [22]. In this study, dinucleotide microsatellites exhibited frequent instability compared to mononucleotide microsatellites perhaps suggesting the occurrence of a distinct form of instability than the one observed in classical mismatch repair (MMR) deficient tumors [25]. A significant proportion (one-third) of tumors exhibited LOH at D9S1748 (*CDKN2A*) consistent with earlier reports [26]. LOH frequency of D2S123 (*hMSH2*), D5S346 (*APC*) and D17S250 (*BRCA1*) observed in our patient cohort appeared to be lower than previous reports [24]. An earlier report from India revealed marginally higher frequency of LOH at *TP53* locus in oral cancer [27], probably due to influence of tumors other than SCCOT.

FHIT harbors one of the most common fragile sites in the genome called FRA3B and is often associated with chromosomal deletions in various cancer cell lines and tumors [28]. P53 inactivation induced genomic instability could be one cause for the association of p53 nuclear stabilization with *FHIT* loss though a similar association with *CDKN2A* LOH was not identified. *FHIT* loss can be expected to be more susceptible to genomic instability given its location within a chromosomal breakpoint region [28]. Strong association of loss of *FHIT* and p53 inactivation in nonsmokers (Table 4) suggests that tumors occurring in tobacco never users with and without p53 inactivation could be distinct entities. Wild type p53 and FHIT are known to have similar roles in inducing apoptosis and cell cycle arrest possibly through Bak and

p21 respectively [29]. Therefore, inactivation of *FHIT* and p53 may facilitate tumor cells to evade apoptosis and escape G0/G1 arrest. A recent report suggests that inactivation of both *FHIT* and p53 may have possible synergistic effect resulting in deregulation of proliferation related genes in lung cancer cell lines and tumors [30], particularly in squamous cell carcinoma subtype of non-small cell lung cancer [31]. Ours is however the first study to report such association in SCCOT (Table 3).

To our knowledge, this is the first report to identify p53 inactivation as an independent prognostic marker for poor survival in SCCOT, though it has been reported in HNSCC [32] and OSCC [33]. Few studies have identified *FHIT* to be a predictor of poor survival in OSCC [34] in HNSCC [35]. However, these studies did not analyze the status of p53 aberrations in the tumors. The association of *FHIT* loss with poor survival is probably a result of association with p53 nuclear stabilization.

Conclusion

Though the study was conducted on a relatively smaller size of samples, it is expected to help in selecting molecular markers for larger studies in the future with more clinical significance. However, this is the most comprehensive molecular genetic study undertaken on Indian SCCOT patients and has identified frequent mutational inactivation of p53 and its significant association with loss of *FHIT*. More importantly, our results show association of wild type p53 and good survival. Genetic aberrations contributing to concomitant *FHIT* loss and p53 stabilization in tumors need to be delineated. It would be interesting to study tumorigenesis pathways contributing to SCCOT in the absence of p53 and *FHIT* inactivation. Given the unique clinico-pathological features associated with SCCOT, this study is an important step towards understanding of this important but hitherto poorly studied HNSCC subtype.

Additional files

Additional file 1: Table S1. Clinico-pathological details of SCCOT patients.

Additional file 2: Table S2. Primers used in the current study.

Additional file 3: Table S3. *TP53* mutations identified in the study.

Additional file 4: Figure S1. Frequency of p53 mutation types observed in this study and in International Agency for Research on Cancer (IARC) *TP53* Database.

Additional file 5: Figure S2. 426-458del33, a novel in-frame deletion identified in *TP53* in SCCOT.

Additional file 6: Table S4. Frequency of EGFR expression, HPV infection and MSI.

Additional file 7: Figure S3. Representative chromatograms depicting MSI.

Abbreviations
SCCT: Squamous cell carcinoma of tongue; SCCOT: Squamous cell carcinoma of oral tongue; HNSCC: Head and neck squamous cell carcinoma; FFPE: Formalin fixed and paraffin embedded; H&E: Hematoxylin and eosin; IHC: Immunohistochemistry; EGFR: Epidermal growth factor receptor; HPV: Human papilloma virus; MSI: Microsatellite instability; LOH: Loss of heterozygosity; MSS: Microsatellite stable; MMR: Mismatch repair; OSCC: Oral squamous cell carcinoma.

Competing interests
All authors declare that they have no competing interests.

Authors' contributions
MDB conceived the study. MDB and RSRA designed the study. RSRA, VK, NAG, SG, SGU, MMA, SD, MR, SR, UKN, MVC acquired data. MDB and RSRA performed statistical analysis. MDB and RSRA prepared manuscript with inputs from all authors. All authors read and approved the final manuscript.

Acknowledgments
The authors thank all patients who consented for the study. RSRA is a registered PhD student of Manipal University, Karnataka, India and is thankful to University Grants Commission (UGC), Govt. of India, for junior and senior research fellowships.

Funding
This study was funded by Indian Council for Medical Research (ICMR) (Grant No. 5/13/129/2009-NCD-III), Council of Scientific and Industrial Research (CSIR), Govt. of India (Grant No. 27(265)/12/EMR-II) and Department of Biotechnology, Govt. of India (a core grant to Centre for DNA Fingerprinting and Diagnostics (CDFD).

Author details
[1]Laboratory of Molecular Oncology, Centre for DNA Fingerprinting and Diagnostics, Nampally, Hyderabad 500001, India. [2]Apollo Hospitals, Jubilee Hills, Hyderabad, India. [3]MNJ Institute of Oncology & Regional Cancer Centre, Red Hills, Hyderabad, India. [4]Nizam's Institute of Medical Sciences, Punjagutta, Hyderabad, India. [5]Omega Hospitals, Jubilee Hills, Hyderabad, India. [6]Currently at National Centre for Cell Science, Ganeshkhind, Pune, India. [7]Currently at Basavatarakam Indo American Cancer Hospital & Research Institute, Hyderabad, India.

References
1. Myers JN, Elkins T, Roberts D, Byers RM: **Squamous cell carcinoma of the tongue in young adults: increasing incidence and factors that predict treatment outcomes.** *Otolaryngol Head Neck Surg* 2000, **122**:44–51.
2. Dahlstrom KR, Little JA, Zafereo ME, Lung M, Wei Q, Sturgis EM: **Squamous cell carcinoma of the head and neck in never smoker-never drinkers: a descriptive epidemiologic study.** *Head Neck* 2008, **30**:75–84.
3. Iype EM, Pandey M, Mathew A, Thomas G, Sebastian P, Nair MK: **Oral cancer among patients under the age of 35 years.** *J Postgrad Med* 2001, **47**:171–176.
4. Sarkaria JN, Harari PM: **Oral tongue cancer in young adults less than 40 years of age: rationale for aggressive therapy.** *Head Neck* 1994, **16**:107–111.
5. Silverman S Jr: **Demographics and occurrence of oral and pharyngeal cancers. The outcomes, the trends, the challenge.** *J Am Dent Assoc* 2001, **132 Suppl**(132 Suppl):7S–11S.
6. Ryott M, Wangsa D, Heselmeyer-Haddad K, Lindholm J, Elmberger G, Auer G, Avall Lundqvist E, Ried T, Munck-Wikland E: **EGFR protein overexpression and gene copy number increases in oral tongue squamous cell carcinoma.** *Eur J Cancer* 2009, **45**:1700–1708.
7. Pandilla Ramaswamy KV, Gowrishankar S, Vamsy CM, Patnaik S, Uppin S, Rao S, Kalidindi N, Regulagadda S, Sundaram C, Srinivasulu M, Vasala A, Bashyam MD: **Distinct genetic aberrations in oesophageal adeno and squamous carcinoma.** *Eur J Clin Invest* 2013, **43**:1233–1239.
8. Raman R, Kotapalli V, Adduri R, Gowrishankar S, Bashyam L, Chaudhary A, Vamsy M, Patnaik S, Srinivasulu M, Sastry R, Rao S, Vasala A, Kalidindi N, Pollack J, Murthy S, Bashyam M: **Evidence for possible non-canonical pathway(s) driven early-onset colorectal cancer in India.** *Mol Carcinog* 2014, **53**(Suppl 1):E181–6.
9. Joerger AC, Fersht AR: **Structural biology of the tumor suppressor p53.** *Annu Rev Biochem* 2008, **77**:557–582.
10. Cho Y, Gorina S, Jeffrey PD, Pavletich NP: **Crystal structure of a p53 tumor suppressor-DNA complex: understanding tumorigenic mutations.** *Science* 1994, **265**:346–355.
11. Kalyankrishna S, Grandis JR: **Epidermal growth factor receptor biology in head and neck cancer.** *J Clin Oncol* 2006, **24**:2666–2672.
12. Peltonen JK, Helppi HM, Paakko P, Turpeenniemi-Hujanen T, Vahakangas KH: **P53 in head and neck cancer: functional consequences and environmental implications of TP53 mutations.** *Head Neck Oncol* 2010, **2**:36.
13. Khan Z, Tiwari RP, Mulherkar R, Sah NK, Prasad GB, Shrivastava BR, Bisen PS: **Detection of survivin and p53 in human oral cancer: correlation with clinicopathologic findings.** *Head Neck* 2009, **31**:1039–1048.
14. Nylander K, Nilsson P, Mehle C, Roos G: **p53 mutations, protein expression and cell proliferation in squamous cell carcinomas of the head and neck.** *Br J Cancer* 1995, **71**:826–830.
15. De Paula AM, Souza LR, Farias LC, Correa GT, Fraga CA, Eleuterio NB, Silveira AC, Santos FB, Haikal DS, Guimaraes AL, Gomez RS: **Analysis of 724 cases of primary head and neck squamous cell carcinoma (HNSCC) with a focus on young patients and p53 immunolocalization.** *Oral Oncol* 2009, **45**:777–782.
16. Feng Z, Hu W, Teresky AK, Hernando E, Cordon-Cardo C, Levine AJ: **Declining p53 function in the aging process: a possible mechanism for the increased tumor incidence in older populations.** *Proc Natl Acad Sci U S A* 2007, **104**:16633–16638.
17. Yemelyanova A, Vang R, Kshirsagar M, Lu D, Marks MA, Shih Ie M, Kurman RJ: **Immunohistochemical staining patterns of p53 can serve as a surrogate marker for TP53 mutations in ovarian carcinoma: an immunohistochemical and nucleotide sequencing analysis.** *Mod Pathol* 2011, **24**:1248–1253.
18. Sorensen DM, Lewark TM, Haney JL, Meyers AD, Krause G, Franklin WA: **Absence of p53 mutations in squamous carcinomas of the tongue in nonsmoking and nondrinking patients younger than 40 years.** *Arch Otolaryngol Head Neck Surg* 1997, **123**:503–506.
19. Lingen MW, Chang KW, McMurray SJ, Solt DB, Kies MS, Mittal BB, Haines GK, Pelzer HJ: **Overexpression of p53 in squamous cell carcinoma of the tongue in young patients with no known risk factors is not associated with mutations in exons 5–9.** *Head Neck* 2000, **22**:328–335.
20. D'Costa J, Saranath D, Dedhia P, Sanghvi V, Mehta AR: **Detection of HPV-16 genome in human oral cancers and potentially malignant lesions from India.** *Oral Oncol* 1998, **34**:413–420.
21. Marur S, D'Souza G, Westra WH, Forastiere AA: **HPV-associated head and neck cancer: a virus-related cancer epidemic.** *Lancet Oncol* 2010, **11**:781–789.
22. Wang Y, Irish J, MacMillan C, Brown D, Xuan Y, Boyington C, Gullane P, Kamel-Reid S: **High frequency of microsatellite instability in young patients with head-and-neck squamous-cell carcinoma: lack of involvement of the mismatch repair genes hMLH1 AND hMSH2.** *Int J Cancer* 2001, **93**:353–360.

23. Glavac D, Volavsek M, Potocnik U, Ravnik-Glavac M, Gale N: **Low microsatellite instability and high loss of heterozygosity rates indicate dominant role of the suppressor pathway in squamous cell carcinoma of head and neck and loss of heterozygosity of 11q14.3 correlates with tumor grade.** *Cancer Genet Cytogenet* 2003, **146**:27–32.

24. Koy S, Plaschke J, Luksch H, Friedrich K, Kuhlisch E, Eckelt U, Martinez R: **Microsatellite instability and loss of heterozygosity in squamous cell carcinoma of the head and neck.** *Head Neck* 2008, **30**:1105–1113.

25. Loukola A, Eklin K, Laiho P, Salovaara R, Kristo P, Jarvinen H, Mecklin JP, Launonen V, Aaltonen LA: **Microsatellite marker analysis in screening for hereditary nonpolyposis colorectal cancer (HNPCC).** *Cancer Res* 2001, **61**:4545–4549.

26. Partridge M, Emilion G, Pateromichelakis S, Phillips E, Langdon J: **Location of candidate tumour suppressor gene loci at chromosomes 3p, 8p and 9p for oral squamous cell carcinomas.** *Int J Cancer* 1999, **83**:318–325.

27. Saranath D, Tandle AT, Deo MG, Mehta AR, Sanghvi V: **Loss of p53 gene as a biomarker of high risk oral leukoplakias.** *Indian J Biochem Biophys* 1997, **34**:266–273.

28. Croce CM, Sozzi G, Huebner K: **Role of *FHIT* in human cancer.** *J Clin Oncol* 1999, **17**:1618–1624.

29. Sard L, Accornero P, Tornielli S, Delia D, Bunone G, Campiglio M, Colombo MP, Gramegna M, Croce CM, Pierotti MA, Sozzi G: **The tumor-suppressor gene *FHIT* is involved in the regulation of apoptosis and in cell cycle control.** *Proc Natl Acad Sci U S A* 1999, **96**:8489–8492.

30. Andriani F, Roz E, Caserini R, Conte D, Pastorino U, Sozzi G, Roz L: **Inactivation of both *FHIT* and p53 cooperate in deregulating proliferation-related pathways in lung cancer.** *J Thorac Oncol* 2012, **7**:631–642.

31. Lee YC, Wu CT, Shih JY, Jou YS, Chang YL: **Frequent allelic deletion at the *FHIT* locus associated with p53 overexpression in squamous cell carcinoma subtype of Taiwanese non-small-cell lung cancers.** *Br J Cancer* 2004, **90**:2378–2383.

32. Mannarini L, Bertino G, Morbini P, Villa C, Benazzo M: **Markers of chemoradiation resistance in patients with locally advanced head and neck squamous cell carcinoma, treated by intra-arterial carboplatin and concurrent radiation.** *Acta Otorhinolaryngol Ital* 2007, **27**:173–180.

33. Perrone F, Bossi P, Cortelazzi B, Locati L, Quattrone P, Pierotti MA, Pilotti S, Licitra L: **TP53 mutations and pathologic complete response to neoadjuvant cisplatin and fluorouracil chemotherapy in resected oral cavity squamous cell carcinoma.** *J Clin Oncol* 2010, **28**:761–766.

34. Kujan O, Oliver R, Roz L, Sozzi G, Ribeiro N, Woodwards R, Thakker N, Sloan P: **Fragile histidine triad expression in oral squamous cell carcinoma and precursor lesions.** *Clin Can Res* 2006, **12**:6723–6729.

35. Tai SK, Lee JI, Ang KK, El-Naggar AK, Hassan KA, Liu D, Lee JJ, Ren H, Hong WK, Mao L: **Loss of *FHIT* expression in head and neck squamous cell carcinoma and its potential clinical implication.** *Clin Can Res* 2004, **10**:5554–5557.

7

Membranous CD24 expression as detected by the monoclonal antibody SWA11 is a prognostic marker in non-small cell lung cancer patients

Michael Majores[1], Anne Schindler[1], Angela Fuchs[1], Johannes Stein[1], Lukas Heukamp[2], Peter Altevogt[3,4] and Glen Kristiansen[1*]

Abstract

Background: Lung cancer is one of the most common malignant neoplasms worldwide and has a high mortality rate. To enable individualized therapy regimens, a better understanding of the molecular tumor biology has still to be elucidated. The expression of the cell surface protein CD24 has already been claimed to be associated with shorter patient survival in non-small cell lung cancer (NSCLC), however, the prognostic value and applicability of CD24 immunostaining in paraffin embedded tissue specimens has been questioned due to the recent acknowledgement of restricted epitope specificity of the commonly used antibody SN3b.

Methods: A cohort of 137 primary NSCLC cases was immunostained with a novel CD24 antibody (clone SWA11), which specifically recognizes the CD24 protein core and the resulting expression data were compared with expression profiles based on the monoclonal antibody SN3b. Furthermore, expression data were correlated to clinico-pathological parameters. Univariate and multivariate survival analyses were conducted with Kaplan Meier estimates and Cox regression, respectively.

Results: CD24 positivity was found in 34 % resp. 21 % (SN3b) of NSCLC with a membranous and/or cytoplasmic staining pattern. Kaplan-Meier analyses revealed that membranous, but not cytoplasmic CD24 expression (clone SWA11) was associated with lympho-nodular spread and shorter overall survival times (both $p < 0.05$). CD24 expression established by SN3b antibodies did not reveal significant clinicopathological correlations with overall survival, neither for cytoplasmic nor membranous CD24 staining.

Conclusions: Membranous CD24 immunoreactivity, as detected with antibody clone SWA11 may serve as a prognostic factor for lymphonodular spread and poorer overall survival. Furthermore, these results corroborate the importance of a careful distinction between membranous and cytoplasmic localisation, if CD24 is to be considered as a potential prognostic biomarker.

Keywords: Non-small cell lung cancer, NSCLC, CD24, Immunohistochemistry, Prognostic marker

* Correspondence: glen.kristiansen@ukb.uni-bonn.de
Michael Majores and Anne Schindler shared first authorship.
[1]Institute of Pathology, University of Bonn, Sigmund-Freud-Str. 25, D-53127 Bonn, Germany
Full list of author information is available at the end of the article

Background

Lung cancer is a major cause of carcinoma related death, being responsible for 17.8 % of all cancer deaths and accounting for more than a million deaths worldwide per year [1]. Despite intense studies to improve therapy options, its prognosis has remained poor with a 5-year overall survival rate of less than 15 % [2].

In the past decade, the largest subgroup of lung cancer, i.e. non-small cell lung cancer (NSCLC), has been subjected to exerted research for a better understanding of the underlying molecular biology of lung cancer. More than ten years ago, CD24 has already been suggested as a novel and promising biomarker for carcinoma progression in NSCLC [3] and several groups have confirmed this finding on protein and transcript level [2, 4]. CD24 is a highly glycosylated protein, that binds to the cell surface through a GPI (glycosyl-phosphatidylinositol)-anchor and functions as a cell adhesion molecule and is involved in cell-cell-interaction via its P-selectin binding site [5]. CD24 has been found to be expressed by pre-B-lymphocytes [5]. It is assumed that CD24-positive cells can attach more easily to platelets and activated endothelial cells [6, 7]. Notably, CD24 has also been observed in many human carcinomas, such as ovarian cancer, renal cell cancer, breast cancer and NSCLC [3, 8–12]. In epithelial ovarian cancer high scores of cytoplasmic CD24 were highly predictive of shorter patient survival times (mean 97.8 vs. 36.5 months), whereas membranous CD24 expression seemed to have no influence on survival times. Interestingly, CD24 positivity (membranous or cytoplasmic) of prostate cancer samples was significantly associated to younger patient age and higher pT stages and a higher 3-year prostate-specific antigen (PSA) relapse rate compared with CD24-negative tumours.

In patients with gallbladder carcinoma, tumors with up-regulation of CD24 revealed lymph node metastasis and lymphovascular invasion more frequently. Moreover, up-regulation of CD24 tended to show deeper invasion depth and higher TNM stage [13]. Together, these findings support CD24 as a prognostic marker for carcinoma progression and poorer survival.

Despite these intriguing findings, major concerns regarding a lack of epitope specificity of the commonly used monoclonal antibody SN3b have been raised [14]. Recent findings indicate that the mAb (monoclonal antibody) SN3b does not bind to the protein core itself, but binds to a glycan structure that decorates the CD24 molecule. On the one hand, this motif is not present on all forms of CD24 and—on the other hand—it can be present in other epitopes irrespective of CD24 [14]. These limitations underline the need for more specific CD24 antibodies, such as the mAb SWA11 antibody that has been suggested to be more specific as it binds to the protein core [14].

As CD24 is a promising biomarker for the risk assessment of disease progression, the goal of the present study was to investigate CD24 expression in NSCLC using the novel, more specific monoclonal antibody (mAb) SWA11. Special emphasis was put on the comparison of SN3b- and SWA11-mediated CD24 detection regarding a) the subcellular distribution of CD24 expression (i.e. membranous versus cytoplasmic expression) and b) its correlation with various clinicopathological features including patient survival times.

Methods

Patient characteristics/ tumor samples

A cohort of 137 primary NSCLC patients, who had undergone surgery between 1995 and 2009 and who were all diagnosed in the Institute of Pathology, University of Bonn, was compiled. Tumor samples were available as formalin-fixed, paraffin-embedded tissue. According to the current WHO classification the NSCLC were classified as adenocarcinoma (AC) ($n = 102$) or squamous cell carcinoma (SCC) ($n = 35$). The male:female ratio (5:2) and mean age at diagnosis (64y; SD +/− 9y; range 24–86y) in our cohort was in accordance with the published epidemiologic distribution [1] (Table 1). No neoadjuvant radiotherapy or chemotherapy were applied before surgery. All cases were subjected to a central review based on the current WHO guidelines [1].

Table 1 Clinicopathological characteristics of the NSCLC cohort

		AC	SCC
		N (%)	N (%)
Tumour stage (pT)			
	1	29 (21.2 %)	5 (3.6)
	2	51 (37.2 %)	23 (16.8 %)
	3	6 (4.4 %)	6 (4.4 %)
	4	1 (0.7 %)	0 (0 %)
Nodal Status (pN)	0	37 (27.0 %)	15 (10.9 %)
	1	15 (10.9 %)	9 (6.6 %)
	2	14 (10.2 %)	3 (2.2 %)
	3	1 (0.7 %)	0 (0.0 %)
Grading (G)	1	5 (3.6 %)	0 (0.0 %)
	2	41 (29.9 %)	16 (11.6 %)
	3	44 (32.1 %)	17 (12.4 %)
Mean age at surgery		64,2	64,56
(median age)		(65)	(67)
Sex (m:w)		68:34	30:5
Median OS (months)		52	24
(SD; 95 % CI [months])		(±23.7; 5.5– 98.5)	(± 12.8;0.0– 49.0)

SD standard deviation; *CI* confidence interval; *n* number of cases; *OS* overall survival

Ethics statement

This study was accomplished under the consent of the independent ethics committee of the University of Bonn (approval number 188/14).

Tissue microarray (TMA) assembly

For construction of the tissue microarrays, suitable areas for extraction of tissue were selected and marked on haematoxylin-eosin (HE) specimen slides. A senior pathologist conducted the microscopic selection of suitable areas. The selected areas were then punched out of the corresponding paraffin donor block and inserted into the recipient block. The tissue arrayer (LD 120 Sm5-x) was purchased from Alphalys, Paris, France. All punch diameters were 0.8 mm (corresponding to an spot area of 0.79 mm^2). Each case was represented by 3 tumor samples and 1 peritumoral non-neoplastic tissue sample.

Immunohistochemistry

Formalin-fixed TMA sections were freshly cut (2–3 μm) and mounted on superfrost specimen slides (Thermo Fisher). Next, dewaxing was carried out with xylene and the tissue sections were gradually rehydrated. Antigen retrieval was achieved by pressure cooking in the autoclave at pH6 and under hyperfrequency wave of 360 W at 125 °C for 8 min. MAb SWA11 was diluted 1:100 and SN3b was diluted 1:50, each using a modul buffer from Medac (TA-250-PM). The immunohistochemical reaction was visualized using the detection system C-DPVB 500 HRP by Medac (all procedures were conducted according to the instructions of the manufacturer).

Positive controls, consisting of tissue samples with known positivity for the antibody, and negative controls (i.e. reactions lacking the primary antibody), were performed in parallel for each TMA slide. Expression intensity was examined in a semiquantitative manner (score 0: no staining, score 1: weak, score 2: moderate and score 3: strong staining). For statistical analyses, cases with moderate to strong expression were bundled in a 'high expression' and cases with negative or weak expression in a 'low expression' group.

Follow-up analyses

Follow-up data were available in 93 cases. Patients suffered from primary malignant tumors of the lung and were subjected to surgical resection or diagnostic sampling between 1995 and 2009 Cases with sufficient availability of formalin-fixed, paraffin-embedded tissue entered the cohort. Survival data were obtained by the analysis of surgical and oncological medical reports as well as written request for data of the local registration offices. The survival time was defined as the time period between the date of surgery and the date of death resp. the date of the documentation as "still alive" at the last available time point.

The median survival of AC cases was 52 months (SD 23.7; 95 % CI: 5.5–98.5; $n = 67$), compared to SCC with 24 months (SD 12; 95 % CI: 0–49.0; $n = 26$). 62 patients died within the follow-up period. The remaining 31 patients were documentes as "still alive" at the last available time point. Only in 13 patients without documentation of death the follow-up period was less than 60 months.

Statistical analysis

For statistical analysis the SPSS software v. 21.0 was used. For evaluation of the correlation between expression of CD24 and clinicopathological parameters Fisher's exact test was used. Univariate survival analysis included Kaplan Meier-analyses with log-rank testing for the estimation of differences in survival times. For multivariate survival analysis, the Cox regression model was used. All cutoff values of significance were set $p < 0.05$ with two-sided testing.

Results

Immunohistochemical detection of CD24 expression using clone SWA11 and SN3b

Using the mAb SWA11, 47 of 137 (34.3 %) NSCLC revealed CD24 expression (either cytoplasmic or membranous) (Table 2). CD24 expression was observed more frequently in adenocarcinomas (AC) than in squamous cell carcinomas (SCC). In AC cytoplasmic expression was observed more frequently than membranous expression. In SCC, both cyptoplasmic and membranous expression was rare. Normal lung parenchyma (i.e. alveolar surface cells) showed no expression of CD24. Bronchial epithelium showed a strong membranous and cytoplasmic staining of the brush border (Fig. 1).

Using the mAb *SN3b*, 29 of 137 (21.2 %) NSCLC revealed CD24 expression (either cytoplasmic or membranous) (Table 2). As above, CD24 expression was observed more frequently in adenocarcinomas (AC) than in squamous cell carcinomas (SCC). However, in contrast to mAb SWA11 cytoplasmic expression was observed less frequently than membranous expression in AC. In SCC, both cytoplasmic and membranous expression was rare. Normal lung parenchyma (i.e. alveolar surface cells) showed a distinct membranous immunoreactivity. Bronchial epithelium revealed both membranous and cytoplasmic staining of CD24.

Correlation between SWA11 and SN3b: As SWA11 and SN3b detect different epitopes, we evaluated the correlation of the immunohistochemical staining patterns. Of 132 NSCLC specimens with matched expression data, only 9 specimens (6.8 %) revealed a concordant CD24 expression. Of these cases, 4 cases revealed a concordant cytoplasmic staining and another 5 cases revealed a concordant membranous CD24 expression. Statistically, no significant correlation between the two mAb could be observed (cc = −0.63, $p = 0.470$; Fisher's exact test $p = 0.665$). The correlation of cytoplasmic and membranous expression (for each

Table 2 Cytoplasmic and membranous expression of CD24

SWA11 (mAb clone)	AC	SCC	SN3b (mAB clone)	AC	SCC
Cytoplasmic	N (%)	N (%)	Cytoplasmic	N (%)	N (%)
0	45 (32.6 %)	19 (13.8 %)	0	76 (55.1 %)	31 (22.5 %)
1	22 (15.9 %)	8 (5.8 %)	1	12 (8.7 %)	1 (0.7 %)
2	17 (12.3 %)	4 (2.9 %)	2	7 (5.1 %)	2 (1.4 %)
3	18 (13.0 %)	4 (2.9 %)	3	1 (0.7 %)	0 (0 %)
	AC	SCC		AC	SCC
Membranous	N (%)	N (%)	Membranous	N (%)	N (%)
0	68 (49.3 %)	21 (15.2 %)	0	64 (46.4 %)	30 (21.7 %)
1	21 (15.2 %)	5 (3.6 %)	1	10 (7.2 %)	2 (1.4 %)
2	8 (5.8 %)	4 (2.9 %)	2	12 (8.7 %)	2 1.4 %)
3	5 (3.6 %)	5 (3.6 %)	3	10 (7.2 %)	0 (0 %)

Staining intensities are determined as follows:
0: negative or equivocal, 1: weak, 2: moderate and 3: strong CD24 staining

antibody) was as follows: cc = 0.475 ($p < 0.05$) for SWA11 ($n = 108$) and cc = 0.140 ($p = 0.11$) for SN3b ($n = 103$).

Survival analyses

Recent studies indicate that CD24 expression is associated with tumor progression and poorer survival rates. Therefore, we performed follow up analyses with a special emphasis on 1) the prognostic value of mAb SWA11 in dependence on subcellular staining characteristics and 2) the prognostic values of different clinicopathological parameters:

Prognostic value of CD24 in Kaplan Meier Analyses

Only membranous CD24 (SWA11) staining revealed significantly poorer survival rates (median overall survival 21 vs. 52 months; $p = 0.005$) as illustrated in Fig. 2. In contrast, cytoplasmic CD24 (SWA11) staining did not affect the survival rates (median OS 34 vs. 35 months; $p = 0.884$) (Table 3). When stratifying the cohort into SCC ($n = 35$) and AC ($n = 102$) in Kaplan Meier analyses, membranous CD24 (SWA11) expression did not affect patients' survival, neither in SCC ($p = 0.243$) nor AC ($p = 0.135$) (Table 3), probably due to the small number of observations (Fisher exact test: $p > 0.05$). After stratification for AC subtypes, membranous CD24 expression (SWA11) showed a tendency towards an association with poorer survival in acinar subtype AC, but failed significance ($p = 0.328$).

CD24 immunoreactivity using the mAb SN3b was not associated with patients' survival: neither the membranous

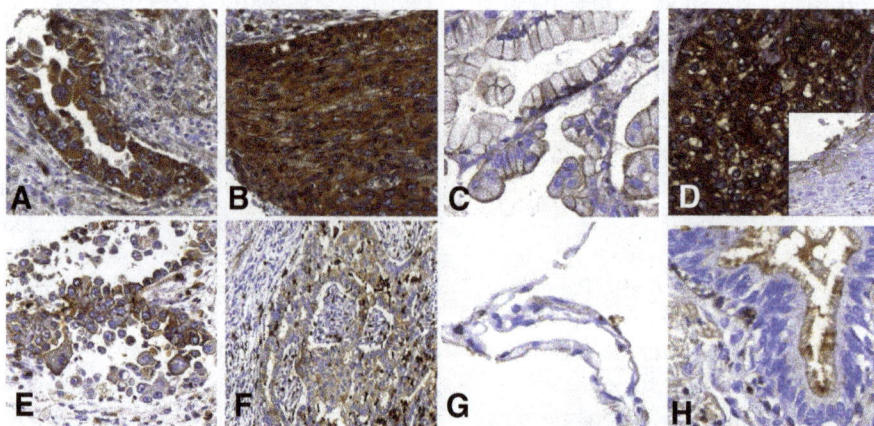

Fig 1 The immunohistochemical characterization reveals membranous and/or cytoplasmic CD24 (mAb SWA11) expression. Strong cytoplasmic CD24 expression is found in a proportion of both AC (**a**) and SCC (**b**, **d**) specimens. Membranous CD24 expression can be pronounced with only scant or even absent cytoplasmic staining as shown in the AC (**c**). Also, both membranous and cytoplasmic CD24 detection can be found in some instances (**d**), the insert is showing the corresponding squamous carcinoma in-situ with membranous staining. Simultaneous membranous and cytoplasmic CD24 expression is also found in AC specimens (**e**, **f**). In normal tissue, alveolar epithelial cells do not express CD24 (**g**), whereas CD24 staining is found at the apical cell membrane of bronchial respiratory epithelia (**h**)

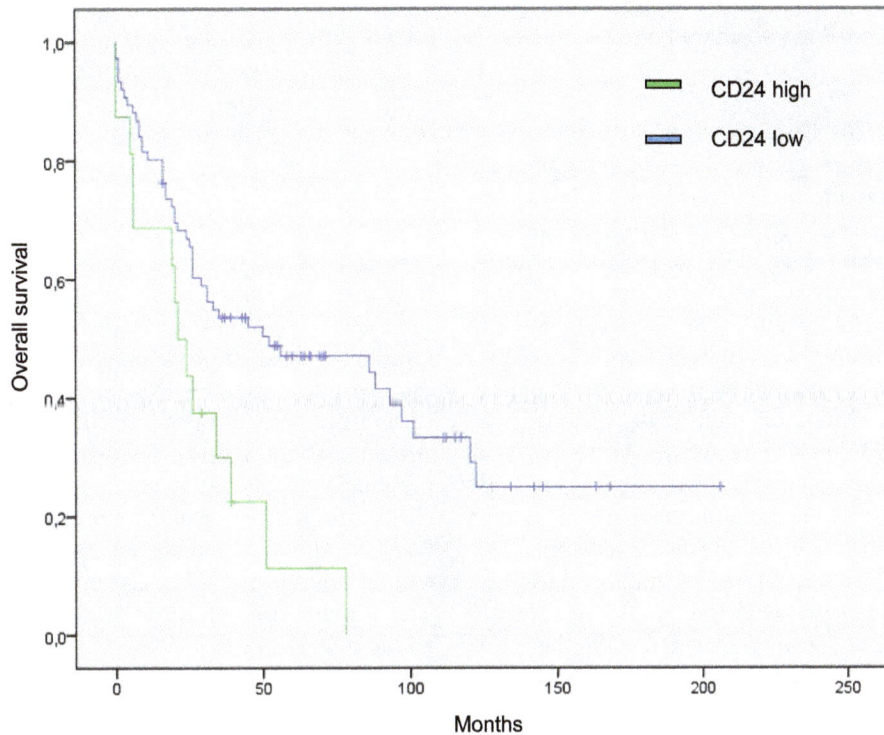

Fig 2 Survival analysis. Kaplan-Meier curves according to SWA11 expression. Cases with moderate to strong expression were bundled in a 'high expression' and cases with negative or weak expression in a 'low expression' group. Membranous expression of CD24 detected by SWA11 proved to be an independent marker for shorter survival times in NSCLC ($p = 0.005$)

Table 3 Univariate survival analysis

SWA11	No. of cases	Mean survival time (months +/− s.e.)	Median survival time (months +/− s.e.)	p-value
Mem CD24				
Negative	76	84.833 +/− 10.395	52.000 +/− 27.030	0.005
Positive	16	27.925 +/− 6.379	21.000 +/− 4.000	
Cyto CD24				
Negative	66	75.209 +/− 10.577	35.000 +/− 12.422	0.884
Positive	26	60.540 +/− 11.551	34.000 +/− 12.196	
Total CD24				
Negative	64	76.972 +/− 10.841	35.000 +/− 13.726	0.633
Positive	28	57.535 +/− 10.895	34.000 +/− 9.303	
SCC				
Mem CD24 negative	16	52.063 +/− 14.668	16.000 +/− 16.000	0.243
Mem CD24 positive	7	21.571 +/− 7.201	24.000 +/− 23.568	
AC				
Mem CD24 negative	59	88.953 +/− 11.631	56.000 +/− 22.885	0.135
Mem CD24 positive	8	39.167 +/− 11.674	21.000 +/− 8.485	
pN0	31	103.641 +/− 14.940	93.000 +/− 28.224	0.012
pN1+	30	54.911 +/− 10.646	26.000 +/− 0.983	

staining pattern ($p = 0.9$), nor the cytoplasmic staining pattern ($p = 0.924$) revealed any significant effect on the overall survival.

Prognostic values of the clinicopathological parameters

To further verify the prognostic values of different clinicopathological parameters, Cox regression analyses were conducted. As expected, positive nodal status (pN > 0) ($p = 0.003$) and disease stage (pT) ($p = 0.006$) were associated with poorer survival rates in univariate analyses (Table 4). Also, membranous CD24 (SWA11) positivity ($p = 0.007$) and histological tumour type ($p < 0.001$) showed a correlation with poorer survival rates. Subjecting the first three criteria to multivariate analyses, only membranous CD24 (SWA11) positivity ($p = 0.014$) and positive nodal status ($p = 0.027$), but not disease stage ($p = 0.185$) maintained independent factors for poorer overall survival (Table 5). In an extended multivariate Cox regression model with inclusion of tumour histology, membranous CD24 expression failed significance, but still showed a trend towards an association with shortened survival times ($p = 0.094$). CD24 expression using the mAb SN3b revealed no association with survival characteristics, neither for total (membranous or cytoplasmic) expression, nor for membranous or cytoplasmic expression alone (all $p > 0.05$, data not shown).

Discussion

In the present study, we have analyzed immunohistochemical staining characteristics and the prognostic value of CD24 expression in NSCLC with a special emphasis on the comparison of the CD24 antibodies SWA11 and SN3b. The most important result of our study is that the prognostic relevance of CD24 is critically dependent on the careful consideration of subcellular compartments and the epitope specificity of the antibody used.

Overall, about one third of the NSCLC cohort revealed a significant CD24 expression (either cytoplasmic or membranous). These results are in line with the findings of other studies. In another NSCLC cohort, CD24 (SN3b) expression was found in 33 % of the samples (87 of 267 cases) [2]. Consistent with those results, we have found similar rates of high CD24 expression levels (35 % of the cases) for SWA11. Originally, we would have

Table 4 Univariate survival analysis according to the Cox regression model (mAb SWA11)

	Beta	HR (hazard ratio)	95 % CI of HR	P-value
SWA11 mem all	0.856	2.353	1.268–4.364	0.007
pN	0.963	2.620	1.389–4.943	0.003
pT	0.844	2.325	1.279–4.224	0.006
Tumour type	0.975	2.651	1.999–3.517	0.000

Table 5 Multivariate survival analysis according to the Cox regression model (mAb SWA11)

	Beta	HR (hazard ratio)	95 % CI of HR	P-value
SWA11 mem all	0.944	2.571	1.211–5.458	0.014
pN	0.737	2.091	1.087–4.021	0.027
pT	0.587	1.799	0.755–4.283	0.185

expected lower rates than those found by Lee et al, as they used the antibody SN3b, that also recognizes yet unidentified other glycoproteins next to CD24. Furthermore, they used whole mount sections instead of tissue microarrays. A possible explanation for rather equal detection rates would be the fact that it has been demonstrated that the epitope recognized by SN3b is indeed present in CD24, but is not found in all glycoforms of CD24 [14]. In contrast to the commonly used mAb SN3b, mAb SWA11 binds to the protein core of CD24 and does not depict other glycan moieties next to CD24. The protein core of CD24 is linear, consisting of the amino acid sequence leucine-proline-alanine (LAP) next to a glycosyl-phosphatidylinositol anchor [15].

CD24 expression has been associated with disease progression and cancer-related death in the majority of malignant tumors [2, 3, 16, 17], although a caveat to these data is that most of these studies are based on the supposedly less specific CD24 clone SN3b. Lee et al demonstrated a significant association between CD24-high expression (SN3b) and shorter patient survival times. Furthermore, Lee and colleagues and ourselves in former studies referred the results to cytoplasmic CD24 expression [2, 3].

In invasive ovarian carcinoma, patients carrying tumors with cytoplasmic CD24 expression showed a significantly shorter mean survival time of 37 months versus patients with tumors without cytoplasmic expression of CD24 (98 months) [16]. Also in NSCLC, expression of CD24 has been claimed to be an independent prognostic marker of shorter patient survival times, especially in AC [3].

Recently, CD24 expression has been addressed as a putative stem cell marker in NSCLC [10]. In that context particular attention has to be paid to the co-expression of CD44. Sterlacci et al. demonstrated that the phenotype CD24−/CD44+ did not show a significant difference in overall survival for the entire NSCLC cohort when compared with the CD24+/CD44 −population. However, when stratified according to histology, AC displaying the putative cancer stem cell (CSC) signature CD24−/CD44+ had a significantly shorter overall survival than CD24+/CD44− AC. However, these findings could not be ascertained as an independent factor, when calculated by multivariable analysis [10]. Since the overwhelming evidence of the protumorigenic properties of CD24 is independent of the CD24low/CD44-high stem cell definition, we focused on

CD24 expression alone and did not include CD44 expression data in the present study.

Our results are only partly consistent with the published data. We were able to demonstrate that membranous staining pattern (using the mAb SWA11) was associated with a poorer overall survival and we revealed an increased risk of lymphonodular spread in the subgroup of CD24-high tumors, being in accordance with the published data. Nonetheless, our results are also partially conflicting with previous immunohistochemical data, as we could not confirm a significant correlation with patient survival for cytoplasmic expression of CD24, neither for SWA11 nor for SN3b.

The underlying biological mechanisms of CD24 promoted tumor progression are still incompletely characterized, although a growing number of studies have contributed to our comprehension [5–7, 17–20]. Expression of CD24 may provide an enhanced capability of tumor cells to adhere to activated endothelial cells mediated by its P-selectin binding site [5] or alter cellular signaling [21]. Aigner and colleagues showed that CD24 functions as a ligand for P-Selectin under physiological flow conditions, using a plate flow chamber assay. In their study, CD24 proved to be necessary for mediation of rolling on P-Selectin, as low expression levels or cleavage of CD24 resulted in inhibition of attachment and rolling, in a breast carcinoma cell line [6]. The precise mechanisms of ligand binding have still to be elucidated. In particular, CD24 does not contain the sulfated tyrosine residue of the P-Selectin glycoprotein ligand 1 (PSGL-1), i.e. another P-Selectin ligand [22]. Another mechanism of CD24 binding focuses on the observed association of CD24 with the sulfate-containing epitope HNK-1 which is also recognized by P-Selectin. This observation may lead to the assumption that HNK-1 mediates CD24 binding [7]. Enhanced disease progression as a result of metastatic spread with poorer survival rates may therefore be reasonable [6, 7]. As known, cells of hematogenously metastasizing tumours attach to platelets in the bloodstream [23–25]. Activated platelets express P-Selectin. Therefore, CD24-positive cells probably attach to activated platelets, containing P-Selectin on their surface, at the point, when the primary tumour invades into the vascular system [6]. Moreover, CD24-mediated tumor propagation has also been associated with an increase of local invasiveness: CD24 mediated invasion of cancer cells has been hypothesized as a result of increased contractile forces as indicated by the findings of A125 human lung cancer cells with different CD24 expression levels using CD24-high and CD24-low transfectants in three-dimensional extracellular matrix (ECM) invasion assays [19]. The percentage of invasive cells and their invasion depth was increased in CD24-high cells compared with CD24-low cells. Conversely,

knockdown of CD24 and of the ß1-integrin subunit in CD24-high cells decreased their invasiveness, indicating that the increased invasiveness is CD24- and ß1-integrin subunit-dependent [19]. Interestingly, besides acting as a ligand for P-Selectin, recently it has been proven that CD24 expression also indirectly stimulates cell adhesion to fibronectin, collagens 1 and 4, and laminin through activation of $\alpha3\beta1$ and $\alpha4\beta1$ integrin activity. Sleeman and colleagues have reported that $\beta1$ integrins colocalize focally with CD24. This suggests a direct interaction between CD24 and $\beta1$-containing integrins. In their study they show that CD24 interacts with c-scr, leading to stabilization of the kinase-active form of c-scr, which is necessary for sufficient activation of integrin adhesion to extracellular matrix components such as fibronectin. Thus, CD24 mediates cell adhesion in a P-Selectin dependent and a P-Selectin independent manner [26]. Next to its influence on cell adhesion, metastasis and on invasion, CD24 also serves as a mediator of proliferation. Apparently, a depletion of CD24 by siRNA leads to a significant decrease of cell numbers in several cell lines as well as to a reduction of their clonogenicity [17]. These experimental results provide a functionally well compatible explanation for the observed clinicopathological correlation of CD24 expression and poorer overall survival resp. increased occurrence of lymphonodular spread in our study.

Notably, CD24 may also provide a promising target for individualized therapy strategies beyond the scope of prediction. For example, CD24 specific antibodies have been applied in the treatment of the transplantation associated B-cell proliferative syndrome [18]. Moreover, mAb SWA11 has recently been shown to have a beneficial effect on anti-cancer treatment when used as addition to gemcitabine treatment in an A549 lung cancer model [20]. Pretreatment with mAb SWA11 led to a significant retardation of carcinoma growth compared to monotherapy with gemcitabine, which was attributed to faster internalisation of tumour antigen-bound therapeutic antibodies and alterations in the intratumoural cytokine milieu. Increased levels of intratumoural chemoattractants such as CXCL9/MIG and CCL2/MCP-1 were observed, in accordance to a heightened infiltration of xenografts by macrophages, possibly gained through the involvement of the antibody-dependent cell-mediated cytotoxicity. [20]

Some parts of our results, however, are conflicting with previous data, as we could not reproduce a significant correlation with patient survival for cytoplasmic expression of CD24 for SWA11. Vice versa, we revealed that only the membranous staining pattern was indicative for poorer overall survival ($p = 0.007$). As a minimal discordance to findings of former NSCLC studies [2, 3], our SWA11 based study could not confirm an especially relevant prognostic value of CD24 for pulmonary adeno-carcinomas. Still, this study demonstrates a small trend towards a subtype-dependent prognostic relevance of membranous CD24 expression. Larger cohorts will be necessary for a more substantial statistical power concerning its prognostic relevance for AC.

Conclusions

In summary, our data provides further evidence for CD24 as a functionally relevant biomarker with prognostic significance in NSCLC. Methodically, our results underline the necessity to choose a specific antibody and to carefully consider subcellular staining differences of CD24 for robust prognostic conclusions. The use of mAb SWA11 should be favoured for a more specific detection of the cell surface protein CD24 as it allows a good visual distinction between membranous and cytoplasmic staining. A distinction between strongly and less strongly stained cells may be challenging in the light of laboratory-specific variations as well as inevitable inter-observer variability. Further studies should clarify, if an adjuvant therapeutic use of CD24 antibodies may have an additive value in cancer treatment.

Abbreviations

NSCLC: Non-small cell lung cancer; GPI: Glycosyl-phosphatidylinositol; PSA: Prostate-specific antigen; mAb: Monoclonal antibody; TMA: Tissue microarray; HE: Haematoxylin-eosin; AC: Adenocarcinomas; SC: Squamous cell carcinomas; LAP: Leucine-proline-alanine; PSGL-1: P-Selectin glycoprotein ligand 1; ECM: Extracellular matrix.

Competing interests

The authors declare that they have no competing interests.

Authors' contributions

MM, GK - conceived the study, analyzed the data, wrote and revised the manuscript, established follow up data.
AS - conducted the study, evaluated immunohistochemistry, analyzed the data, wrote and revised the manuscript, generation of tissue microarrays, established follow up data.
AF, JS, LH - provided tumor samples, read and revised the paper, established follow up data, generation of tissue microarrays.
PA - provided SWA11-antibody, analyzed the data, read and revised the manuscript.

Acknowledgements

We are greatly indebted to Susanne Steiner for excellent technical assistance.

Author details

[1]Institute of Pathology, University of Bonn, Sigmund-Freud-Str. 25, D-53127 Bonn, Germany. [2]New Pathology, Cologne, Germany. [3]Skin Cancer Unit, German Cancer Research Center (DKFZ), Heidelberg, Germany. [4]Department of Dermatology, Venereology and Allergology University Medical Center Mannheim, Ruprecht-Karl University of Heidelberg, Mannheim, Germany.

References

1. Siegel R, Naishadham D, Jemal A. Cancer statistics, 2013. CA Cancer J Clin. 2013;63(1):11–30.
2. Lee HJ, Choe G, Jheon S, Sung SW, Lee CT, Chung JH. CD24, a novel cancer biomarker, predicting disease-free survival of non-small cell lung carcinomas: a retrospective study of prognostic factor analysis from the viewpoint of forthcoming (seventh) new TNM classification. J Thorac Oncol. 2010;5(5):649–57.
3. Kristiansen G, Schluns K, Yongwei Y, Denkert C, Dietel M, Petersen I. CD24 is an independent prognostic marker of survival in nonsmall cell lung cancer patients. Br J Cancer. 2003;88(2):231–6.
4. Györffy G, Surowiak S, Budczies B, Lanczky L. Online Survival Analysis Software to Asses the Prognostic Value of Biomarkers Using Transcriptomic Data in Non-Small-Cell Lung Cancer. PLOS One. 2013;18(8(12)):e82241.
5. Sammar M, Aigner S, Hubbe M, Schirrmacher V, Schachner M, Vestweber D, et al. Heat-stable antigen (CD24) as ligand for mouse P-selectin. Int Immunol. 1994;6(7):1027–36.
6. Aigner S, Ramos CL, Hafezi-Moghadam A, Lawrence MB, Friederichs J, Altevogt P, et al. CD24 mediates rolling of breast carcinoma cells on P-selectin. Faseb J. 1998;12(12):1241–51.
7. Aigner S, Sthoeger ZM, Fogel M, Weber E, Zarn J, Ruppert M, et al. CD24, a mucin-type glycoprotein, is a ligand for P-selectin on human tumor cells. Blood. 1997;89(9):3385–95.
8. Burgos-Ojeda D, Wu R, McLean K, Chen Y, Talpaz M, Yoon E, et al. CD24+ Ovarian Cancer Cells Are Enriched for Cancer-Initiating Cells and Dependent on JAK2 Signaling for Growth and Metastasis. Mol Cancer Ther. 2015;14(7):1717–27.
9. Rostoker R, Abelson S, Genkin I, Ben-Shmuel S, Sachidanandam R, Scheinman EJ, et al. CD24+ cells fuel rapid tumor growth and display high metastatic capacity. Breast Cancer Research. 2015;17:78.
10. Sterlacci MD, Savic S, Fiegl M, Obermann E, Tzankov A. Putative Stem Cell Markers in Non-Small-Cell-Lung Cancer A Clinicopathologic Characterization. J Thorac Oncol. 2014;9:41–9.
11. Stuelten CH, Mertins SD, Busch JI, Gowens M, Scudiero DA, Burkett MW, et al. Complex Display of Putative Tumor Stem Cell Markers in the NCI60 Tumor Cell Line Panel. Stem Cells. 2010;28:649–60.
12. Wang G, Zhang Z, Ren Y. TROP-1/Ep-CAM and CD24 are potential candidates for ovarian cancer therapy. Int J Clin Exp Pathol. 2015;8(5):4705–14.
13. Song SP, Zhang SB, Liu R, Yao L, Hao YQ, Liao MM, et al. NDRG2 down-regulation and CD24 up-regulation promote tumor aggravation and poor survival in patients with gallbladder carcinoma. Med Oncol. 2012;29(3):1879–85.
14. Kristiansen G, Machado E, Bretz N, Rupp C, Winzer KJ, Konig AK, et al. Molecular and clinical dissection of CD24 antibody specificity by a comprehensive comparative analysis. Lab Invest. 2010;90(7):1102–16.
15. Weber E, Lehmann HP, Beck-Sickinger AG, Wawrzynczak EJ, Waibel R, Folkers G, et al. Antibodies to the protein core of the small cell lung cancer workshop antigen cluster-w4 and to the leucocyte workshop antigen CD24 recognize the same short protein sequence leucine-alanine-proline. Clin Exp Immunol. 1993;93(2):279–85.
16. Kristiansen G, Denkert C, Schluns K, Dahl E, Pilarsky C, Hauptmann S. CD24 is expressed in ovarian cancer and is a new independent prognostic marker of patient survival. Am J Pathol. 2002;161(4):1215–21.
17. Smith SC, Oxford G, Wu Z. The Metastasis Associated Gene CD24 Is Regulated by Ral GTPase and Is Mediator of Cell Proliferation and Survival in Human Cancer. Cancer Research. 2006;66(4):1917–22.
18. Benkerrou M, Jais JP, Leblond V, Durandy A, Sutton L, Bordigoni P, et al. Anti-B-cell monoclonal antibody treatment of severe posttransplant B-lymphoproliferative disorder: prognostic factors and long-term outcome. Blood. 1998;92(9):3137–47.
19. Mierke CT, Bretz N, Altevogt P. Contractile forces contribute to increased glycosylphosphatidylinositol-anchored receptor CD24-facilitated cancer cell invasion. J Biol Chem. 2011;286(40):34858–71.
20. Salnikov AV, Bretz NP, Perne C, Hazin J, Keller S, Fogel M, et al. Antibody targeting of CD24 efficiently retards growth and influences cytokine milieu in experimental carcinomas. Br J Cancer. 2013;108(7):1449–59.
21. Bretz N, Salnikov A, Perne C, Keller S, Wang X, Mierke C, et al. CD24 controls Src/STAT3 activity in human tumors. Cell Mol Life Sci. 2012;69(22):3863–79.
22. Needham LK, Schnaar RL. The HNK-1 reactive sulfoglucuronyl glycolipids are ligand for L-selectin and P-selectin. Proc Natl Acad Sci USA. 1993;90:1359.
23. Gasic GJ. Role of plasma, platelets, and endothelial cells in tumour metastasis. Cancer Metastasis Rev. 1984;3:99–144.
24. Grigani G, Pacchiarini L, Pagliarino M. The possible role of blood platelets in tumour growth and dissemination. Haematologica. 1986;71:245–55.
25. Honn KV, Tang DG, Crissman JD. Platelets and cancer metastasis-a causal relationship. Cancer Metastasis Rev. 1992;11:325–251.
26. Sleeman JP, Baumann P, Cremers N, Kroese F, Gertraud O, Chiquet-Ehrismann R, et al. CD24 Expression Causes the Aquisition of Multiple Cellular Properties Associated with Tumor Growth and Metastasis. Cancer Research 2005. 2005;65(23):10783–93.

8

Histological findings in infants with Gastrointestinal food allergy are associated with specific gastrointestinal symptoms; retrospective review from a tertiary centre

Neil Shah[1,3*†], Ru-Xin Melanie Foong[1†], Osvaldo Borrelli[1], Eleni Volonaki[1], Robert Dziubak[1], Rosan Meyer[1], Mamoun Elawad[1] and Neil J. Sebire[2]

Abstract

Background: Gastrointestinal food allergy (GIFA) occurs in 2 to 4 % of children, the majority of whom are infants (<1 year of age). Although endoscopy is considered the gold standard for diagnosing GIFA, it is invasive and requires general anaesthesia. Therefore, we aimed to investigate whether in infants with GIFA, gastrointestinal symptoms predict histological findings in order to help optimise the care pathway for such patients.

Methods: All infants <1 year of age over a 20 year period who underwent an endoscopic procedure gastroscopy or colonoscopy for GIFA were evaluated for the study. Symptoms at presentation were reviewed and compared with mucosal biopsy histological findings, which were initially broadly classified for study purposes as "Normal" or "Abnormal" (defined as the presence of any mucosal inflammation by the reporting pathologist at the time of biopsy).

Results: Of a total of 1319 cases, 544 fitted the inclusion criteria. 62 % of mucosal biopsy series in this group were reported as abnormal. Infants presenting with diarrhoea, rectal (PR) bleeding, irritability and urticaria in any combination had a probability >85 % (OR > 5.67) of having abnormal histological findings compared to those without. Those with isolated PR bleeding or diarrhoea were associated with 74 % and 68 % probability (OR: 2.85 and 2.13) of an abnormal biopsy, respectively. Conversely, children presenting with faltering growth or reflux/vomiting showed any abnormal mucosal histology in only 50.8 % and 45.3 % (OR: 1.04 and 0.82) respectively.

Conclusions: Food allergy may occur in very young children and is difficult to diagnose. Since endoscopy in infants has significant risks, stratification of decision-making may be aided by symptoms. At least one mucosal biopsy demonstrated an abnormal finding in around half of cases in this selected population. Infants presenting with diarrhoea, PR bleeding, urticaria and irritability are most likely to demonstrate abnormal histological findings.

Keywords: Endoscopy, Infant, Food allergy, Biopsy, Histopathology, Eosinophil

Background

Gastrointestinal food allergy (GIFA) is increasing in prevalence and usually affects very young children [1]. Approximately 2-4 % of children between the ages of 0-3 years are diagnosed with food allergy [2, 3] and up to 60 % of these children display gastrointestinal symptoms

such as abdominal pain, poor appetite, vomiting and diarrhoea. Other children may present with symptoms affecting skin, such as eczema, catarrhal problems or even anaphylaxis. Clinically, symptoms are often very pronounced and warrant investigations to eliminate other diagnoses before food allergy is considered [2, 4, 5]. Normally, the mucosal barrier in the gastrointestinal (GI) tract develops an "oral tolerance" to food antigens ingested [6]. However, in children with food allergy, this mechanism is believed to fail, resulting in allergic sensitisation and elicitation of allergy-type responses [6, 7]. This reaction, which

* Correspondence: neil.shah@gosh.nhs.uk
†Equal contributors
[1]Paediatric Gastroenterology Department, Great Ormond Street Hospital, London WC1N 3JH, United Kingdom
[3]Institute of Child Health/UCL, London WC1N 1EH, UK
Full list of author information is available at the end of the article

can manifest as a wide range of different symptoms, can be classified as immunoglobulin E (IgE)-mediated allergy, non-IgE mediated allergy or mixed IgE and non-IgE allergy [8]. Gastrointestinal food allergies (GIFA) are generally considered as non-IgE mediated, but eosinophilic dominant gastrointestinal disorders may be mixed IgE and non-IgE allergies. The most common age of presentation of non-IgE mediated allergies affecting the gut is in children under the age of one year, with cow's milk, soy protein, hens' egg and wheat being the most frequent causative foods [2, 4, 5, 9, 10].

The immunopathology of non-IgE mediated GIFA is still not fully understood, which makes diagnosis and management difficult, often requiring an elimination diet followed by food challenge [8, 11]. Endoscopy and biopsy has become increasingly important, with some considering endoscopic biopsy as the gold standard since it is relatively objective and may provide information regarding possible mechanisms. [4, 7] For example, in eosinophilic oesophagitis, the histological appearance defines the diagnosis [12]. However, endoscopy for very young children is often limited to specialised centres and involves general anaesthesia, requiring administration by paediatric anaesthetists, and procedural risks such as intestinal perforation [13, 14]. There are no studies investigating gastrointestinal symptoms in relation to histological features in infant GIFA [15]. Hence, the aim of this study was to investigate whether specific symptoms are associated with abnormal histological findings in endoscopic biopsies obtained from children with GIFA in order to optimise care pathway decision making.

Methods

Routinely collected data was reviewed from children under the age of one-year referred to a tertiary paediatric gastroenterology centre during the study period (June 1987 to August 2007), who had undergone endoscopic biopsy. Jejunal biopsies performed by the now historical procedure of Crosby capsule (common in the early years of our study) were excluded, and we also excluded children biopsied for other indications unrelated to GIFA. For all cases clinical symptoms were assessed in relation to histopathological findings based on contemporaneous biopsy reports. A single researcher extracted data according to predefined objective criteria.

All biopsies were reported by specialist paediatric histopathologists from the same tertiary centre. For the purposes of this study, histopathological findings were coded as either "Normal" or "Abnormal" (presence of any significant abnormal finding at any biopsy site including acute or chronic inflammation, with or without increased mucosal eosinophil density [16], or other pathologies such as partial villous atrophy or *Helicobacter pylori* see Fig. 1). Chronic inflammation with predominantly excess mucosal eosinophil density was considered most suggestive of food allergy in this cohort of young children [12, 17, 18].

Data were analysed using IBM SPSS Statistics for Windows, Version 22 (Armonk, NY). Continuous variables

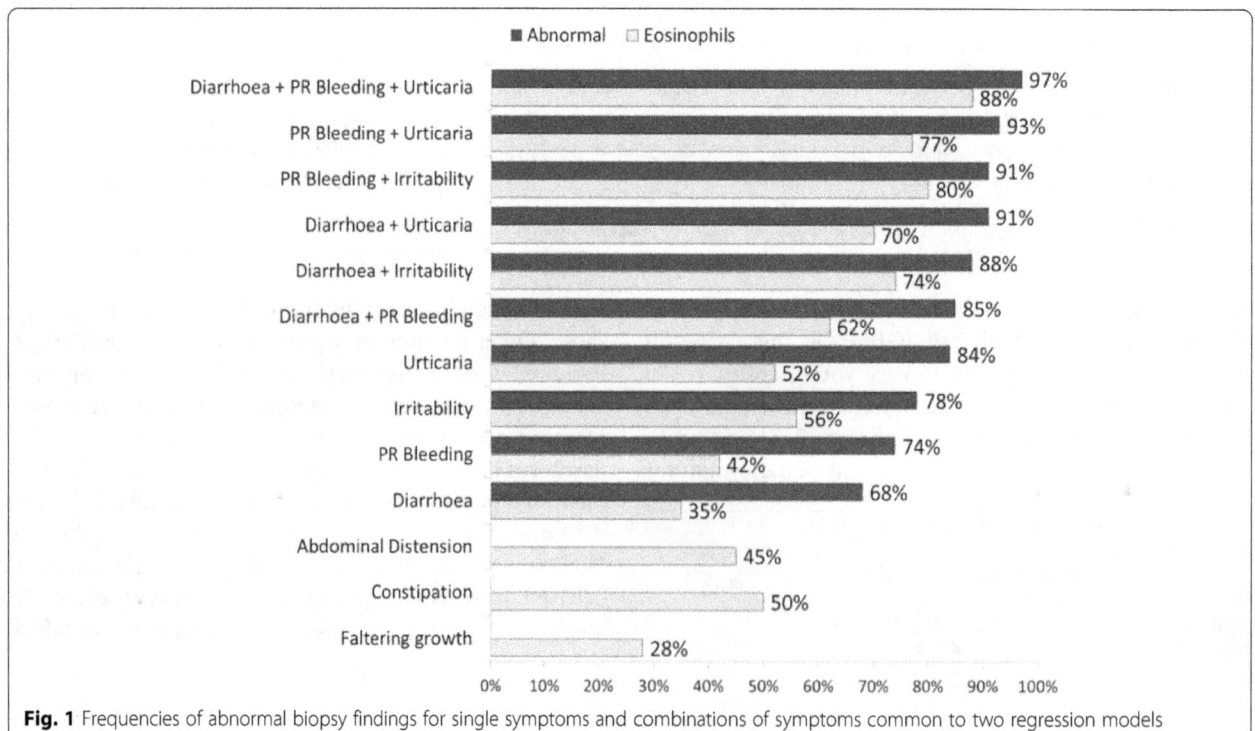

Fig. 1 Frequencies of abnormal biopsy findings for single symptoms and combinations of symptoms common to two regression models

were presented as medians with interquartile ranges and categorical variables as frequencies and percentages. Mann-Whitney U test and chi-square test were used to examine the differences between groups.

For all symptoms in isolation (in cases when the patient presented with only one symptom) Positive Predictive Values (PPV) of abnormal biopsy findings were calculated. Multiple logistic regression was used to investigate the relationship between biopsy findings and symptoms with adjustment for potential confounders of age and gender. Based on logistic regression models, probabilities of abnormal biopsy findings were calculated for combinations of symptoms using the median age. Goodness of fit of logistic regression models was based on Hosmer-Lemeshow test. All tests were two-tailed and significance level was set to 0.05. The study was approved by the local Research Ethics Committee (Bloomsbury REC). All data was retrospective and identified by study number only and individual patient consent was not required for data inclusion. The study conformed to the Helsinki declaration regarding research performance.

Results

Of 1319 infants undergoing endoscopic biopsies, 318 were excluded due to insufficient clinical information, 265 due to being Crosby capsule biopsies and 60 due to specific non GIFA indications (congenital diarrhoea, autoimmune enteropathy, graft-versus-host disease, tufting enteropathy and disaccharidase deficiency), leaving 676 patients who met the inclusion criteria. Some patients had multiple endoscopies and repeat biopsies, 122 in total, which were also excluded and only the initial presentation biopsy included. 554 endoscopic biopsy series were therefore included. Fifty-one per cent (285/554) were male, median age 7 months (IQR = 0.2-12 months). Overall, 62 % (344/554) had abnormal mucosal biopsy findings. The median age of those with abnormal biopsy was significantly lower than those with normal findings (median 6.6 months versus median 7.5 months, P < 0.001).

The most common presenting symptoms as indications for endoscopy were reflux/vomiting (40 %), faltering growth (37 %), diarrhoea (35 %) and rectal (PR) bleeding (12 %). 309 (56 %) patients presented with one symptom, 190 (34 %) with two, 49 (9 %) with three and six patients (1 %) with four symptoms. Positive predictive values (PPV) for symptoms based on the patients who presented with one symptom ($n = 309$) are shown in Table 1.

Diarrhoea was associated with a significantly greater frequency of abnormal histological findings than faltering growth (70.8 % vs. 50.8 %, $p = 0.018$) or reflux (70.8 % vs. 45.3 %, $p = 0.001$). PR bleeding was associated with a significantly greater rate of abnormal histological findings than faltering growth (74.2 % vs. 50.8 %, $p = 0.031$) or reflux (74.2 % vs. 45.3 %, $p = 0.004$). There were no significant differences between the frequency of abnormal biopsies between those presenting with diarrhoea and PR Bleeding, ($p = 0.728$) or those presenting with reflux and faltering growth, ($p = 0.484$).

Multiple logistic regression models were used to assess the frequency of any abnormal biopsy findings with combinations of symptoms (Hosmer-Lemeshow $p = 0.373$), as well as the probability of increased mucosal eosinophil density (Hosmer-Lemeshow $p = 0.413$), adjusted for differences in age and gender. Diarrhoea ($p < 0.001$), PR bleeding ($p < 0.01$), irritability ($p < 0.05$) and urticaria ($p < 0.05$) were significantly associated with both abnormal biopsy and excess eosinophils (Table 2). The site, Oesophagus, stomach, duodenum or colon, of the abnormal findings are shown in Table 3. Faltering growth, constipation and abdominal distension were also predictors of finding eosinophils in a biopsy ($p < 0.05$, $p < 0.01$, $p < 0.05$ respectively; Table 2). Age was an important confounding factor as we found a higher probability of an abnormal biopsy in younger children. Among others, reflux/vomiting was a poor predictor; therefore it was excluded from the models. Similarly, gender was not a significant confounding factor.

Specific symptom combinations were more likely to have biopsies with excess eosinophils present. For example, children who presented with a combination of diarrhoea, PR bleeding and urticaria had an 88 % frequency of excess eosinophils.

Discussion

This is the first large study to examine whether specific symptoms at presentation in very young children are associated with abnormal endoscopic biopsy findings in children being assessed for GIFA. The findings demonstrate that younger infants are more likely to have abnormal mucosal histological findings, and those presenting with specific combinations of symptoms are associated with high frequency of abnormal mucosal biopsy findings, including increased mucosal eosinophil density. In the current patient population, first presentation of GI symptoms occurred at around five months of age. However, it is likely that this represents a highly selected group referred to a specialist centre who are likely to have been experiencing more severe symptoms and hence were evaluated earlier in life than the general population and were all deemed to have symptoms of sufficient severity to warrant endoscopic examination. The risks of undergoing a general anaesthetic procedure and associated potential complications involved in performing endoscopy in very young infants as well as the impact on families are important considerations when deciding on whether to perform an endoscopy [13, 14, 19].

Table 1 Positive Predictive Values (PPV) of abnormal mucosal biopsies in infants being assessed for GIFA based on a single presenting gastrointestinal symptom based on 309/554 patients who presented with one symptom only

	Number	Percent	Isolated increased mucosal eosinophil density	PPV	Any abnormal biopsy	PPV
			n		n	
Reflux/vomiting	117	37.9 %	19	16.2 %	53	45.3 %
Diarrhoea	72	23.3 %	30	41.7 %	51	70.8 %
Faltering growth	61	19.7 %	19	31.1 %	31	50.8 %
PR Bleeding	31	10.0 %	16	51.6 %	23	74.2 %
Haematemesis	7	2.3 %	1	14.3 %	4	57.1 %
Constipation	6	1.9 %	3	50.0 %	3	50.0 %
Feeding difficulties	4	1.3 %	0	0.0 %	0	0.0 %
Irritability	4	1.3 %	1	25.0 %	2	50.0 %
Anaemia	2	0.6 %	0	0.0 %	0	0.0 %
Hypoalbuminaemia	2	0.6 %	0	0.0 %	2	100.0 %
Abdominal distension	2	0.6 %	1	50.0 %	1	50.0 %
Recurrent Abdominal pain	1	0.3 %	0	0.0 %	1	100.0 %

The most common symptoms were diarrhoea, reflux/vomiting, PR bleeding and faltering growth. Of these, if isolated, infants presenting with diarrhoea or PR bleeding, had an approximate 70 % probability of a histologically abnormal biopsy. However, infants who presented with combinations of diarrhoea, PR bleeding, irritability and urticaria were both more likely to have abnormal biopsy findings and also more likely to demonstrate increased mucosal eosinophil density. For example, almost 90 % of those presenting with diarrhoea and irritability had an abnormal biopsy. There were few patients who presented with irritability in isolation (1.3 %). However, it is possible that parents and clinicians underreport this symptom especially in the presence of other more common and recognisable symptoms. [20, 21] The frequency of an abnormal biopsy was lower for infants presenting with reflux/vomiting (45 %) and faltering growth (51 %).

Food allergic diagnoses are classified according to the site and severity of inflammation, which influences the presenting symptoms. With gastrointestinal mucosal disease that is identified by endoscopic biopsy there is a close spatial relationship of inflammatory mediators known to be released by mucosal inflammatory cells and enteric nerves [2]. The exact mechanisms of the manifestations of gastrointestinal symptoms are slowly being unravelled with the concept of paracrine immune interaction on the enteric nervous system, being known as a neuro-immune interaction [22, 23] leading to the disturbed motility and symptoms seen in GIFA such as reflux, diarrhoea or constipation. Much workstill needs to be done to fully explain how these symptoms develop and respond to dietary or anti-inflammatory measures.

Limitations of the study are related to the retrospective nature of data collected over a long time period with possible associated variation in the clinical suspicion of GIFA and management of such infants by endoscopic examination and biopsy. In GIFA, despite adherence to the diagnosis only being made by clinicians in out unit

Table 2 Multiple logistic regression models for association with abnormal mucosal biopsies in infants being assessed for GIFA

Variables in the model	Regression model for excess eosinophils in biopsy		Regression model for any Abnormal Biopsy	
	B	p-value	B	p-value
Constant	−0.96	0.001	0.49	0.05
Age (months)	−0.07	0.033	−0.06	0.041
Urticaria	1.50	0.007	1.59	0.038
Irritability	1.69	<0.001	1.22	0.018
PR Bleeding	1.12	< 0.001	1.00	0.002
Diarrhoea	0.79	< 0.001	0.71	< 0.001
Constipation	1.42	0.002	n/a	n/a
Abdominal Distension	1.24	0.045	n/a	n/a
Faltering growth	0.49	0.016	n/a	n/a

Table 3 Symptoms related to the site of abnormal findings in cases with only a single site affected

	Oesophagus (n = 61)	Percent	Stomach (n = 16)	Percent	Duodenum (n = 50)	Percent	Colon (n = 44)	Percent
Reflux/Vomiting	44	72 %	5	31 %	19	38 %	15	34 %
FTT	18	30 %	5	31 %	26	52 %	18	41 %
Diarrhoea	5	8 %	6	38 %	19	38 %	18	41 %
PR Bleeding	3	5 %	0	0 %	5	10 %	10	23 %
Constipation	0	0 %	2	13 %	3	6 %	8	18 %
Anaemia	0	0 %	0	0 %	0	0 %	2	5 %
Feed Diff	2	3 %	2	13 %	3	6 %	2	5 %
Mouth Ulcers	0	0 %	0	0 %	0	0 %	0	0 %
Rash	1	2 %	0	0 %	3	6 %	2	5 %
Irritability	2	3 %	1	6 %	4	8 %	5	11 %
Haematemesis	6	10 %	3	19 %	1	2 %	0	0 %
Hypoalbuminaemia	0	0 %	1	6 %	2	4 %	1	2 %
Abd. Distension	1	2 %	0	0 %	1	2 %	5	11 %
RAP	1	2 %	0	0 %	0	0 %	3	7 %

following elimination diet of major dietary antigens (Diary, egg, soya and wheat usually) with clinical improvement and subsequent reappearance of symptoms on rechallenge, the diagnosis remains subjective. The symptoms can be delayed and is unblended and subject to parental reporting. Furthermore, even with such a large dataset, for the purposes of this study we have classified mucosal biopsy findings broadly into normal versus abnormal, (with the only subcategory being those with apparently isolated increased mucosal eosinophil density at any site since this has been suggested as the most characteristic feature of GIFA) [12, 24]. More detailed sub-analysis of the relationship between other specific histological findings and their combinations with symptoms is not possible in this dataset and much larger numbers of cases, all of whom undergo multiple biopsies from small and large intestinal sites, would be required, but is unlikely to be available.

The clinical decision regarding whether an infant requires endoscopic examination and biopsy for diagnosis of food allergy can be difficult, since the procedure in this age group requires general anaesthesia with associated risks. The current data demonstrates that specific symptom patterns at presentation are associated with varying yield of abnormal mucosal histological findings, in particular, infants who experience diarrhoea, PR bleeding, irritability and urticaria having a high frequency of abnormal biopsies. This information may aid the decision making process for young children presenting with probable food allergy.

Conclusions

Gastrointestinal food allergy (GIFA), may present with a wide variety of symptoms in the first year of life and specific symptom patterns at presentation are associated with varying yield of abnormal mucosal histological findings at endoscopic biopsy. Infants who experience diarrhoea, PR bleeding, irritability and urticaria have a high frequency of abnormal gastrointestinal mucosal biopsies, including prominent mucosal eosinophils.

Competing interests
Dr Shah has performed consultancy work for Mead Johnson Nutrition, unrelated to this project. The other authors declare that they have no competing interests and have not received reimbursements, fees, funding, or salary from an organization that may in any way gain or lose financially from the publication of this manuscript, either now or in the future.

Authors' contributions
NS, ME and NJS conceived and planned the study. RMF, EV, RD and RM performed the data extraction and analysis. All authors participated in drafting of the manuscript and read and approved the final manuscript.

Acknowledgements
NJS is part supported by an NIHR Senior Investigator award and the NIHR GOSH BRC. This report is independent research and the views expressed in this publication are those of the authors and not necessarily those of the NHS, the NIHR or the Department of Health.

Author details
[1]Paediatric Gastroenterology Department, Great Ormond Street Hospital, London WC1N 3JH, United Kingdom. [2]Histopathology Department, Great Ormond Street Hospital, London, United Kingdom. [3]Institute of Child Health/UCL, London WC1N 1EH, UK.

References
1. Prescott SL, Pawankar R, Allen KJ, et al. A global survey of changing patterns of food allergy burden in children. World Allergy Organ J. 2013;6:21.
2. Meyer R, Schwarz C, Shah N. A Review of the Diagnosis and Management of Food-induced Gastrointestinal Allergies. Curr Allergy Clin Immunol. 2012;25:10–7.
3. Venter C, Pereira B, Voigt K, et al. Prevalence and cumulative incidence of food hypersensitivity in the first 3 years of life. Allergy. 2008;63:354–9.

4. Maloney J, Nowak-Wegrzyn A. Educational clinical case series for pediatric allergy and immunology: Allergic proctocolitis, food protein-induced enterocolitis syndrome and allergic eosinophilic gastroenteritis with protein-losing gastroenteropathy as manifestations of non-IgE-mediated cow's milk allergy. Pediatr Allerg Immunol. 2007;18:360–7.

5. Meyer R, Fleming C, Dominguez-Ortega G, et al. Manifestations of food protein induced gastrointestinal allergies presenting to a single tertiary paediatric gastroenterology unit. World Allergy Organ J. 2013;6:13–6.

6. Dupont C. Food allergy: recent Advances in Pathophysiology and Diagnosis. Ann Nutr Metab. 2011;59:8–18.

7. Vickery BP, Chin S, Burks AW. Pathophysiology of Food Allergy. Pediatr Clin North Am. 2011;58:363–76.

8. Boyce JA, Assaad A, Burks AW, et al. Guidelines for the Diagnosis and Management of Food Allergy in the United States: Summary of the NIAID-Sponsored Expert Panel Report. Nutr Res. 2011;31:61–75.

9. Husby S. Food Allergy as Seen by a Paediatric Gastroenterologist. J Ped Gast Nutr. 2008;47:S49–52.

10. Fogg MI, Spergel JM. Management of food allergies. Expert Opin Pharmacother. 2003;4:1025–37.

11. Sicherer SH, Sampson HA. Food Allergy. J Allergy Clin Immunol. 2010;125:S116–25.

12. Liacouras CA, Furuta GT, Hirano I, et al. Eosinophilic esophagitis: Updated consensus recommendations for children and adults. J Allergy Clin Immunol. 2011;128:3–20.

13. Jimenez SG, Catto-Smith AG. Impact of day-case gastroscopy on children and their families. J Gast Hepatol. 2008;23:379–84.

14. Ammar MS, Pfefferkorn MD, Croffie JM, et al. Complications after outpatient upper GI endoscopy in children: 30-day follow-up. Am J Gastroenterol. 2003;98:1508–11.

15. Volonaki E, Sebire NJ, Borrelli O, et al. Gastrointestinal Endoscopy and Mucosal Biopsy in the First Year of Life: Indications and Outcome. J Pediatr Gastro Nutr. 2012;55:62–5.

16. Sebire NJ, Ramsay A, Smith VV, Malone M, Risdon RA. Lamina propria eosinophil density in paediatric gastrointestinal mucosal biopsies. J Pathol. 2002;198:25a.

17. Papadopoulou A, Koletzko S, Heuschkel R, et al. Management guidelines of Eosinophilic Esophagitis in Childhood. J Pediatr Gastrol Nutr. 2014;58:107–88.

18. Atkins D, Furuta GT. Mucosal immunology, eosinophic esophagitis, and other intestinal inflammatory diseases. J Allergy Clin Immunol. 2010;125:S255–61.

19. Melville D, da Silva MS, Young J, et al. Postprocedural effects of gastrointestinal endoscopy performed as a day case procedure in children: implications for patient and family education. Gastroenterology Nursing. 2007;30:426–34.

20. National Institute for Health and Care Excellence (NICE). CG116 Food allergy in children and young people: NICE guideline 2012 http://guidance.nice.org.uk/CG116

21. Venter C, Brown T, Shah N, et al. Diagnosis and management of non-IgE-mediated cow's milk allergy in infancy – a UK primary care practical guide. Clin Transl Allergy. 2013;3:23.

22. Chandrasekharan B, Nezami BG, Srinivasan S. Emerging neuropeptide targets in inflammation: NPY and VIP. Am J Physiol Gastrointest Liver Physiol. 2013;304:G949–57.

23. Wood JD. Enteric neuroimmunophysiology and Pathophysiology. Gastroenterol. 2004;127:635–57.

24. Tunis MC, Marshall JS. Toll-Like Receptor 2 as a Regulator of Oral Tolerance in the Gastrointestinal Tract. Mediators Inflamm. 2014; 606383.

9

Histopathological characterization of corrosion product associated adverse local tissue reaction in hip implants: a study of 285 cases

Benjamin F. Ricciardi[1], Allina A. Nocon[2], Seth A. Jerabek[1], Gabrielle Wilner[3], Elianna Kaplowitz[3], Steven R. Goldring[3], P. Edward Purdue[3] and Giorgio Perino[4*]

Abstract

Background: Adverse local tissue reaction (ALTR), characterized by a heterogeneous cellular inflammatory infiltrate and the presence of corrosion products in the periprosthetic soft tissues, has been recognized as a mechanism of failure in total hip replacement (THA). Different histological subtypes may have unique needs for longitudinal clinical follow-up and complication rates after revision arthroplasty. The purpose of this study was to describe the histological patterns observed in the periprosthetic tissue of failed THA in three different implant classes due to ALTR and their association with clinical features of implant failure.

Methods: Consecutive patients presenting with ALTR from three major hip implant classes ($N = 285$ cases) were identified from our prospective Osteolysis Tissue Database and Repository. Clinical characteristics including age, sex, BMI, length of implantation, and serum metal ion levels were recorded. Retrieved synovial tissue morphology was graded using light microscopy. Clinical characteristics and features of synovial tissue analysis were compared between the three implant classes. Histological patterns of ALTR identified from our observations and the literature were used to classify each case. The association between implant class and histological patterns was compared.

Results: Our histological analysis demonstrates that ALTR encompasses three main histological patterns: 1) macrophage predominant, 2) mixed lymphocytic and macrophagic with or without features of associated with hypersensitivity/allergy or response to particle toxicity (eosinophils/mast cells and/or lymphocytic germinal centers), and 3) predominant sarcoid-like granulomas. Implant classification was associated with histological pattern of failure, and the macrophagic predominant pattern was more common in implants with metal-on-metal bearing surfaces (MoM HRA and MoM LHTHA groups). Duration of implantation and composition of periprosthetic cellular infiltrates was significantly different amongst the three implant types examined suggesting that histopathological features of ALTR may explain the variability of clinical implant performance in these cases.

Conclusions: ALTR encompasses a diverse range of histological patterns, which are reflective of both the implant configuration independent of manufacturer and clinical features such as duration of implantation. The macrophagic predominant pattern and its mechanism of implant failure represent an important subgroup of ALTR which could become more prominent with increased length of implantation.

Keywords: Adverse local tissue reaction, Corrosion products, Revision arthroplasty, Synovial inflammation, Metal-on-metal total hip replacement, Hip resurfacing

* Correspondence: perinog@hss.edu
[4]Department of Pathology and Laboratory Medicine, Hospital for Special Surgery, 535 East 70th Street, New York, NY 10021, USA
Full list of author information is available at the end of the article

Background

The introduction over the past two decades of alternative bearing surfaces, in particular a new generation of metal-on-metal (MoM) bearing, and increased modularity at the head-neck and neck-stem tapers has attempted to reduce wear debris formation at the bearing surface, risk of dislocation, and improve accurate reproduction of leg length, offset, and version [1–3]. These modifications have had unintended consequences, although clinical concerns regarding formation of corrosion products were raised; in particular, increased rates of adverse periprosthetic soft tissue reactions reported across a diverse spectrum of implant configurations [4–9]. These failures have resulted in extensive soft tissue necrosis, injury to the hip abductors, increased revision complications, and significant patient morbidity [8, 10–12].

Early studies described an unusual pattern of periprosthetic soft tissue inflammation with mixed macrophagic and lymphocytic infiltrates, variable tissue necrosis, vascular wall changes, and cytoplasmic inclusions of uncertain composition in the macrophages, which was collectively described as aseptic lymphocyte dominated vasculitis associated lesion (ALVAL) [13–15]. The formation of corrosion products at modular junctions and/or bearing surface and subsequent penetration into the periprosthetic soft tissue have been a common feature associated with the reaction [5, 16–18]. More recent studies have focused on characterizing the lymphocytic infiltrate, noting mixed interstitial and perivascular B- and T-cell populations with formation of germinal centers or sarcoid-like granulomas in subsets of patients [17, 19, 20].

Unlike the early reports that focused primarily on aspects of lymphocytic infiltrate and necrosis, subsequent studies suggested that the histological spectrum of these reactions, named adverse local tissue reaction (ALTR) or adverse reaction to implant debris (ARMD) is more diverse than originally appreciated, and lymphocyte rich infiltrate with significant necrosis represents only a subset of these cases [17, 20, 21]. In particular, a subgroup of patients with neo-synovial florid macrophagic infiltrate containing wear debris with no or minimal lymphocytic component in their periprosthetic tissue has been described in these studies, although its contribution to implant failure has not been well characterized. It is critical to identify the full spectrum of ALTR failures because different histological subtypes may have unique needs for longitudinal clinical follow-up and complication rates after revision arthroplasty.

In the present study, we report the histological features of 285 cases of ALTR from a large, diverse group of hip implants that includes three major classes: metal-on-metal (MoM) hip resurfacing arthroplasty (HRA), MoM large head total hip arthroplasty (THA), and non-

MoM THA with cobalt/chrome (CoCr) dual modular neck. Histopathological analysis of the periprosthetic tissue across the three classes of implants was performed to answer the following research questions: 1. What are the histopathological patterns of soft tissue failure in ALTR; 2. What is the association between implant class and different histopathological features of ALTR; 3. What is the association of histopathological findings with clinical features of implant failure.

Methods

Patients

All patients who underwent revision hip arthroplasty between June 2011 and December 2014 implanted with a prosthetic device of the above mentioned classes of implants at risk of ALTR were identified retrospectively from the prospective Osteolysis/Adverse Local Reaction Tissue Database and Repository at our institution (Fig. 1). These patients were all eligible for inclusion in the current study [$N = 303$]. Exclusion criteria included infection diagnosed in compliance with the criteria reported by the International Consensus Meeting on periprosthetic joint infection and accepted by the Centers for Disease Control [22] [$N = 3$] with 5 out of 5, 6 out of 6, and 5 out of 5 intraoperative positive cultures, insufficient tissue retrieval for comparative pathologic examination (less than 5 tissue sections and more than 75 % tissue necrosis at light microscopy examination on all slides examined) [$N = 13$], and two cases for non-ALTR related post-operative complications with histological examination: periprosthetic fracture [$N = 1$] and recurrent dislocation [$N = 1$]. The exclusion of these patients left a total of 285 cases for inclusion in this study. In addition, 18 cases were identified with a post-operative unexpected diagnosis of ALTR in conventional MoP implants without dual modular neck that were not consented for inclusion in our registry prospectively and were not eligible for enrollment in the current study.

Patients were divided into three groups based on the design of their implant. Previous work has shown that implant design influences both clinical and pathologic manifestations of ALTR [17]. The three major implant classes examined were: 1. MoM HRA group; 2. MoM large head ($\geq$36 mm) THA with or without cobalt chromium (CoCr) metallic adapter sleeve (MoM LHTHA group); and 3. Metal-on-polyethylene (MoP), ceramic-on-polyethylene (CoP), or ceramic-on-ceramic (CoC) bearing surface with femoral heads <36 mm and (CoCr) dual modular neck (Non-MoM DMNTHA). These represent the most common implant classes that have resulted in ALTR in case reports and case series [5, 23–27]. Demographic data (age, sex, body mass index, duration of implantation, duration of symptoms, implant type) were recorded for each patient when available. The onset of

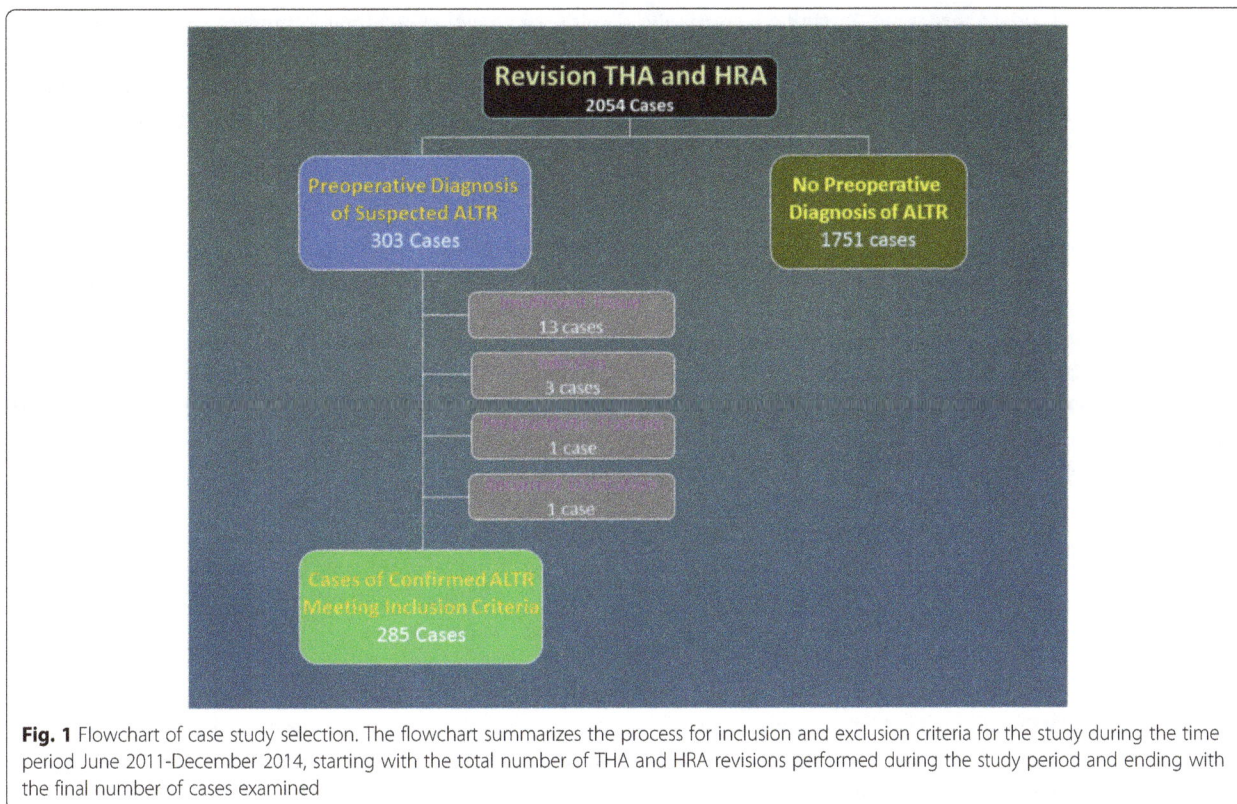

Fig. 1 Flowchart of case study selection. The flowchart summarizes the process for inclusion and exclusion criteria for the study during the time period June 2011-December 2014, starting with the total number of THA and HRA revisions performed during the study period and ending with the final number of cases examined

symptoms was assessed via questionnaire at the time of revision surgery. Symptoms included increasing pain around the hip and mechanical symptoms such as "grinding sensation". Other symptoms such as discomfort around the hip, although frequent in the Non-MoM DMNTHA group were not considered positive unless progression to pain was recorded before revision. Preoperative serum cobalt and chromium levels were obtained by quantitative inductively coupled plasma-mass spectrometry at the operating surgeons' discretion (ARUP Laboratories, Salt Lake City, Utah). Ethical committee approval was obtained prior to this study and all patients had an informed consent obtained in writing for inclusion in the registry (Institutional Review Board, Hospital for Special Surgery, Protocol Number 26085).

Tissue collection and sampling

Tissue collection and sampling for all patients was performed as previously described [17]. Briefly, patients suspected of having ALTR underwent magnetic resonance imaging (MRI) with multi-acquisition variable-resonance image combination (MAVRIC) scan to further reduce susceptibility artifact. Areas of inflammation were identified preoperatively on MRI when available, and used as guidance for tissue sampling by the operating surgeon.

Samples were taken from multiple regions around the hip joint including the periprosthetic pseudocapsule, bursal synovium, and adjacent skeletal muscle when necessary and labeled accordingly. Acetabular and femoral bone samples, core biopsies of osteolytic areas, and/or reamings were collected at the discretion of the operating surgeon to evaluate possible bone marrow involvement when suitable. Extensive sampling was performed at macroscopic examination with care to the orientation of the specimens, including necrotic areas and/or friable, loose material. Femoral heads from resurfacing specimens were separated from the metallic cup at surgery when possible and extensively sampled or subject to multiple biopsies when retrieved in situ. The mean number of individual surgical specimens between the groups was not different [DMN cohort was 4.3 (SD 1.5), for the MoM THA cohort was 3.5 (1.6), and for the resurfacing cohort 3.5 (1.3); $p > 0.05$]. Extensive samples between 5 and 15 tissue blocks containing one or two histological sections were taken depending on the available tissue for each specimen.

Histological analysis

Histological analysis was performed as previously described [17]. Briefly, all sections were processed and embedded with standard procedures, stained routinely with hematoxylin-eosin. Cases were scored for this study by an experienced musculoskeletal pathologist (GP) and a surgeon trained in examining periprosthetic tissue from revision hip arthroplasty (BFR). Investigators were blinded from clinical patient characteristics. All cases were examined by both observers. Disagreement was handled by consensus between the two observers. This method of grading and assessment has been reported in previous publication [17] and also validated for intraobserver variability [28]. The ALVAL scoring system proposed by Campbell et al, which was previously used as correlative index with MRI imaging analysis, was recorded for each case [13, 28].

Histological sections were examined for synovial structure, cellularity, macrophage particle content, and bone marrow involvement using a previously described scoring system [17] and summarized in Table 1. Results were expressed as the percentage of samples containing the selected feature. All patients enrolled in our registry over the same time period with a diagnosis of aseptic loosening due to osteolysis with conventional MoP implants without dual modular neck (MoP OLTHA) were subject to the same tissue collection, histological analysis, and scored to serve as non-ALTR controls for pathological data [$N = 31$].

Histological patterns
Several histological patterns have been observed in ALTR in previous studies [13, 17, 20, 21, 29, 30]. We divided these into four broad groups based on these previous studies: 1) predominantly macrophagic pattern with absent or minimal lymphocytic response, 2) mixed inflammatory pattern, macrophagic and lymphocytic with variable presence of plasma cells, eosinophils, and mast cells, and 3) granulomatous pattern, predominant or associated with the mixed inflammatory pattern; and 4) predominantly lymphocytic pattern with absence of macrophagic component [Table 2]. The macrophagic pattern represents a group of patients with an adverse

soft tissue reaction resulting in implant failure with minimal lymphocytic infiltration [20, 30, 31]. The mixed inflammatory group is divided into two subsets: (A) with and (B) without lymphocytic germinal centers usually associated with tall endothelial cell venules and/or mast cell/eosinophilic infiltrate because the A subset may identify patients with distinct immunologic response [13, 15, 19, 29]. The third group has prominent formation of sarcoid-like granulomas, defined as a nodular collection of epithelioid macrophages with multinucleated giant cells and lymphocytic cuffing associated with large aggregates of corrosion products particles and a mixed macrophagic/lymphocytic infiltrate, possibly representing a subset of patients with distinctive macrophagic features [20, 29]. The fourth group shows perivascular/interstitial lymphocytic infiltrate without macrophagic component [21]. Patients in each implant class were classified based on the predominant histological pattern seen at light microscopy. The rate of appearance of each pattern was compared between the different implant classes.

Statistics
All demographic and histological variables were compared across the three implant classes. Descriptive statistics are presented as medians and ranges for continuous variables and as frequencies and percentages for categorical variables. Continuous variables were assessed using the Kruskall-Wallis test. Histological patterns amongst the different implant classes were compared using the Fischer's exact test. A multinomial logistic regression was performed in order to identify possible predictive factors for the development of the scale of ALTR severity as described in the Campbell's score. Bonferroni correction was used for pairwise comparisons of histological data adjusted for multiple comparisons.

Results
Demographic results
Implant designs that resulted in cases of ALTR in this study are shown in Table 3. Patients in the HRA group

Table 1 Histological grading system used for all cases of ALTR

Synovial Structure	Cellularity	Macrophage Content	Bone and Bone Marrow Involvement
Synovial Layer Loss (Present, Absent)	Macrophages (Grade 0–3)	Polyethylene Particles (Present, Absent)	Necrosis (Present, Absent)
Cell Exfoliation (Present, Absent)	Lymphocytes (Grade 0–4)	Metal Particles (Present, Absent)	Macrophages (Present, Absent)
Soft Tissue Necrosis (Present, Absent)	Stromal Cells (Grade 1–3)	Corrosion Products (None, Intracellular, Extracellular)	Reactive Lymphocytic Aggregates (Present, Absent)
Vascular Wall Changes (Present, Absent)	Neutrophils (Present, Absent)		Germinal Centers (Present, Absent)
Granulomas (Present, Absent)	Plasma Cells (Grade 0–2)		
	Eosinophils (Present, Absent)		

Table 2 Histological patterns analyzed in hip replacement failures due to ALTR

Histological Pattern	Characteristics
Macrophagic Pattern	Macrophagic infiltrate (grade ≥ 1) without or with minimal evidence of interstitial and/or perivascular lymphocytic infiltrate (<grade 1)
Mixed Macrophagic and Lymphocytic Pattern w/wo Plasmacytic Component	Macrophagic (grade ≥ 1) and lymphocytic (grade ≥ 1) infiltrate
Without Presence of Germinal Centers or Eosinophils	
With Presence of Germinal Centers or Eosinophils	
Granulomatous Pattern	Any pattern with predominant presence of sarcoid-like granulomas
Lymphocytic Pattern	Interstitial and/or perivascular lymphocytic infiltrate without evidence of macrophagic infiltrate

were younger in age at time of revision relative to the other implant classes (Table 4). Total implantation time was shortest in the Non-MoM DMNTHA group [median 28 months (range 6–65)], and these patients had a significantly shorter duration of implantation relative to the MoM HRA group [median 48 months (range 5–120); $p < 0.001$] and the MoM LHTHA groups [median 60 months (range 23–132); $p < 0.001$] (Table 4). Duration of symptoms prior to revision did not differ between the different implant classes (Table 4). Preoperative serum cobalt and chromium ion levels were increased in the MoM

Table 3 Retrieved implants with failure due to ALTR

Non-MoM DMNTHA	Number of Hips
Rejuvenate (Stryker, Kalamazoo, MI)	111
ABG II (Stryker, Kalamazoo, MI)	5
SMF (Smith and Nephew, London, UK)	3
Redapt (Smith and Nephew, London, UK)	2
OTI/Encore R-120 (DJO Surgical, Austin, TX)	1
Aesculap Hip Replacement (Aesculap, Hazelwood, MO)	1
MoM HRA	
Birmingham Hip Resurfacing (Smith and Nephew, London, UK)	36
Cormet Hip Resurfacing (Corin Group, Cirencester, UK)	5
Conserve Hip Resurfacing (Wright Medical Technology, Arlington, TN)	2
ASR Hip Resurfacing (Depuy/Synthes, Warsaw, IN)	1
MoM LHTHA	
Birmingham Hip Replacement (Smith and Nephew, London, UK)	44
ASR Hip Replacement (Depuy/Synthes, Warsaw, IN)	22
Pinnacle Ultramet (Depuy/Synthes, Warsaw, IN)	19
Durom/Metasul (Zimmer, Warsaw, IN)	10
M2a Magnum (Biomet, Warsaw, IN)	8
Profemur (Wright Medical Technology, Arlington, TX)	6
Metal on Metal Bearing S-ROM (Depuy/Synthes, Warsaw, IN)	4
Conserve Hip Replacement (Wright Medical Technology, Arlington, TN)	4
Cormet Hip Replacement (Corin Group, Cirencester, UK)	1

HRA and MoM LHTHA groups relative to the Non-MoM DMNTHA group (Table 4). Head sizes were larger in the MoM bearing surface groups (HRA and LHTHA) relative to the Non-MoM DMNTHA group.

Histological patterns

A summary of the histological patterns seen in each of the three implant classes is shown in Table 5.

The macrophagic pattern is characterized by flat to papillary hypertrophic neo-synovium with a variable amount of macrophagic infiltrate and exfoliation of necrotic forms with absence or presence of giant cells containing fine globular and/or irregular aggregates of greenish corrosion products of variable dimension with or without particles of needle-shaped and/or irregular conventional black metallic debris and absent or minimal interstitial and/or perivascular lymphocytic infiltrate (Fig. 2a and b). A thick layer of necrosis is usually not present, although infarction of the neo-synovial papillae or a thin layer of superficial necrosis/infarction can be focally present along with variable foci of foamy macrophages. This pattern was seen in 41 % of cases of MoM HRA failures, but was less common in the other two implant classes (MoM LHTHA, 11 % of cases; Non-MoM DMNTHA, 6 % of cases) (Table 5).

The mixed macrophagic and lymphocytic pattern is characterized by a superficial layer of macrophages with or without an interstitial lymphocytic component, a layer of tissue necrosis/infarction of variable thickness or a band of desmoplastic fibrosis, a variable deep perivascular lymphocytic infiltrate, and macrophages containing fine globular and/or irregular aggregates of greenish corrosion products with or without particles of needle-shaped and/or irregular conventional black metallic debris (Fig. 2c and d). A subset of the mixed macrophagic and lymphocytic pattern shows features usually associated with hypersensitivity/allergy reactions, such as focal or diffuse eosinophilic infiltrate and presence of a large number of mast cells in association with particle-laden macrophages and/or perivascular lymphocytic infiltrate with formation of germinal centers (Fig. 2e and f). Implants with non-MoM bearing surfaces had increased mixed pattern

Table 4 Demographic characteristics from all three major implant classes

	Non-MoM DMNTHA (N = 120 patients)	MoM HRA (N = 44 patients)	MoM LHTHA (N = 113 patients)
Age (years)	66 (47–87)*	56 (43–75)*	60 (31–84)*
Sex (% female)	64 %	58 %	54 %
Body Mass Index	28 (17–43)^	25 (18–36)^	26 (19–59)
Implantation Time (months)	28 (6–65)°	48 (5–120)°	60 (23–132)°
Symptom Duration (months)	9 (0–60)	12 (0–63)	18 (0–60)
Serum Cobalt	7 (0–169)#	16 (1–115)#	13 (4–16)#
Serum Chromium	1 (0–64)§	14 (1–160)§	60 (23–132)§
Head Size	28 (22–52)¶	46 (38–52)¶	46 (36–64)¶
Cup Size	52 (38–64)	52 (46–58)	52 (48–64)

All values are given as median (range)
*$p < 0.005$ for the MoM HRA group compared to the other two groups
^$p < 0.05$ for the MoM HRA group compared to the non-MoM DMNTHA group ($p = 0.005$)
°$p < 0.05$ for the non-MoM-DMN THA group compared to the MoM HRA group ($p < 0.001$) and the MoM LHTHA group ($p < 0.001$)
#$p < 0.05$ for the non-MoM DMNTHA group compared to the MoM HRA group ($p = 0.042$)
§$p < 0.05$ for the MoM HRA and the MoM LHTHA groups compared to the non-MoM DMNTHA group ($p < 0.001$) and the MoM HRA group compared to the MoM LHTHA group ($p = 0.026$)
¶$p < 0.05$ for the MoM HRA ($p < 0.001$) and the MoM LHTHA ($p < 0.001$) groups compared to the non-MoM DMNTHA group

with hypersensitivity features as a percent of total failures (Non-MoM DMNTHA 32 %) versus implant classes with a MoM bearing surface (HRA 11 % of cases and LHTHA 22 % of cases) (Table 5).

The granulomatous pattern is characterized by predominant isolated or confluent granulomas composed of centrally located large aggregates of particulate corrosion products lined or contained by multinucleated giant cells surrounded by a nodular infiltrate of epithelioid macrophages lined by lymphocytic cuff of variable thickness with or without presence of a plasmacytic component (Fig. 2g and h). A granulomatous pattern was most commonly seen in the Non-MoM DMNTHA (16 % of cases) versus the other two implant classes (Table 5).

A significant association ($p < 0.001$) was found with length of implantation and histological classification on univariate analysis, with longer durations of implantation associated with a macrophagic pattern of failure and shorter durations of implantation associated with granulomatous or a mixed pattern with eosinophils and/or germinal centers. Duration of patient symptoms was not associated with histological classification in univariate analysis ($p = 0.16$).

Morphology results

A summary of morphologic findings among the three classes of implants and the control group is shown in Table 6.

Macrophage distributions were significantly different between the three implant classes, and the MoM HRA group had the highest percentage of cases of grade 3 macrophage distribution (95 % of cases) versus MoM LHTHA (65 % of cases; $p = 0.007$) and the Non-MoM DMNTHA (42 % of cases; $p = 0.007$) (Table 6). Compared with the MoP OLTHA group, the MoM HRA and MoM LHTHA had similar macrophage distributions ($p = 0.14$) (Table 6). Non-MoM DMNTHA had decreased macrophage distributions relative to the MoP OLTHA group ($p = 0.007$) (Table 6). Soft tissue necrosis was more common in the Non-MoM DMNTHA (53 % of cases) relative to the other implant classes (32 % in the MoM LHTHA [$p = 0.0048$], 11 % in the MoM HRA group; $p = 0.007$) (Table 6).

Focal or diffuse macrophagic involvement of the bone marrow was observed in the MoM HRA, MoM LHTHA, and the Non-MoM DMNTHA implants (Table 6). More cases of osteolysis/massive particle laden macrophagic infiltration within retrieved periprosthetic bone samples were seen in the MoM HRA relative to the other implant classes (Table 6). Examination of some of the femoral heads retrieved from failed hip resurfacing implants showed florid particle-laden macrophagic infiltrate in the neo-synovium and massive infiltration of the bone marrow with formation of macroscopically evident,

Table 5 Distribution of the histological patterns in the three implant classes

Implant class	Macrophagic pattern	Mixed Pattern w/o hypersensitivity features	Mixed Pattern w/Hypersensitivity Features	Granulomatous pattern	Lymphocytic pattern
Non-MoM DMNTHA	6	46	32	16	0
MoM HRA	41	48	11	0	0
MoM LHTHA	11	62	22	5	0

All values are expressed as a percentage of total cases of each histological pattern for a specific implant class

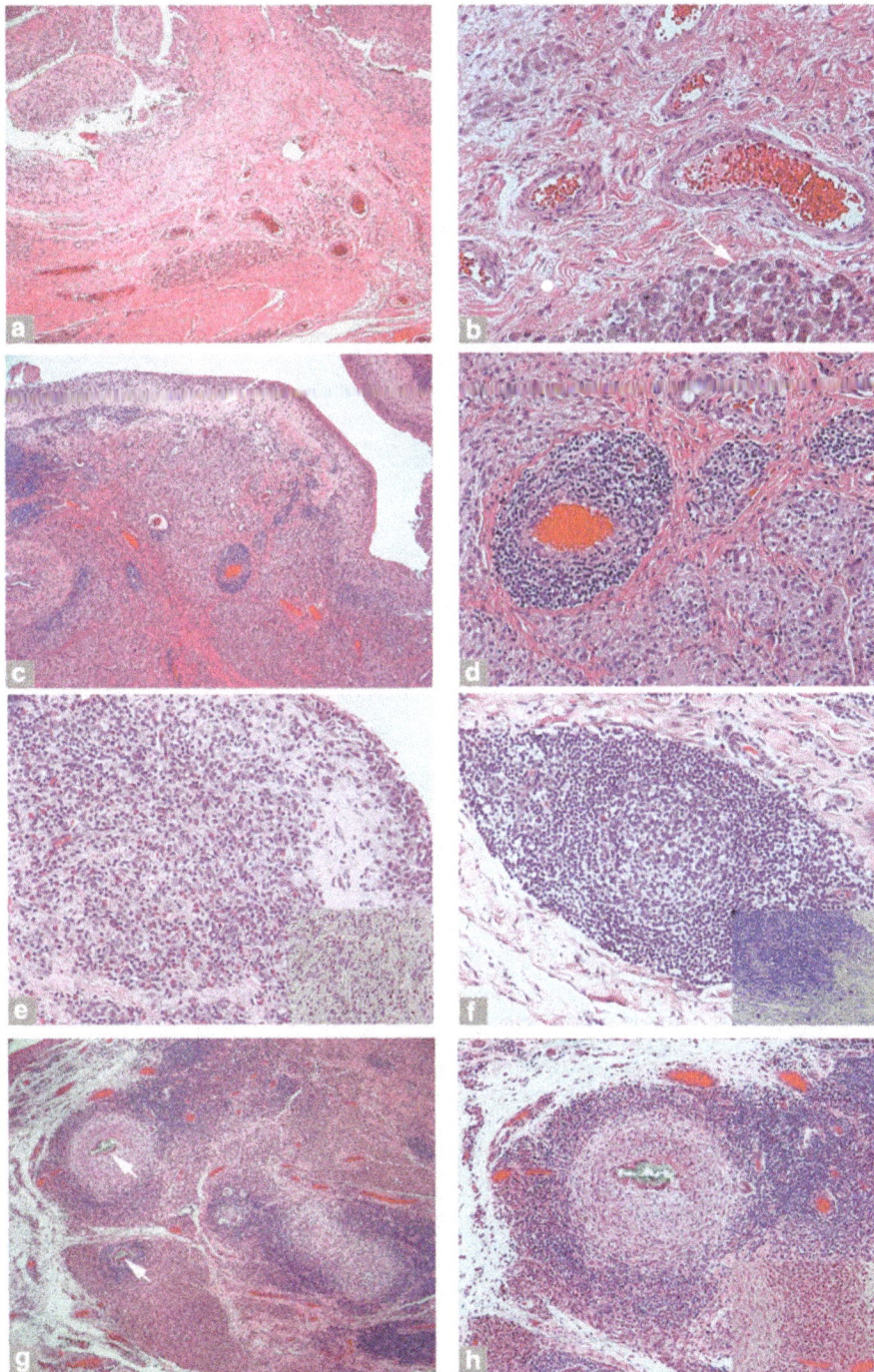

Fig. 2 Histological patterns of ALTR. *Macrophagic pattern*: **a** Papillary neo-synovium with macrophagic infiltrate and underlying vascular layer (H-E x50). **b** Vascular layer without lymphocytic infiltrate and cluster of particle laden macrophages, white arrow (H-E x400). *Mixed macrophagic and lymphocytic pattern*: **c** Neo-synovium with superficial macrophagic layer and desmoplastic band, white arrow, and perivascular lyphocytic infiltrate (H-E x50). **d** Perivascular lymphocytic infiltrate associated with large clusters of particle laden macrophages (H-E x200). *Subset of the mixed pattern with heightened immunological features*: **e** Neo-synovium with florid interstitial lymphocytic and eosinophilic infiltrate (H-E x200) and association of eosinophils with particle laden macrophages (inset, H-E x400). **f** Perivascular lymphocytic infiltrate with germinal center (H-E x200) associated with numerous mast cells (inset, Toluidine Blue x400). *Granulomatous pattern*: **g** Multiple sarcoid-like granulomas with central aggregate of corrosion products, white arrow (H-E x100). **h** Granuloma at higher power with central collection of epithelioid macrophages and occasional giant cells (H-E x200) and plasmacytic component with binucleated forms admixed with particle laden macrophages (inset, H-E x400)

Table 6 Significant differences in histological findings from all three implant classes and the control group

	Non-MoM DMN**THA** (N = 123 hips)	MoM HRA (N = 44 hips)	MoM LHTHA (N = 118 hips)	MoP OLTHA (N = 31 hips)
Synovial Structure				
Synovial Layer Loss (%)	99	89	99	16.1
Soft Tissue Necrosis (%)	53‡	11‡	32‡	0‡
Sarcoid-like Granulomas (%)	16*	0*	5*	0
Campbell Score (median)	8§	5§	6§	-
Cellularity				
Macrophages (% Grade 1, Grade 2, Grade 3)	7, 51, 42^	0, 5, 95^	1, 34, 65^	3, 16, 81^
Lymphocytes (% Grade 1, Grade 2, Grade 3, Grade 4)	7, 29, 34, 24°	25, 18, 11, 7 °	25, 31, 23, 10°	10, 0, 0, 0°
Plasma Cells (% Grade 1, Grade 2)	26, 18	11, 9	29, 18	0, 0
Eosinophils (%)	20	9	17	0
Macrophage Content				
Polyethylene Particles (%)	2	0	0	80
Metallic Particles (%)	8#	39#	30#	65#
Corrosion Products (%)	95	100	99	0
Large Aggregates	74¶	11¶	63¶	0¶
Bone and Bone Marrow	N = 58	N = 44	N = 36	N = 0
Necrosis (%)	47	11	23	-
Macrophage Infiltration (%)	57	67	73	-
Germinal Centers (%)	12	2	3	-
Osteolysis (# cases)	4	9	4	-

All values for synovial structure, macrophage content, eosinophils, cell distributions, and bone and bone marrow content expressed as percentage of cases with each morphologic feature
*$p = 0.013$ for Non-MoM DMNTHA versus MoM LHTHA and MoM HRA
^$p = 0.007$ for OL versus Non-MoM DMNTHA; $p = 0.007$ for MoM HRA versus MoM LHTHA; MoM HRA versus Non-MoM DMNTHA, and Non-MoM DMNTHA versus MoM LHTHA
°$p = 0.007$ for significant difference in distributions of lymphocyte grade between all implant classes except MoM LHTHA versus MoM HRA ($p = 0.0023$)
#$p = 0.007$ for OL versus MoM LTHA and Non-MoM DMNTHA; $p = 0.007$ for Non-MoM DMNTHA versus MoM HRA and MoM LHTHA
§$p < 0.001$ for significant difference in Campbell score between ALTR implant classes
‡$p = 0.007$ for OL versus Non-MoM DMNTHA, MoM LHTHA; $p = 0.007$ for MoM HRA versus Non-MoM DMNTHA; $p = 0.009$ MoM HRA versus MoM LHTHA; $p = 0.0048$ MoM LHTHA versus Non-MoM DMNTHA
¶$p = 0.011$ for OL versus MoM HRA; $p = 0.007$ OL versus Non-MoM DMNTHA and MoM LHTHA; $p = 0.007$ for MoM HRA versus MoM LHTHA and Non-MoM DMNTHA; $p = 0.026$ MoM LHTHA versus Non-MoM DMNTHA

macrophage-lined pseudocystic cavities (Fig. 3a, arrow) with marked exfoliation of necrotic forms (Fig. 3b). Macrophages containing greenish particles of corrosion products (Fig. 3b, inset and 3c) sometimes in association with black particles of conventional metallic debris (Fig. 3e and 3f) were observed streaming from the adjacent neo-synovium and infiltrating the bone marrow forming massive aggregates (Fig. 3f) or small clusters and single forms in the fatty marrow (Fig. 3g) or pushing underneath the orthopedic cement border lined by giant cells (Fig. 3c). In some cases, these were associated with large lymphocytic aggregates (Fig. 3h) or without lymphocytic reaction (Fig. 3d). The presence or absence of lymphocytic infiltrate in the bone marrow usually corresponded to the response seen in the neo-synovial membrane.

In the MoM LHTHA, a significant amount of necrotic debris containing macrophagic forms was observed in the metallic femoral head groove of a range of implant manufacturers (Fig. 4a and 4e), deposited from exfoliation of macrophagic viable/necrotic forms containing particles of corrosion products with or without conventional metallic debris (Fig. 4g) from thickened neo-synovial membrane with or without papillary features (Fig. 4b and 4f). Free aggregates of irregular green particles of corrosion products were found in synovial fluid (Fig. 4h, arrow) and in larger aggregates entrapped in necrotic cellular debris (Fig. 4d, arrow).

Lymphocyte distributions were significantly different between the three implant classes, and the MoM HRA group had the lowest percentage of cases of grade 3 and 4 lymphocyte distributions (18 % of cases) relative to the Non-MoM DMNTHA (58 % of cases; $p = 0.0007$), the MoM LHTHA (33 % of cases; $p = 0.0027$) (Table 6). All three ALTR groups had increased lymphocyte distributions relative to the MoP OLTHA group ($p = 0.007$; Table 6). Eosinophils were least common in the MoM HRA (9 % of cases) relative to the Non-MoM DMNTHA

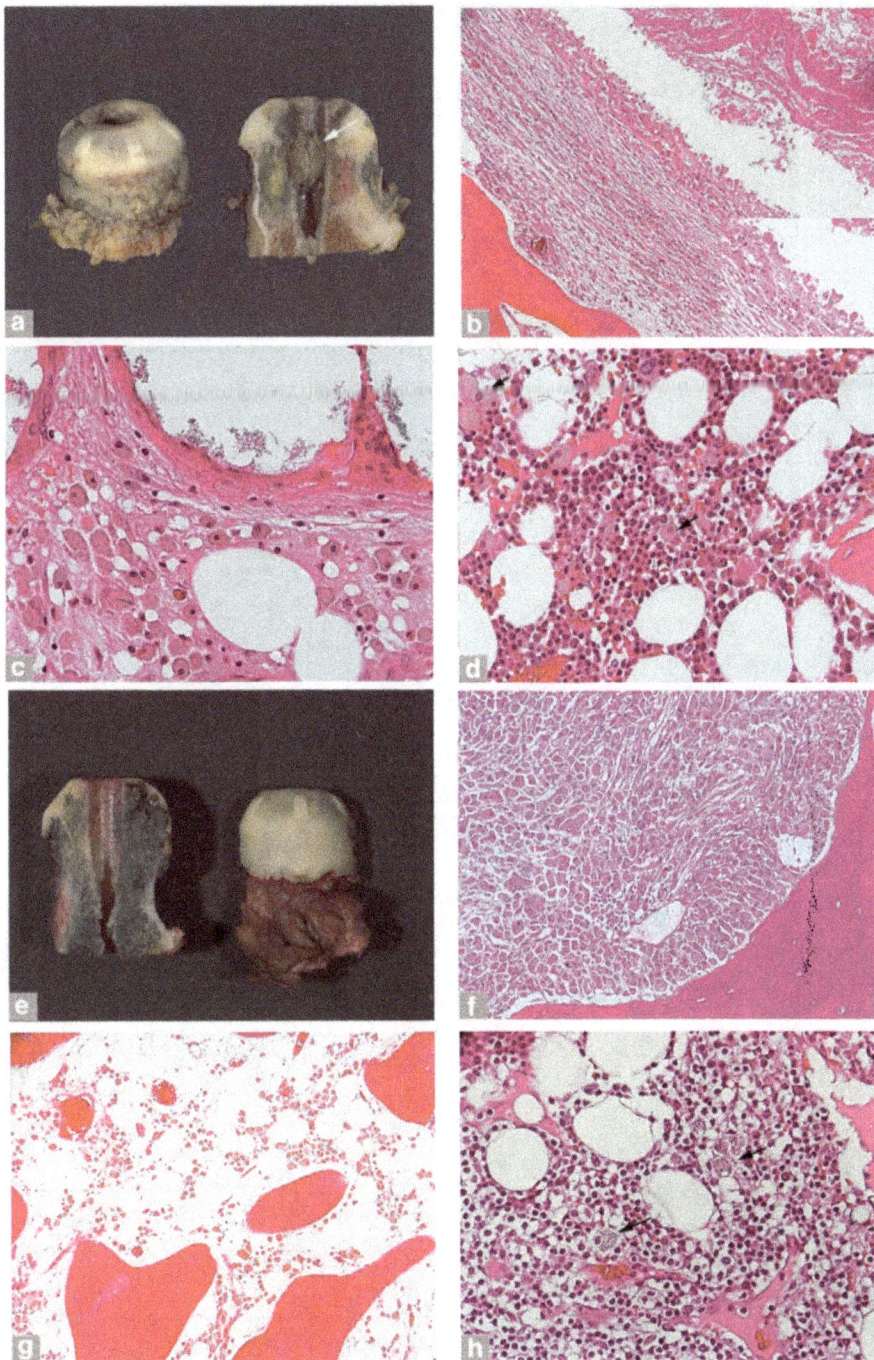

Fig. 3 Osteolysis features in the MoM RHA group. **a** Femoral head with orthopedic cement cap lined by papillary neo-synovium and showing osteolytic cavity involving the central groove of the metallic stem, white arrow (Smith and Nephew Birmingham, implantation time 48 months). **b** Content of the osteolytic cavity composed of particle laden macrophages with central exfoliation of necrotic forms in the right upper corner (H-E x100) and detail of the cavity lining cell layer containing greenish corrosion products in inset (x400). **c** Particle laden macrophagic infiltrate under the orthopedic cement cap lined by multinucleated giant cells (H-E x400). **d** Hematopoietic marrow with particle laden macrophages without evidence of lymphocytic reaction (H-E x400). **e** Femoral head with orthopedic cement cap lined by papillary neo-synovium with charcoal grey bone marrow, secondary to diffuse permeation by macrophagic infiltrate with metallic wear content (Smith and Nephew Birmingham, implantation time 78 months). **f** Massive macrophagic infiltrate in bone marrow containing greenish particles of corrosion products and black particles of abrasion metallic wear without evidence of osteoclastic activity (H-E x200). **g** Seeding of particle-laden macrophages in fatty marrow indicative of increased motility (H-E x100). **h** Large aggregate of lymphocytes positive for T-cell (CD3) and B-cell (CD20) marker (not shown) with interspersed particle laden macrophages, black arrows (H-E x 400)

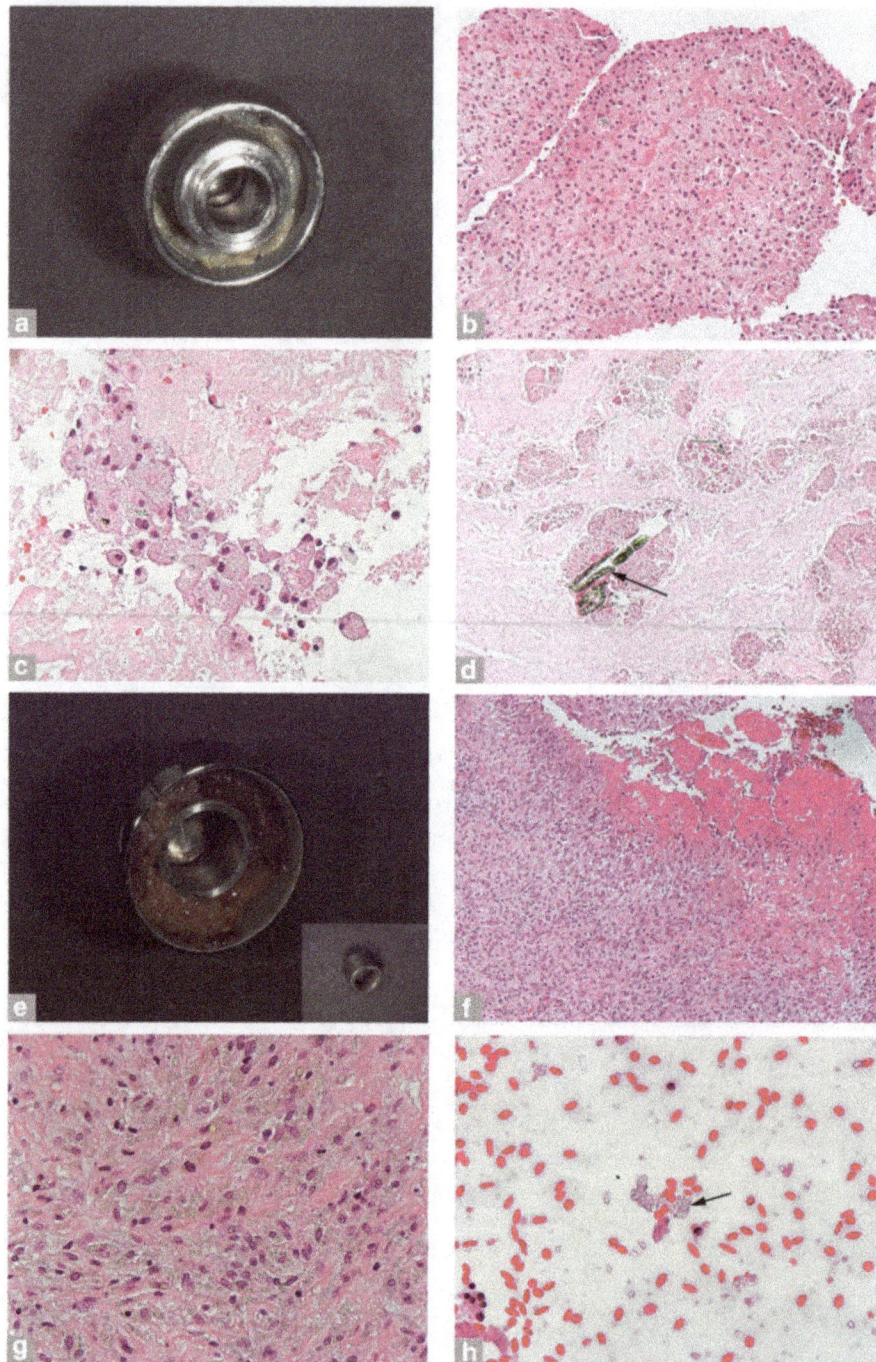

Fig. 4 Features of macrophagic pattern in the MoM LHTHA group. **a** Metallic femoral head and inserted metallic adapter sleeve (MAS) with groove filled with dense necrotic cellular debris (DePuy ASR, implantation time 61 months). **b** Papillary neo-synovium with florid macrophagic infiltrate and superficial exfoliation of necrotic forms (H-E x200). **c** Mixture of viable and necrotic particle laden macrophages of necrotic cellular debris shown in (A). **d** Necrotic cellular debris with entrapped large aggregates of greenish particulate corrosion products, black arrow (H-E x400). **e** Metallic femoral head and separate MAS (inset) with groove filled with dense necrotic cellular debris (Smith and Nephew Birmingham, implantation time 44 months). **f** Neo-synovium with florid macrophagic infiltrate and marked exfoliation of necrotic cellular debris (H-E x100). **g** Detail of the macrophgic infiltrate containing globular and irregular aggregates of greenish particulate corrosion products (H-E x400). **h** Cluster of aggregates of pale green corrosion products particles detected in smeared synovial fluid pellet spun at 3,000 rpm x 15 min (H-E x 400)

(20 % of cases) and MoM LHTHA (17 % of cases), however without reaching significance ($p = 0.26$) (Table 6).

The observation of particles of conventional metallic debris was less common in the Non-MoM DMN THA (8 % of cases) relative to the MoM HRA (39 % of cases; $p < 0.0001$), the MoM LHTHA (30 % of cases) ($p < 0.0001$). Corrosion products were seen in either intracellular and/or extracellular locations in almost all cases in each group (Table 6). Extracellular aggregates of these corrosion products were less common in the MoM HRA group (11 % of cases) relative to the Non-MoM DMNTHA (74 % of cases; $p = 0.007$) and the MoM LHTHA (63 % of cases; $p = 0.007$) (Table 6). Examples of large aggregates are shown in two Non-MoM DMNTHAs (Fig. 5a and 5e) with similar histological appearance in the neo-synovial membrane (Fig. 5b and 5f). The large aggregates of particles of corrosion products with plate-like, stratified configuration were present on implant components (Fig. 5a, inset and 5e, lower inset), detachable from the surface (Fig. 5h), or embedded in periprosthetic tissue with breakdown in multinucleated giant cells (Fig. 5c and 5d) with or without a granulomatous histological pattern irrespective of implant bearing surface (Fig. 5g and 5d). Sarcoid-like granulomas were more likely to be present in the Non-MoM DMNTHA (16 % of cases) than in the MoM LHTHA (5 % of cases; $p = 0.013$) and MoM HRA (0 % of cases; $p = 0.013$) (Table 6).

Median Campbell (ALVAL) score was lower in implants with MoM bearing surfaces (MoM HRA, median score 5 and LHTHA, median score 6 relative to the Non-MoM DMNTHA, median score 8 ($p < 0.001$). A multinomial logistic regression was performed in order to examine the association between preoperative demographic variables (age, sex, BMI, implant type, duration of symptoms, duration of implantation) with Campbell's ALVAL score at revision. After adjustment, age ($p = 0.010$) and implant type ($p = 0.002$) were the only variables independently associated with Campbell's ALVAL score at revision. The MoM HRA group was an independent factor for a lower score at revision, using MoM bearing surfaces as a reference.

Discussion

The occurrence of ALTR has been described in cases series for all three classes of implants analyzed in our study [4, 5, 13–15, 24, 27, 30, 32–46]. Recent reports have shown that the histological patterns of ALTR are more diverse than the original description of ALVAL and this complexity may result in different mechanisms of failure, which can have clinical implications for patient surveillance and outcomes after revision arthroplasty [13, 17, 20, 21, 29, 46]. The purposes of this study were to describe the frequency of different histopathological patterns of soft tissue failure in ALTR, their association with different implant class, and the association

of histopathological findings with clinical features of implant failure.

Our histological analysis demonstrates that ALTR encompasses a range of histological patterns ranging from purely macrophagic to mixed lymphocytic and macrophagic with or without features of associated with hypersensitivity (eosinophils/mast cells and/or lymphocytic germinal centers), and predominant sarcoid-like granulomas as previously described [13, 17, 19–21, 29, 46]. This is the largest study to the best of our knowledge to classify the histological patterns of ALTR across a diverse range of implants and its association to their clinical performance.

Macrophagic pattern

Our results confirm that a macrophage predominant pattern of soft tissue failure exists in ALTR as previously reported, and it occurs more commonly in implants with MoM bearing surfaces [20, 21, 29]. We hypothesize that this is related to surface corrosion generating nanoparticle size wear debris unique to this bearing surface, as originally observed and later characterized by transmission and scanning microscopy [15, 18]. Phagocytosis/pinocytosis of metallic nanoparticle debris into cytoplasmic phagosomes with subsequent release of metallic ions has been shown to produce high level of oxidative stress in macrophages, resulting in a marked increase in reactive oxygen species promoting protein carbonylation, a well-known consequence of cellular oxidative stress, leading to a loss of biological function and ultimately cell death [47]. This process may be accelerated and enhanced by the addition of corrosion wear particles generated at the head-neck taper surface through the interposition of a CoCr metallic adapter sleeve. A proposed mechanism of implant failure of ALTR with the macrophagic pattern due to soft tissue and bone involvement exemplified for a MoM LHTHA is illustrated in Fig. 6. We hypothesize that massive corrosion product-associated macrophage apoptosis, exfoliation of necrotic cellular debris and phagocytized secondary wear particles into the joint fluid alters the bearing surface lubrication in implants with a MoM bearing surface. This failure mechanism would be difficult to replicate in any in-vitro tribology system or constructed tribocorrosion test apparatus [48, 49]. These alterations of the tribological film may lead to accelerated corrosion of the bearing surface and formation of abrasion-induced metallic wear. Clinically, this process may manifest as patient-reported mechanical symptoms that develop years after implantation along with increased serum metallic ion levels as the bearing surface is no longer properly lubricated. Previous studies have also shown that elevated metal ion levels occur due to implant misalignment; however, implant positioning does not account for many clinical failures, and this mechanism could provide an alternative explanation [50].

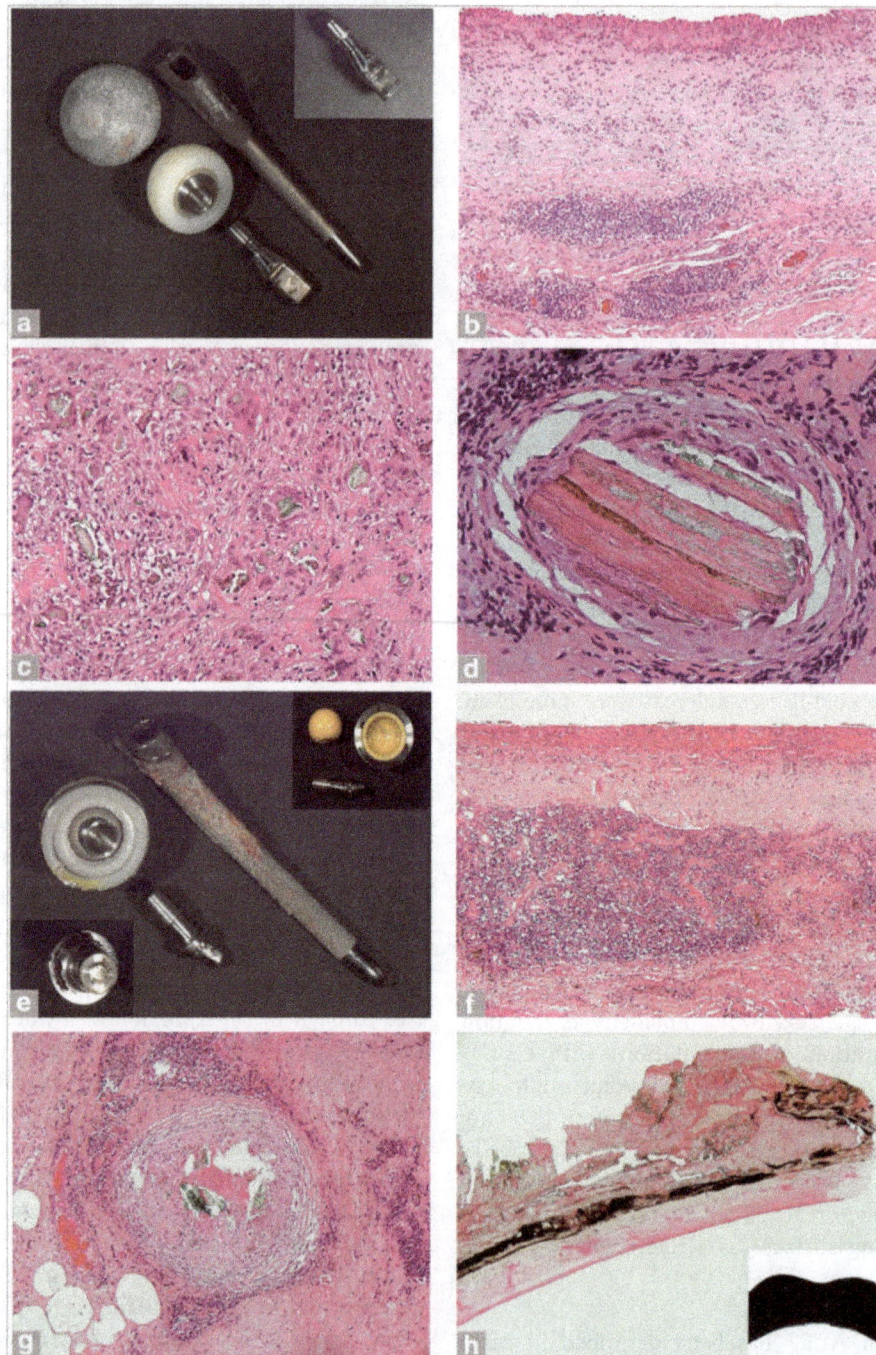

Fig. 5 Features of corrosion products in the Non-MoM DMNTHA group. **a** MoP THA with CoCr dual exchangeable neck (inset) with corrosion on distal male taper (Stryker Rejuvenate, implantation time 20 months). **b** Neo-synovium showing superficial layer of macrophagic infiltrate and deep lymphocytic infiltrate (H-E x100). **c** Giant cell reaction without formation of granulomas to large aggregates of greenish and corrosion products (H-E x200). **d** Large aggregate of corrosion products with plate-like structure suggestive of layering of corrosion (greenish) and blood (reddish) products (H-E x400). **e** MoP THA with CoCr dual exchangeable neck with original CoC bearing surface and neck (inset, right upper corner) and second revision neck (inset, lower corner) with corrosion products on the male geared surface (OTI Encore, implantation time at first revision 36 months and at second revision 44 months from first revision). **f** Neo-synovium of first revision showing superficial layer of macrophagic infiltrate and dense layer of lymphocytic infiltrate (H-E x100). **g** Sarcoid-like granulomatous reaction with central green aggregates of corrosion products of second revision (H-E x100). **h** Large aggregate of layered corrosion products detached from the dual exchangeable neck (H-E x100) with scalloped shape of the gearing surface (inset)

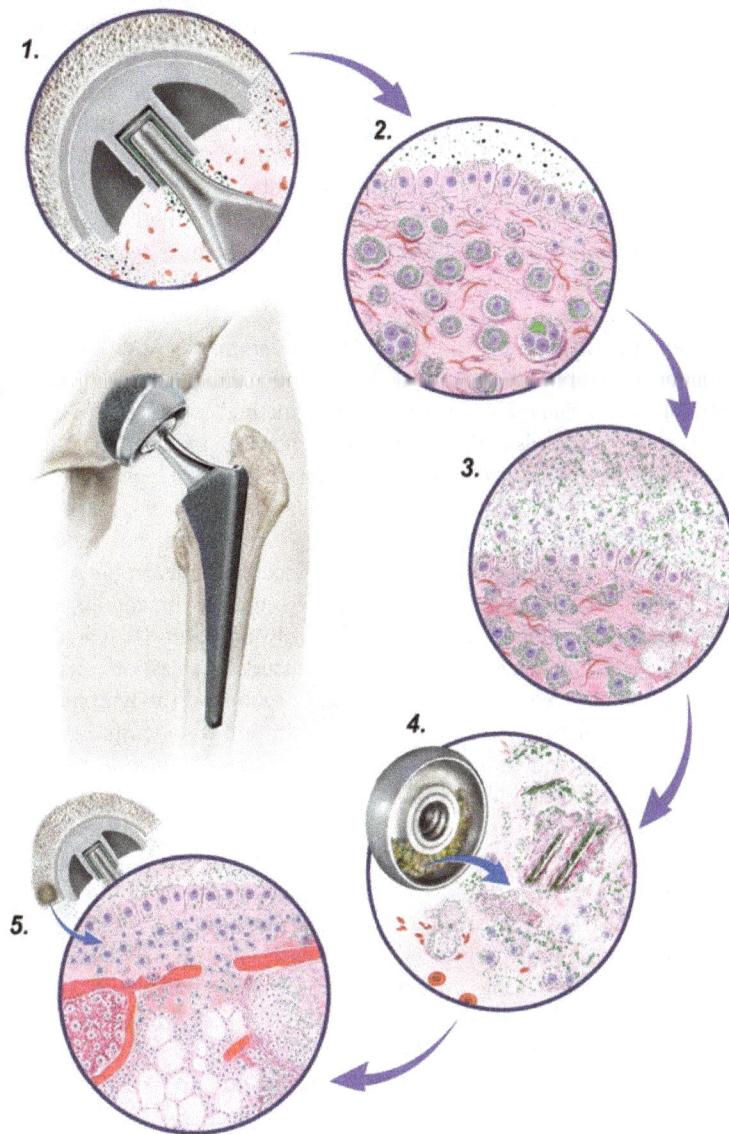

Fig. 6 Phases of macrophagic pattern of ALTR in MoM LHTHA prosthesis. *Circle 1:* Nano-scale particles generated at the bearing surface by sliding tribocorrosion and nano and micron-scale at the metallic adapter sleeve-femoral neck surface by fretting/crevice corrosion where larger aggregates are formed. Conventional abrasion metallic wear can also be generated at the bearing surface by edge loading and/or neck junction at any time of implantation. *Circle 2:*
Phagocytosis/pinocytosis of particulate material by neo-synovial superficial and deep layer macrophages with multinucleated giant cells containing large
particulate aggregates. *Circle 3:* Massive apoptosis of neo-synovial particle-laden macrophages through oxidative stress with formation of degenerated foamy forms (right side) and release of necrotic cellular debris and secondary particles of corrosion products/abrasion metallic particles with disruption of cytoplasmic phagosomes. *Circle 4:* Accumulation of viable macrophages, necrotic cellular debris, red blood cells, and entrapped small and large aggregates of primary and secondary particles of corrosion products in the femoral head groove with substantial increase in thickness of the synovial fluid and subsequent modification of its lubrication properties. *Circle 5:* Bone marrow involvement by neo-synovial particle-laden macrophagic infiltrate through resorptive osteoblastic activity and direct invasion through cortical gaps with formation of osteolytic cavity (right side), diffuse seeding of the fatty marrow (middle area), and involvement of the hematopoietic marrow (left side)

The occurrence of macrophagic bone marrow infiltrate with or without associated histological evidence of osteolysis in the MoM HRA class may be explained by three different mechanisms: 1. The well-studied osteoclastic activation; 2. Increased macrophagic motility with mass burden necrosis and formation of pseudocystic cavities in the acetabular and/or femoral bones; 3. Penetration of corrosion particles and viable macrophages pushed by lubrication fluid pressure during motion. This component of the ALTR has been overlooked, but could become clinically significant with extended time of implantation and corrosion wear particle generation, especially for MoM HRA and MoM LHTHA groups [51, 52].

Mixed macrophagic/lymphocytic pattern

Similar to previous studies, we found a mixed lymphocytic and macrophagic pattern to be common in ALTR however, within this group, the range of cellular infiltrates and tissue morphology suggests that individual variation exists within this pattern. Specifically, we have found the presence of mast cells/eosinophils and/or formation of lymphocytic germinal centers usually associated with tall endothelial cell venules in a subset of patients within this group. Mast cells are difficult to be identified in a crowded inflammatory background with conventional histology, although their presence has been previously demonstrated by immunohistochemistry [17]. The increased presence of mast cells, eosinophilic infiltrate, and lymphocytic germinal centers may be an expression of hypersensitivity/allergy to particulate conventional metallic or corrosion debris in certain subsets of patients. Previous authors have noted a weak correlation between wear characteristics and soft tissue response in a subgroup of patients with ALTR [29, 39]. Subsets of patients with evidence of neo-synovial tertiary lymphoid organs or sarcoid-like granulomas have been noted by previous authors, and these all may represent patient-specific variable immune responses to particulate corrosion debris [17, 19, 20]. Identification of patients with hypersensitivity to metal debris in joint replacement remains controversial because skin patch testing and lymphocyte transformation testing does not reliably predict patient-specific implant performance [53–55]. Systemic toxicity such as cardiomyopathy, neuropathy, and dermatological manifestations has been reported in limited case series, and these findings are typically associated with very high serum ion levels, particularly cobalt [56]. Recent work has shown a prominent up-regulation of interferon gamma associated chemokine expression in ALTR with a mixed lymphocytic and macrophagic pattern [57]. Activation of hypoxia-inducible factor secondary to cellular oxidative stress has also been implicated in this process [47, 58, 59]. Further studies on the molecular signaling pathways involved in ALTR are critical.

Similar to other non-specific foreign body responses, a pure lymphocytic pattern was not observed in our study, and macrophagic phagocytosis of wear particles is a key initial event. This activation of the innate immune system may or may not be associated with subsequent involvement of an adaptive immune response, which may in turn lead to further macrophagic recruitment [29]. We believe that the absence of particle laden macrophages in some reported cases may be related to tissue sampling rather than true absence of such cells from the affected tissues [21].

Granulomatous pattern

The granulomatous pattern was observed in both THA groups with variable frequency and not in the MoM HRA group. We hypothesize that it requires the presence of large aggregates of particulate corrosion products, which is seldom present in the MoM HRA group. This pattern represents a distinctive patient-dependent macrophagic response which might be similar to the granulomatous reaction observed in sarcoidosis and triggered by exposure to various microbial agents.

Use of Campbell's ALVAL scoring system

Currently, the Campbell's ALVAL score has been the primary method to assess ALTR in the periprosthetic soft tissue, showing good correlation with MRI studies [28, 60]. Using multinomial logistic regression, we found that implant configuration was associated with the Campbell's ALVAL score. In particular, hip resurfacing was associated with a lower score at revision for ALTR. In our experience the use of the score has limitations in ALTR because it is focused primarily on necrosis, scored twice in the synovial lining and tissue organization sections with a maximum of 3 points each, and the lymphocytic infiltrate, which is given a maximum of 4 points in a total maximum score of 10 [13]. The predominantly macrophagic pattern of soft tissue failure would produce low Campbell's ALVAL scores due to no or minimal lymphocytic infiltrate and no necrosis, but can still result in soft tissue arthroplasty failure. There is no grading of the macrophagic exfoliation and no consideration for macrophagic involvement with or without associated osteolysis in the femoral/acetabular bone marrow, which may have significant clinical implications for implant performance.

Public health implications

Our study suggests that the histological analysis of periprosthetic tissue in cases of ALTR can provide information that may be useful for longitudinal monitoring of implants. For example, we found that mixed lymphocytic and granulomatous subtypes were associated with shorter durations of implantation and were more common in the MoM LHTHA and Non-MoM DMNTHA with a known occurrence of taper corrosion [5, 7–9, 27, 61, 62]. In contrast, the predominantly macrophagic pattern is more common in the MoM HRA group which generates nano-size corrosion/conventional metallic debris particles only at bearing surface.

The association between histological classification and time to revision may have clinical implications because implants with high number of patients with mixed macrophagic/lymphocytic pattern may fail earlier due to formation of pseudotumors with soft tissue necrosis, and this has resulted in implant recalls, such as the Stryker Rejuvenate and ABGII models. Implants with predominant macrophagic pattern, may fail at medium-long implantation time at an undetermined rate due to changes in the tribological lubrication process and/or macrophagic driven osteolysis. This unpredictable risk at the present time would call for a follow-up program with a frequency and modalities to be determined coupled with studies aiming at identifying biological and cellular factors associated with this type of adverse reaction [52, 63].

Our analysis showed that similar patterns of ALTR were present in implant classes of similar configuration and material composition independent of the manufacturer. This suggests the need for prompt observation and monitoring of any class of implants exhibiting a pattern of early failure with immediate reporting of sentinel cases to regulatory agencies/implant registries with the aim of avoiding high rates of complications for a large number of patients. Additionally, our results have made a case for the inclusion of the pathology report of revision cases in hospital based, regional, and national implant registries as an important and valuable tool in assessing modalities of implant failures along with the implementation of an international consensus classification, as the one recently reported for the periprosthetic soft tissue [64].

Study limitations

We acknowledge several limitations with the current study. The first and most important is that our analysis is based on our hospital osteolysis/adverse local reaction tissue and repository database, which depends on the patient population admitted to the hospital and histological examination at surgical implant revision end-point. Our hospital serves as a tertiary referral center for revision arthroplasty cases; therefore, we cannot determine the overall class or device-specific implant performance from our data. The second is the attempt to reconstruct the natural history of the adverse reaction based on a single observation at the time of implant revision, although partially compensated for by the extensive tissue sampling. The third is the absence of the following sets of clinical data: a. physical activity pre and post-operative, although it has shown a weak correlation to elevated serum metal ion levels, suggesting that activity-related bearing surface wear plays only a minor role in elevated serum cobalt or chromium levels [65, 66]; b. pre and post-operative bone density, which may influence the occurrence/rate of implant mechanical loosening/osteolysis especially in the female population which requires a sophisticated method for proper assessment, such as high-spatial-resolution bone densitometry with dual-energy X-ray absorptiometric region-free analysis [67], which is not currently performed as standard of care at our institution; c. wear analysis by biomechanics examination of the metal-on-metal implants for surface roughness, although retrieval analysis and blood metal

measurements contribution to the understanding of ALTR has been previously addressed in a comprehensive review and no clear dose–response relationship between wear and ALTR could be established [68].

Conclusions

ALTR encompasses a diverse range of histological patterns, which are reflective of both the implant configuration independent of manufacturer and clinical features such as duration of implantation. The predominant macrophagic pattern and its mechanism of implant failure represent an important subgroup of ALTR which could become more prominent with increased length of implantation. Further studies should characterize the physical and chemical characteristics of wear particles and the molecular characteristics of the generation and development of these different histological patterns of ALTR and relevant mechanisms of failure in different implant classes and/or specific devices.

Abbreviations

THA: Total hip arthroplasty; ALVAL: Aseptic lymphocyte dominated vasculitis associated lesion; ALTR: Adverse local tissue reaction; ARMD: Adverse reaction to metallic debris; MoP: Metal-on-polyethylene; CoP: Ceramic-on-polyethylene; DMN: Dual modular neck; MoM: Metal-on-metal; LHTHA: Large head THA; HRA: Hip resurfacing arthroplasty.

Competing interests

The authors declare they have no competing interests.

Authors' contributions

BFR – data collection, pathological analysis, data interpretation, manuscript preparation. AAN – statistical analysis, manuscript preparation. SAJ – assist with data interpretation, manuscript preparation. GW – patient enrollment, data collection. EK – patient enrollment, data collection. SRG – assist with data interpretation and study conception, manuscript preparation. PEP – assist with data interpretation and study conception, manuscript preparation. GP – study conception, patient enrollment, pathological analysis, data interpretation, manuscript preparation. All authors read and approved the final manuscript.

Acknowledgements

We would like to acknowledge the surgeons of the Adult Reconstruction and Joint Replacement Service at the Hospital for Special Surgery for providing periprosthetic tissue for this study; Irina Shuleshko and Yana Bronfman for technical assistance in histology preparation; Philip Rusli for technical assistance for preparation of the manuscript; and Randal McKenzie of McKenzie Illustrations for preparation of the medical illustration.

Author details

[1]Department of Orthopedic Surgery, Hospital for Special Surgery, New York, NY, USA. [2]Healthcare Research Institute, Hospital for Special Surgery, New York, NY, USA. [3]Division of Research, Hospital for Special Surgery, New York, NY, USA. [4]Department of Pathology and Laboratory Medicine, Hospital for Special Surgery, 535 East 70th Street, New York, NY 10021, USA.

References

1. Amstutz HC, Grigoris P. Metal on metal bearings in hip arthroplasty. Clin Orthop Relat Res. 1996;329(Suppl):S11–34.
2. Srinivasan A, Jung E, Levine BR. Modularity of the femoral component in total hip arthroplasty. J Am Acad Orthop Surg. 2012;20(4):214–22.

3. Werner PH, Ettema HB, Witt F, Morlock MM, Verheyen CC. Basic principles and uniform terminology for the head-neck junction in hip replacement. Hip Int. 2015;25(2):115–9.

4. Jacobs JJ, Gilbert JL, Urban RM. Corrosion of metal orthopaedic implants. J Bone Joint Surg Am. 1998;80(2):268–82.

5. Cooper HJ, Urban RM, Wixson RL, Meneghini RM, Jacobs JJ. Adverse local tissue reaction arising from corrosion at the femoral neck-body junction in a dual-taper stem with a cobalt-chromium modular neck. J Bone Joint Surg Am. 2013;95(10):865–72.

6. Khair MM, Nam D, DiCarlo E, Su E. Aseptic lymphocyte dominated vasculitis-associated lesion resulting from trunnion corrosion in a cobalt-chrome unipolar hemiarthroplasty. J Arthroplasty. 2013;28(1):196.e11–4.

7. Mao X, Tay GH, Godbolt DB, Crawford RW. Pseudotumor in a well-fixed metal-on-polyethylene uncemented hip arthroplasty. J Arthroplasty. 2012; 27(3):493.e13–7.

8. Munro JT, Masri BA, Duncan CP, Garbuz DS. High complication rate after revision of large-head metal-on-metal total hip arthroplasty. Clin Orthop Relat Res. 2014;472(2):523–8.

9. Witt F, Bosker BH, Bishop NE, Ettema HB, Verheyen CC, Morlock MM. The relation between titanium taper corrosion and cobalt-chromium bearing wear in large-head metal-on-metal total hip prostheses: a retrieval study. J Bone Joint Surg Am. 2014;96(18):e157.

10. Beaver Jr WB, Fehring TK. Abductor dysfunction and related sciatic nerve palsy, a new complication of metal-on-metal arthroplasty. J Arthroplasty. 2012;27(7):1414.e13–5.

11. Kayani B, Rahman J, Hanna SA, Cannon SR, Aston WJ, Miles J. Delayed sciatic nerve palsy following resurfacing hip arthroplasty caused by metal debris. BMJ Case Rep. 2012;2012.

12. Wyles CC, Van Demark 3rd RE, Sierra RJ, Trousdale RT. High rate of infection after aseptic revision of failed metal-on-metal total hip arthroplasty. Clin Orthop Relat Res. 2014;472(2):509–16.

13. Campbell P, Ebramzadeh E, Nelson S, Takamura K, De Smet K, Amstutz HC. Histological features of pseudotumor-like tissues from metal-on-metal hips. Clin Orthop Relat Res. 2010;468(9):2321–7.

14. Davies AP, Willert HG, Campbell PA, Learmonth ID, Case CP. An unusual lymphocytic perivascular infiltration in tissues around contemporary metal-on-metal joint replacements. J Bone Joint Surg Am. 2005;87:18–27.

15. Willert HG, Buchhorn GH, Fayyazi A, Flury R, Windler M, Köster G, et al. Metal-on-metal bearings and hypersensitivity in patients with artificial hip joints. A clinical and histomorphological study. J Bone Joint Surg Am. 2005;87:28–36.

16. Huber M, Reinisch G, Trettenhahn G, Zweymüller K, Lintner F. Presence of corrosion products and hypersensitivity-associated reactions in periprosthetic tissue after aseptic loosening of total hip replacements with metal bearing surfaces. Acta Biomater. 2009;5(1):172–80.

17. Perino G, Ricciardi BF, Jerabek SA, Martignoni G, Wilner G, Maass D, Goldring SR, Purdue PE. Implant based differences in adverse local tissue reaction in failed total hip arthroplasties: a morphological and immunohistochemical study. BMC Clin Pathol. 2014;14:39.

18. Xia Z, Kwon YM, Mehmood S, Downing C, Jurkschat K, Murray DW. Characterization of metal-wear nanoparticles in pseudotumor following metal-on-metal hip resurfacing. Nanomedicine. 2011;7(6):674–81.

19. Mittal S, Revell M, Barone F, Hardie DL, Matharu GS, Davenport AJ, et al. Lymphoid aggregates that resemble tertiary lymphoid organs define a specific pathological subset in metal-on-metal hip replacements. PLoS One. 2013;8(5):e63470.

20. Natu S, Sidaginamale RP, Gandhi J, Langton DJ, Nargol AV. Adverse reactions to metal debris: histopathological features of periprosthetic soft tissue reactions seen in association with failed metal on metal hip arthroplasties. J Clin Pathol. 2012;65(5):409–18.

21. Berstock JR, Baker RP, Bannister GC, Case CP. Histology of failed metal-on-metal hip arthroplasty; three distinct sub-types. Hip Int. 2014;24(3):243–8.

22. Enayatollahi MA, Parvizi J. Diagnosis of infected total hip arthroplasty. Hip Int. 2015;25(4):294–300.

23. Fehring TK, Odum S, Sproul R, Weathersbee J. High frequency of adverse local tissue reactions in asymptomatic patients with metal-on-metal THA. Clin Orthop Relat Res. 2014;472(2):517–22.

24. Junnila M, Seppänen M, Mokka J, Virolainen P, Pölönen T, Vahlberg T, et al. Adverse reaction to metal debris after Birmingham hip resurfacing arthroplasty. Acta Orthop. 2015;86(3):345–50.

25. Kiran M, Boscainos PJ. Adverse reactions to metal debris in metal-on-polyethylene total hip arthroplasty using a titanium-molybdenum-zirconium-iron alloy stem. J Arthroplasty. 2015;30(2):277–81.

26. Meyer H, Mueller T, Goldau G, Chamaon K, Ruetschi M, Lohmann CH. Corrosion at the cone/taper interface leads to failure of large-diameter metal-on-metal total hip arthroplasties. Clin Orthop Relat Res. 2012;470(11):3101–8.

27. Mokka J, Junnila M, Seppänen M, Virolainen P, Pölönen T, Vahlberg T, et al. Adverse reaction to metal debris after ReCap-M2A-Magnum large-diameter-head metal-on-metal total hip arthroplasty. Acta Orthop. 2013;84(6):549–54.

28. Nawabi DH, Gold S, Lyman S, Fields K, Padgett DE, Potter HG. MRI predicts ALVAL and tissue damage in metal-on-metal hip arthroplasty. Clin Orthop Relat Res. 2014;472(2):471–81.

29. Grammatopoulos G, Pandit H, Kamali A, Maggiani F, Glyn-Jones S, Gill HS, Murray DW, Athanasou N. The correlation of wear with histological features after failed hip resurfacing arthroplasty. J Bone Joint Surg Am. 2013;95:e81.

30. Mahendra G, Pandit H, Kliskey K, Murray D, Gill HS, Athanasou N. Necrotic and inflammatory changes in metal-on-metal resurfacing hip arthroplasties. Acta Orthop. 2009;80:653–9.

31. Jacobs JJ, Urban RM, Gilbert JL, Skipor AK, Black J, Jasty M, et al. Local and distant products from modularity. Clin Orthop Relat Res. 1995;319:94–105.

32. Barrett WP, Kindsfater KA, Lesko JP. Large-diameter modular metal-on-metal total hip arthroplasty: incidence of revision for adverse reaction to metallic debris. J Arthroplasty. 2012;27(6):976–83.e1.

33. Fabi D, Levine B, Paprosky W, Della Valle C, Sporer S, Klein G, et al. Metal-on-metal total hip arthroplasty: causes and high incidence of early failure. Orthopedics. 2012;35(7):e1009–16.

34. Gill IP, Webb J, Sloan K, Beaver RJ. Corrosion at the neck-stem junction as a cause of metal ion release and pseudotumour formation. J Bone Joint Surg Br. 2012;94(7):895–900.

35. Hasegawa M, Yoshida K, Wakabayashi H, Sudo A. Prevalence of adverse reactions to metal debris following metal-on-metal THA. Orthopedics. 2013; 36(5):e606–12.

36. Hinsch A, Vettorazzi E, Morlock MM, Rüther W, Amling M, Zustin J. Sex differences in the morphological failure patterns following hip resurfacing arthroplasty. BMC Med. 2011;9:113.

37. Langton DJ, Joyce TJ, Jameson SS, Lord J, Van Orsouw M, Holland JP, et al. Adverse reaction to metal debris following hip resurfacing: the influence of component type, orientation and volumetric wear. J Bone Joint Surg Br. 2011;93(2):164–71.

38. Langton DJ, Sidaginamale R, Lord JK, Nargol AV, Joyce TJ. Taper junction failure in large-diameter metal-on-metal bearings. Bone Joint Res. 2012;1(4): 56–63.

39. Matthies A, Underwood R, Cann P, Ilo K, Nawaz Z, Skinner J, et al. Retrieval analysis of 240 metal-on-metal hip components, comparing modular total hip replacement with hip resurfacing. J Bone Joint Surg Br. 2011;93(3):307–14.

40. Meftah M, Haleem AM, Burn MB, Smith KM, Incavo SJ. Early corrosion-related failure of the rejuvenate modular total hip replacement. J Bone Joint Surg Am. 2014;96(6):481–7.

41. Molloy DO, Munir S, Jack CM, Cross MB, Walter WL, Walter Sr WK. Fretting and corrosion in modular-neck total hip arthroplasty femoral stems. J Bone Joint Surg Am. 2014;96(6):488–93.

42. Nassif NA, Nawabi DH, Stoner K, Elpers M, Wright T, Padgett DE. Taper design affects failure of large-head metal-on-metal total hip replacements. Clin Orthop Relat Res. 2014;472(2):564–71.

43. Pandit H, Glyn-Jones S, McLardy-Smith P, Gundle R, Whitwell D, Gibbons CL, et al. Pseudotumours associated with metal-on-metal hip resurfacings. J Bone Joint Surg Br. 2008;90(7):847–51.

44. Silverton CD, Jacobs JJ, Devitt JW, Cooper HJ. Midterm results of a femoral stem with a modular neck design: clinical outcomes and metal ion analysis. J Arthroplasty. 2014;29(9):1768–73.

45. Vundelinckx BJ, Verhelst LA, De Schepper J. Taper corrosion in modular hip prostheses: analysis of serum metal ions in 19 patients. J Arthroplasty. 2013; 28(7):1218–23.

46. Phillips EA, Klein GR, Cates HE, Kurtz SM, Steinbeck M. Histological characterization of periprosthetic tissue responses for metal-on-metal hip replacement. J Long Term Eff Med Implants. 2014;24(1):13–23.

47. Scharf B, Clement CC, Zolla V, Perino G, Yan B, Elci SG, et al. Molecular analysis of chromium and cobalt-related toxicity. Sci Rep. 2014;4:5729.

48. Rieker CB, Schön R, Konrad R, Liebentritt G, Gnepf P, Shen M, et al. Influence of the clearance on in-vitro tribology of large diameter metal-on-metal articulations pertaining to resurfacing hip implants. Orthop Clin North Am. 2005;36(2):135–42. vii.

49. Mathew MT, Runa MJ, Laurent M, Jacobs JJ, Rocha LA, Wimmer MA. Tribocorrosion behavior of CoCrMo alloy for hip prosthesis as a function of

loads: a comparison between two testing systems. Wear. 2011;271(9–10): 1210–9.

50. Hart AJ, Skinner JA, Henckel J, Sampson B, Gordon F. Insufficient acetabular version increases blood metal ion levels after metal-on-metal hip resurfacing. Clin Orthop Relat Res. 2011;469(9):2590–7.

51. Asaad A, Hart A, Khoo MM, Ilo K, Schaller G, Black JD, Muirhead-Allwood S. Frequent femoral neck osteolysis with Birmingham mid-head resection resurfacing arthroplasty in young patients. Clin Orthop Relat Res. 2015; 473(12):3770–8.

52. Mont MA, Cherian JJ. CORR insights(®): frequent femoral neck osteolysis with Birmingham mid-head resection resurfacing arthroplasty in young patients. Clin Orthop Relat Res. 2015;473(12):3779–80.

53. Hallab NJ, Anderson S, Stafford T, Glant T, Jacobs JJ. Lymphocyte responses in patients with total hip arthroplasty. J Orthop Res. 2005;23(2):384–91.

54. Kwon YM, Thomas P, Summer B, Pandit H, Taylor A, Beard D, et al. Lymphocyte proliferation responses in patients with pseudotumors following metal-on-metal hip resurfacing arthroplasty. J Orthop Res. 2010; 28(4):444–50.

55. Thyssen JP, Menné T. Metal allergy–a review on exposures, penetration, genetics, prevalence, and clinical implications. Chem Res Toxicol. 2010;23(2): 309–18.

56. Bradberry SM, Wilkinson JM, Ferner RE. Systemic toxicity related to metal hip prostheses. Clin Toxicol (Phila). 2014;52(8):837–47.

57. Kolatat K, Perino G, Wilner G, Kaplowitz E, Ricciardi BF, Boettner F, et al. Adverse local tissue reaction (ALTR)associated with corrosion products in metal-on-metal and dual modular neck total hip replacements is associated with upregulation of interferon gamma-mediated chemokine signaling. J Orthop Res. 2015;33(10):1487–97.

58. Nyga A, Hart A, Tetley TD. Importance of the HIF pathway in cobalt nanoparticle-induced cytotoxicity and inflammation in human macrophages. Nanotoxicology. 2015;13:1–13.

59. Vanlangenakker N, Vanden Berghe T, Vandenabeele P. Many stimuli pull the necrotic trigger, an overview. Cell Death Differ. 2012;19(1):75–86. Epub 2011 Nov 11. Review.

60. Burge AJ, Gold SL, Lurie B, Nawabi DH, Fields KG, Koff MF, et al. MR imaging of adverse local tissue reactions around rejuvenate modular dual-taper stems. Radiology. 2015;1:141967.

61. Barry J, Lavigne M, Vendittoli PA. Evaluation of the method for analyzing chromium, cobalt and titanium ion levels in the blood following hip replacement with a metal-on-metal prosthesis. J Anal Toxicol. 2013;37(2):90–6.

62. DeMartino I, Assini JB, Elpers ME, Wright TM, Westrich GH. Corrosion and fretting of a modular hip system: a retrieval analysis of 60 rejuvenate stems. J Arthroplasty. 2015;30(8):1470–5.

63. Hart AJ, Sabah SA, Henckel J, Lloyd G, Skinner JA. Lessons learnt from metal-on-metal hip arthroplasties will lead to safer innovation for all medical devices. Hip Int. 2015;25(4):347–54.

64. Krenn V, Morawietz L, Perino G, Kienapfel H, Ascherl R, Hassenpflug GJ, et al. Revised histopathological consensus classification of joint implant related pathology. Pathol Res Pract. 2014;210(12):779–86.

65. Heisel C, Silva M, Skipor AK, Jacobs JJ, Schmalzried TP. The relationship between activity and ions in patients with metal-on-metal bearing hip prostheses. J Bone Joint Surg Am. 2005;87(4):781–7.

66. Khan M, Kuiper JH, Richardson JB. The exercise-related rise in plasma cobalt levels after metal-on-metal hip resurfacing arthroplasty. J Bone Joint Surg Br. 2008;90(9):1152–7.

67. Morris RM, Yang L, Martín-Fernández MA, Pozo JM, Frangi AF, Wilkinson JM. High-spatial-resolution bone densitometry with dual-energy X-ray absorptiometric region-free analysis. Radiology. 2015;274(2):532–9.

68. Campbell PA, Kung MS, Hsu AR, Jacobs JJ. Do retrieval analysis and blood metal measurements contribute to our understanding of adverse local tissue reactions? Clin Orthop Relat Res. 2014;472(12):3718–27.

10

Length of prostate biopsies is not necessarily compromised by pooling multiple cores in one paraffin block: an observational study

Teemu T Tolonen[1,2*], Jorma Isola[2], Antti Kaipia[3,4], Jarno Riikonen[4], Laura Koivusalo[3,5], Sanna Huovinen[1], Marita Laurila[1], Sinikka Porre[1], Mika Tirkkonen[1] and Paula Kujala[1]

Abstract

Background: Individually submitted prostatic needle biopsies are recommended by most guidelines because of their potential advantage in terms of core quality. However, unspecified bilateral biopsies are commonly submitted in many centers. The length of the core is the key quality indicator of prostate biopsies. Because there are few recent publications comparing the quality of 12 site-designated biopsies versus pooled biopsies, we compared the lengths of the biopsies obtained by both methods.

Methods: The material was obtained from 471 consecutive subjects who underwent prostatic needle biopsy in the Tampere University Hospital district between January and June 2013. Biopsies from 344 subjects fulfilled the inclusion criteria. The total number of cores obtained was 4047. The core lengths were measured on microscope slides. Extraprostatic tissue was subtracted from the core length.

Results: The aggregate lengths observed were 129.5 ± 21.8 mm (mean $\pm$ SD) for site-designated cores and 136.9 ± 26.4 mm for pooled cores (p = 0.09). The length of the core was 10.8 ± 1.8 mm for site-designated cores and 11.4 ± 2.2 mm for pooled cores (p = 0.87). The median length for pooled cores was 11 mm (range 5 mm – 18 mm). For individual site-designated cores, the median length was 11 mm (range 7 mm –15 mm). The core length was not correlated with the number of cores embedded into one paraffin block (r = 0.015). There was no significant difference in cancer detection rate (p = 0.62).

Conclusions: Our results suggest that unspecified bilateral biopsies do not automatically lead to reduced core length. We conclude that carefully embedded multiple (three to nine) cores per block may yield cores of equal quality in a more cost-efficient way and that current guidelines favoring individually submitted cores may be too strict.

Keywords: Prostate cancer, Prostatic needle biopsies, Biopsy quality, Guidelines

Background

The diagnosis of prostatic adenocarcinoma is based on the histopathological findings obtained from prostatic needle biopsies. There is a lot of debate on the best protocol for submitting and labeling of prostate biopsies. According to several current guidelines, individual site-designated biopsies submitted in separate vials are preferred, as they are thought to give better quality samples in terms of tissue fragmentation as well as core length [1,2]. However, it is a common practice to submit unspecified bilateral biopsies both in the U.S. and in Europe [3,4]. The length of the biopsy core is the key quality indicator of a successful biopsy, which influences cancer detection rates and the estimation of prognostic parameters [5-7]. Currently, the recommended procedure is to take five to six biopsies from each side [1,2]. Specifically, additional laterally targeted biopsies have been shown to detect 31% more cancers when compared to the sextant biopsy protocol [5]. The role of augmented biopsy protocols is still controversial. It has been suggested that there is no advantage to taking extended

* Correspondence: teemu.tolonen@fimlab.fi
[1]Department of Pathology, Fimlab Laboratories, Tampere University Hospital, Tampere, Finland
[2]Department of Cancer Biology, Institute of Biomedical Technology, University of Tampere, Tampere, Finland
Full list of author information is available at the end of the article

(20 cores) or saturation biopsies (24 cores) in the initial biopsy [8,9]. However, a recent meta-analysis has shown that initial diagnostic saturation biopsies may be warranted for patients with low PSA-values or high-volume prostates [10].

In terms of biopsy quality, it has been suggested that up to three cores could be safely embedded in one paraffin block without compromising the biopsy quality [11]. Currently, approximately half of the pathology laboratories in Europe receive unspecified bilateral biopsies together with individually submitted targeted biopsies from a distinct nodule, while only 40% of laboratories receive all biopsies in separate vials [4]. In the U.S., it is slightly more common to submit site-designated biopsies [3]. Compared to pooled biopsies, a submission of 12 site-designated biopsy cores by the urologist increases the workload for pathology laboratories. The advantage of site-designated biopsies is that localization information is spared, which is important for active surveillance follow-up protocols and helps the urologist to plan surgeries. The quality of needle biopsies is operator dependent, but the main result (i.e., how the tissue looks on a slide) is also dependent upon the pathology laboratory [12]. A recent guideline by the pathology committee of the European Randomized Study of Screening for Prostate Cancer (ERSPC) highlights the importance of special techniques in processing and (pre-)embedding for preserving the quality of the biopsy [13]. Such techniques include the use of sponges to flatten the cores during fixation and dehydration, and the use of metal tampers for the embedding process.

The aim of this study was to determine whether there is a quality difference between site-designated individually embedded and unspecified bilateral (pooled) biopsies, using core length as the main quality indicator and cancer detection rate as a secondary measure. It was hypothesized, that pooling samples in the same biopsy container and resulting paraffin block does not affect the quality of the biopsy. Pooling biopsies reduces the workload of laboratory technicians and pathologists, so if pooled samples are of similar quality than site-designated biopsies, it would be possible to get the same results with less effort.

Methods

The study was approved by the Ethical Committee of Tampere University Hospital (TAUH), reference number R03203. The material was obtained from 471 consecutive prostate biopsies submitted to Fimlab Laboratories for evaluation during a half year period from January to June 2013. The biopsies were taken in the Tampere University Hospital (TAUH) district by several urologists under standard operating procedure. All the obtained prostate biopsies were evaluated with the following

inclusion criteria: 1) the biopsy was reported by one of our five uropathologists (ML, MT, SH, PK, TT), 2) the biopsies were comprised of either 12 individually submitted cores or bilateral pooled biopsies submitted in two formalin vials (plus an extra vial containing one core from a distinct nodule in some cases), and 3) all cores were measured in millimeters and reported in a standardized manner (see later section). Biopsies from 344 subjects fulfilled the inclusion criteria and yielded a total number of 4047 biopsy cores. All of the accepted site-designated biopsies consisted of a set of 12 biopsy containers with a single biopsy inside, except for one case in which only 11 containers were submitted because there were erroneously two biopsies in one vial. A total of 127 cases were excluded. Although it met the inclusion criteria, one case with 12 individually processed cores containing only 20 mm intraprostatic tissue was excluded as a statistical outlier. The inclusion procedure is presented schematically in Figure 1.

All biopsies were taken transrectally with ultrasonography guidance using an 18-gauge needle biopsy gun with an 18-mm sample notch (Bard peripheral vascular, Temple, AZ, U.S.A., ref no. MC 1825) and a side-fire probe. Biopsies were put into vials containing 10% neutral-buffered formalin straight from the biopsy needle. Biopsies from a single patient were transported to our laboratory either in 12 separate vials or in two vials containing several biopsy cores (median number of cores per container was six). The number of submitted vials depended on how the urologist performed the prostate biopsy. All biopsies were processed in Fimlab Laboratories, Tampere University Hospital, in Tampere, Finland.

Site-designated individual biopsies were transferred to separate tissue cassettes in which they were straightened (not stretched) and flattened between sponges during standard dehydration and microwave processing. Pooled biopsies from one vial were treated equally but remained pooled (e.g., multiple straightened cores were sandwiched between sponges into one cassette). Two to four sections were cut from the individual cores and transferred to one slide, depending on the technologist's visual impression. Because pooled biopsies may have more planar variation inside the paraffin blocks, they were cut on four levels which resulted in the generation of two slides. The blocks were not cut through and step sections were not collected because our current protocol offers residual material for potential immunostaining in most cases.

The lengths of the biopsy cores were collected from pathology reports. For individually processed biopsies, the lengths were reported for each biopsy core in millimeters. The 12 loci of individual biopsies were standardized as follows: 1–3 were right lateral base, mid and apex, 4–6 were right medial base, mid and apex, 7–9

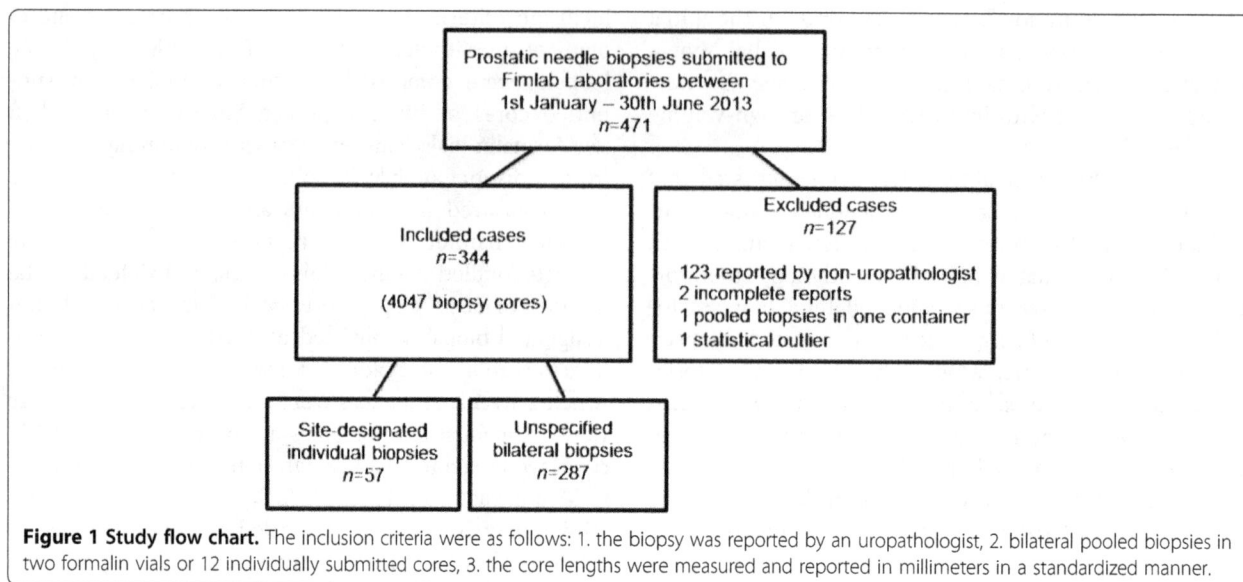

Figure 1 Study flow chart. The inclusion criteria were as follows: 1. the biopsy was reported by an uropathologist, 2. bilateral pooled biopsies in two formalin vials or 12 individually submitted cores, 3. the core lengths were measured and reported in millimeters in a standardized manner.

were left lateral base, mid and apex, and 10–12 were left medial base, mid and apex, respectively. The current scheme for site-specific needle biopsies in the TAUH district is presented in Figure 2. In the case of multiple biopsies per paraffin block, the information regarding the number of biopsies in the block and the total length of the biopsies in millimeters was required. Separately submitted additional cores targeting a region of palpable resistance were excluded from the length measurements but were included in the cancer detection rate. The length of the core and the possible length of the cancerous tissue were measured from hematoxylin-eosin (H&E) -stained slides either under a light microscope as multiples of 4x/10x objectives visual field diameter or by a liner, depending on the extent of the cancer. According to our standardized protocol, extraprostatic tissue was subtracted from the total core length to obtain the most accurate percentage of cancer. Tissue was considered extraprostatic when containing obvious fat or loose mesenchymal tissue that was distinct from the (pseudo)capsule. For cancerous prostates, a standardized scoring table was applied. The recorded parameters included primary and secondary Gleason patterns, the number of positive cores/total number of cores, cancer length/total length, the percentage of cancer, high grade prostatic intraepithelial neoplasia, and perineural invasion. The microscopic appearance of slides with individually embedded and pooled biopsies are represented in Figure 3.

Statistical analysis

Data were analyzed using a two-tailed Wilcoxon-Mann–Whitney test to compare aggregate and single biopsy length means and a two-tailed Fisher's exact test to compare cancer detection rates. The impact of the number of cores embedded in a single paraffin block on the mean length of cores in the corresponding block was tested using Pearson's correlation coefficient analysis. Statistical significance was considered at $p < 0.05$.

Results

Individual site-designated biopsies were submitted to our laboratory in 57 (16.6%) cases, and non-specified (pooled) bilateral biopsies were submitted in 287 (83.4%) cases. Of the pooled biopsies, exactly six plus six cores from the right and left sides were obtained 188 (65.5%) times. More than 12 biopsies were submitted in 38 (13.2%) cases, and less than 10 biopsies were submitted in 18 (6.2%) cases. The minimum number of biopsy cores per subject was 6 (n = 1), and the maximum number was 15 (n = 7).

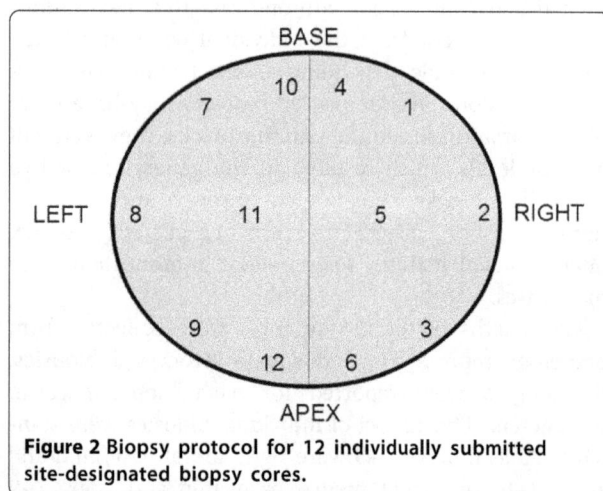

Figure 2 Biopsy protocol for 12 individually submitted site-designated biopsy cores.

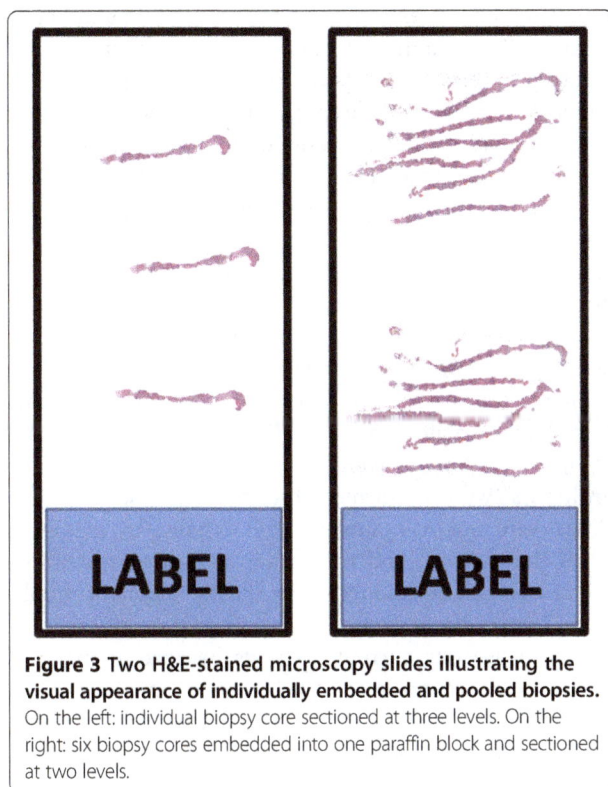

Figure 3 Two H&E-stained microscopy slides illustrating the visual appearance of individually embedded and pooled biopsies. On the left: individual biopsy core sectioned at three levels. On the right: six biopsy cores embedded into one paraffin block and sectioned at two levels.

The mean aggregate length of all biopsy cores from one subject was 133.6 ± 29.9 mm (mean $\pm$ SD). No statistically significant difference in the mean aggregate lengths was noted between site-designated and pooled $(6 + 6)$ biopsies or between benign and malignant biopsies (Table 1).

The average core length was 11.4 ± 2.2 mm for pooled biopsies and 10.8 ± 1.8 mm for individually processed cores (p = 0.87). The median length for pooled cores was 11 mm (range 5 mm - 18 mm). For individual site-designated cores the median length was 11 mm (range 7 mm - 15 mm). Because the number of biopsy cores in the vials varied from 1 to 9, we also tested whether increasing the number of cores in a paraffin block would have an adverse effect on the mean length of the cores

Table 1 Comparison of aggregate lengths of the biopsy cores

	n	Aggregate length, mm (mean ± SD)
All	344	133.6 ± 29.9
Site-designated	57	129.5 ± 21.8[1]
Pooled 6 + 6	188	136.9 ± 26.4[1]
Benign	151	132.7 ± 29.3[2]
Malignant	193	134.2 ± 30.4[2]

[1]No statistically significant difference was noted between 12 site-designated cores and unspecified bilateral (6 + 6) cores, p = 0.09.
[2]No statistically significant difference was noted between benign and malignant cases, p = 0.25.

as one might expect. However, no correlation was noted (Table 2).

The overall cancer detection rate was 55.8%. Adenocarcinoma was detected in 28/57 (49.1%) cases with site-designated biopsies and in 164/287 (57.1%) cases with pooled biopsies (p = 0.62).

Discussion

A recent survey regarding the handling of prostate biopsies by the European Network for Uropathologists (ENUP) showed that there is a wide diversity among European pathology centers in the handling of prostate biopsy specimens [4]. The number of biopsy cores taken, the number of cores in a formalin vial, and the (pre-)embedding methods are all variable. Multiple biopsies per vial (and paraffin block) were used in approximately half of the centers that participated in the survey, which is not recommended due to a presumption that tissue quality will be compromised. In our study, there was no difference in the lengths of biopsies regardless of whether they were processed individually or pooled. Furthermore, cancer detection rates were approximately equal between the groups. The slightly lower cancer detection rate noted in individually processed biopsies may be related to the different indications for a biopsy procedure between the groups. However, the observed overall cancer detection rate of 55.8% is quite high. Previously, in a Finnish prostate cancer screening study conducted as a part of the European Randomized Study of Screening for Prostate Cancer (ERSPC), the observed cancer detection rate at a PSA cutoff level of 4 µg/l was found to be 27% [14].

There are several possible reasons for the high cancer detection rate observed in this study. The population included in the study has a relatively high PSA screening frequency due to the prostate cancer screening trial.

Table 2 The impact of the number of biopsy cores embedded into one paraffin block to the mean length of cores in the corresponding block[1]

No. of cores in paraffin block	*n*	Length of cores, mm (mean ± SD)
1	684	10.8 ± 1.8
3	8	12.9 ± 2.1
4	20	10.6 ± 2.7
5	75	11.0 ± 2.9
6	417	11.5 ± 2.4
7	40	11.8 ± 2.5
8	10	11.5 ± 2.1
9	2	11.1 ± 1.2

[1]The length of biopsies was not correlated to the number of cores in the block, r = 0.015.

Some of the patients may have PSA data going back to the start of screening trial in 1996, which has lead to a higher threshold for taking biopsies. Also, the PSA value is no longer considered the only indication for taking a prostate biopsy; more significance is given to the value of free PSA per total PSA. Another reason for the high cancer detection rate may be that some of biopsies are taken from patients in an active follow-up. Finally, there might be skewness in the results due to the inclusion criteria. Benign biopsies are not always reported with the same accuracy as cancer cases, and this inaccuracy in reporting of biopsy length may have disqualified some benign cases from inclusion in this study. Also, urgent cases with a high suspicion of cancer are more likely to be reported by one of the uropathologists conducting the study, which may increase the overall cancer detection percentage.

Our results suggest that the problems encountered with multiple biopsies in one container can be overcome by special tissue pre-embedding methods, including straightening and flattening the cores between sponges before tissue processing and by paying attention to the laboratory technologist's education. According to the ERSPC pathology committee's newest guidelines, up to three cores can be safely embedded in a single paraffin block without significant tissue loss [13]. Our results suggest that the maximum number of cores that can safely be embedded in a single paraffin block may be a matter of technique – if one is able to embed single cores well enough, why would it not work for the core next to it? In fact, in one of our earlier experiments, we embedded twelve biopsies in one paraffin block and obtained a satisfactory visual appearance. However, the technique was abandoned because there were two obvious disadvantages: the orientation of the biopsies in the paraffin block needed to be diagonal instead of longitudinal which made sectioning more difficult, and the tips of the cores stayed outside of the staining area of the automated immunostaining system due to their marginal position.

According to Bostwick et al., the mean length of prostate biopsies in Western Europe was 13.1 mm at the entry level of their study [12]. In the present study, the mean length of the core was shorter (11.4 mm). However, the aforementioned values are not comparable because in our study extraprostatic tissue was subtracted to obtain the most accurate percentage of cancer tissue possible.

It is likely that the most important advantage of individually embedded biopsies is not the biopsy core quality but rather the spared locus information. This is an important issue in selected cases, and site-designated biopsies should be encouraged. On the other hand, the use of multiple biopsies per vial (and paraffin block) is

supported by less extensive laboratory loading and better facilities for immunohistochemistry. Our medium-sized laboratory receives biopsies from approximately 1000 patients per year. Widespread use of site-designated biopsies would annually increase the number of paraffin blocks by approximately 10,000, which increases the workload for the pathology laboratory throughout various steps including processing, embedding, sectioning and analyzing. Roughly estimated this would take approximately 80 working days for sectioning only and would increase the time pathologists spend analyzing and reporting prostate biopsies (Figure 4).

There are several limitations in the present study. First, the prostate biopsies, although taken with same equipment, may have variations due to different urologists who performed the biopsies. Second, the slides were not re-evaluated. Additionally, by digitizing all of the material and measuring core areas instead of the lengths of the biopsies, the quality indicator would have been more accurate. In the present study we preferred to use our current methods because at the moment there are no area-based prognostic nomograms available, and measuring the actual tissue from histological slides is the gold standard. Third, the subtraction of extraprostatic tissue is somewhat subjective. However,

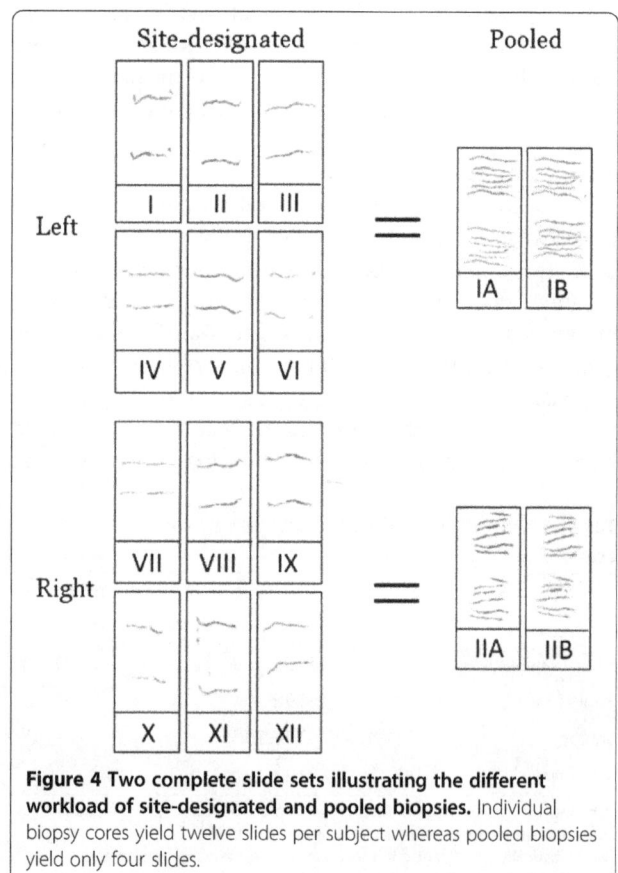

Figure 4 Two complete slide sets illustrating the different workload of site-designated and pooled biopsies. Individual biopsy cores yield twelve slides per subject whereas pooled biopsies yield only four slides.

this subjectivity should be equally transferred to both types of specimens. Finally, the amount of site-designated individual biopsies only represented 17% of the studied cases and the imbalance between the groups may cause unreliability in the final results. As a limitation of this study, it must be pointed out, that this study only shows the situation in our facility and to determine the real impact in a clinical context, a multicenter study would describe the overall situation of prostate biopsies better. Our aim was simply to determine whether there were fundamental differences in favor of either method.

Conclusions

The number of submitted vials depends on how the urologist performs the prostate biopsy. We have received both individually submitted and pooled biopsies for several years without noticing an obvious difference in their quality. However, the workload for laboratory technologists and pathologists is substantially higher for site-designated individually embedded biopsy cores. In our material, we did not find evidence regarding the superior quality of the individually submitted and embedded biopsies. We conclude that the current recommendations favoring site-designated biopsies may be too strict - the guidelines should probably recommend a result rather than a process.

Competing interests
The authors declare that they have no competing interests.

Authors' contributions
TT was responsible for the conception, study design and implementation of the project and drafted the manuscript. JI, AK and JR participated in the conception and design of the study. JI, LK and AK helped to draft the manuscript. TT, SH, ML, SP, MT and PK participated in the analysis of the data. JI and TT performed the statistical analysis. All authors read and approved the final manuscript.

Acknowledgements
The authors would like to thank Fimlab Laboratories, Tampere University Hospital, Satakunta Hospital and University of Tampere for enabling and funding parts of the research. The authors also thank the urologists of Tampere University Hospital district, who submitted the studied biopsies, and the skilful and dedicated laboratory personnel of pathology laboratory of Fimlab Laboratories.

Author details
[1]Department of Pathology, Fimlab Laboratories, Tampere University Hospital, Tampere, Finland. [2]Department of Cancer Biology, Institute of Biomedical Technology, University of Tampere, Tampere, Finland. [3]Department of Surgery, Satakunta Hospital district, Pori, Finland. [4]Department of Urology, Tampere University Hospital, Tampere, Finland. [5]Department of Materials Science, Tampere University of Technology, Tampere, Finland.

References
1. Epstein JI, Allsbrook Jr WC, Amin MB, Egevad LL. The 2005 International Society of Urological Pathology (ISUP) Consensus Conference on Gleason Grading of Prostatic Carcinoma. Am J Surg Pathol. 2005;29:1228–42.
2. Heidenreich A, Bellmunt J, Bolla M, Joniau S, Mason M, Matveev V, et al. EAU guidelines on prostate cancer. Part 1: screening, diagnosis, and treatment of clinically localised disease. Eur Urol. 2011;59:61–71.
3. Iczkowski KA, Bostwick DG. Sampling, submission, and report format for multiple prostate biopsies: a 1999 survey. Urology. 2000;55:568–71.
4. Varma M, Berney DM, Algaba F, Camparo P, Compérat E, Griffiths DFR, et al. Prostate needle biopsy processing: a survey of laboratory practice across Europe. J Clin Pathol. 2013;66:120–3.
5. Eichler K, Hempel S, Wilby J, Myers L, Bachmann LM, Kleijnen J. Diagnostic value of systematic biopsy methods in the investigation of prostate cancer: a systematic review. J Urol. 2006;175:1605–12.
6. Iczkowski KA, Casella G, Seppala RJ, Jones GL, Mishler BA, Qian J, et al. Needle core length in sextant biopsy influences prostate cancer detection rate. Urology. 2002;59:698–703.
7. Öbek C, Doğanca T, Erdal S, Erdoğan S, Durak H. Core length in prostate biopsy: size matters. J Urol. 2012;187:2051–5.
8. Jones JS, Patel A, Schoenfield L, Rabets JC, Zippe CD, Magi-Galluzzi C. Saturation technique does not improve cancer detection as an initial prostate biopsy strategy. J Urol. 2006;175:485–8.
9. Irani J, Blanchet P, Salomon L, Coloby P, Hubert J, Malavaud B, et al. Is an extended 20-core prostate biopsy protocol more efficient than the standard 12-core? A randomized multicenter trial. J Urol. 2013;190:77–83.
10. Jiang X, Zhu S, Feng G, Zhang Z, Li C, Li H, et al. Is an initial saturation prostate biopsy scheme better than an extended scheme for detection of prostate cancer? A systematic review and meta-analysis. Eur Urol. 2013;63:1031–9.
11. Bertaccini A, Fandella A, Prayer-Galetti T, Scattoni V, Galosi AB, Ficarra V, et al. Systematic development of clinical practice guidelines for prostate biopsies: a 3-year Italian project. Anticancer Res. 2007;27:659–66.
12. Bostwick DG, Qian J, Drewnowska K, Varvel S, Bostwick KC, Marberger M, et al. Prostate needle biopsy quality in reduction by dutasteride of prostate cancer events study: worldwide comparison of improvement with investigator training and centralized laboratory processing. Urology. 2010;75:1406–10.
13. Van der Kwast T, Bubendorf L, Mazerolles C, Raspollini MR, Van Leenders GJ, Phil C-G, et al. Guidelines on processing and reporting of prostate biopsies: the 2013 update of the pathology committee of the European Randomized Study of Screening for Prostate Cancer (ERSPC). Virchows Arch. 2013;463:367–77.
14. Mäkinen T. The Finnish population-based prostate cancer screening trial: a clinical perspective. Tampere: Tampere University Press; 2008.

11

Tannic acid label indicates abnormal cell development coinciding with regeneration of renal tubules

Will W Minuth[*†] and Lucia Denk[*†]

Abstract

Background: Stem/progenitor cells are in the focus of research as a future therapeutic option to stimulate regeneration in diseased renal parenchyma. However, current data indicate that successful seeding of implanted stem/progenitor cells is prevented by harmful interstitial fluid and altered extracellular matrix. To find out possible parameters for cell adaptation, the present investigation was performed.

Methods: Renal stem/progenitor cells were mounted in an artificial interstitium for perfusion culture. Exposure to chemically defined but CO_2-independent culture media was tested during 13 days. Cell biological features were then analyzed by histochemistry, while structural details were investigated by transmission electron microscopy after conventional and improved fixation of specimens.

Results: Culture of renal stem/progenitor cells as well in Leibovitz's L-15 Medium as CO_2 Independent Medium shows in fluorescence microscopy spatial development of numerous tubules. Specimens of both media fixed by conventional glutaraldehyde exhibit in electron microscopy a homogeneous cell population in developed tubules. In contrast, fixation by glutaraldehyde including tannic acid illuminates that dispersed dark marked cells of unknown function are present. The screening further demonstrates that the dark cell type does not comply with cells found in embryonic, maturing or matured renal parenchyma.

Conclusions: The actual data show that development of abnormal cell features must be taken into account, when regeneration of renal tubules is simulated under in vitro conditions.

Background

Numerous papers published during the last years illustrate that an implantation of stem/progenitor cells appears as an innovative therapeutic alternative to treat acute and chronic renal failure [1,2]. However, critical reading of related literature also elucidates that this approach still moves more in a phase of basic research than in sound clinical trials. One of the obstacles is the minimal survival of implanted stem/progenitor cells limiting in turn successful regeneration of parenchyma [3].

Further on, implantation of stem/progenitor cells for regeneration of diseased renal parenchyma is not done with a simple injection but is only one of the links in an

unexpected complex biomedical process. Literature informs, for example, that stem/progenitor cells can be principally administered via the arterial or venous vessel system, by punctual injections into diseased parenchyma or by seeding in the space left between the organ capsule and the outer parenchyma [4,5]. The various results illustrate that irrespective of applied implantation technique the expectations have not been achieved yet.

One has further to consider that before and during implantation stem/progenitor cells naturally occur within a special niche environment or are kept in the beneficial atmosphere of an individual culture medium [6,7]. However, when an implantation is performed, the environment for stem/progenitor cells drastically changes. Exposure to degenerating epithelia, altering extracellular matrix, unbalanced electrolytes, growth factors, interleukins and hormones supports inflammation but does not

* Correspondence: will.minuth@vkl.uni-regensburg.de;
lucia.denk@vkl.uni-regensburg.de
[†]Equal contributors
Department of Molecular and Cellular Anatomy, University of Regensburg,
University Street 31, D-93053 Regensburg, Germany

promote development of implanted cells [8-11]. The small fraction of surviving stem/progenitor cells has to migrate then to the molecular site of necessary restoration for turning the harmful environment into an atmosphere pushing repair of parenchyma. But how can it be realized, when stimulating interstitial fluid and attractive extracellular matrix are lacking. In this situation it appears that from stem/progenitor cells is required more than they can really perform.

To investigate developmental capacity in relation to environmental stress under in vitro conditions, renal stem/progenitor cells can be mounted in a pad consisting of a polyester fleece [5,12,13]. In this scenario the fibers of the fleece mimic extracellular matrix, while the space between acts as a reservoir for interstitial fluid. For controlled culture the artificial interstitium is then placed in a perfusion container, where contained cells are provided with always fresh nutrition and respiratory gas by a constant transport of medium.

In the present set of experiments renal stem/progenitor cells were exposed to media containing different buffer systems stabilized against atmospheric air. Influence on developmental capacity was then recorded by cell biological methods and transmission electron microscopy. The actual data demonstrate for the first time that regenerated tubules contain beside normal also abnormal epithelial cells. Comparisons show that described abnormal cells are not contained in embryonic, maturing or matured renal parenchyma.

Methods
Preparation of renal stem/progenitor cells
Care, use of animals and performed experiments are in accordance with the Animal Ethics Committee, University of Regensburg, Regensburg, Germany. Kidneys from one-day old New Zealand rabbits (Seidl, Oberndorf, Germany) were isolated under sterile conditions and cut into a ventral and dorsal half as earlier described [14]. Then the fibrous organ capsule was stripped off by fine forceps to obtain a constantly thin layer of stem/progenitor cell niches adherent to the explant. Applying this method embryonic tissue of up to 1 cm in square can be isolated.

Offering an artificial interstitium
To analyze development of renal tubules an isolated embryonic tissue layer containing numerous stem/progenitor niches was mounted in an artificial interstitium as it was earlier described [5,13]. Briefly, the isolated tissue was placed between punched out layers (5 and 13 mm in diameter) of polyester fleece (I7, Walraf, Grevenbroich, Germany) and mounted inside a Minusheet® tissue carrier (Minucells and Minutissue, Bad Abbach, Germany) (Figure 1a). The tissue carrier was transferred

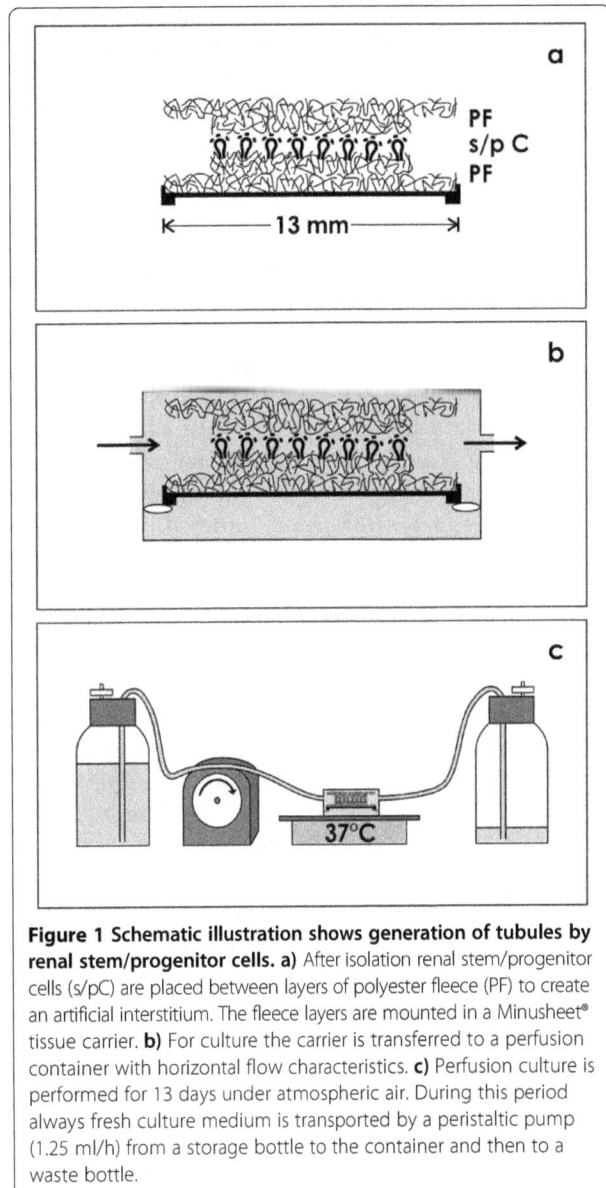

Figure 1 Schematic illustration shows generation of tubules by renal stem/progenitor cells. a) After isolation renal stem/progenitor cells (s/pC) are placed between layers of polyester fleece (PF) to create an artificial interstitium. The fleece layers are mounted in a Minusheet® tissue carrier. **b)** For culture the carrier is transferred to a perfusion container with horizontal flow characteristics. **c)** Perfusion culture is performed for 13 days under atmospheric air. During this period always fresh culture medium is transported by a peristaltic pump (1.25 ml/h) from a storage bottle to the container and then to a waste bottle.

to a perfusion culture container with horizontal flow characteristics (Figure 1b). Then for a period of 13 days always fresh culture medium was continuously transported at a rate of 1.25 ml/h with an IPC N8 peristaltic pump (Ismatec, Wertheim, Germany) (Figure 1c). To work independently from a CO_2-incubator, all of the culture experiments were performed under atmospheric air on a thermo plate (Medax-Nagel, Kiel, Germany) at 37°C.

Chemical defined culture media
For the present experiments chemical defined Leibovitz's L-15 Medium (Nr. 31415–029, 34 cultured specimens) and CO_2 Independent Medium (Nr. 18045–054, 43 cultured specimens) all including Phenolred (GIBCO/

Invitrogen, Karlsruhe, Germany) were applied. Infections were prevented by adding an antibiotic-antimycotic cocktail (1%, GIBCO/Invitrogen). Development of tubules was induced by application of aldosterone (1×10^{-7} M, Fluka, Taufkirchen, Germany) as it was earlier described [5]. The pH of 7.4 under atmospheric air is stable in CO_2 Independent Medium. To obtain this pH in Leibovitz's L-15 Medium, N-2-Hydroxyethylpiperazine-N-2-Ethane Sulfonic Acid (HEPES; GIBCO/Invitrogen) was added by titration.

Histochemistry on generated tubules

After run of a perfusion culture experiment the polyester fleeces 13 mm in diameter with adherent renal tubules were fixed in 70% ethanol for whole mount label. Before labeling the specimens were washed several times with phosphate buffered saline (PBS, pH 7.5) and incubated for 30 minutes with blocking solution (PBS, 10% horse serum from GIBCO/Invitrogen, 1% bovine serum albumin from Serva, Heidelberg, Germany). Then the undiluted antibody anti-cytokeratin 19 (TROMA III, Developmental Studies Hybridoma Bank DSHB, Iowa, USA) was applied for one hour. After washing with 1% BSA in PBS the specimens were incubated for 45 minutes with goat-anti-rat-IgG-rhodamine (Jackson Immunoresearch Laboratories, West Grove, USA) diluted 1:50 in PBS containing 1% BSA. Following several washes with PBS the labeled specimens were analyzed using a CM12 confocal laser scanning microscope (Zeiss, Oberkochen, Germany). Fluorescence images were taken with a digital camera at a standard exposure time and thereafter processed with Corel DRAW Graphic Suite X5 (Corel Corporation, Otawa, Canada). In parallel, screening for renal cell features was performed with fluorescent lectins such as BPL (Bauhinia Purpurea Lectin), GSL (Griffonia Simplicifolia Lectin), LTL (Lotus Tetragonolobus Lectin), WGA (Wheat Germ Agglutinin), DBA (Dolichos Biflorus Agglutinin), PNA (Peanut Agglutinin) and SBA (Soybean Agglutinin) all from Vector (Burlingame, USA).

Transmission electron microscopy (TEM)

The polyester fleeces 5 mm in diameter containing generated tubules were harvested after 13 days of culture and cut in four parts. Kidneys were surgically removed and then prepared. To obtain a correct orientation of parenchyme along the cortico-medullary axis of lining collecting ducts, tissue blocks between both organ poles were specifically excised as it was performed earlier [15].

In the present investigation specimens were analyzed after conventional fixation in glutaraldehyde (GA) and after improved contrasting by GA solution including tannic acid as it was earlier described [14,16].

For fixation the following solutions were used:

1. Specimens for control: 5% GA (Serva) buffered with 0.15 M sodium cacodylate, pH 7.4.
2. Specimens for improved contrast with tannic acid: 5% GA buffered with 0.15 M sodium cacodylate, pH 7.4 + 1% tannic acid (Sigma-Aldrich Chemie, München, Germany).

Primary fixation was performed for 1 day at room temperature. After several washes with 0.15 M sodium cacodylate the samples were postfixed in the same buffer but additionally containing 1% osmium tetroxide (Science Services, München, Germany). Then specimens were washed with sodium cacodylate buffer and dehydrated in graded series of ethanols.

Finally, specimens were embedded in Epon (Fluka, Taufkirchen, Germany), which was polymerized at 60°C for 48 h. Semithin and ultrathin sections were made with a diamond knife on an ultramicrotome EM UC6 (Leica, Wetzlar, Germany).

Semithin sections of specimens fixed by glutaraldehyde were stained with Richardson solution, while specimens fixed by glutaraldehyde including tannic acid were analyzed without further staining. Analysis of semithin sections was performed with an Axioscope microscope (Zeiss). Images were taken with a digital camera (AxioCam MRC, Zeiss) and thereafter processed with Corel DRAW Graphic Suite X5 (Corel Corporation).

Ultrathin sections were collected onto slot grids coated with 1.5% Pioloform (Plano, Wetzlar, Germany) and contrasted using 1% uranyl acetate and lead citrate as it was earlier described [17]. Analysis of ultrathin sections was performed at 80 kV using an EM 902 transmission electron microscope (Zeiss).

Definition of cells within the renal stem/progenitor cell niche

For the presented experiments embryonic parenchyma derived from the outer cortex of neonatal rabbit kidney was analyzed containing renal stem/progenitor cell niches. The nomenclature of previously published papers was used [18].

Results

During the process of implantation stem/progenitor cells are transferred from a beneficial culture medium to the inflammatory environment of diseased parenchyma. To obtain first basic information, if such a harsh transition can be balanced to a certain degree, renal stem/progenitor cells were embedded in a polyester fleece as a substitute for interstitial extracellular matrix and exposed to chemically defined media. In the present series the influence of CO_2-stabilized culture media on tubule development was tested.

Fluorescence microscopy on generated tubules

After 13 days of perfusion culture whole mount label was performed on harvested specimens to analyze the degree of spatial development of regenerated tubules (Figure 2). As well in series with CO_2 Independent Medium (Figure 2a) as in series with Leibovitz's L-15 Medium (Figure 2b) confocal fluorescence microscopy points out that numerous tubules labeled by TROMA III are developing between the polyester fibers of the artificial interstitium. Further can be seen that generated tubules of both CO_2 Independent Medium (Figure 2c) and Leibovitz's L-15 Medium (Figure 2d) show an epithelium with prismatic cells. In selected cross and longitudinal sections a lumen and a continuously developed basal lamina is visible.

Fluorescence microscopy also elucidates that SBA label illustrates numerous collecting duct tubules developing between the polyester fibers of the artificial interstitium. This marker indicates that most probably collecting duct tubules are contained as it was earlier described (no figure) [5,13]. To recognize features typical for proximal tubule cells binding of further lectins was tested. Astonishingly, only a barely visible reaction on single tubules was found in series labeled by BPL, while no label was detected in series with GSL, LTL and WGA. In none of the cases label on single cells within the tubule epithelium was registered (no figure).

Light microscopical analysis

In the following set of experiments semithin sections were produced to obtain more information about morphological details of tubule cells generated in CO_2 Independent Medium (Figure 3a,c,e) and Leibovitz's L-15 Medium (Figure 3b,d,f).

Specimens fixed in conventional glutaraldehyde show after staining with Richardson solution that numerous tubules are present within the artificial interstitium (Figure 3a,b). In series with either CO_2 Independent Medium (Figure 3a) or Leibovitz's L-15 Medium (Figure 3b) cross sections illustrate that a single layer of a homogeneous cell population with a basal lamina is bordering a lumen. Differences in morphological quality of cells cannot be recognized. In several cases the lumen is filled with apoptotic cells and a luminal matrix as it is known from other developing epithelia [19]. Vacuoles in the cytoplasm of generated tubule cells are rare. This result indicates that toxic effects or non appropriate chemical compounds are obviously not present in selected culture media.

In contrast, specimens fixed in glutaraldehyde containing tannic acid show after culture with CO_2 Independent Medium (Figure 3c,e) and Leibovitz's L-15 Medium (Figure 3d,f) a completely different cell pattern as compared to series fixed in conventional glutaraldehyde (Figure 3a,b). Fixation by glutaraldehyde including tannic acid reveals that two different phenotypes of tubules are contained within the artificial interstitium. While the one type of tubules shows a homogeneously composed bright cell population (T^B), the second type exhibits a heterogeneously composed epithelium consisting of dark and bright cells ($T^{D/B}$). Thus, fixation of

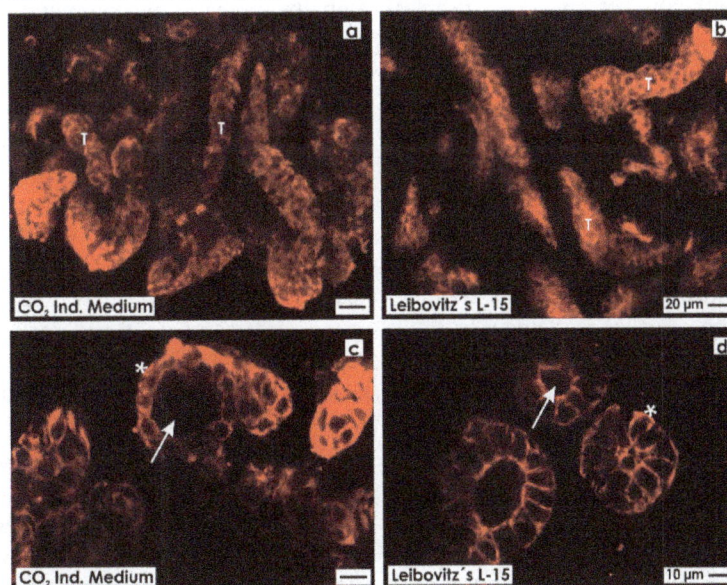

Figure 2 Confocal fluorescence microscopy on whole mount species labeled for cytokeratin 19 (Troma III) to analyze spatial distribution of generated tubules. As well in **(a)** CO_2 Independent Medium and **(b)** Leibovitz's L-15 Medium development of numerous tubules (T) is observed within the artificial interstitium. **c,d)** Higher magnification depicts that label is detected on all of analyzed cells. Further generated tubules contain a simple epithelium with prismatic cells bordering a lumen (arrow) and a basal lamina (asterisk).

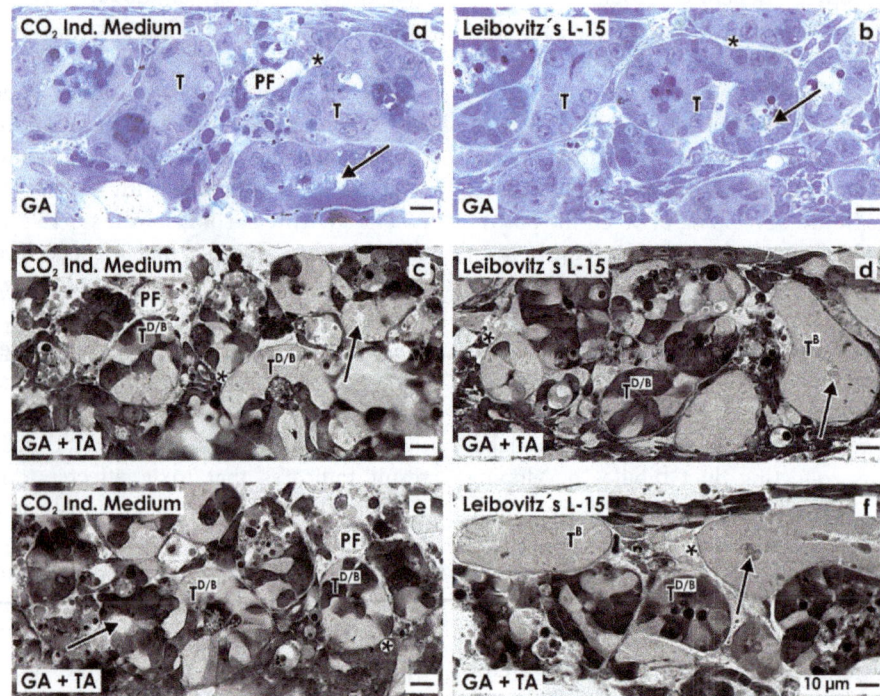

Figure 3 Light microscopy on semithin sections demonstrates numerous tubules (T) generated between fibers of the polyester fleece (**PF**). Development of tubules is observed in series with (**a,c,e**) CO_2 Independent Medium and (**b,d,f**) Leibovitz's L-15 Medium. Generated tubules exhibit a lumen (arrow) and a basal lamina (asterisk). **a,b** Fixation of specimens in conventional glutaraldehyde followed staining by Richardson solution shows tubules with an inconspicuously looking homogeneous cell population. In contrast, specimens generated in (**c,e**) CO_2 Independent Medium or (**d,f**) Leibovitz's L-15 Medium but fixed by glutaraldehyde containing tannic acid show tubules with a dark and bright cell population ($T^{D/B}$) or tubules containing only bright cells (T^B).

specimens in glutaraldehyde including tannic acid demasks hidden details and illuminates a heterogeneously composed cell population in the epithelium of generated tubules (Figure 3c,e and d,f).

TEM on generated tubules fixed by glutaraldehyde

To obtain more information about the heterogeneous cell population, transmission electron microscopy (TEM) was performed (Figure 4).

Specimens generated in CO_2 Independent Medium (Figure 4a) or Leibovitz's L-15 Medium (Figure 4b) fixed in conventional glutaraldehyde show tubules containing a polarized epithelium with intact morphology. In both cases the cytoplasm is looking inconspicuously. The luminal side of cell faces a lumen occasionally filled with apoptotic cells and some luminal matrix. The basal side of the epithelial cells rests on a continuously developed basal lamina.

In contrast, samples generated in CO_2 Independent Medium (Figure 4c,e) or Leibovitz's L-15 Medium (Figure 4d,f) fixed with glutaraldehyde including tannic acid show tubules including a polarized epithelium with intact morphology. Tubule segments were found, where bright cells dominate, while in other segments an equal number of bright and dark cells is visible. In both series

the cytoplasm looks intact. In screened cases the luminal plasma membrane of cells is bordering a lumen. Finally, the basal plasma membrane is in contact with a continuously developed basal lamina consisting of a lamina rara, lamina densa and lamina fibroreticularis.

Higher magnifications of series with CO_2 Independent Medium (Figure 4e) and Leibovitz's L-15 Medium (Figure 4f) illustrate that between the luminal and lateral plasma membranes as well on bright as dark cells an intact tight junction complex is developed. This finding is a hint that a physiological sealing is established between neighboring cells. Further the intercellular space between bright and dark cells is not pathologically extended but appears to be narrow. In all of analyzed cases a close basal slit is found at the contact site between the basal and lateral plasma membranes. On the lateral plasma membranes only few interdigitating microvilli respectively folds are found.

For control, to find out whether newly detected dark cells in generated tubules (Figure 4c-f) have similarities with a related cell population in renal parenchyma, a further screening by transmission electron microscopy was performed (Figure 5).

Specimens fixed by conventional glutaraldehyde illustrate a stem/progenitor cell niche in the outer cortex of

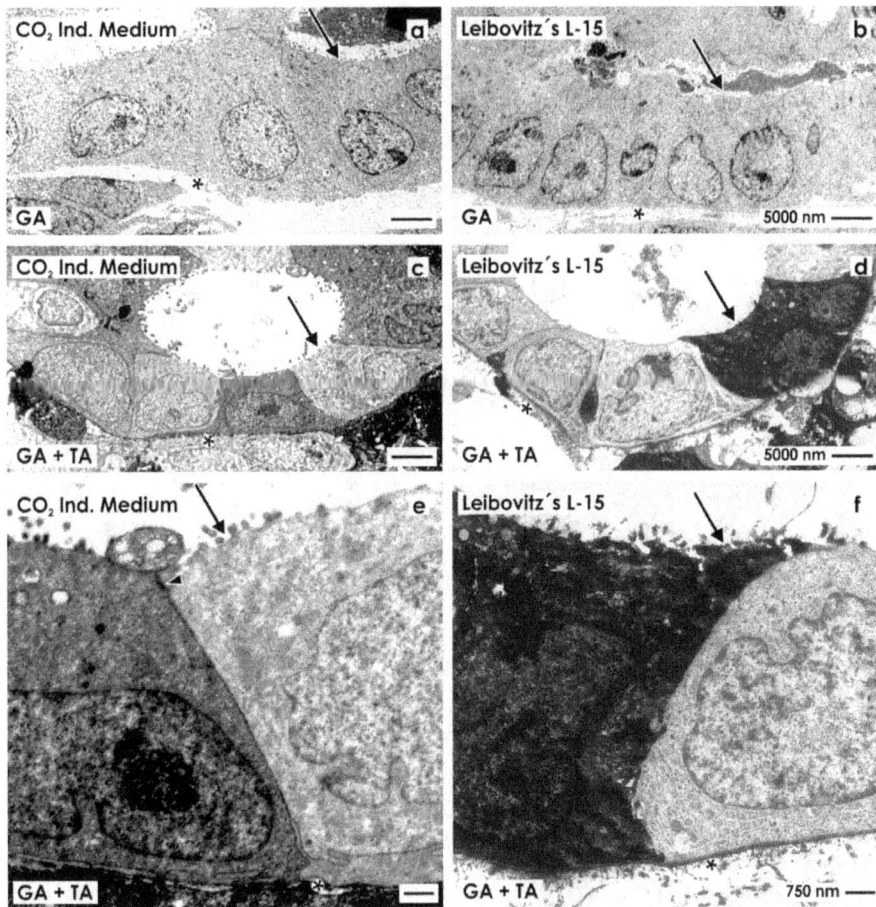

Figure 4 Transmission electron microscopy of renal tubules generated in (a,c,e) CO₂ Independent Medium and (b,d,f) Leibovitz's L-15 Medium for 13 days. Specimens fixed by **(a,b)** conventional glutaraldehyde show only bright tubule cells. In contrast, specimens fixed in **(c-f)** glutaraldehyde containing tannic acid reveal a heterogeneously composed epithelium consisting of bright and dark cells. **e,f)** High magnification shows intact bright and dark cells. The apical plasma membrane faces a lumen (arrow), while the basal side rests on a basal lamina (asterisk). Luminal and lateral plasma membranes are separated by a tight junction (arrow head).

neonatal kidney. In the center the tip of an ureteric bud derived collecting duct (CD) ampulla can be recognized (Figure 5a). Contained epithelial stem/progenitor cells are separated from mesenchymal stem/progenitor cells by a noticeably bright interstitial interface. The stem/progenitor cell niche as a whole is covered by few cell layers of the organ capsule. At the lateral side of the CD ampulla condensed mesenchymal cells are visible performing a mesenchymal-epithelial transition to develop into a renal vesicle, Comma- and then a S-shaped body as first visible signs of nephron development. Without exception all of demonstrated cells show the same light staining profile.

At the neck of an ampulla the collecting duct tubule matures. At this site the primary development of well known light 'Principal (P) Cells' and somewhat darker labeled 'Intercalated (IC) Cells' can be seen (Figure 5c). As compared to light 'Principal Cells' neighboring 'Intercalated Cells' can be recognized by a slightly increased

grey label of cytoplasm and by a barely increased amount of mitochondria. In so far 'Intercalated Cells' within the kidney do not appear to be identical with the dark cell type found in generated tubules (Figure 4c-f).

Further on, neonatal rabbit kidney fixed by glutaraldehyde including tannic acid was analyzed. Within the tip of a CD ampulla contained epithelial stem/progenitor cells are recognized. At the interstitial interface between the basal aspect of a CD ampulla and surrounding mesenchymal stem/progenitor cells intense label of tannic acid can be seen as it was described earlier (Figure 5b) [15]. Most important, in none of the cases label of tannic acid can be seen within the cytoplasm of cells. At the lateral side of a CD ampulla the label for tannic acid decreases so that the interstitial space at this site is free of label. Finally, at the neck of a collecting duct ampulla maturing 'Principal Cells' and 'Intercalated Cells' can be recognized. A slightly different grey label within the cytoplasm makes the difference (Figure 5d).

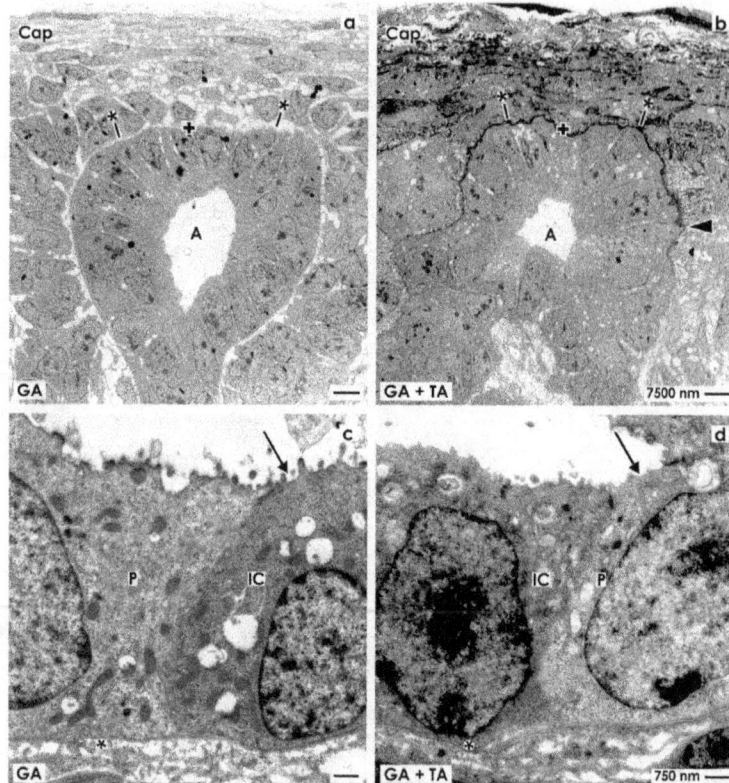

Figure 5 Transmission electron microscopy of the stem/progenitor cell niche in neonatal rabbit kidney after fixation of specimens by (a,c) conventional glutaraldehyde and (b,d) glutaraldehyde including tannic acid. **a)** Neither in a collecting duct ampulla (A) nor in surrounding mesenchymal stem/progenitor cells or organ capsule (Cap) a dark cell type is detected. The epithelial-mesenchymal interface is bright (asterisk with bar). The basal aspect of a CD ampulla is marked by a cross. **c)** At the ampulla neck maturation of light 'Principal Cells' and grey 'Intercalated Cells' is seen. **b)** Fixation of specimens in glutaraldehyde including tannic acid shows intense label at the epithelial-mesenchymal interface (asterisk with bar) as it was earlier described [15]. **d)** Label of tannic acid is lost at the lateral side of the ampulla (arrow head). Neither in embryonic, maturing or matured renal parenchyma dark cells within a tubule epithelium are present.

Most important, after fixation in glutaraldehyde containing tannic acid the dark cells found in generated tubules could neither detected in the embryonic, maturing or matured parenchyma of the kidney. Further comparing earlier immunohistochemical profiles with tannic acid labeled cells in none of the cases a coincidence was found. Thus, neither in glomeruli, proximal, intermediate or distal portions of the nephron a comparable cell type was seen. In so far the dark cell type found in generated tubules has to be ascribed to abnormal development (Figure 4c-f).

Discussion

Implantation of stem/progenitor cells into renal parenchyma appears as an attractive option to cure in future acute and chronic renal failure [20,21]. Although the concept sounds convincing, but a solid therapeutic basis is until now not in sight. Reasons for it are manifold comprising an up to date ineffective implantation technique, a suboptimal seeding and only a minimal survival of stem/progenitor cells in diseased renal parenchyma [22].

The injection of stem/progenitor cells into diseased parenchyma is the prerequisite to start the process of regeneration. However, the targeted application expects from stem/progenitor cells a complex adaption. During isolation their special niche environment is exchanged against a more or less suitable culture medium [5,23]. The situation becomes especially critical after infusion respectively injection. In contrast to the niche stem/progenitor cells are yet exposed to harmful interstitial fluid and altered extracellular matrix within diseased renal parenchyma [24-28]. In this unphysiological surrounding stimulating extracellular matrix and biochemical signals are missing sustaining normally stemness, proliferation, differentiation and development. Although all of these environmental conditions are poor, stem/progenitor cells have to seed and start with restoration. Thus, the challenge for the next future is consequently to elaborate an implantation technique that achieves on the one hand a protection against the unphysiological atmosphere in diseased parenchyma and supports on the other hand the initial seeding.

To gather basic data about environmental tolerance and individual physiological needs renal stem/progenitor cells were kept for the present investigation in advanced perfusion culture (Figure 1) [5]. For protection stem/progenitor cells were embedded in a fleece pad serving as an artificial interstitium [13]. Applying this concept the fibers of the polyester fleece mimic intact extracellular matrix, while the space between acts as a reservoir containing fresh interstitial fluid. Providing permanently fresh culture medium this technique produces a constant environment including a stable pH for a prolonged period of time. By varying experimental parameters developmental capacity of contained renal stem/progenitor cells can be tested. In a further step it is envisaged to implant the polyester pad under the renal organ capsule as a buffering reservoir for contained stem/progenitor cells.

In the actual series of experiments renal stem/progenitor cells were exposed to CO_2 Independent Medium (Figure 2a,c) and Leibovitz's L-15 Medium (Figure 2b,d). Although different in chemical composition, in both experimental series intense TROMA III label illustrates spatial development of numerous tubules within the artificial interstitium. Also semithin sections of specimens demonstrate occurrence of numerous tubules between fibers of the polyester fleece (Figure 3). Finally cross sections reveal that in regenerated tubules a lumen and a basal lamina are contained.

Most interestingly, the kind of fixation displays quite new results. Specimens fixed by conventional glutaraldehyde exhibit an epithelium with a homogeneous cell population (Figure 3a,b). In contrast, fixation of specimens in glutaraldehyde containing tannic acid illustrates that tubules contain a heterogeneously composed epithelium consisting of bright and dark cells (Figure 3c,f). This important finding points out that conventional fixation by glutaraldehyde does not show all morphological details, while fixation by glutaraldehyde including tannic acid unmasks hidden morphological features.

Stem/progenitor cells cultured in CO_2 Independent Medium (Figure 4a,c,e) and Leibovitz's L-15 Medium (Figure 4b,d,f) show after fixation by glutaraldehyde that nucleus and cytoplasm of generated tubule cells appear normal. Intact mitochondria are orientated more to the basal than to the apical cell side of the cell. The apical and lateral plasma membranes were found in all cases to be separated by a tight junction complex. The lateral plasma membranes form narrow slits at the basal side speaking for an intact side to side contact of cells as it is found within the kidney. Further the basal plasma membrane of epithelial cells rests on a continuously developed basal lamina. In so far morphological analysis suggests that tubules generated in series with CO_2 Independent Medium and Leibovitz's L-15 Medium appear

to be similar to renal tubule epithelium. In contrast, transmission electron microscopy displays also substantial inequalities. While after fixation with conventional glutaraldehyde a homogeneous tubule epithelium is seen consisting only of bright cells (Figure 4a,b), fixation by glutaraldehyde including tannic acid illustrates a heterogeneously composed epithelium consisting of bright and dark cells (Figure 4e-f). This observation was made as well in series with CO_2 Independent Medium (Figure 4c,e) as in Leibovitz's L-15 Medium (Figure 4d,f).

To obtain more information about identity, the dark cell type was searched in the rabbit kidney (Figure 5). Consequently, embryonic, maturing and matured parenchyma in neonatal kidney was investigated after fixation with conventional glutaraldehyde (Figure 5a,c) and by fixation with glutaraldehyde including tannic acid (Figure 5b,d). However, neither in the proximal tubule, the intermediate tubule, the distal, connecting or collecting duct tubule a dark cell type was registered. Only the known type of 'Intercalated Cells' in the connecting tubule and collecting duct epithelium was detected [29,30]. The primary development of an 'Intercalated Cell' can be seen in the neck of a ureteric bud derived collecting duct ampulla (Figure 5c,d). Thus, the dark cell type found in regenerated tubules fixed by glutaraldehyde containing tannic acid cannot be detected within the normal kidney.

A key question is whether illustrated darkly labeled tubule cells show features of normal development or whether up to date unknown pathological characteristics are contained. Formation of an excess of vacuoles as an indicator for cytotoxicity was not observed. In transmission electron microscopy it was further detected that the luminal cell border is clear so that the dark cells do not exhibit a luminal matrix. During tubulogenesis such a material is normally secreted by the surrounding epithelial cells to coordinate alterations in shape resulting in a correct lumen dimension [19]. Consequently, the lack of luminal matrix speaks for a differentiated cell. Moreover, in the illustrated dark cell type signs of programmed cell death (PCD) such as apoptosis or necroptosis cannot be recognized [31]. Finally, the intact appearance including integration within the epithelium indicates maintenance of differentiation. In so far the presently shown dark cell type found in generated tubules is unique and has to be ascribed to abnormal cell development.

Conclusions

In the present experiments renal stem/progenitor cells were isolated to investigate regeneration of tubules under advanced in vitro conditions. The actual data exhibit that the kind of fixation for transmission electron microscopy displays quite new results. Specimens fixed by conventional glutaraldehyde exhibit an epithelium with a homogeneous cell population. In contrast, fix-ation of specimens in glutaraldehyde containing tannic acid illustrates that tubules contain a heterogeneously composed epithelium consisting of bright and dark cells. This important finding points out that conven-tional fixation by glutaraldehyde does not show all morphological details, while fixation by glutaraldehyde including tannic acid unmasks hidden morphological features.

Competing interests
The authors declare no competing interests.

Authors' contributions
WWM coordinated the experiments, performed perfusion culture, analyzed specimens in fluorescence microscopy and interpreted results in transmission electron microscopy, designed the figure presentations and wrote the manuscript. LD isolated renal stem/progenitor cells, prepared media and the artificial interstitium, performed histochemical experiments, made special fixation, embedding, semi- and ultrathin sections and analysis in transmission electron microscopy. Further she made all works dealing with figure presentation. Both authors read and approved the final manuscript.

Acknowledgements
The authors thank the Institute of Molecular and Cellular Anatomy, University of Regensburg for financial support and technical assistance.

References
1. Herrera M, Mirotsou M: **Stem cells: potential and challenges for kidney repair.** *Am J Physiol Renal Physiol* 2014, **306:**F12–F23.
2. Harari-Steinberg O, Metsuyanim S, Omer D, Gnatek Y, Gershon R, Pri-chen S, Ozdemir DD, Lerenthal Y, Noiman T, Ben-Hur H, Vaknin Z, Schneider DF, Aronow BJ, Goldstein RS, Hohenstein P, Dekel B: **Identification of human nephron progenitors capable of generation of kidney structures and functional repair of chronic renal disease.** *EMBO Mol Med* 2013, **5:**1556–1568.
3. Burst V, Pütsch F, Kubacki T, Völker LA, Bartram MP, Müller RU, Gillis M, Kurschat CE, Grundmann F, Müller-Ehmsen J, Benzing T, Teschner S: **Survival and distribution of injected haematopoietic stem cells in acute kidney injury.** *Nephrol Dial Transplant* 2013, **28:**1131–1139.
4. Wang Y, He J, Pei X, Zhao W: **Systematic review and meta-analysis of mesenchymal stem/stromal cells therapy for impaired renal function in small animals.** *Nephrology* 2013, **18:**201–208.
5. Minuth WW, Denk L: **Initial steps to stabilize the microenvironment for implantation of stem/progenitor cells in diseased renal parenchyma.** *Transplant Technol* 2013, **1:**2.
6. Morigi M, Benigni A: **Mesenchymal stem cells and kidney repair.** *Nephrol Dial Transplant* 2013, **28:**788–793.
7. Stine RR, Matunis EL: **Stem cell completion: finding balance in the niche.** *Trends Cell Biol* 2013, **23**(8):357–364.
8. Bonventre JV, Yang L: **Cellular pathophysiology of ischemic acute kidney injury.** *J Clin Invest* 2011, **121**(11):4210–4221.
9. Lee DW, Faubel S, Edelstein CL: **Cytokines in acute kidney injury (AKI).** *Clin Nephrol* 2011, **76**(3):165–173.
10. Miyamoto T, Carrero JJ, Stenvinkel P: **Inflammation as a risk factor and target for therapy in chronic kidney disease.** *Curr Opinion Nephrol Hypertens* 2011, **20**(6):662–668.
11. Chiang CK, Tanaka T, Nangaku M: **Dysregulated oxygen metabolism of the kidney by uremic toxins: review.** *J Ren Nutr* 2012, **22**(1):77–80.
12. Roessger A, Denk L, Minuth WW: **Potential of stem/progenitor cell cultures within polyester fleeces to regenerate renal tubules.** *Biomaterials* 2009, **30**(22):3723–3732.
13. Minuth WW, Denk L, Gruber M: **Search for chemically defined culture medium to assist initial regeneration of diseased renal parenchyma after stem/progenitor cell implantation.** *Int J Stem Cell Res Transplant* 2013, **1:**202.
14. Minuth WW, Denk L: **Interstitial interfaces show marked differences in regenerating tubules, matured tubules and the renal stem/progenitor cell niche.** *J Biomed Mater Res A* 2012, **100**(5):1115–1125.
15. Minuth WW, Denk L: **Structural links between the renal stem/progenitor cell niche and the organ capsule.** *Histochem Cell Biol* 2014, **141**(5):459–471.
16. Minuth WW, Denk L: **Illustration of extensive extracellular matrix at the epithelial-mesenchymal interface within the renal stem/progenitor cell niche.** *BMC Clin Pathol* 2012, **12:**16.
17. Minuth WW, Denk L, Meese C, Rachel R, Roessger A: **Ultrastructural insights in the interface between generated renal tubules and a polyester interstitium.** *Langmuir* 2009, **25**(8):4621–4627.
18. Minuth WW, Denk L, Miess C, Glashauser A: **Peculiarities of the extracellular matrix in the interstitium of the renal stem/progenitor cell niche.** *Histochem Cell Biol* 2011, **136**(3):321–334.
19. Luschnig S, Uv A: **Luminal matrices: an inside view on organ morphogenesis.** *Exp Cell Res* 2014, **321**(1):64–70.
20. Winyard PJ, Price KL: **Experimental renal progenitor cells: repairing and creating kidneys?** *Pediatr Nephrol* 2013, **29**(4):665–672.
21. de Almeida DC, Donizetti-Oliviera C, Barbosa-Costa P, Origassa CS, Camara NO: **In search of mechanisms associated with mesenchymal stem cell-based therapies for acute kidney injury.** *Clin Biochem Rev* 2013, **34**(3):131–144.
22. Alagesan S, Griffin MD: **Autologous and allogenic mesenchymal stem cells in organ transplantation: what do we know about their safety and efficacy?** *Curr Opin Organ Transplant* 2014, **19**(1):65–72.
23. Gattazzo F, Urciuolo A, Bonaldo P: **Extracellular matrix: a dynamic microenvironment for stem cell niche.** *Biochim Biophys Acta* 2014, **1840**(8):2506–2519.
24. Barak H, Huh SH, Chen S, Jeanpierre C, Martinovic J, Parisot M, Bole-Feysot C, Nitschke P, Salomon R, Antignac C, Ornitz DM, Kopan R: **FGF9 and FGF20 maintain the stemness of nephron progenitors in mice and man.** *Dev Cell* 2012, **22**(6):1191–1207.
25. Carroll TJ, Das A: **Defining the signals that constitute the nephron progenitor niche.** *J Am Soc Nephrol* 2013, **24**(6):873–876.
26. Ahn SY, Kim Y, Kim ST, Swat W, Miner JH: **Scaffolding proteins DLG1 and CASK cooperate to maintain the nephron progenitor population during kidney development.** *J Am Soc Nephrol* 2013, **24:**1127–1138.
27. Hilliard SA, Yao X, El-Dahr SS: **Mdm2 is required for maintenance of the nephrogenic niche.** *Dev Biol* 2014, **387**(1):1–14.
28. Kopan R, Chen S, Little M: **Nephron progenitor cells: shifting the balance of self-renewal and differentiation.** *Curr Top Dev Biol* 2014, **107:**293–331.
29. Satlin LM, Matsumoto T, Schwartz GJ: **Postnatal maturation of rabbit collecting duct. III Peanut lectin-binding intercalated cells.** *Am J Physiol* 1992, **262:**F199–F208.
30. Al-Aqati Q: **Cell biology of the intercalated cell in the kidney.** *FEBS Lett* 2013, **587**(13):1911–1914.
31. Li X, Guo M, Shao Y: **Ultrastructural observations of programmed cell death during metanephric development in mouse.** *Microscopy Res Technique* 2013, **76:**467–475.

12

Primary Burkitt lymphoma of the thyroid gland: case report of an exceptional type of thyroid neoplasm and review of the literature

Mohamed Allaoui[1]*, Ilias Benchafai[2], El Mehdi Mahtat[3], Safae Regragui[3], Adil Boudhas[1], Mustapha Azzakhmam[1], Mohammed Boukhechba[1], Abderrahmane Al Bouzidi[1] and Mohamed Oukabli[1]

Abstract

Background: Primary thyroid lymphoma is an uncommon pathological entity that accounts for only 1 to 5 % of all thyroid malignancies. Primary Burkitt lymphoma of the thyroid gland is very rare. This article presents the first Moroccan case of a primary BL of the thyroid to be reported in the literature to date.

Case presentation: We describe here a case of a 70-year-old male who developed a rapidly enlarging thyroid gland with progressive symptoms of compression. Core biopsy confirmed the diagnosis of Burkitt lymphoma. The patient died of septic shock, 2 weeks after the first cycle of appropriate therapeutic chemotherapy.

Conclusions: This presentation emphasizes the importance of considering lymphoma when dealing with a thyroid mass, as its management is different from that of other thyroid pathologies, and affords an opportunity to review a very rare type of primary thyroid lymphoma.

Keywords: Burkitt lymphoma, Thyroid gland, Chemotherapy

Background

Primary Burkitt lymphoma (BL) of the thyroid gland is a very uncommon pathological entity with a few isolated case reports in adult patients [1, 2].

This highly aggressive malignancy arises from B-lymphoid cells. It presents usually as a rapidly expanding thyroid mass causing compressive symptoms.

To the best of our knowledge, this article reports the first Moroccan case of a primary BL of the thyroid to be reported in the literature to date.

BL should be promptly recognized because its management is quite different from the treatment of other neoplasms of the thyroid gland. Moreover, this disease is quite curable if diagnosed early and treated appropriately.

* Correspondence: allaoui.m1@gmail.com
[1]Department of Pathology, Military General Hospital Mohammed V, Mohammed V Souissi University - Faculty of Medicine and Pharmacy of Rabat, Hay Riad, Rabat 10000, Morocco
Full list of author information is available at the end of the article

Case presentation

A 70-year-old male presented a rapidly expanding mass of the neck associated with history of airway compression symptoms; progressive dyspnea and dysphonia lasting for 4 weeks, in a context of apyrexia and impairment of general condition. The patient was admitted to the hospital because of increasing dyspnea and urgently received a tracheostomy.

A biopsy of the cervical mass was carried out and the histological examination showed diffuse infiltration of the thyroid gland by a monotonous population of atypical intermediate-sized lymphoid cells (Fig. 1). These last possess scanty amphophilic to basophilic cytoplasm with centrally located nuclei of irregular shape, displaying dispersed basophilic chromatin, and frequent apoptotic figures (Fig. 2). Scattered tingible body type macrophages were also present. Little residual thyroid follicles and some areas of necrosis was observed.

Immunohistochemical staining was then performed and the tumour cells were positive for CD20, CD10 and

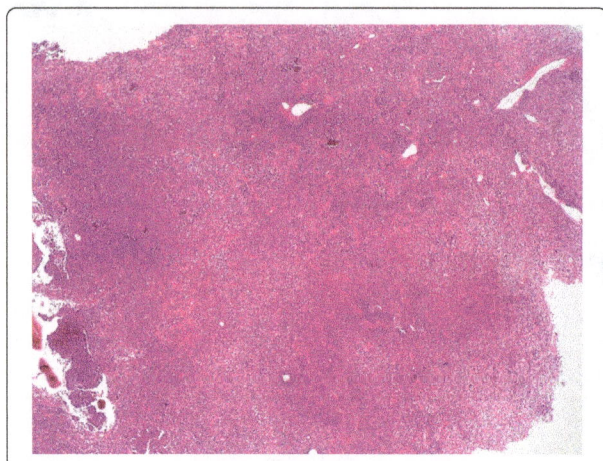

Fig. 1 Low magnification showing a diffuse infiltration of atypical lymphoid cells in the thyroid gland (haematoxylin & eosin stain, ×50)

BCL6. Ki-67 showed proliferation index approaching 100 %. CD3 and CD5 stained the background T cells (Fig. 3). Immunoreactivity for Epstein-Barr virus (EBV) was negative. The diagnosis of BL was confirmed on fluorescence in situ hybridisation that showed tumour cell positivity for the t (8; 14) translocation. Bone marrow examination was normal.

The patient was transferred to the Clinical Haematology department. On physical examination, he was apyretic and hemodynamically stable with a cervical armouring by a huge mass of hard consistency. Neurological examination shows no sensorimotor deficits.

Other systemic examinations were normal, without any palpable lymphadenopathy or organomegaly.

The computerized tomography (CT) scan showed a heterogeneous process of the thyroid gland measuring 10.5 × 8.2 × 6.5 cm in size, extending up towards the

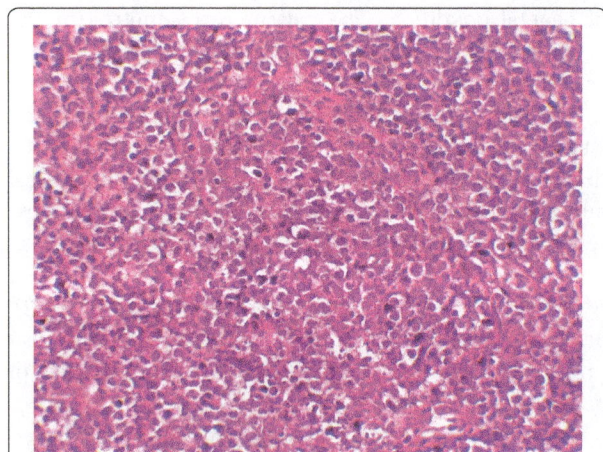

Fig. 2 Higher magnification showing a monotonous population of intermediate-sized lymphoid cells with scant dark blue cytoplasm, small cytoplasmic vacuoles and tingible-body macrophages (haematoxylin & eosin stain, ×400)

laryngeal region, infiltrating the right vocal cord and reducing the laryngeal lumen (Fig. 4).

The thoraco-abdominal CT scan showed no other localization.

The examination of the cephalorachidian liquid showed no central nervous system involvement. The patient was diagnosed with thyroidal Burkitt lymphoma, stage I of Murphy [3].

After cardiac, renal and liver functions assessment, the patient received chemotherapy according to the LMBA02 protocol [4], group A (Age > 60 years, no CNS nor bone marrow involvement), with a first course of COP (Cyclophosphamide, Vincristine and Prednisone) and intrathecal Methotrexate, followed a week after by a course of R-COPADEM (Rituximab at day 0 and day 6, Cyclophosphamide day 2,3 and 4, Prednisone from day 1 to 5, Doxorubicineat day 2, high dose Methotrexate at day 1 with folic acid rescue from day 2 to day 6 and intrathecal chemotherapy at day 2 and day 6).

At day 15 of chemotherapy, the patient developed febrile neutropenia, refractory to broad-spectrum antibiotics and antifungals. The evolution was marked by the installation of a septic shock with acute respiratory distress syndrome that led to his transfer to intensive care unit where he was intubated and ventilated. The patient died 2 days after.

Discussion

Primary thyroid lymphoma (PTL) is defined as a lymphoma involving only the thyroid gland or the thyroid gland and adjacent (regional) neck lymph nodes, without contiguous spread or distant metastases from other areas of involvement at diagnosis [5].

PTL is an uncommon pathological entity that accounts for only 1 to 5 % of all thyroid malignancies, comprises approximately 2 % of all malignant extra nodal lymphomas and which predominantly originate from B lymphocytes [5, 6].

The common histological subtypes are diffuse large B-cell lymphoma and mucosa-associated lymphoid tissue (MALT) lymphoma [6–9]. Primary Burkitt lymphoma of the thyroid is very rare with a few isolated case reports (Table 1) [1–3, 10, 11].

Burkitt lymphoma is a highly aggressive disease that is endemic in Africa and sporadic in other parts of the world. The endemic variant is associated with Epstein-Barr virus.

BL was one of the first tumours shown to have a chromosomal translocation that activates an oncogene (c-MYC) [12, 13].

Normally, the thyroid gland does not contain native lymphoid tissue, therefore, the intrathyroid lymphoid tissue that causes thyroid lymphoma comes from the migration of lymphoid tissue into the thyroid during an

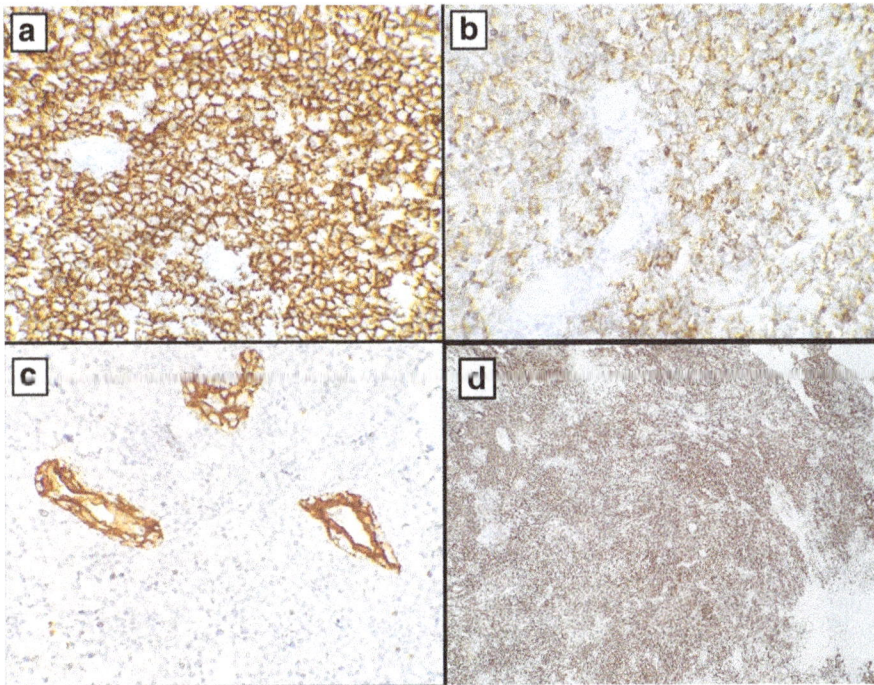

Fig. 3 Immunohistochemical staining revealed the expression of CD20 (**a**) and CD10 (**b**) by the neoplastic cells. Keratin highlights the lymphoepithelial lesions (**c**). Ki-67 immunostaining showed a high proliferation index (**d**)

inflammatory or immunologic process. The most common condition resulting in lymphoid migration is autoimmune thyroiditis (i.e., Hashimoto's thyroiditis) [14–16]. Large adult population-based as well as retrospective clinicopathological case series suggest that primary thyroid Non-Hodgkin lymphoma NHL typically occur in middle to older-aged persons and have a predilection for females (it have also shown that patients with chronic lymphocytic thyroiditis have a greater risk of subsequently developing thyroid lymphoma when compared to age and gender matched normal individuals) [5, 6, 16–21].

Clinically, lymphomas originating in the thyroid can frequently mimic anaplastic thyroid carcinoma in that both have similar clinical characteristics of rapid growth, which might be associated with compression symptoms dyspnea, dysphagia, pain and hoarseness of voice [2, 22–25].

Ultrasonography is generally the initial diagnostic modality used in the workup of thyroid enlargement and nodules. Although nonspecific, there are certain characteristics that

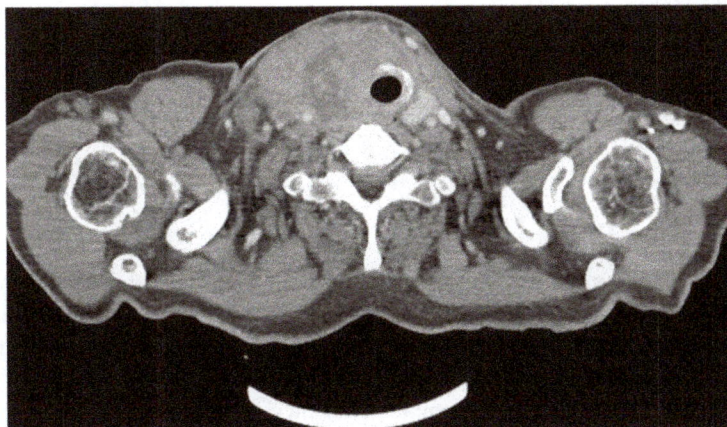

Fig. 4 CT showing a large heterogeneous mass of the thyroid gland

Table 1 Clinical and pathological characteristics of patients with primary Burkitt lymphoma of the thyroid gland in the literature

Author	Age (year)	Sex	Clinical presentation	Size of tumor (cm)	Histology	Translocation type	Treatment	Follow-up time (month)	Evolution
Our case	70	M	Rapidly expanding mass of the neck associated with airway compression symptoms	10.5	Burkitt lymphoma	t (8; 14)	chemotherapy according to the LMBA02 protocol; with a first course of COP and intrathecal Methotrexate, followed by a course of R-COPADEM.	Patient died	The patient died of septic shock, 2 weeks after the first cycle of chemotherapy
Camera et al. [2010] [1]	56	M	Incidental discovery of a large left thyroid lobe nodule on CT	4.9	Burkitt-like large B–cell lymphoma		Left lobe thyroidectomy. After diagnosis, The patient was treated with 8 cycles of intensive chemotherapy (cyclophosphamide, vincristine, doxorubicine, and dexamethasone)	1	Reduction of all lesions with improvement of symptoms.
Kalinyak et al. [2006] [2]	53	M	Tracheal compressive symptoms from a rapidly expanding thyroid mass	6	Burkitt lymphoma		Rituxan and CHOP therapy, changed to hyper-CVAD-R chemotherapy. The patient also received a single dose of intrathecal methotrexate	27	Patient free of disease after end of treatment
Kandil et al. [2012] [10]	60	F	Rapidly expanding thyroid mass with airway compression and difficulty in swallowing	8.7	Burkitt-like lymphoma (B-cell lymphoma, unclassifiable)		Rituximab, Cyclophosphamide, Mensa, Vincristine and Doxorubicin		Successfully treated with 1 cycle of appropriate therapeutic chemotherapy
Cooper et al. [2014] [14]	14	M	Large predominantly left-sided firm thyroid swelling, with a 3-month history of malaise, lethargy, and weight loss	6.7	Burkitt lymphoma	t (8; 14)	COP and prednisolone followed by 2 courses of COPADM, prednisolone and two courses of CYM chemotherapy. This was accompanied by intrathecal chemotherapy	36	Disease free 3 years after end of treatment
Yildiz et al. [2012] [22]	31	M	Rapidly enlarging mass on the fore neck	4	Burkitt lymphoma		R-Hyper-CVAD therapy	6	PET-CT scans performed after chemotherapy and at the 6-month follow-up were normal
Mweempwa et al. [2013] [24]	58	F	Background of benign goiter presented with a rapidly enlarging thyroid mass, causing dysphagia and dyspnea	8	Burkitt lymphoma	t (8; 14)	Modified Magrath protocol for Burkitt's lymphoma, low risk disease, which involved having 3 cycles of R-CODOX-M	4	Complete resolution of the tumour mass, 4 weeks after end of treatment
Liying et al. [2014] [30]	8	M	Mass in the right anterior neck with difficulty in swallowing	4	Burkitt lymphoma	t (8; 14)	Right lobe thyroidectomy. After diagnosis, the patient underwent alternate R-B-NHL-BFM-90-A and R-B-NHL-BFM-90-B treatment, for 4 cycles each	48	After 4 years of follow-up, the patient appears well and remains free of disease

suggest PTL, based essentially upon ultrasound findings of internal echoes, borders, and posterior echoes. For example, Enhanced posterior echoes help in distinguishing lymphoma from other types of thyroid lesions [26, 27].

Once PTL is suspected based upon clinical presentation and ultrasound findings, the next step in diagnosis is biopsy. Traditionally, open surgical biopsy was felt to

be necessary to differentiate thyroid lymphoma from thyroiditis and anaplastic carcinoma. However, with recent advances in immunophenotypic analysis, the accuracy of fine-needle aspiration (FNA) has improved. These advances in diagnosis of PTL mirror those seen with systemic lymphomas with a reported accuracy rate of FNA of 80–100 %. Nevertheless, there are still challenges in

FNA diagnosis of thyroid lymphoma, particularly due to the histological similarities with thyroiditis and the high coincidence of these pathologies within the same gland, which results in increased false-negative rates from sampling error [26].

Histologically, the tumour cells of BL are medium-sized cells (nuclei similar or smaller to those of histiocytes) and show a diffuse monotonous pattern of growth. The cells appear to be cohesive but sometimes exhibit squared-off borders of retracted cytoplasm. The nuclei are round with finely clumped and dispersed chromatin, with multiple basophilic medium-sized, paracentrally situated nucleoli. The cytoplasm is deeply basophilic and usually contains lipid vacuoles. The tumour has an extremely high proliferation fraction (many mitotic figures) as well as a high fraction of apoptosis. A "starry sky" pattern is usually present, which is imparted by numerous benign macrophages that have ingested apoptotic tumour cells [28].

In Burkitt lymphoma, the tumour cells express moderate to strong levels of membrane IgM with light chain restriction and B-cell-associated antigens (CD19, CD20 and CD22), CD10, BCL6, c-MYC and CD38. The neoplastic cells are usually negative or only weakly positive for BCL2 and are uniformly TdT and MUM-1/IRF-4 negative. Nearly 100 % of the cells are positive for Ki67. There are very few admixed T-cells [12, 28–30]. In the present case, the immunophenotype of the atypical lymphoid cells was consistent with these features.

Burkitt lymphoma is characterized at the molecular level by a reciprocal translocation involving the *c-MYC* proto-oncogene, which normally resides on chromosome 8q24. The most common translocation in Burkitt lymphoma is a t (8;14) (q24;q32), which results in the translocation of *c-MYC* to the B-cell heavy-chain gene locus on chromosome 14q32. This translocation occurs in approximately 80 % of Burkitt lymphoma cases regardless of the clinical setting. Other variant translocations involve the translocation of *c-MYC* to the kappa light chain locus on chromosome 2, t (2;8) (p12;q24), which occurs in approximately 15 % of cases, and translocation of *c-MYC* to the lambda light-chain locus on chromosome 22, t (8;22) (q24;q11), which occurs in approximately 5 % of cases [12, 28, 31].

In addition, it has been confirmed that the occurrence of BL is associated with viral infections, particularly EBV infection. However, the EBV detection rates in different subtypes of BL also vary [32]. EBV infection is detected in the vast majority of endemic BL and ~30 % of sporadic BL [12, 30, 32].

Treatment of Burkitt lymphoma in most centers is guided by the FAB LMB study (cooperative study between the Children's Cancer Group, the Societé Francaise d'Oncologie Pediatrique, and the UK Children's Cancer Study Group) [33, 34]. The former consists of initial cytoreduction with cyclophosphamide, prednisolone, and vincristine, followed by more intensive chemotherapy in varying combinations containing doxorubicin, alkylators, vincristine, etoposide and therapy directed to eradicate or to prevent CNS disease such as high dose methotrexate [3, 12].

Aggressive high-dose therapy is needed for adult Burkitt lymphoma. However, interpretation of response is difficult because most studies of this approach have been done with a single protocol in mainly young adults. The regimen generally used in the UK and USA is cyclophosphamide, vincristine, doxorubicin, and highdose methotrexate alternating with ifosfamide, etoposide, and high-dose cytarabine [12].

The use of a less toxic dose adjusted EPOCH (etoposide, prednisone, vincristine, cyclophosphamide, adriamycin) plus rituximab (DA-REPOCH) led to an event free survival of 96 % and an overall survival of 100 % with a median follow up to 86 months in a small study that included 19 HIV negative patients [35]. The use of rituximab (anti-CD20) in primary therapy has been assessed and a randomized clinical trial including 257 patients demonstrated that the addition of rituximab to the LMB regimen improved the event free survival and the overall survival without adding more toxicities [4].

Conclusions

In summary, the current study presents a case of sporadic primary BL of the thyroid occurring in a seventy-year-old male, which exhibited the typical morphological features and immunophenotype of BL and which, to the authors' knowledge, is the first case of BL of the thyroid gland to be reported in Morocco. We also emphasize here the importance of considering lymphoma when dealing with a thyroid mass, as its management is different from that of other thyroid pathologies and delaying treatment has an impact on prognosis.

Abbreviations

BL: Burkitt lymphoma; CT: computerized tomography; EBV: epstein-barr virus; PTL: primary thyroid lymphoma.

Competing interests

The authors declare that they have no competing interests.

Authors' contributions

MA, IB, EMM, SR and MA analyzed and interpreted the patient data, drafted the manuscript and made the figures. MA, AB, MB and MO performed the histological examination and proposed the study. MA, AAB and MO made substantial contributions to conception and design, and revised the manuscript. All authors of this paper have read and given final approval of the version to be published.

Author details

[1]Department of Pathology, Military General Hospital Mohammed V, Mohammed V Souissi University - Faculty of Medicine and Pharmacy of Rabat, Hay Riad, Rabat 10000, Morocco. [2]Department of Clinical Haematology, Military General Hospital Mohammed V, Mohammed V Souissi University - Faculty of Medicine and Pharmacy of Rabat, Hay Riad, Rabat 10000, Morocco. [3]Department of Otorhinolaryngology, Military General Hospital Mohammed V, Mohammed V Souissi University - Faculty of Medicine and Pharmacy of Rabat, Hay Riad, Rabat 10000, Morocco.

References

1. Camera A, Magri F, Fonte R, et al. Burkitt-like lymphoma infiltrating a hyperfunctioning thyroid adenoma and presenting as a hot nodule. Thyroid. 2010;20(9):1033–6.
2. Kalinyak JE, Kong CS, McDougall IR. Burkitt's lymphoma presenting as a rapidly growing thyroid mass. Thyroid. 2006;16(10):1053–7.
3. Murphy SB. Classification, staging and end results of treatment of childhood non- Hodgkin's lymphomas: dissimilarities from lymphomas in adults. Semin Oncol. 1980;7:332–9.
4. Ribrag V, Koscielny S, Bouabdallah K, et al. Addition of rituximab improves outcome of HIV negative patients with Burkitt lymphoma treated with the LMBA protocol: results of the randomized intergroup (GRAALL-lysa) LMBA02 protocol [abstract]. Blood. 2012;120(21):Abstract 685.
5. Derringer GA, Thompson LD, Frommelt RA, Bijwaard KE, Heffess CS, Abbondanzo SL. Malignant lymphoma of the thyroid gland: a clinicopathologic study of 108 cases. Am J Surg Pathol. 2000;24:623e39.
6. Pedersen RK, Pedersen NT. Primary non-Hodgkin's lymphoma of the thyroid gland: a population based study. Histopathology. 1996;28(1):25–32.
7. Earnest LM, Cooper DS, Sciubba JJ, Tufano RP. Thyroid MALT lymphoma in patients with a compressive goiter. Head Neck. 2006;28(8):765–70.
8. Yang L, Wang A, Zhang Y, Mu Y. 12 cases of primary thyroid lymphoma in China. J Endocrinol Investig. 2015;38(7):739–44.
9. Alzouebi M, Goepel JR, Horsman JM, et al. Primary thyroid lymphoma: the 40 year experience of a UK lymphoma treatment centre. Int J Oncol. 2012;40(6):2075–80.
10. Kandil E, Safah H, Noureldine S, et al. Burkitt-like lymphoma arising in the thyroid gland. Am J Med Sci. 2012;343(1):103–5.
11. Ha CS, Shadle KM, Medeiros LJ, Wilder RB, Hess MA, Cabanillas F, et al. Localized non-Hodgkin lymphoma involving the thyroid gland. Cancer. 2001;91:629e35.
12. Molyneux EM, Rochford R, Griffin B, Newton R, Jackson G, Menon G, Harrison CJ, Israels T, Bailey S. Burkitt's lymphoma. Lancet. 2012;379(9822):1234–44.
13. Jaff ES. The 2008 WHO classification of lymphomas: implications for clinical practice and translational research. Hematology Am Soc Hematol Educ Program. 2009;1:523–31.
14. Cooper K, Gangadharan A, Arora RS, Shukla R, Pizer B. Burkitt lymphoma of thyroid gland in an adolescent. Case Rep Pediatr. 2014;2014(187467):3.
15. Ansell SM, Grant CS, Habermann TM. Primary thyroid lymphoma. Semin Oncol. 1999;26(3):316–23.
16. Widder S, Pasieka JL. Primary thyroid lymphomas. Curr Treat Options Oncol. 2004;5:307e13.
17. Holm LE, Bloomgren H, Lowhagen T. Cancer risks in patients with chronic lymphocytic thyroiditis. N Engl J Med. 1985;312:601–4.
18. Matsuzuka F, Miyauchi A, Katayama S, Narabayashi I, Ikeda H, Kuma K, Sugawara M. Clinical aspects of primary thyroid lymphoma: diagnosis and treatment based on our experience of 119 cases. Thyroid. 1993;3(2):93–9.
19. Isaacson PG. Lymphoma of the thyroid gland. Curr Top Patyhol. 1997;91:1e14.
20. Kossev P, Livolsi V. Lymphoid lesions of the thyroid: review in light of the revised Europeane American lymphoma classification and upcoming World Health Organization classification. Thyroid. 1999;9:1273e80.
21. Saxena A, Alport EC, Moshynska O, Kanthan R, Boctor MA. Clonal B cell populations in a minority of patients with Hashimoto's thyroiditis. J Clin Pathol. 2004;57:1258e63.
22. Yildiz I, Sen F, Toz B, et al. Primary Burkitt's lymphoma presenting as a rapidly growing thyroid mass. Case Rep Oncol. 2012;5(2):388–93.
23. Sarinah B, Hisham AN. Primary lymphoma of the thyroid: diagnosis and therapeutic considerations. Asian J Surg. 2010;33(1):20–4.
24. Mweempwa A, Prasad J, Islam S. A rare neoplasm of the thyroid gland. N Z Med J. 2013;126(1369):75–8.
25. Albert S. Primary Burkitt lymphoma of the thyroid. Ear Nose Throat J. 2013;92(12):E1–2.
26. Stein SA, Wartofsky L. Primary thyroid lymphoma: a clinical review. J Clin Endocrinol Metab. 2013;98(8):3131–8.
27. Ota H, Ito Y, Matsuzuka F, et al. Usefulness of ultrasonography for diagnosis of malignant lymphoma of the thyroid. Thyroid. 2006;16:983–7.
28. Swerdlow SH, Campo E, Harris NL, et al. WHO classification of tumours of haematopoietic and lymphoid tissues. Lyon: IARC Press; 2008.
29. Chuang SS, Ye H, Du MQ, Lu CL, Dogan A, Hsieh PP, Huang WT, Jung YC. Histopathology and immunohistochemistry in distinguishing Burkitt lymphoma from diffuse large B-cell lymphoma with very high proliferation index and with or without a starry–sky pattern: a comparative study with EBER and FISH. Am J Clin Pathol. 2007;128(4):558–64.
30. Liying Z, Lanxiang G, Guang L, Luping W, Chunwei X, Lin L, Yuwang T, Huiru F, Zhe G. Primary Burkitt's lymphoma of the thyroid without Epstein-Barr virus infection: a case report and literature review. Oncol Lett. 2014;7(5):1519–24.
31. Hecht JL, Aster JC. Molecular biology of Burkitt's lymphoma. J Clin Oncol. 2000;18(21):3707–21.
32. Queiroga EM, Gualco G, Chioato L, Harrington WJ, Araujo I, Weiss LM, Bacchi CE. Viral studies in Burkitt lymphoma: association with Epstein Barr virus but not HHV 8. Am J Clin Patho. 2008;130:186–92.
33. Patte C, Philip T, Rodary C, et al. High survival rate in advanced-stage B-cell lymphomas and leukemias without CNS involvement with a short intensive polychemotherapy: results from the French pediatric oncology society of a randomized trial of 216 children. J Clin Oncol. 1991;9(1):123–32.
34. Patte C, Auperin A, Michon J, et al. The Societe Francaise d'Oncologie pediatrique LMB89 protocol: highly effective multiagent chemotherapy tailored to the tumor burden and initial response in 561 unselected children with B-cell lymphomas and L3 leukemia. Blood. 2001;97:3370–79.
35. Dunleavy K, Pittaluga S, Shovlin M, et al. Low-intensity therapy in adults with Burkitt's lymphoma. N Engl J Med. 2013;369(20):1915–25.

13

Extracellular vesicles: potential applications in cancer diagnosis, prognosis, and epidemiology

Mukesh Verma[*], Tram Kim Lam, Elizabeth Hebert and Rao L Divi

Abstract

Both normal and diseased cells continuously shed extracellular vesicles (EVs) into extracellular space, and the EVs carry molecular signatures and effectors of both health and disease. EVs reflect dynamic changes that are occurring in cells and tissue microenvironment in health and at a different stage of a disease. EVs are capable of altering the function of the recipient cells. Trafficking and reciprocal exchange of molecular information by EVs among different organs and cell types have been shown to contribute to horizontal cellular transformation, cellular reprogramming, functional alterations, and metastasis. EV contents may include tumor suppressors, phosphoproteins, proteases, growth factors, bioactive lipids, mutant oncoproteins, oncogenic transcripts, microRNAs, and DNA sequences. Therefore, the EVs present in biofluids offer unprecedented, remote, and non-invasive access to crucial molecular information about the health status of cells, including their driver mutations, classifiers, molecular subtypes, therapeutic targets, and biomarkers of drug resistance. In addition, EVs may offer a non-invasive means to assess cancer initiation, progression, risk, survival, and treatment outcomes. The goal of this review is to highlight the current status of information on the role of EVs in cancer, and to explore the utility of EVs for cancer diagnosis, prognosis, and epidemiology.

Keywords: Cancer, Diagnosis, Epidemiology, Extracellular vesicles, Exosomes, Microvesicles

Introduction
Conventional biomarkers and circulating biomarkers
Living cells secrete a large number of endocytic or plasma membrane vesicle including exosomes, microvesicles (MVs), and apoptotic bodies into extracellular space [1-3] called extracellular vesicles (EVs). Different names are reported in the literature for EVs, such as exosomes, ectosomes, oncosomes, apoptotic bodies, microparticles, and microvesicles (MVs) [3]. Based on intracellular origin or biogenesis, two major classes of EVs are reported: exosomes and MVs [4].

The exosomes, nano-particle size (30–100 nm) vesicles with a buoyant density of 1.13 – 1.19 g/cm³, are shed by both healthy and diseased cells. Exosomes are derived from the endolysosomal pathway and originate from the endosomal compartment called multivesicular bodies. Lee et al. reported that EVs may be generated by mesenchymal stem cells and their involvement in suppressing angiogenesis [5]. Other cell types, such as platelets,

neutrophils, reticulocytes, macrophages, megakaryocytes, monocytes, B and T cells, mast cells, and endothelial cells, release EVs [6].

The microvesticles are generated by budding from the plasma membrane. The microvesicles are 100–1000 nm in size and originate from budding and fusion of plasma membrane into extracellular space, and share several similarities with the parental cells, including having membrane lipids, receptors, and several types of nucleic acids and proteins [1,7-10].

In general, the molecular composition of each EV closely mimics the parental cell or tissue and contains growth factors, receptors, proteases, adhesion molecules, microRNAs (miRNAs), proteins, and lipids [1,7,8]. Several studies reported the presence of numerous bioactive proteins, nucleic acids, lipids and other biomolecules in the EVs [1,11,12]. Caby et al. demonstrated that EVs contain tetraspanin molecules such as CD9, CD63, and CD81; class I and class II major histocompatibility complex (MHC) molecules; and lysosomal-associated membrane protein-2 (LAMP-2) [7]. Thakur et al. demonstrated the presence of double stranded DNA (representing whole

* Correspondence: vermam@mail.nih.gov
Epidemiology and Genomics Research Program, Division of Cancer Control and Population Sciences, National Cancer Institute, National Institutes of Health, Rockville, MD 20850, USA

genome) inside exosomes isolated from myeloid leukemia, colorectal carcinoma, and melanoma cells [13].

Cancer development is a multistep and multifactorial process that includes uncontrolled growth, resistance to apoptosis, genetic and epigenetic changes, and alterations in the surrounding microenvironment. These changes include the development of EVs and some have speculated that EVs can be potentially used as biomarkers for disease diagnosis, prognosis, and epidemiology [3,4,14-19]. Generally biomarkers indicate the turbulence in the normal biological status that contributes to carcinogenesis. Currently, a number of biomarkers, mostly from circulating cells, are used in diagnosing cancer [15-19], epidemiology [20-23], and treatment follow up [24-26]. Many of the existing biomarkers offer insufficient information about the tissue origin and thus it is difficult to use them in targeted therapy [16]. In turn, this significantly limits their utility in both research and the clinical setting.

Inherent characteristics of EVs may make them ideal next-generation biomarkers for the 21st century research and therapy. The involvement of EVs in intracellular communication and the dynamic nature of their composition, for example, have allowed investigators to explore their tumor-modulating potential [1,4,27-29]. It has been shown that the quantity and composition of EVs changes during cancer development [1,3,30]. For example, Baran et al. reported elevation of number of EVs in gastric cancer patients and the number correlated with the stage of cancer development [31]. Increased expression of CCR6 and Her-2/neu was also observed in plasma samples from patients with advanced stage of the disease. Levels of PTEN present inside exosomes isolated from prostate cancer patients correlated with the development of disease and used for prostate cancer diagnosis [32]. Furthermore, EVs have excellent biodistribution and biocompatibility [33]; these qualities make them ideal for use in drug delivery and distribution. The fact that EVs contain functional nucleic acids suggests that they are like viral particles [34].

EVs have been found in several biofluids including amniotic fluid [35], breast milk [36], bronchoalveolar lavage [37], cerebro-spinal fluid [38], malignant ascites [39], plasma [40], saliva [41] and urine [42]. The ubiquity of EVs in the biofluids, coupled with the fact that they reflect the composition of their parent cells, offer a unique platform for population-based research. It is biologically plausible that EVs could contribute significantly and prospectively to the characterization of normal versus disease states. For example, in epidemiologic research it is challenging and in some cases not feasible to collect multiple biospecimens prior to the development of a disease in large prospective cohort studies. With EVs, epidemiologists could obtain a serial collection of biofluids containing EVs via a non-invasive or minimally invasive

approach from both controls and cases. Morphological, molecular and functional analysis of these EV-riched biofluids could be conducted and expand our understanding of cancer risk and development. Investigators have shown differential molecular profiles of EVs in cancer patients' sera/plasma from breast [43-46], prostate [32,47-50], lung [51], liver [52], gastric [53], glioblastoma [54,55], KSHV-associated malignancies [56]; and urine from prostate [57-59].

Table 1 presents a list of tumor types in which EVs have been reported, and Table 2 provides a list of biospecimens in which EVs may be isolated for diagnosis, prognosis, and epidemiology. Viaud et al. and other groups proposed using EVs as a cell-free vaccine in therapeutics [5,60].

Review
EV biogeneration
There are two main pathways of exosomal generation, endocytic and exocytic. According to the endocytic pathway, exosomes are formed in a two step process and are released from the plasma membrane via the endosomal sorting complex required for transport (ESCRT) [61]. The second pathway is ESCRT independent and require sphingolipid (ceramide) [62], tetraspanins [63], and heat shock proteins [64]. Ghossoub et al. characterized proteins such as GTPase ADP ribosylation factor 6 (ARF6) and its effector phospholipase D2 (PLD2) involved in biogenesis of exosomes [65]. These two proteins control budding of intraluminal vesicles into multivesicular bodies. Few other proteins involved in biogenesis process include TSG101 [66,67], Rab5 [68], Rab7 [69], Vps4, and Vps36 [70]. Among them TSG101 is an integral part of the ESCRT (this complex includes ESCRT-0, ESCRT-I, ESCRT-II, ESCRT-III, ALIX, and TSG101 [71]). ALIX promotes intraluminal budding of vesicles in endosomes upon interaction with syntenin which is the cytoplasmic adapter of heparin sulfate proteoglycan receptor [72].

Different types of EVs are generated from endosomes and during maturation of the endosomes they accumulate intraluminal vesicles. Protein sorting in these vesicles depends on monoubiquitination and the endosomal sorting complex required for transport. mRNA recruitment is guided by a zip code in the 3'UTR, and miRNA by physical and functional coupling of RNA-induced silencing complexes (RISCs). MV as opposed to exosomes synthesis involves an increase in cytosolic Ca++, which activates different pathways, resulting in depolymerization of the actin cytoskeleton and, finally, the release of MVs [6]. In HPV-positive cells, silencing of the E6/E7 proteins resulted in alterations in the number and composition of MVs [73]. MVs from HPV-positive cells contained higher levels of survivin and anti-apoptotic proteins compared to HPV-negative cells. In lung cancer, MVs are released in circulation and in pleural effusion due to lung cancer [3].

Table 1 Extracellular vesicles' analysis in different tumor types

Cancer types	Comments	References
Bladder cancer	Exosomes from urine contain the angiogenesis-promoting protein EDIL-3	[99]
Breast cancer	Microvesicle numbers and the amount of focal adhesion kinase and EGFR in plasma fractions were associated with different stages of breast cancer	[89]
Colorectal cancer	Proteomic analysis was conducted on EVs from colorectal cancer cells	[103]
Gastric cancer	Proteomic analysis was conducted on EVs from gastric cancer patients	[31]
Glioblastoma	Microvesicle RNA biomarkers of glioblastoma multiforme were identified	[29,55]
Head and neck cancer	Exosomes and microvesicles from patient saliva were used for diagnosis	[104]
Lung cancer	Proteins isolated from microvesicles in pleural effusions due to lung cancer were characterized to identify diagnostic markers	[3]
Melanoma	Proteomic analysis was conducted on exosomes from melanoma patients were used for	[105]
Ovarian cancer	Exosomes from ovarian cancer patients contain different sets of proteins and miRNAs compared to exosomes from normal subjects; the amount of circulating exosomes was 4 times higher in patients	[1,2,92,93,106]
Pancreatic cancer	EVs were used in diagnosing pancreatic cancer	[30]
Prostate cancer	Urine exosomes expressed higher levels of PCA-3 and TMPRSS2-ERG	[58]

About 900 MV specific proteins were identified from pleural effusion of nonsmall cell lung cancer patients. These proteins were different from EV proteins isolated from patients with other cancer types. Park et al. developed bioinformatics tools and identified pathologically-significant proteins from those 912 MV specific proteins from lung cancer patients [3]. Ostrowski et al. demonstrated the role of Rab27a and Rab27 b in exosome secretion pathway [74].

EV functions

Various biological roles have been proposed for EVs, including disposal of superfluous or harmful cellular content, emission of signaling and regulatory molecules for cell-cell communication and functional modification, propagation of pathogens, stimulation or inhibition of the immune system, antigen presentation, and many more [4,75]. EVs are involved in both beneficial and pathological functions. EVs can be used in cancer diagnosis and prognosis precisely because the function of the original cell can be extrapolated by examining EV composition (proteins, mRNAs, miRNAs, non-coding RNAs, lipids, and other molecules) in body fluids. Kahlert et al. demonstrated the presence of double stranded DNA in serum collected from pancreatic cancer patients [9]. DNA isolated from these EVs was used to detect p53 and KRAS mutations. Collectively, EVs were not shown to contain mitochondrial, nuclear, or endoplasmic reticulum proteins [76,77]. Exosomes, specifically, do not contain most of the ribosomal RNAs and contain mainly mRNAs and miRNAs [58]. EVs can interact with target cells directly via cell surface receptors, or can be internalized by target cells via membrane fusion or endocytosis [78]. Once EV-associated signaling molecules are recognized, the target cell's function is modified or regulated.

EV isolation and analysis of the contents

Table 3 shows the methods that are used for isolating extracellular vesicles. Obtaining pure exosomes is critical for preserving the physicochemical and functional characteristics of the exosomes. Most frequently used and accepted method for enriching EVs is ultracentrifugation

Table 2 Biofluids/biospecimens used to isolate extracellular vesicles for cancer diagnosis, prognosis, and epidemiology

Biospecimen	Comments	References
Ascites	Used in diagnosing ovarian cancer and determining its aggressiveness	[39]
Blood and plasma	Used in diagnosing ovarian cancer and breast cancer	[89,93]
Breast milk	Exosomes were isolated from breast milk	[36]
Mesenchymal stem cells	Suppression of angiogenesis shown in tumor cells mediated by miR-16 isolated from exosomes	[5]
Pregnancy-associated sera	Exosomes were isolated in different stages of pregnancy	[107]
Saliva	Exosomes and MVs found in patient saliva	[104]
Stem cells	Renal stem cells contained MVs with angiogenesis-specific mRNAs and miRNAs	[94]
Tissues	Ovarian cancer tissues were used to isolate exosomes and then in isolating miRNAs from them	[1,14]
Urine	Urine was used to isolate exosomes and in analyzing proteins by MS or transcriptome analysis	[58,99]

Table 3 Methods for isolating extracellular vesicles (EVs)

EV Isolation Method	Sample	~ Time required for isolation	Reference/Company
Deferential centrifugation	Serum, urine and cell culture supernatant	2-15 h	[79]
Deferential centrifugation	Cell culture supernatant or saliva	2-15 h	[108,109]
Density gradient centrifugation	Cell culture supernatant	24 h	[80]
Sequential membrane filtration	Cell culture supernatant and biofluids	24 h	[81,110]
Nanomembrane	Urine	<2 h	[82]
Size exclusion chromatography	Plasma	20 min	[111]
Microfluidics	Cell culture supernatant	-	[112]
Nanoshearing	Cell culture supernatant and serum	-	[46]
ExoCap	Cell culture supernatant and biofluids	30 min	MBL International
ExomiR	Cell-free biofluids' exosomal RNA	20 min	Bioo Scientific
Exo-spin	Cell culture supernatant, urine and saliva	3 h	Cell Guidance Systems
ExoQuick	Serum, plasma, ascites, urine, CSF and cell culture supernatant	2-15 h	System Bioscinces
miRCURY	Serum, plasma, cells, urine and CSF	2 h	Exiqon
Total exosome isolation	Cell culture supernatant and biofluids	2 h	Life Technologies
PureExo	Serum, plasma and cell culture supernatant	2 h	101Bio
ME Kit based on Vn96 peptide binding to heat shock proteins on exosomes	Serum, plasma, urine, cell culture supernatant	30 min	New England Peptide
Streptavidin-biotin-specific antibody to a known antigen on exosome	Cell culture supernatant	>12 h	Life Technologies
Anti-tetraspanin antibody-magnetic bead based	Cell culture supernatant	>12 h	Life Technologies
Anti-EpCAM-antibody magnetic bead based	Cell culture supernatant	>4 h	Life Technologies

[79] followed by density gradient centrifugation [80], however, these procedures are laborious and time consuming (2–24 h). Moreover, protein aggregates may co-precipitate with exosomes and there is a possibility of labile biomolecules being degraded during the long centrifugation steps. Another limitation is that these methods do not offer size separation. Alternatively, size based filtration is another approach for fractionating and obtaining exosome-rich preparations [81,82]. These filter-based methods are quick (<2 h) at isolating exosomes; nevertheless, they have been shown to isolate nano-particle size RNA-protein complexes and chylomicrons whose size (100–350 nm) is similar to the exosomes as well, thus raising concerns about contamination. Currently, polyethylene glycol or other polymers based precipitation is being extensively commercialized as an alternative to isolating exosomes. These precipitation methods are quick (~2 h), but non-specific because they are known to also isolate non-exosome biomolecules and cellular debris. Additionally, affinity methods based on capture of exosomes using peptides or antibodies are being used as specific methods.

The current technologies are thus limited, and moving forward, simpler methods are needed. Improved methods must be able to combine isolation of pure exosomes and analysis, since the existing methods are not perfect and yield varying compositions and quality of exosomes. Microfluidics combined with biosensors, employing biological or biomimetic capture agents, may quickly isolate total or specific exosomes and facilitate faster and cheaper analysis of exosomal cargo. This technology may advance our understanding of EVs, and increase EVs utility in research and therapy.

Methods to characterize EVs are emerging and developing. Extracellular vesicles have been routinely characterized using transmission electron microscopy (TEM), florescence microscopy or flow cytometry [83]. There are several limitations to TEM. It is expensive and requires specialized experience, the sensitivity of the fluorescence microscopy is not optimal for nano-micro vesicle characterization. Nanoparticle tracking analysis (NTA), designed to measure the size and concentration of EVs, is based on flow cytometry. NTA has been reported to be used for analyzing circulating EVs [84]. Wei et al. established a method called electric field induced release and measurement (EFIRM) for simultaneously disrupting and releasing exosomal RNA/biomarkers for on-site monitoring [85]. They have adapted the method for blood and saliva [85]. A multiplexed microfluidic device for specific capture and detection of exosomal contents using nanoshearing technology, based on a tunable alternating current electrohydrodynamic (ac-EHD) methodology, was used for measuring human epidermal growth factor receptor 2 (HER2) and PSA in human samples [46]. Ueda et al. developed anti-CD9 antibody-coupled to highly porous monolithic silica microtips for exosome extraction from multiple clinical samples, and applied it to measure exosomal proteins by mass spectrometry in serum samples from lung cancer patients [51].

Recent estimates indicate that 1 ml serum (or comparable amounts of other biofluids) is sufficient to analyze EV miRNAs and proteins [30]. Park et al. isolated 912 proteins from MVs from the pleural effusion of non-small lung cancer patients by applying nuclear magnetic resonance mass spectrometry (NMR-MS) followed by SDS-PAGE [3]. The composition of MVs from these lung cancer patients was different than MVs from other malignancies such as breast, prostate, and colon cancers. Further characterization of these proteins (mainly lung-enriched surface antigens and proteins related to epidermal growth factor receptor [EGFR] signaling) indicated their potential in lung cancer diagnosis. Ovarian cancer ascites were isolated by centrifuging malignant ascites to remove cells, followed by sucrose gradient centrifugation [39]. The pelleted vesicles were further characterized by gelatin zymography [86]. Ascite-derived exosomes exhibit gelatinolytic activity, and gelatinases increase tumor progression [87]. Analysis of EV proteins was achieved by liquid chromatography combined with matrix-assisted laser ionization/desorption time of flight mass spectrometry (LC-MALDI-TOF MS) [88]. Specific MV proteins, such as focal adhesion kinase and EGFR, from breast cancer patient sera were characterized by Western blotting [89].

Pathological functions of exosomes and utility in cancer research

In response to pathological alterations, cells communicate with each other by secreting a heterogeneous mixture of vesicles (including MVs and exosomes) with different compositions. Pegtel et al. demonstrated that miRNAs present in the exosomes isolated from Epstein-Barr Virus (EBV)-infected cells could release their miRNA (and induce silencing of specific genes) when kept in contact with surrounding uninfected B cells [90]. Whether EVs are released from the infected host or infectious agent, information from the analysis of EVs may facilitate their use as biomarkers for diagnosis. The EV content analysis also will promote understanding of host-infectious agent interaction to enable effective vaccine design and development of novel therapeutics [91].

Using EVs to diagnose cancer

EVs' contents reflect the content of the cells (both stromal and tumor) from which they originate. EVs could be used as biomarkers for diagnosis or to predict or monitor a patient's response to treatment. It has been demonstrated, at least in the case of ovarian cancer, that the profiling of miRNAs isolated from circulating exosomes is similar to exosomes present in tissue [14]. This suggests that circulating exosomes can be used as a surrogate for tissue miRNAs, and exosome-derived miRNA profiling can be used as a diagnostic biomarker for ovarian cancer.

Differential prevalence of EVs has been identified in varying tumor types (Table 1) which could be exploited for future research. For example, diagnostic biomarkers for ovarian cancer are currently unknown and approximately 70% of ovarian cancer cases are diagnosed at an advanced stage. Emerging evidence suggests that exosome biomarkers may be useful in ovarian cancer screening [2]. Specifically, Went et al. showed that the amount of circulating exosomes released from tissues is four times higher in ovarian cancer patients than in normal subjects [92]. Liang et al. characterized the proteomic and genomic profiling of ovarian cancer exosomes [2]. This study showed that epithelial cell adhesion molecule (EpCAM), CD24, and miRNAs are present in the exosomes. These contents may serve as additional biomarkers for use in diagnosing ovarian cancer. Since EpCAM overexpression was reported to be correlated with epithelial cell proliferation, a technology using microbeads coated with EpCAM antibodies may be used for isolating ovarian cancer exosomes for further analysis [93]. Taylor et al. demonstrated that exosomal miRNA profiling can be used as diagnostic biomarkers for ovarian cancer [14]. This study showed that a group of miRNAs (miR-21, miR-141, miR-200a, miR-200b, miR-200c, miR-205, and miR-214) present in the exosomes possessed characteristics similar to those isolated from ovarian tissue. Furthermore, higher levels of these miRNAs are correlated with advanced ovarian cancer [14].

In addition to exosomes, the diagnostic promise also holds for microvesicles in several malignancies. Elevated levels of MVs were reported in sera from breast cancer patients compared to normal individuals [89]. In renal cancer, MVs containing different miRNAs and mRNAs were released from renal cancer stem cells, and their role in tumor vascularization has been proposed [94,95]. To identify an EV biomarker for glioblastoma multiforme, serum MVs were analyzed by microarray expression analysis, and a group of RNAs that are upregulated or downregulated in this tumor type was identified [29,55]. Transcriptome analysis of urine exosomes from prostate cancer patients showed higher levels of PCA-3 and TMPRSS2-ERG when compared with controls [58]. Because prostate cancer tissue is heterogeneous in its phenotypes, a biopsy taken from a specific site may not represent the overall tumor malignancy status, including tumor-specific variants, mutations, and levels of mRNAs and miRNAs for diagnosing prostate cancer. Transcriptome analysis of circulating vesicles, however, may be representative of prostate cancer malignancy status.

Using EVs to determine cancer aggressiveness

Identification of cancer aggressiveness is an important marker in prognosis. There is promising evidence that EVs can be capitalized for this purpose [96]. For example, in ovarian cancer, higher levels of CD24 indicate worst prognosis and reduce patient survival rates [97]. A study showed that levels of EpCAM and CD24 present in exosomes were correlated with the aggressiveness of ovarian cancer [39]. In that study, Runz and colleagues isolated ascites-derived exosomes from ovarian cancer patients. They found that cytoplasmic localization of CD24 occurred in tumors with high invasive potential. In melanoma, exosomes isolated from metastatic cells were capable of making primary tumor aggressive by permanently converting bone marrow progenitors [96]. Proteins involved in regulation of membrane trafficking and exosome formation, such as RAB1A, RAB5B, RAB7, and RAB27A, were highly expressed in these melanoma cells. In bladder cancer, exosomes isolated from the urine of high-grade bladder cancer patients had higher levels of EDIL-3, a molecule that promotes angiogenesis, compared to exosomes from healthy individuals [98,99]. The line of evidence extends to hepatocellular carcinoma where EDIL-3 was shown to be overexpressed in tumors [100]. EDIL-3 plays a role in tumor progression. Receptor tyrosine kinase MET mediates exosome mediated metastatic behavior in the melanoma mice model. When Met expression was reduced in exosomes, the pro-metastatic behavior of bone marrow cell also diminished [96].

Using EVS for therapeutic purposes

As mentioned earlier, applying EVs in therapeutics as a cell-free vaccine was proposed by Viaud et al. and others [5,60]. Advantages of EVs include that they are non-living and easily recovered from biological fluids. These are bioavailable vehicles that are well tolerated; targetable to specific tissues; resistant to metabolic processes; and, most-importantly, membrane-permeable. EVs are considered ideal candidates for delivery of miRNAs/small interfering RNAs (siRNAs), or drugs that otherwise would be degraded rapidly. Potential applications of EVs in cancer therapeutics also were proposed recently [4]. EVs can be loaded with a selective combination of drugs for delivery with minimal issues related to immunity and passing the blood–brain barrier [101]. EVs are stable in the blood and can deliver functional RNAs to host cells. For personalized medicine, EVs collected from one individual can be enriched, mixed with a drug(s), and given back to the same individual without causing immunity-related issues. EVs from tumors carry tumor

antigens and present them to T cells, priming them to induce the anti-tumor response and resulting in tumor cell death [27,28]. Using EVs, especially nanovesicles, in cell-free cancer vaccines also has been proposed [101]. EVs are capable of priming the immune system to recognize tumor-specific antigens and initiate an appropriate immunologic response toward the abnormal cancer cell while leaving the normal surrounding cells unchanged.

Potential utility of EVs for population-based research

Beyond clinical and therapeutic usefulness, EVs can be exploited for population-based research in several ways. For example, the bioavailability of EVs (from milk, urine, blood, serum, etc.) may be capitalized for epidemiologic research in which longitudinal studies are difficult to conduct using tissue biospecimens. EVs offer a non-invasive and almost continuous access to circulating information on the disease state in epidemiologic investigations. In addition, cancer epidemiologists may use EVs to investigate whether the characteristics of EVs may be influenced by exposure to certain carcinogenic factors (e.g., smoking, physical activity, obesity). In turn, EVs may be used as biomarkers in epidemiologic studies to characterize the mechanistic underpinnings and follow up on findings from association studies. There is evidence to support EVs utility. Data from a study by Xu et al. [102] showed that arsenic-transformed human bronchial epithelial cells release exosomal miR-21 that subsequently stimulated normal neighboring cells. These data suggest that neoplastic cell-to-normal cell communication mediated by an exosomal miRNA may be involved in carcinogenesis induced by exogenous factors.

Challenges and potential solutions

Although the concentration of EVs increases in cancer, the methods for EV isolation tend to be time-consuming and yield samples that need further purification. These factors, together with the high costs currently associated with this process, may limit research—particularly in epidemiologic studies in which thousands of samples are analyzed. Therefore, further improvements in EV isolation, purification, and content analysis are required. Further, current isolation technologies make it difficult to distinguish different EV subpopulations. This explains the broad use of the term "EVs" in publications instead of specific types of EVs (e.g., exosomes and MVs). Contamination from RNA-protein complexes, protein aggregates, and other micro particles may affect the results. Therefore, there is a need for technologies which can isolate highly pure EVs for downstream analysis (transcriptomics, miRnomics, proteomics).

Because of the multifunctional nature of EVs, it is important to understand the balance between healthy and oncogenic EV signaling. One way to use EVs for therapeutic purposes is to remove these vesicles to prevent metastasis and tumorigenesis. However, the technical and financial challenges involved in removing EVs have prevented the clinical implementation of this technique to date. Technological improvements being made may change this in near future.

At times, MVs released from a specific organ site exhibit the properties of drug resistance by carrying multidrug resistance (MDR) proteins [6]. There is a need to understand how EV biosynthesis and/or intercellular communication can be altered so that EVs can be used for targeted therapies. Research also is needed to evaluate whether therapies that target the uptake of tumor-derived EVs by recipient cells are specific enough to prevent side effects. A better understanding of the molecular mechanisms that underlie EV biosynthesis and their physiological relevance also is needed.

Conclusions

Despite the challenges cited above, the scientific community is interested in these tissue-derived vesicles and their multiple roles and functions. EVs hold great promise for cancer diagnosis and treatment. Likewise, there are many potential uses of EVs in cancer research and epidemiology.

Abbreviations

EGFR: Epidermal growth factor receptor; EpCAM: Epithelial cell adhesion molecule; ESCRT: Endosomal sorting complex required for transport; EVs: Evesicles; mRNA: messenger RNA; miRNA: microRNA; MVs: Microvesicles.

Competing interests

The authors declare that they have no competing interests.

Authors' contributions

All authors contributed in planning, developing, and writing the manuscript. All authors read and approved the final manuscript.

Acknowledgements

We are thankful to Joanne Brodsky of Scientific Consulting group (SCG) for reading the manuscript and providing comments.

References

1. Beach A, Zhang HG, Ratajczak MZ, Kakar SS. Exosomes: an overview of biogenesis, composition and role in ovarian cancer. J Ovarian Res. 2014;7(1):14.
2. Liang B, Peng P, Chen S, Li L, Zhang M, Cao D, et al. Characterization and proteomic analysis of ovarian cancer-derived exosomes. J Proteomics. 2013;80C:171–82.
3. Park JO, Choi DY, Choi DS, Kim HJ, Kang JW, Jung JH, et al. Identification and characterization of proteins isolated from microvesicles derived from human lung cancer pleural effusions. Proteomics. 2013;13(14):2125–34.
4. Vader P, Breakefield XO, Wood MJ. Extracellular vesicles: emerging targets for cancer therapy. Trends Mol Med. 2014;20(7):385–93.
5. Lee JK, Park SR, Jung BK, Jeon YK, Lee YS, Kim MK, et al. Exosomes derived from mesenchymal stem cells suppress angiogenesis by down-regulating VEGF expression in breast cancer cells. PLoS One. 2013;8(12):e84256.
6. Jorfi S, Inal JM. The role of microvesicles in cancer progression and drug resistance. Biochem Soc Trans. 2013;41(1):293–8.
7. Caby MP, Lankar D, Vincendeau-Scherrer C, Raposo G, Bonnerot C. Exosomal-like vesicles are present in human blood plasma. Int Immunol. 2005;17(7):879–87.
8. Ren Y, Yang J, Xie R, Gao L, Yang Y, Fan H, et al. Exosomal-like vesicles with immune-modulatory features are present in human plasma and can induce CD4+ T-cell apoptosis in vitro. Transfusion. 2011;51(5):1002–11.
9. Kahlert C, Melo SA, Protopopov A, Tang J, Seth S, Koch M, et al. Identification of double-stranded genomic DNA spanning all chromosomes with mutated KRAS and p53 DNA in the serum exosomes of patients with pancreatic cancer. J Biol Chem. 2014;289(7):3869–75.
10. Pisetsky DS, Gauley J, Ullal AJ. Microparticles as a source of extracellular DNA. Immunol Res. 2011;49(1–3):227–34.
11. Mathivanan S, Fahner CJ, Reid GE, Simpson RJ. ExoCarta 2012: database of exosomal proteins, RNA and lipids. Nucleic Acids Res. 2012;40(Database issue):D1241–4.
12. Simpson RJ, Kalra H, Mathivanan S. ExoCarta as a resource for exosomal research. J Extracellular Vesicles. 2012;1:1–7.
13. Thakur BK, Zhang H, Becker A, Matei I, Huang Y, Costa-Silva B, et al. Double-stranded DNA in exosomes: a novel biomarker in cancer detection. Cell Res. 2014;24(6):766–9.
14. Taylor DD, Gercel-Taylor C. MicroRNA signatures of tumor-derived exosomes as diagnostic biomarkers of ovarian cancer. Gynecol Oncol. 2008;110(1):13–21.
15. Cen P, Ni X, Yang J, Graham DY, Li M. Circulating tumor cells in the diagnosis and management of pancreatic cancer. Biochim Biophys Acta. 2012;1826(2):350–6.
16. Jin T, Peng H, Wu H. Clinical value of circulating liver cancer cells for the diagnosis of hepatocellular carcinoma: a meta-analysis. Biomed Rep. 2013;1(5):731–6.
17. Mockelmann N, Laban S, Pantel K, Knecht R. Circulating tumor cells in head and neck cancer: clinical impact in diagnosis and follow-up. Eur Arch Otorhinolaryngol. 2014;271(1):15–21.
18. Ren C, Chen H, Han C, Jin G, Wang D, Wang D, et al. Detection and molecular analysis of circulating tumor cells for early diagnosis of pancreatic cancer. Med Hypotheses. 2013;80(6):833–6.
19. Saad F, Pantel K. The current role of circulating tumor cells in the diagnosis and management of bone metastases in advanced prostate cancer. Future Oncol. 2012;8(3):321–31.
20. Boffetta P. Biomarkers in cancer epidemiology: an integrative approach. Carcinogenesis. 2010;31(1):121–6.
21. Fader AN, Arriba LN, Frasure HE, von Gruenigen VE. Endometrial cancer and obesity: epidemiology, biomarkers, prevention and survivorship. Gynecol Oncol. 2009;114(1):121–7.
22. Verma M. Epigenome-Wide Association Studies (EWAS) in cancer. Curr Genomics. 2012;13(4):308–13.
23. Verma M, Patel P, Verma M. Biomarkers in prostate cancer epidemiology. Cancers. 2011;3(4):3773–98.
24. Grotenhuis AJ, Vermeulen SH, Kiemeney LA. Germline genetic markers for urinary bladder cancer risk, prognosis and treatment response. Future Oncol. 2010;6(9):1433–60.
25. Kesisis G, Kontovinis LF, Gennatas K, Kortsaris AH. Biological markers in breast cancer prognosis and treatment. J BUON. 2010;15(3):447–54.
26. Pasche B, Grant SC. Non-small cell lung cancer and precision medicine: a model for the incorporation of genomic features into clinical trial design. JAMA. 2014;311(19):1975–6.
27. Cho JA, Yeo DJ, Son HY, Kim HW, Jung DS, Ko JK, et al. Exosomes: a new delivery system for tumor antigens in cancer immunotherapy. Int J Cancer. 2005;114(4):613–22.
28. Schorey JS, Bhatnagar S. Exosome function: from tumor immunology to pathogen biology. Traffic. 2008;9(6):871–81.
29. Skog J, Wurdinger T, van Rijn S, Meijer DH, Gainche L, Sena-Esteves M, et al. Glioblastoma microvesicles transport RNA and proteins that promote tumour growth and provide diagnostic biomarkers. Nat Cell Biol. 2008;10(12):1470–6.
30. Zoller M. Pancreatic cancer diagnosis by free and exosomal miRNA. World J Gastrointest Pathophysiol. 2013;4(4):74–90.
31. Baran J, Baj-Krzyworzeka M, Weglarczyk K, Szatanek R, Zembala M, Barbasz J, et al. Circulating tumour-derived microvesicles in plasma of gastric cancer patients. Cancer Immunol Immunother. 2010;59(6):841–50.
32. Gabriel K, Ingram A, Austin R, Kapoor A, Tang D, Majeed F, et al. Regulation of the tumor suppressor PTEN through exosomes: a diagnostic potential for prostate cancer. PLoS One. 2013;8(7):e70047.

33. Smyth T, Kullberg M, Malik N, Smith-Jones P, Graner MW, Anchordoquy TJ. Biodistribution and delivery efficiency of unmodified tumor-derived exosomes. J Control Release. 2015;199:145–55.

34. Izquierdo-Useros N, Puertas MC, Borras FE, Blanco J, Martinez-Picado J. Exosomes and retroviruses: the chicken or the egg? Cell Microbiol. 2011;13(1):10–7.

35. Keller S, Rupp C, Stoeck A, Runz S, Fogel M, Lugert S, et al. CD24 is a marker of exosomes secreted into urine and amniotic fluid. Kidney Int. 2007;72(9):1095–102.

36. Admyre C, Johansson SM, Qazi KR, Filen JJ, Lahesmaa R, Norman M, et al. Exosomes with immune modulatory features are present in human breast milk. J Immunol. 2007;179(3):1969–78.

37. Prado N, Marazuela EG, Segura E, Fernandez-Garcia H, Villalba M, Thery C, et al. Exosomes from bronchoalveolar fluid of tolerized mice prevent allergic reaction. J Immunol. 2008;181(2):1519–25.

38. Street JM, Barran PE, Mackay CL, Weidt S, Balmforth C, Walsh TS, et al. Identification and proteomic profiling of exosomes in human cerebrospinal fluid. J Transl Med. 2012;10:2–7.

39. Runz S, Keller S, Rupp C, Stoeck A, Issa Y, Koensgen D, et al. Malignant ascites-derived exosomes of ovarian carcinoma patients contain CD24 and EpCAM. Gynecol Oncol. 2007;107(3):563–71.

40. Grant R, Ansa-Addo E, Stratton D, Antwi-Baffour S, Jorfi S, Kholia S, et al. A filtration-based protocol to isolate human plasma membrane-derived vesicles and exosomes from blood plasma. J Immunol Methods. 2011;371(1–2):143–51.

41. Ogawa Y, Kanai-Azuma M, Akimoto Y, Kawakami H, Yanoshita R. Exosome-like vesicles with dipeptidyl peptidase IV in human saliva. Biol Pharm Bull. 2008;31(6):1059–62.

42. Pisitkun T, Shen RF, Knepper MA. Identification and proteomic profiling of exosomes in human urine. Proc Natl Acad Sci U S A. 2004;101(36):13368–73.

43. Olimon-Andalon V, Aguilar-Lemarroy A, Ratkovich-Gonzalez S, Uribe-Lopez A, Mariscal-Ramirez I, Delgadillo-Cristerna R et al. Proapoptotic CD95L levels in normal human serum and sera of breast cancer patients. Tumour biology : the journal of the International Society for Oncodevelopmental Biology and Medicine 2015:23-28.

44. Khan S, Bennit HF, Turay D, Perez M, Mirshahidi S, Yuan Y, et al. Early diagnostic value of survivin and its alternative splice variants in breast cancer. BMC Cancer. 2014;14:176.

45. Eichelser C, Stuckrath I, Muller V, Milde-Langosch K, Wikman H, Pantel K, et al. Increased serum levels of circulating exosomal microRNA-373 in receptor-negative breast cancer patients. Oncotarget. 2014;5(20):9650–63.

46. Vaidyanathan R, Naghibosadat M, Rauf S, Korbie D, Carrascosa LG, Shiddiky MJ, et al. Detecting exosomes specifically: a multiplexed device based on alternating current electrohydrodynamic induced nanoshearing. Anal Chem. 2014;86(22):11125–32.

47. Khan S, Jutzy JM, Valenzuela MM, Turay D, Aspe JR, Ashok A, et al. Plasma-derived exosomal survivin, a plausible biomarker for early detection of prostate cancer. PLoS One. 2012;7(10):e46737.

48. Lazaro-Ibanez E, Sanz-Garcia A, Visakorpi T, Escobedo-Lucea C, Siljander P, Ayuso-Sacido A, et al. Different gDNA content in the subpopulations of prostate cancer extracellular vesicles: apoptotic bodies, microvesicles, and exosomes. Prostate. 2014;74(14):1379–90.

49. Mizutani K, Terazawa R, Kameyama K, Kato T, Horie K, Tsuchiya T, et al. Isolation of prostate cancer-related exosomes. Anticancer Res. 2014;34(7):3419–23.

50. Bryant RJ, Pawlowski T, Catto JW, Marsden G, Vessella RL, Rhees B, et al. Changes in circulating microRNA levels associated with prostate cancer. Br J Cancer. 2012;106(4):768–74.

51. Ueda K, Ishikawa N, Tatsuguchi A, Saichi N, Fujii R, Nakagawa H. Antibody-coupled monolithic silica microtips for highthroughput molecular profiling of circulating exosomes. Sci Rep. 2014;4:6232.

52. Sugimachi K, Matsumura T, Hirata H, Uchi R, Ueda M, Ueo H, et al. Identification of a bona fide microRNA biomarker in serum exosomes that predicts hepatocellular carcinoma recurrence after liver transplantation. Br J Cancer. 2015;112:532–8.

53. Loei H, Tan HT, Lim TK, Lim KH, So JB, Yeoh KG, et al. Mining the gastric cancer secretome: identification of GRN as a potential diagnostic marker for early gastric cancer. J Proteome Res. 2012;11(3):1759–72.

54. Manterola L, Guruceaga E, Gallego Perez-Larraya J, Gonzalez-Huarriz M, Jauregui P, Tejada S, et al. A small noncoding RNA signature found in exosomes of GBM patient serum as a diagnostic tool. Neuro Oncol. 2014;16(4):520–7.

55. Noerholm M, Balaj L, Limperg T, Salehi A, Zhu LD, Hochberg FH, et al. RNA expression patterns in serum microvesicles from patients with glioblastoma multiforme and controls. BMC Cancer. 2012;12:22.

56. Chugh PE, Sin SH, Ozgur S, Henry DH, Menezes P, Griffith J, et al. Systemically circulating viral and tumor-derived microRNAs in KSHV-associated malignancies. PLoS Pathog. 2013;9(7):e1003484.

57. Neeb A, Hefele S, Bormann S, Parson W, Adams F, Wolf P, et al. Splice variant transcripts of the anterior gradient 2 gene as a marker of prostate cancer. Oncotarget. 2014;5(18):8681–9.

58. Nilsson J, Skog J, Nordstrand A, Baranov V, Mincheva-Nilsson L, Breakefield XO, et al. Prostate cancer-derived urine exosomes: a novel approach to biomarkers for prostate cancer. Br J Cancer. 2009;100(10):1603–7.

59. Lu Q, Zhang J, Allison R, Gay H, Yang WX, Bhowmick NA, et al. Identification of extracellular delta-catenin accumulation for prostate cancer detection. Prostate. 2009;69(4):411–8.

60. Viaud S, Ullrich E, Zitvogel L, Chaput N. Exosomes for the treatment of human malignancies. Horm Metab Res. 2008;40(2):82–8.

61. Johnstone RM, Adam M, Hammond JR, Orr L, Turbide C. Vesicle formation during reticulocyte maturation. Association of plasma membrane activities with released vesicles (exosomes). J Biol Chem. 1987;262(19):9412–20.

62. Frydrychowicz M, Kolecka-Bednarczyk A, Madejczyk M, Yasar S, Dworacki G. Exosomes - structure, biogenesis and biological role in non-small-cell lung cancer. Scand J Immunol. 2015;81(1):2–10.

63. van Niel G, Charrin S, Simoes S, Romao M, Rochin L, Saftig P, et al. The tetraspanin CD63 regulates ESCRT-independent and -dependent endosomal sorting during melanogenesis. Dev Cell. 2011;21(4):708–21.

64. Sahu R, Kaushik S, Clement CC, Cannizzo ES, Scharf B, Follenzi A, et al. Microautophagy of cytosolic proteins by late endosomes. Dev Cell. 2011;20(1):131–9.

65. Ghossoub R, Lembo F, Rubio A, Gaillard CB, Bouchet J, Vitale N, et al. Syntenin-ALIX exosome biogenesis and budding into multivesicular bodies are controlled by ARF6 and PLD2. Nat Commun. 2014;5:3477.

66. Calistri A, Munegato D, Toffoletto M, Celestino M, Franchin E, Comin A, et al. Functional interaction between the ESCRT-I component TSG101 and the HSV-1 tegument ubiquitin specific protease. J Cell Physiol. 2014;12:3–9.

67. Chamontin C, Rassam P, Ferrer M, Racine PJ, Neyret A, Laine S, et al. HIV-1 nucleocapsid and ESCRT-component Tsg101 interplay prevents HIV from turning into a DNA-containing virus. Nucleic Acids Res. 2015;43(1):336–47.

68. Beloribi S, Ristorcelli E, Breuzard G, Silvy F, Bertrand-Michel J, Beraud E, et al. Exosomal lipids impact notch signaling and induce death of human pancreatic tumoral SOJ-6 cells. PLoS One. 2012;7(10):e47480.

69. Stenmark H. Rab GTPases as coordinators of vesicle traffic. Nat Rev Mol Cell Biol. 2009;10(8):513–25.

70. Bishop N, Woodman P. ATPase-defective mammalian VPS4 localizes to aberrant endosomes and impairs cholesterol trafficking. Mol Biol Cell. 2000;11(1):227–39.

71. Thery C, Boussac M, Veron P, Ricciardi-Castagnoli P, Raposo G, Garin J, et al. Proteomic analysis of dendritic cell-derived exosomes: a secreted subcellular compartment distinct from apoptotic vesicles. J Immunol. 2001;166(12):7309–18.

72. Baietti MF, Zhang Z, Mortier E, Melchior A, Degeest G, Geeraerts A, et al. Syndecan-syntenin-ALIX regulates the biogenesis of exosomes. Nat Cell Biol. 2012;14(7):677–85.

73. Honegger A, Leitz J, Bulkescher J, Hoppe-Seyler K, Hoppe-Seyler F. Silencing of human papillomavirus (HPV) E6/E7 oncogene expression affects both the contents and the amounts of extracellular microvesicles released from HPV-positive cancer cells. Int J Cancer. 2013;133(7):1631–42.

74. Ostrowski M, Carmo NB, Krumeich S, Fanget I, Raposo G, Savina A, et al. Rab27a and Rab27b control different steps of the exosome secretion pathway. Nat Cell Biol. 2010;12(1):19–30. sup pp 11–13.

75. Lee TH, D'Asti E, Magnus N, Al-Nedawi K, Meehan B, Rak J. Microvesicles as mediators of intercellular communication in cancer–the emerging science of cellular 'debris'. Semin Immunopathol. 2011;33(5):455–67.

76. Kowal J, Tkach M, Thery C. Biogenesis and secretion of exosomes. Curr Opin Cell Biol. 2014;29C:116–25.

77. Thery C, Zitvogel L, Amigorena S. Exosomes: composition, biogenesis and function. Nat Rev Immunol. 2002;2(8):569–79.

78. Al-Nedawi K, Meehan B, Micallef J, Lhotak V, May L, Guha A, et al. Intercellular transfer of the oncogenic receptor EGFRvIII by microvesicles derived from tumour cells. Nat Cell Biol. 2008;10(5):619–24.

79. Thery C, Amigorena S, Raposo G, Clayton A. Isolation and characterization of exosomes from cell culture supernatants and biological fluids. Current protocols in cell biology / editorial board, Juan S Bonifacino [et al.] 2006, Chapter 3:Unit 3 22. Pp. 1-24

80. Jeppesen DK, Hvam ML, Primdahl-Bengtson B, Boysen AT, Whitehead B, Dyrskjot L, et al. Comparative analysis of discrete exosome fractions obtained by differential centrifugation. J Extracellular Vesicles. 2014;3:25011.

81. Heinemann ML, Ilmer M, Silva LP, Hawke DH, Recio A, Vorontsova MA, et al. Benchtop isolation and characterization of functional exosomes by sequential filtration. J Chromatogr A. 2014;1371C:125–35.

82. Sigdel TK, Ng YW, Lee S, Nicora CD, Qian WJ, Smith RD, et al. Perturbations in the urinary exosome in transplant rejection. Front Med. 2014;1:57.

83. Moldovan L, Batte K, Wang Y, Wisler J, Piper M. Analyzing the circulating microRNAs in exosomes/extracellular vesicles from serum or plasma by qRT-PCR. Methods Mol Biol. 2013;1024:129–45.

84. Dragovic RA, Southcombe JH, Tannetta DS, Redman CW, Sargent IL. Multicolor flow cytometry and nanoparticle tracking analysis of extracellular vesicles in the plasma of normal pregnant and pre-eclamptic women. Biol Reprod. 2013;89(6):151.

85. Wei F, Yang J, Wong DT. Detection of exosomal biomarker by electric field-induced release and measurement (EFIRM). Biosens Bioelectron. 2013;44:115–21.

86. Lunter PC, van Kilsdonk JW, van Beek H, Cornelissen IM, Bergers M, Willems PH, et al. Activated leukocyte cell adhesion molecule (ALCAM/CD166/MEMD), a novel actor in invasive growth, controls matrix metalloproteinase activity. Cancer Res. 2005;65(19):8801–8.

87. Bjorklund M, Koivunen E. Gelatinase-mediated migration and invasion of cancer cells. Biochim Biophys Acta. 2005;1755(1):37–69.

88. Welton JL, Khanna S, Giles PJ, Brennan P, Brewis IA, Staffurth J, et al. Proteomics analysis of bladder cancer exosomes. Mol Cell Proteomics. 2010;9(6):1324–38.

89. Galindo-Hernandez O, Villegas-Comonfort S, Candanedo F, Gonzalez-Vazquez MC, Chavez-Ocana S, Jimenez-Villanueva X, et al. Elevated concentration of microvesicles isolated from peripheral blood in breast cancer patients. Arch Med Res. 2013;44(3):208–14.

90. Pegtel DM, Cosmopoulos K, Thorley-Lawson DA, van Eijndhoven MA, Hopmans ES, Lindenberg JL, et al. Functional delivery of viral miRNAs via exosomes. Proc Natl Acad Sci U S A. 2010;107(14):6328–33.

91. Ranganathan S, Garg G. Secretome: clues into pathogen infection and clinical applications. Genome Med. 2009;1(11):113.

92. Went PT, Lugli A, Meier S, Bundi M, Mirlacher M, Sauter G, et al. Frequent EpCam protein expression in human carcinomas. Hum Pathol. 2004;35(1):122–8.

93. Lim LP, Lau NC, Garrett-Engele P, Grimson A, Schelter JM, Castle J, et al. Microarray analysis shows that some microRNAs downregulate large numbers of target mRNAs. Nature. 2005;433(7027):769–73.

94. Atala A. Re: Microvesicles released from human renal cancer stem cells stimulate angiogenesis and formation of lung premetastatic niche. J Urol. 2012;187(4):1506–7.

95. Grange C, Tapparo M, Collino F, Vitillo L, Damasco C, Deregibus MC, et al. Microvesicles released from human renal cancer stem cells stimulate angiogenesis and formation of lung premetastatic niche. Cancer Res. 2011;71(15):5346–56.

96. Peinado H, Aleckovic M, Lavotshkin S, Matei I, Costa-Silva B, Moreno-Bueno G, et al. Melanoma exosomes educate bone marrow progenitor cells toward a pro-metastatic phenotype through MET. Nat Med. 2012;18(6):883–91.

97. Aktas IY, Bugdayci M, Usubutun A. Expression of p16, p53, CD24, EpCAM and calretinin in serous borderline tumors of the ovary. Turk Patoloji Dergisi. 2012;28(3):220–30.

98. Street JM, Yuen PS, Star RA. Bioactive exosomes: possibilities for diagnosis and management of bladder cancer. J Urol. 2014;192(2):297–8.

99. Beckham CJ, Olsen J, Yin PN, Wu CH, Ting HJ, Hagen FK, et al. Bladder cancer exosomes contain EDIL-3/Del1 and facilitate cancer progression. J Urol. 2014;192(2):583–92.

100. Sun JC, Liang XT, Pan K, Wang H, Zhao JJ, Li JJ, et al. High expression level of EDIL3 in HCC predicts poor prognosis of HCC patients. World J Gastroenterol. 2010;16(36):4611–5.

101. Natasha G, Gundogan B, Tan A, Farhatnia Y, Wu W, Rajadas J, et al. Exosomes as Immunotheranostic Nanoparticles. Clin Ther. 2014;36(6):820–9.

102. Xu Y, Luo F, Liu Y, Shi L, Lu X, Xu W, et al. Exosomal miR-21 derived from arsenite-transformed human bronchial epithelial cells promotes cell proliferation associated with arsenite carcinogenesis. Arch Toxicol. 2014;2:31–5.

103. Choi DS, Lee JM, Park GW, Lim HW, Bang JY, Kim YK, et al. Proteomic analysis of microvesicles derived from human colorectal cancer cells. J Proteome Res. 2007;6(12):4646–55.

104. Principe S, Hui AB, Bruce J, Sinha A, Liu FF, Kislinger T. Tumor-derived exosomes and microvesicles in head and neck cancer: implications for tumor biology and biomarker discovery. Proteomics. 2013;13(10–11):1608–23.

105. Abastado JP. The next challenge in cancer immunotherapy: controlling T-cell traffic to the tumor. Cancer Res. 2012;72(9):2159–61.

106. Giusti I, D'Ascenzo S, Dolo V. Microvesicles as potential ovarian cancer biomarkers. Biomed Res Int. 2013;2013:703048.

107. Taylor DD, Akyol S, Gercel-Taylor C. Pregnancy-associated exosomes and their modulation of T cell signaling. J Immunol. 2006;176(3):1534–42.

108. Lasser C, Eldh M, Lotvall J. Isolation and characterization of RNA-containing exosomes. JoVE. 2012;59:e3037.

109. Michael A, Bajracharya SD, Yuen PS, Zhou H, Star RA, Illei GG, et al. Exosomes from human saliva as a source of microRNA biomarkers. Oral Dis. 2010;16(1):34–8.

110. Tauro BJ, Greening DW, Mathias RA, Ji H, Mathivanan S, Scott AM, et al. Comparison of ultracentrifugation, density gradient separation, and immunoaffinity capture methods for isolating human colon cancer cell line LIM1863-derived exosomes. Methods. 2012;56(2):293–304.

111. Boing AN, van der Pol E, Grootemaat AE, Coumans FA, Sturk A, Nieuwland R. Single-step isolation of extracellular vesicles by size-exclusion chromatography. Journal of extracellular vesicles 2014,3.

112. Santana SM, Antonyak MA, Cerione RA, Kirby BJ. Microfluidic isolation of cancer-cell-derived microvesicles from hetergeneous extracellular shed vesicle populations. Biomed Microdevices. 2014;16(6):869–77.

14

Implant based differences in adverse local tissue reaction in failed total hip arthroplasties: a morphological and immunohistochemical study

Giorgio Perino[1*], Benjamin F Ricciardi[2], Seth A Jerabek[2], Guido Martignoni[3], Gabrielle Wilner[4], Dan Maass[4], Steven R Goldring[4] and P Edward Purdue[4]

Abstract

Background: Adverse local tissue reaction (ALTR) is characterized by periprosthetic soft tissue inflammation composed of a mixed inflammatory cell infiltrate, extensive soft tissue necrosis, and vascular changes. Multiple hip implant classes have been reported to result in ALTR, and clinical differences may represent variation in the soft tissue response at the cellular and tissue levels. The purpose of this study was to describe similarities and differences in periprosthetic tissue structure, organization, and cellular composition by conventional histology and immunohistochemistry in ALTR resulting from two common total hip arthroplasty (THA) implant classes.

Methods: Consecutive patients presenting with ALTR from two major hip implant classes (N = 54 patients with Dual-Modular Neck implant; N = 14 patients with Metal-on-Metal implant) were identified from our prospective Osteolysis Tissue Database and Repository. Clinical characteristics including age, sex, BMI, length of implantation, and serum metal ion levels were recorded. Retrieved synovial tissue morphology was graded using light microscopy and cellular composition was assessed using immunohistochemistry.

Results: Length of implantation was shorter in the DMN group versus MoM THA group (21.3 [8.4] months versus 43.6 [13.8] months respectively; p < 0.005) suggesting differences in implant performance. Morphologic examination revealed a common spectrum of neo-synovial proliferation and necrosis in both groups. Macrophages were more commonly present in diffuse sheets (Grade 3) in the MoM relative to DMN group (p = 0.016). Perivascular lymphocytes with germinal centers (Grade 4) were more common in the DMN group, which trended towards significance (p = 0.066). Qualitative differences in corrosion product morphology were seen between the two groups. Immunohistochemistry showed features of a CD4 and GATA-3 rich lymphocyte reaction in both implants, with increased ratios of perivascular T-cell relative to B-cell markers in the DMN relative to the MoM group (p = 0.032).

Conclusion: Our results demonstrate that both implant classes display common features of neo-synovial proliferation and necrosis with a CD4 and GATA-3 rich inflammatory infiltrate. Qualitative differences in corrosion product appearance, macrophage morphology, and lymphocyte distributions were seen between the two implant types. Our data suggests that ALTR represents a histological spectrum with implant-based features.

Keywords: Adverse local tissue reaction, Corrosion products, Revision arthroplasty, Synovial inflammation

* Correspondence: perinog@hss.edu
[1]Department of Pathology, Hospital for Special Surgery, 535 East 70th Street, New York, NY 10021, USA
Full list of author information is available at the end of the article

Background

Modifications in bearing surface modularity and stem designs in total hip replacement (THA) were introduced in the past two decades with the goal of reducing the incidence of aseptic loosening and instability [1,2]. One of these modifications included the metal-on-metal (MoM) bearing surface, which was combined with a metallic adapter sleeve for large heads in the early 2000s. The rationale for the revival of this bearing surface included a reduction in volumetric wear and osteolysis compared to conventional metal-on-polyethylene bearings (MoP), decreased impingement throughout range of motion, and decreased rates of dislocation [1]. A second modification to increase modularity in THA was the introduction of the dual-modular neck. This provided surgeons with increased reconstructive options to potentially match each patient's anatomy and permit the use of a MoP or ceramic-on-polyethylene (CoP) bearing surface [2].

The unintended consequence of these implant modifications has been an increasing number of new interacting surfaces of different biomaterials, subject to short-term mechanical and no biologic testing before worldwide marketing and use [3]. This has resulted in increased MoM implant failures due to a distinct type of cellular/tissue reaction, originally reported as aseptic lymphocyte dominated vasculitis-associated lesions (ALVAL), now collectively referred in the literature as adverse local tissue reactions (ALTR) or adverse reaction to metallic debris (ARMD) [4-12]. Previous histological analyses of retrieved periprosthetic tissue have shown evidence of corrosion products, metallic debris generated by abrasion and/or surface fatigue, extensive soft tissue necrosis, combined macrophagic and lymphocytic infiltrate with variable plasmacytic and eosinophilic components, and vascular wall changes [5,13-19]. A comprehensive review describing features of periprosthetic inflammation to wear debris has been addressed in a recent review article by Gallo et al. [20]. The constellation of pathologic findings observed in response to MoM implants was encompassed under the acronym ALVAL by Willert et al. to illustrate the unique lymphocytic component and probable vascular changes not seen in other typical modes of THA failure such as osteolysis or infection [14]. Failure due to ALTR has predominantly been attributed and described for MoM bearing surfaces, but evidence of head-neck and neck-stem corrosion in modular implants has been reported to result in ALTR [4,9-12,21-23].

We hypothesized that corrosion products, as previously described in the literature, generated at different contact surfaces of THA implants could be the defining factor of ALTR irrespective of the bearing surface, and these differences would be reflected in the histologic and immunohistochemical profiles of retrieval tissue between different implant types [5,7,11]. In order to investigate this hypothesis, we compared the morphologic and immunohistochemical characteristics from retrieved periprosthetic tissue using two separate classes of implants: 1) MoM bearing surface and a metallic adapter sleeve at the head-neck taper junction and 2) conventional bearing surface (metal-on-polyethylene or metal-on-ceramic) with a dual-modular neck with tapers at the head-neck and neck-stem junctions. The purposes of this study were to analyze implant-based similarities and differences in: 1. Periprosthetic tissue structure, organization, corrosion product morphology, and cellular composition by conventional histology; and 2. Cellular composition by immunohistochemistry.

This is the first study to describe the morphologic and immunohistochemical similarities and differences between ALTR associated with different implant classes. Our results demonstrate that implant design can affect corrosion product morphology and the periprosthetic tissue pathology, and indicate that the interaction between implant design and host biology can have important clinical consequences in surveillance and outcomes of hip orthopedic implants in the future.

Methods

Patients

Between April 2012 and June 2013, all patients with the diagnosis of ALTR based on histological analysis were identified retrospectively from the Osteolysis Tissue Database and Repository at the Hospital for Special Surgery. This prospective database collects demographics, selected clinical data, periprosthetic tissue, and biological fluid (serum, synovial fluid) from all consenting patients undergoing revision THA with suspected ALTR. Ethical committee approval was obtained prior to this study (Institutional Review Board, Hospital for Special Surgery, Protocol Number 26085). Two groups of patients were selected, representing the two major implant classes resulting in ALTR: the Dual-Modular Neck group (DMN) had a MoP or CoP bearing surface with a dual-modular neck (cobalt-chromium-molybdenum, CoCrMo) and TMZF (titanium, molybdenum, zirconia, iron) stem (Stryker, Rejuvenate) [N = 55 hips, 54 patients], and the MoM THA group had a MoM bearing surface (CoCrMo) with a metallic adapter sleeve (CoCrMo) at the head-neck junction and titanium stem (Smith & Nephew, Birmingham THA) [N = 18 hips, 14 patients]. All polyethylene used in the DMN implant was second-generation highly cross-linked polyethylene (X3, Stryker Corporation). Exclusion criteria included previous revision arthroplasty, positive intraoperative cultures, and insufficient tissue retrieval for comparative pathologic examination (less than 5 tissue sections and more than 75% tissue necrosis at light microscopy examination on all slides examined). These two implants were selected because they are examples of recently marketed modular implants with a sufficient number of cases in our institution to allow an in-depth morphologic and immunohistochemical analysis. Preoperative serum cobalt and chromium levels were obtained by quantitative inductively coupled plasma-mass spectrometry at the operating surgeons' discretion (ARUP Laboratories, Salt Lake City, Utah). Acetabular and stem components were recorded for each implant.

Tissue collection and sampling

All patients suspected of having ALTR at our institution undergo magnetic resonance imaging (MRI) with multi-acquisition variable-resonance image combination (MAVRIC) scan to further reduce susceptibility artifact [24]. Findings suggestive of ALTR include bulky synovitis, extracapsular disease, tendon/intramuscular edema, and capsular avulsion [24]. Periprosthetic tissue sampling in revision cases for the implants included in the database has been standardized in our institution since September 2011, when the first cases of the two series of patients described in this report were observed. Areas of inflammation were identified preoperatively on MRI, and used as guidance for tissue sampling by the operating surgeon. Samples were taken from multiple regions around the hip joint including the periprosthetic pseudocapsule, bursal synovium, and adjacent skeletal muscle when necessary and labeled accordingly. The use of cautery was minimized to avoid compromising the tissue for histologic and molecular analysis. Additionally, acetabular and femoral bone samples, core biopsies of osteolytic areas, and/or reamings were sent separately to evaluate possible bone marrow involvement when suitable. Separate tissue samples identified by location were sent to the microbiology laboratory to rule out infection and, if sizable, retrieved after culture preparation for further histological analysis.

The project research coordinator (DM, GW) harvested biological samples with presence of the pathologist (GP) to assure consistency among all the surgeons contributing cases to the database. The tissue was retrieved fresh in labeled tissue cups from the sterile area as soon as possible and kept on ice. One pathologist (GP) performed frozen section by sampling of the fresh tissue in order to assess viability and cell composition and when feasible, a representative tissue sample was processed for RNA isolation for future investigations. Remaining tissue samples were provided between two and six sites surrounding the implant. Extensive sampling was performed at macroscopic examination with care to the orientation of the specimens, including necrotic areas and/or friable, loose material. Acetabular reaming was also collected, osteolytic areas were sampled when present, and cancellous bone was also scraped from the femoral stem and/or the acetabular shell when possible. The number of paraffin blocks containing one or two tissue sections processed per case varied from 7 to 14, to minimize sampling error due to necrosis and to ensure valuable representation of the viable tissue. Photographs of each implant and selected gross tissue specimens were taken.

Histologic analysis

All sections were processed and embedded with standard procedures, stained routinely with hematoxylin-eosin, and examined by an experienced musculoskeletal pathologist (GP) to assess the presence of ALTR. A range of 7 – 14 sections were examined per case depending on tissue availability. Cases were scored by one investigator experienced in examining periprosthetic tissue from revision THA (GP), one experienced surgical pathologist (GM), and a third investigator trained for three months on 100 archival hip revision cases with a full spectrum of adverse reactions (BR). Investigators were blinded from clinical patient characteristics. Discrepancies in scoring were resolved by consensus agreement. The ALVAL scoring system proposed by Campbell et al., which was previously used at our institution as correlative index with MRI imaging analysis, was recorded for each case [16,25-27].

Histological sections were examined for the presence (Y) or absence (N) of synovial lining loss/hyperplasia, partial or full thickness necrosis of the neo-synovial membrane and subsynovial soft tissue, cell exfoliation, vascular wall changes, high endothelial cell venules (HEV), granulomas (sarcoidosis-like with or without central necrosis), and skeletal muscle inflammatory infiltrate (Table 1). Semi-quantitative evaluation was undertaken for grading of the macrophages [28]. Macrophages were graded on a 0–3 scale (absent, occasional, clusters, diffuse/sheets). Total lymphocytes were graded as interstitial (band-like) and/or perivascular. Perivascular lymphocytes were graded according to average lymphoctic cuff thickness using a Zeiss Axioskop 40 calibrated reticule and scored as described by Natu et al. on a 0–4 scale with absence or presence of germinal centers [17]. Neutrophils were graded on a 0–2 scale [(absent, occasional, focally numerous (>5 cells x 10 HPF)]. Plasma cells were graded on a 0–2 scale [(absent, occasional, or numerous (>10 cells per HPF)]. Eosinophils were graded on a 0–1 scale (absent or present), stromal cell cellularity was graded on a 1–3 scale (slight, moderate, marked). Results were expressed as the percentage of samples containing the selected feature.

Macrophage content (polyethylene, metal, and ceramic particles) was graded according to the method used for metallic particles by Natu et al. [17] (Table 1). Presence of intracellular corrosion products was recorded and extracellular aggregates were graded on a 0–1 scale (absent or present). Presence of hemosiderin deposits and/or suture material was recorded.

Table 1 Morphologic comparison of synovial structure, cellularity, macrophage content, and bone marrow involvement between the Dual-Modular Neck and the Metal-on-Metal (MoM) total hip arthroplasty (THA) groups

Morphologic characteristic	Dual-Modular Neck THA (N = 55 hips)	MoM THA (N = 18 hips)	P value
Synovial structure	Cases (%)	Cases (%)	
Synovial layer loss	96.4	100.0	
Synovial layer hyperplasia	78.2	77.8	
Cell exfoliation	87.3	94.4	
Necrosis	65.5	61.1	
Vascular wall changes	18.2	16.7	
High endothelial cell venules	14.5	16.7	
Granulomas	18.2	11.1	0.482
Cellularity			
Macrophages			0.016*
Grade 1	16.4	5.6	
Grade 2	30.9	5.6	
Grade 3	50.9	88.9	
Lymphocytes			0.066#
Grade 1	1.8	16.7	
Grade 2	9.1	5.6	
Grade 3	52.7	61.1	
Grade 4	34.5	16.7	
Stromal Cells			0.593
Grade 1	27.3	38.9	
Grade 2	50.9	44.4	
Grade 3	16.4	11.1	
Neutrophils	10.9	11.1	
Plasma cells sparse	32.7	38.9	
Plasma cells numerous	20.0	22.2	
Eosinophils	32.7	33.3	
Macrophage content			
Polyethylene particles	1.8	0.0	
Metallic particles	1.8	33.3	<0.005*
Corrosion products	100	100	
Intracellular distribution	Sparse	Diffuse	
Intracellular morphology	Irregular	Globular + Irregular	
Extracellular corrosion aggregates	72.7	66.7	0.662
Bone/bone marrow			
Necrosis	47.1	28.6	
Macrophage infiltration	47.1	100.0	

Table 1 Morphologic comparison of synovial structure, cellularity, macrophage content, and bone marrow involvement between the Dual-Modular Neck and the Metal-on-Metal (MoM) total hip arthroplasty (THA) groups *(Continued)*

Benign lymphocytic aggregates	35.3	28.6	
Germinal centers	17.6	0.0	

*Statistically significant at p < 0.05 for Dual-Modular Neck versus MoM THA.
#trend towards statistical significance p < 0.10 for Dual-Modular Neck versus MoM THA.
Morphologic Characteristics of Synovial Tissue from Dual-Modular Neck and MoM THA Groups.

Bone marrow sections were evaluated for the presence (Y) or absence (N) of necrosis of bone and marrow cellular elements, macrophage infiltration, and benign lymphocytic aggregates with or without presence of germinal centers. Results were expressed as a percentage of patients displaying each morphologic feature.

Immunohistochemistry

Fifteen cases for each of the DMN and MoM THA groups were analyzed by immunohistochemistry. The cases from the larger DMN group were selected to be representative of the spectrum of histological patterns observed as described in the results section. Conventional immunohistochemistry was performed using standard techniques on consecutive sections (GM). Heat-induced antigen retrieval was performed using a microwave oven and 0.01 mol/L of citrate buffer. All samples were processed using a sensitive 'Bond polymer Refine' detection system in an automated Bond immunohistochemistry instrument (Vision-Biosystem, Menarini, Florence, Italy). Antibody dilutions and source are shown in Table 2. Commercially available monoclonal antibodies were used and each batch was tested by titration for optimal dilution on both internal and external controls. Macrophage markers were CD68 (all macrophages) and CD163 (M2 macrophages) [29,30]. The lymphocytic response was assessed by expression of CD20 for B cells and CD3, CD4, and CD8 for T cells. Expression of T-bet, GATA3, and FOXP3 was used as marker for transcription factors for Th1, Th2, and Treg cells to sub-classify the T cell distribution [31-33]. High endothelial cell venules were identified as CD123 positive cells. Mast cells were identified as CD117 positive cells [34].

Semiquantitative analysis was performed for evaluation of macrophage, mast cell, and HEV distributions. Evaluation of CD68 and CD163 stained sections were graded as +, ++, and +++ by three investigators (GP, GM, BR) blinded to the clinical data. CD117 staining was assessed from 0-2 [absent, occasional, numerous (>5 forms per HPF)]. Granzyme immunohistochemistry and the presence

Table 2 Description of antibodies and dilutions utilized for immunohistochemistry

Antibody	Clone	Source	Dilution
CD3	SP7	THERMO SC.	1:150
CD4	4B12	NOVOCASTRA	1:150
CD8	C8/144B	DAKO	1:200
CD20	L26	NOVOCASTRA	1:100
CD68	PG-M1	DAKO	1:50
CD123	7G3	BD Phamingen	1:100
CD163	10D6	NOVOCASTRA	1:200
GATA-3	L50-823	BD Phamingen	1:150
FOXP3	221D/D3	SEROTEC	1:200
T-bet	4B10	SANTA CRUZ	1:100
Granzyme	GrB-7	MONOSAN	1:100
CD117	T595	NOVOCASTRA	1:10

Antibody Sources and Dilutions for Immunohistochemistry.

of CD123 positive HEVs were assessed by the presence (Y) or absence (N) of positive cells.

A quantitative analysis (Bioquant Osteo, Bioquant Image Analysis Corporation, Nashville, TN) was performed on all sections to evaluate lymphocytic distributions in both perivascular and interstitial regions. Two perivascular and two interstitial areas on each slide were randomly selected and evaluated at high power (×400), and lymphocytes with positive stain were counted manually by two investigators blinded to the clinical characteristics (BR, GP). The results were expressed as percentage of positive cells per mm^2. The same areas from consecutive sections were chosen for each stain, ensuring consistency in area of evaluation. The ratios between CD20:CD3, CD4:CD8, and GATA3:T-bet on the same sections were then calculated. The CD20: CD3, CD4:CD8, and GATA3:T-bet were described as a > 2:1, 1:1, or > 1:2 ratio.

A comparison control group of periprosthetic tissue was used for immunohistochemistry. For the control group (N = 17), average age was 63.5 years (standard deviation 14.0) and 71% were females. These included three cases (N = 3) of osteoarthritis with variable amount

of lymphoplasmacytic infiltrate without clinical diagnosis of rheumatic disease, three cases of periprosthetic osteolysis from polyethylene/metallic wear debris in standard THA, and three (N = 3) cases of MoM implants not examined in our series (1 resurfacing, 2 MoM THA). Average time of implantation was 30 months in these patients. Additionally, we examined all cases of preoperative native synovial tissue (time zero) available for patients in our series with ALTR and identified five cases (N = 5) with variable perivascular lymphoplasmacytic infiltrate to provide a baseline comparison. These cases underwent the same pathologic and immunohistochemical evaluation as the ALTR cases in this study. Two archival cases of pelvic lymph nodes in patients with history of total hip replacement served as negative and positive immunohistochemistry controls.

Statistics

Categorical variables were reported as frequencies and percentages and compared between the DMN and MoM THA groups by chi-square tests. Continuous variables were summarized as means and standard deviations and compared between groups with independent samples t-tests. In cases where data was not normally distributed, a Mann–Whitney U test was utilized. All statistical tests were two-sided and p-values less than 0.05 were considered statistically significant. Statistical analyses were performed with SAS version 9.3 (SAS Institute, Cary, NC).

Results

Clinical demographics

Demographics for patients that met study criteria are summarized in Table 3. Patients were older in the DMN group (N = 55 hips in 54 patients) versus the MoM THA group (p = 0.03) (Table 3). Mean time to revision was earlier in the DMN group versus MoM THA group (21.3 [8.4] months versus 43.6 [13.8] months respectively; p < 0.005) (Table 3). Serum cobalt and chromium levels were increased in the MoM THA relative to the DMN group, however, only the chromium level in unilateral cases reached statistical significance (Table 4).

Table 3 Demographic data for the Dual-Modular Neck and Metal-on-Metal (MoM) total hip arthroplasty (THA) groups

Demographic factor	Dual-Modular Neck THA N = 54 patients N = 55 hips	MoM THA N = 14 patients N = 18 hips	P Value
Age (years)	67.3 (range 47 – 87)	58.6 (range 31–75)	0.03*
Female (%)	59.3	64.3	0.79
BMI (mean [SD])	27.1 (4.8)	26.6 (4.3)	0.72
Time to revision (mean [SD])	21.3 (8.4)	43.6 (13.8)	<0.005*
Campbell score (mean [SD])	8.1 (1.9)	7.4 (1.6)	0.15

SD: standard deviation. *statistically significant at p < 0.05 for Dual-Modular Neck versus MoM THA.
Demographic Factors in the Dual-Modular Neck and MoM THA Groups.

Table 4 Preoperative serum cobalt and serum chromium levels in patients with unilateral or bilateral arthroplasties in the Dual-Modular Neck or Metal-on-Metal (MoM) total hip arthroplasty (THA) groups

	Dual-Modular Neck THA	MoM THA	P value
Serum Cobalt (ng/mL)			
Unilateral (N = 43, N = 6)	7.5 (5.6)	29.0 (54.4)	0.581
Bilateral (N = 3, N = 5)	16.8 (1.5)	23.8 (21.2)	1.0
Serum Chromium (ng/mL)			
Unilateral (N = 43, N = 6)	1.2 (1.4)	11.0 (16.4)	0.004*
Bilateral (N = 3, N = 5)	2.9 (1.5)	14.6 (14.2)	0.142

Data represented as mean (standard deviation) for all values.
Preoperative Serum Ion Levels in the Dual-Modular Neck and MoM THA Groups.
*statistically significant at p < 0.05 for Dual-Modular Neck versus MoM THA.

Histological analysis

Histologic examination of the retrieved tissues showed similar development of ALTR in both implants (Figures 1 and 2). Development of a reactive neo-synovial membrane ranging from flat/micropapillary, especially in bursal specimens, to florid papillary hypertrophy, ranging from coarse to polypoidal configuration, with a variable amount of stromal cell proliferation and hyperplasia of the lining layer was observed in both series (Figures 1A and 2A). The lining layer of the neo-synovium was predominantly formed by macrophages with exfoliation of viable and necrotic elements with occasional formation of a distinct eosinophilic border of coagulative necrosis, previously described in the literature as adherent fibrinous exudates (Figures 1B and 2B). An underlying band of dense sclerosis/fibroplasia and abundant macrophagic exfoliation was more commonly seen in the MoM THA (Figures 1B and 2B). Superficial perivascular lymphocytic infiltrate associated with particle-laden macrophages was commonly observed (Figures 1C and 2C). Detachment of the superficial layer or of cell contents with macrophages at different stages of degeneration (foamy elements) of the papillary projections was also observed in the MoM THA, contributing to the formation of a dense creamy fluid occasionally filling the groove of the metallic femoral head (Figure 2D). Florid papillary hypertrophy with a distribution of the inflammatory infiltrate similar to those seen in rheumatologic disorders was occasionally seen in the DMN group (Figure 1D). Tissue necrosis/infarction of variable thickness of the neo-synovial membrane, possibly reflecting more advanced stages of the reaction, was observed in 61.1% and 65.5% of cases in the MoM THA and DMN groups respectively (Table 1; Figures 1E and 2E). A deep layer of mixed macrophagic and lymphocytic infiltrate with variable number of plasma cells and eosinophils was seen in both implants (Table 1; Figures 1F and 2F). Deep perivascular lymphocytic infiltrate with formation of germinal centers and CD123 positive tall endothelial cell venules containing lymphocytes was also seen in both implants (Table 1; Figure 2G with inset). Other vascular changes were observed: the most frequent was a variable amount of non-specific myointimal proliferation of vessels with stenosis of the lumen but without identifiable luminal fibrinous exudate, thrombi, and wall damage. Occasionally onion skin pattern was present, albeit focal without evidence of a diffuse distribution in any case. Formation of sarcoidosis-like granulomas with giant cells with distinct positivity for CD123 (interleukin-3) and lymphoctic cuffing associated with the presence of corrosion products was observed in both groups (Figure 1G with inset). Higher grades of macrophagic infiltrate were seen in the MoM THA (p = 0.016) (Table 1). In contrast, higher grades of lymphocytic infiltrate were seen in the DMN group, and this trended towards significance (p = 0.066) (Table 1).

Bone marrow involvement was observed in both implants when sampled, with cell necrosis and macrophagic-lymphocytic infiltrate with associated osteoclastic activity (Figures 1H) or with benign lymphocytic aggregates associated with particle-laden macrophages (Table 1 and Figure 2H).

Evaluation of corrosion products

Corrosion products with morphologies similar to those described in previous studies were seen in many cases in both implant types, with the exception of retrieved tissues with extensive necrosis of the superficial neo-synovial layer, in which case it was not possible to adequately assess the samples [5,11,35,36] (Figure panel 3; A-D, DMN implant; E-H. MoM THA implant). Large aggregates of corrosion products were seen in the soft tissues in both implants (66.7% versus 72.7% for MoM THA and the DMN groups respectively). A crystal-like appearance of the corrosion products with formation of flat sheets in both implant types was seen, often with alternating green and red layers on H-E staining (Figures 3A,B,E). In other areas, these larger aggregates were fragmented, and these irregular particles of variable size were engulfed within multi-nucleated giant cells and mononuclear macrophages either in soft tissue (Figure 3C) or bone marrow (Figure 3D). We confirmed the origin of these corrosion products from the implants by embedding loose black

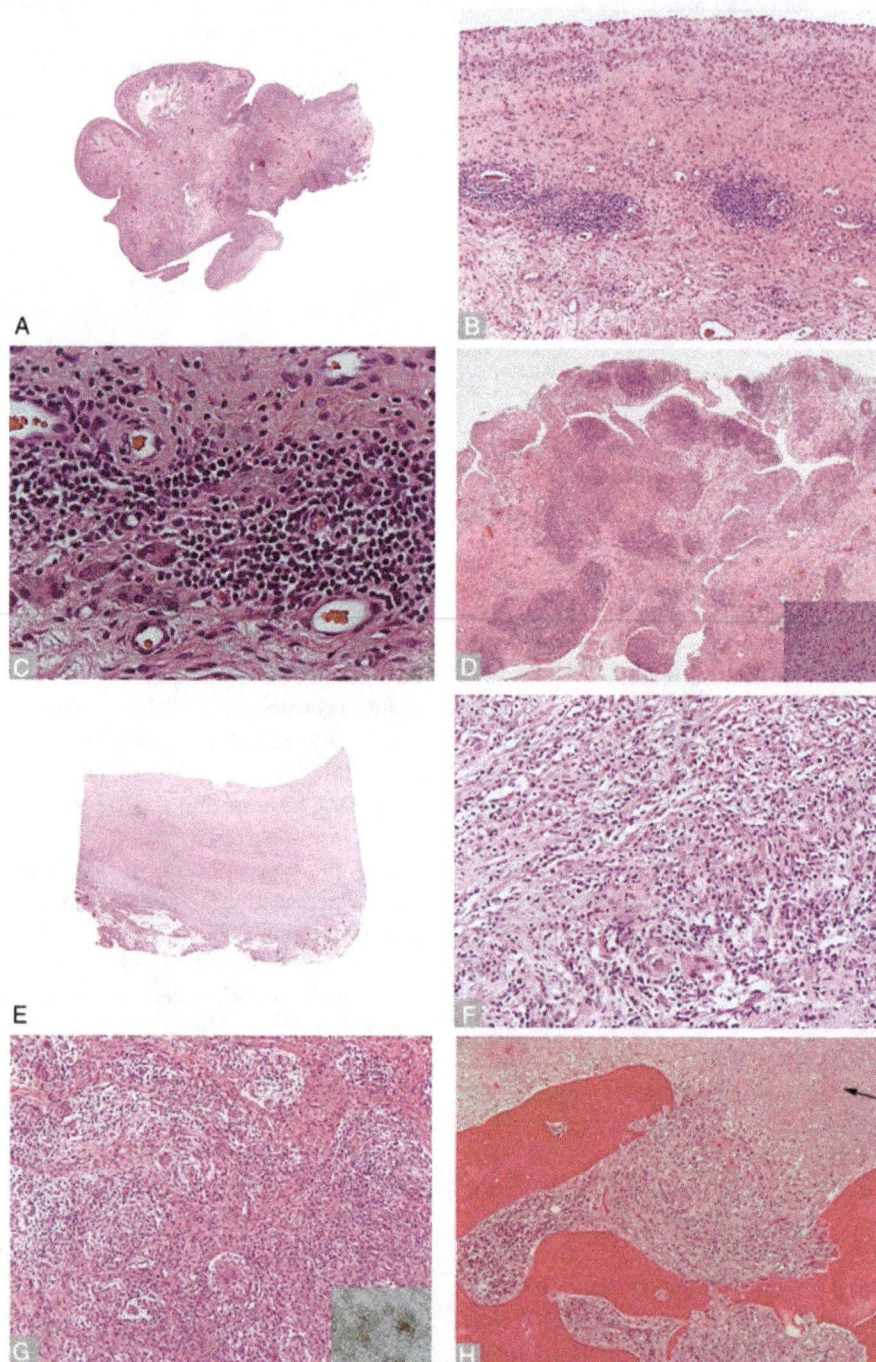

Figure 1 Histopathologic images from Dual-Modular Neck group. A) Periprosthetic neosynovium with polypoid hypertrophy (whole mount).
B) Neo-synovial membrane with lining layer composed of macrophages, marked stromal sclerosis, and perivascular lymphocytic infiltrate (x100).
C) Perivascular lymphocytic infiltrate associated with particle-laden macrophages (x400). **D)** Papillary synovium with marked perivascular
lymphocytic infiltrate (x40) associated to giant cells containing corrosion products (inset x400). **E)** Late stage of adverse reaction with thick layer
of necrosis/infarction and deep seated inflammatory infiltrate (whole mount). **F)** Band-like inflammatory infiltrate composed of macrophages,
lymphocytes, plasma cells, and eosinophils (x400). **G)** Granulomatous pattern composed of small granulomas with multi-nucleated giant cells and
lymphocytic cuffing (x100). **H)** Bone marrow involvement with area of necrosis (black arrow) and mixed macrophagic and lymphocytic infiltrate
with resorptive osteoclastic activity (x100).

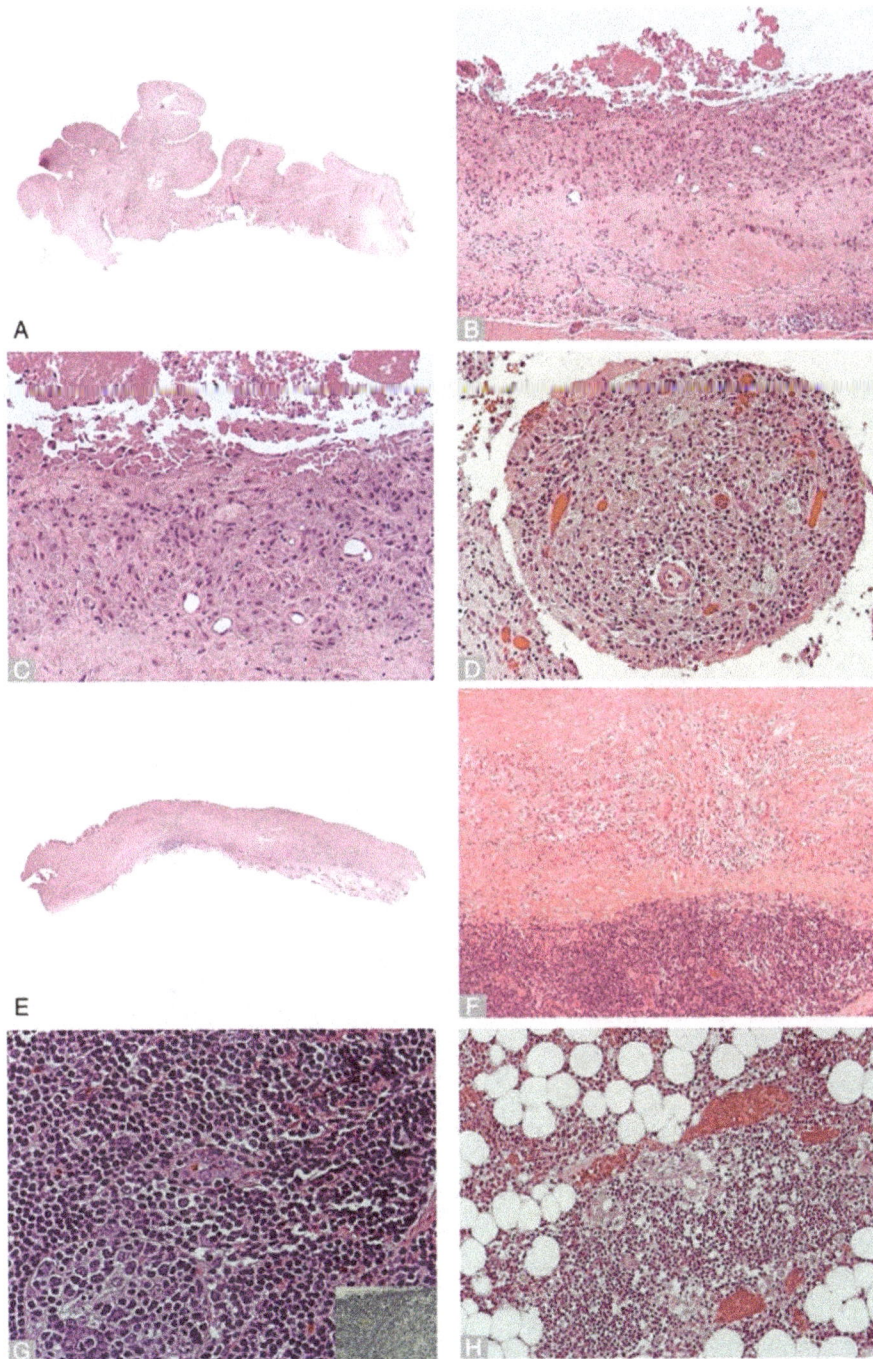

Figure 2 Histopathologic images from MoM THA group A) Periprosthetic neo-synovium with polypoid hypertrophy (whole mount). **B)** Superficial macrophagic infiltrate with exfoliation of necrotic elements without significant lymphocytic response (x100). **C)** Corrosion product-laden macrophages with exfoliation of viable and necrotic elements (x200). **D)** Synovial papilla with particle-laden macrophages at different stages of degeneration with foamy elements (x200). **E)** Late stage of reaction with thick layer of necrosis and deep seated inflammatory infiltrate (whole mount). **F)** Band-like mixed inflammatory infiltrate and deep perivascular lymphocytic infiltrate (x100). **G)** Evidence of germinal center formation (lower left corner) and tall endothelial cell venule (x400) with positive staining for CD123 (inset x400). **H)** Bone marrow with benign reactive lymphocytic aggregate mixed with particle-laden macrophages (x200).

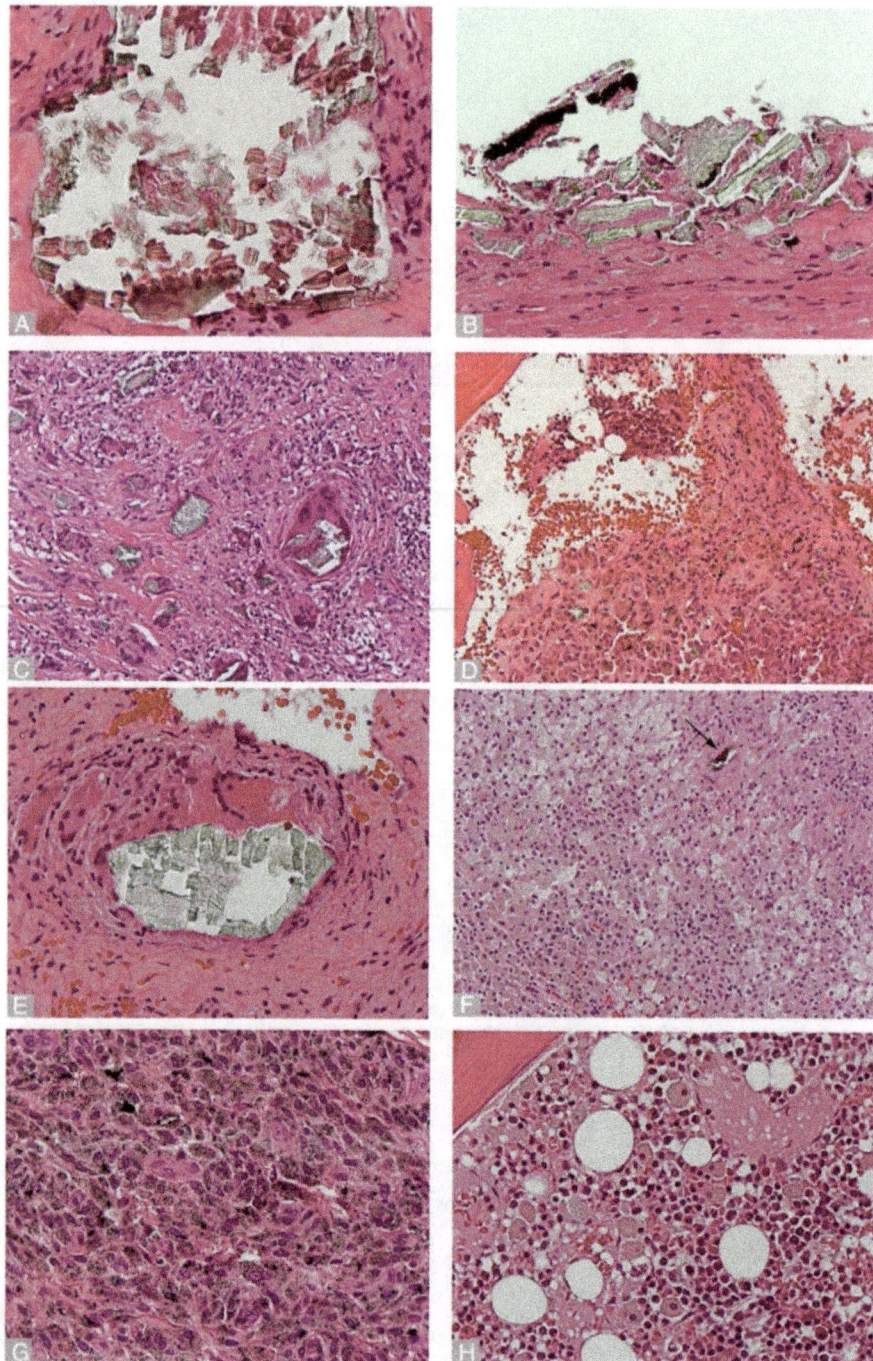

Figure 3 Histopathology of corrosion products in Dual-Modular Neck and MoM THA groups. Dual Modular Neck : **A)** Large fragments of layered corrosion products with crystal-like configuration (x400). **B)** Large aggregate of green oxidized corrosion product with plated crystal-like configuration (x400). **C)** Fragmentation of corrosion material from **(B)** engulfed into multinucleated giant cells (x200). **D)** Macrophages containing small and large particles of corrosion products infiltrating the bone marrow. MoM THA: **E)** Large aggregate of green crystal-like corrosion material surrounded by giant cells (x400). **F)** Macrophages containing corrosion products with many foamy elements and one giant cell containing larger aggregate, black arrow (x200). **G)** Macrophagic infiltrate containing predominantly globular particles of corrosion products and irregular black particles of metallic abrasion debris (x400). **H)** Hematopoietic marrow infiltrated with many macrophages containing green particles of corrosion products of variable size (x200).

debris from the taper junctions of both implants in paraffin and obtaining H-E sections, which revealed similar morphology to those observed in the periprosthetic soft tissue of the same cases.

In contrast to these irregular extracellular aggregates, the intracellular content of the macrophages showed distinct differences between the two groups: in the DMN group the cells contained scattered irregular greenish particles which were present in large amount only in areas close to the large aggregates (Figure 3C); moreover particles were difficult to identify in the deep inflammatory layer in the cases with marked necrosis. In the MoM THA group, larger macrophages were observed, containing cytoplasmic globular particles ranging from golden brown to greenish, similar in morphology to cases of resurfacing with the same bearing surface, and scattered irregular particles. Additionally, in the MoM THA, black, irregular metallic particles were seen along

with green corrosion products within the macrophages, suggesting different origins and/or compositions of metallic debris being produced in this implant type (Figure 3G). In contrast, the DMN implant did not have a metal-on-metal bearing surface, and abrasion metallic particles were not identified at light microscopy (Table 1). Bone marrow involvement of these larger aggregates and corrosion product-containing macrophages was observed in cases of both implant types if bone samples were available (Figure 3D,H).

Immunohistochemistry

Both implant types had significant macrophagic infiltrates expressing CD68 and CD163 in all samples examined, with higher intensity of the latter (Figures 4A and B). Both implants displayed a mixed perivascular lymphocytic infiltrate, with increased T cell to B cell ratios in the DMN group relative to the MoM THA (Table 5; p = 0.032). In

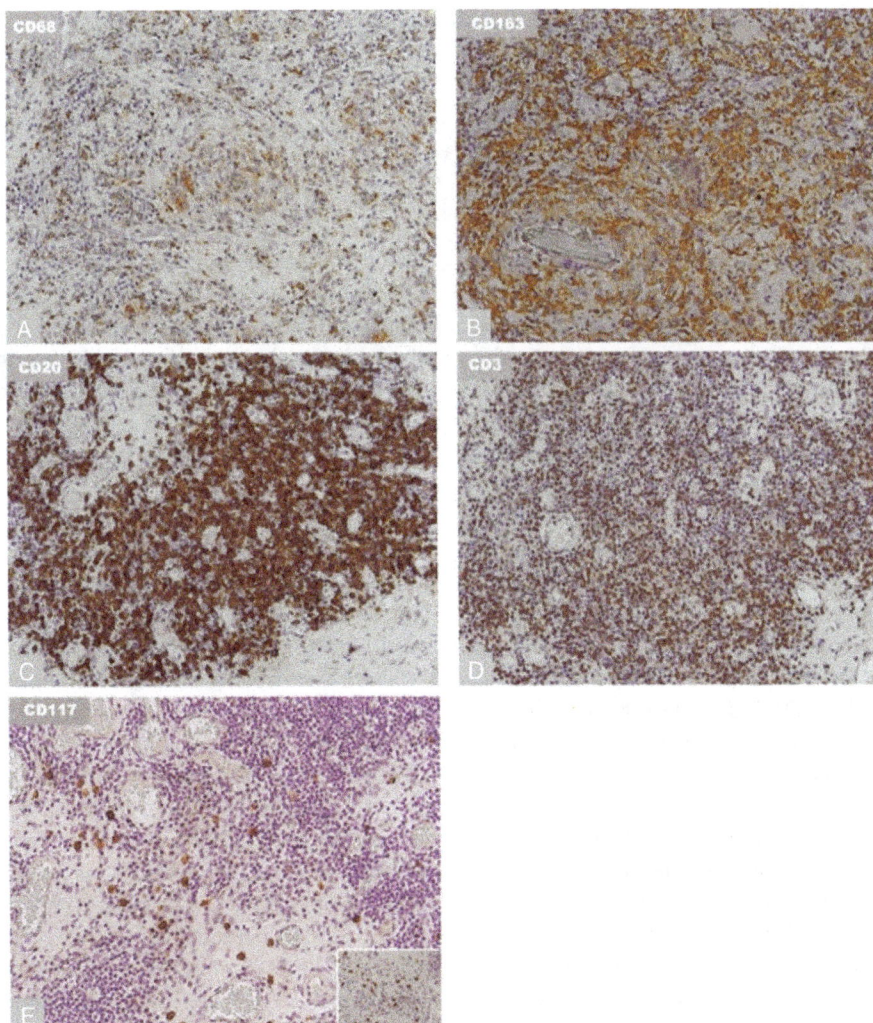

Figure 4 Immunohistochemistry in the Dual-Modular Neck and MoM THA groups (all 200X magnification). Macrophage positivity for **A)** CD68 and **B)** CD163. Perivascular lymphocytic infiltrate with **C)** CD20 positivity, **D)** CD3 positivity, and **E)** interstitial CD117 positive mast cells.

Table 5 Immunhistochemistry comparison between Dual-Modular Neck and the Metal-on-Metal (MoM) total hip arthroplasty (THA) groups

	Perivascular region			Interstitial region		
	Dual-Modular Neck THA (N = 15)	MoM THA (N = 12)	P value	Dual-Modular Neck THA (N = 15)	MoM THA (N = 12)	P value
CD20:CD3			*0.032			0.35
1:2	46.1%	0%		85.7%	66.7%	
1:1	30.8%	25.0%		14.3%	25.0%	
2:1	23.1%	75.0%		0%	8.3%	
CD4:CD8						
1:2	15.4%	14.3%	0.964	50.0%	16.7%	0.189
1:1	23.1%	28.6%		35.7%	66.7%	
2:1	61.5%	57.1%		14.3%	16.7%	
GATA3:Tbet						
1:2	0%	0%	1.00	0%	0%	0.42
1:1	0%	0%		38.5%	22.2%	
2:1	100%	100%		61.5%	77.8%	

All values listed as percentage of cases representing qualitative grade for each antibody. *statistically significant at p < 0.05 for Dual-Modular Neck versus MoM THA.

Immunohistochemistry Characteristics of Synovial Tissue from Dual-Modular Neck and MoM THA Groups.

the interstitial regions, both implants had T cell predominant lymphyocytic infiltrates. The majority of patients had a mixed population of CD4 and CD8 positive T cells, with CD4 cells being more numerous in most cases in perivascular regions (Figures 5A and B; Table 5). In interstitial regions, a subset of patients in both implant types had increased CD8 positive cell density relative to CD4, however, there was no significant difference between the implant types in CD4 to CD8 ratio (p = 0.189). Further lymphocytic sub-classification showed increased number of GATA3 positive expression relative to T-bet in all samples examined (Figures 5C and D; Table 5). FOXP3 positive lymphocytes were frequently present in lymphocyte-rich regions in both implant groups, and were graded as numerous in 47% and 25% of cases in the DMN and MoM THA respectively (Figure 5E). Immunohistochemistry for granzyme showed increased presence of positive cells in the DMN group relative to the MoM THA (27% versus 0% of cases respectively), and this trended towards significance (p = 0.053). Staining for CD117 showed a variable number of mast cells, ranging from occasional to numerous (>5 cells per HPF) in interstitial and perivascular regions in both implant groups (Figure 4E).

Examination of control samples of retrieved revision tissues from patients with polyethylene-induced osteolysis showed no lymphocytic infiltration in any cases and a similar staining pattern for the macrophagic markers CD68 and CD163. A similar distribution of CD20:CD3, CD4:CD8, and GATA3:T-bet was seen in perivascular regions in the synovium from patients with osteoarthritis with excessive synovial chronic inflammatory infiltrate. We had the unique opportunity to evaluate native,

preoperative synovial tissue from five patients in our series who subsequently developed ALTR after their total hip arthroplasty. A comparison of their native synovium with synovium after revision for ALTR showed similar lymphocytic distributions, including the presence of a CD4, GATA3 predominant perivascular lymphocytic infiltrate. Synovial necrosis was not identified in these pre-operative groups, although mild hyperplasia of the lining layer was observed. Similarly, in cases of ALTR with other MoM implants, a similar CD4 and GATA3 predominant lymphocytic infiltrate was seen.

Histologic patterns

Three distinct histologic patterns were identified at light microscopy in this series: 1) a predominantly macrophagic pattern with absent or minimal lymphocytic response, 2) mixed inflammatory pattern, macrophagic and lymphocytic with variable presence of plasma cells, eosinophils, and mast cells, and 3) granulomatous pattern, predominant or associated with the inflammatory pattern. The predominantly macrophagic group represented a group of patients with an adverse soft tissue reaction resulting in implant failure with minimal lymphocytic activation [16,18,37]. The mixed inflammatory pattern was subdivided into those with (A) or without (B) germinal centers because this may stratify patients based on variation of the immune response [15,17,19]. The third group had prominent formation of sarcoidosis-like granulomas in the presence of a mixed or macrophagic infiltrate, and this may represent a subset of patients with particular macrophage characteristics [15,17]. In our series, a macrophagic pattern of ALTR was seen in

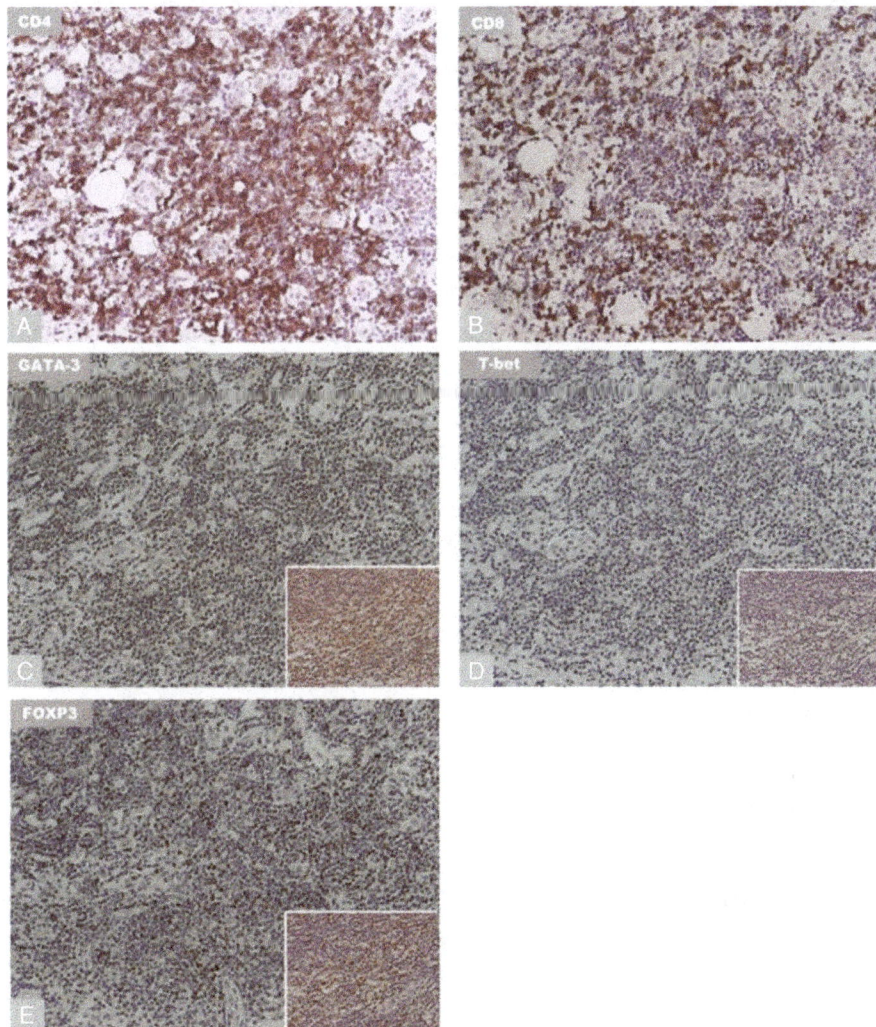

Figure 5 Immunohistochemistry in the Dual-Modular Neck and MoM THA groups (all 200X magnification). Perivascular lymphocytic infiltrate demostrates **A)** CD4 positivity and **B)** CD8 positivity. Further subclassification of perivascular lymphocytes shows **C)** T cell GATA-3 positivity, **D)** T cell T-bet positivity, and **E)** T cell FOXP3 positivity.

0% and 5.2% of cases of ALTR in the DMN and the MoM THA respectively with absent or minimal lymphocytic response (Table 6). The second, and most common, subtype was the mixed inflammatory pattern. An increased percentage of cases with germinal centers were seen in the DMN group (Table 6). Granulomatous pattern was seen more commonly in the DMN group (Table 6). In the inflammatory and granulomatous groups, ALVAL with necrosis was observed in certain cases.

Discussion

Failure due to ALTR has previously been described for MoM bearing surfaces and modular junctions at the head-neck and neck-stem [4,9-14,21-23,35,38,39]. The purposes of this study were to compare implant-based differences in periprosthetic tissue structure, organization, corrosion product morphology, and cellular composition by conventional histology and immunohistochemistry in ALTR resulting from two common implant configurations. Our results demonstrate that similarities between these two implants included spectrum of histologic patterns, composition of the inflammatory infiltrate, and presence of corrosion products. Differences between these implant types included macrophage and lymphocyte distributions, and corrosion product morphology. This is the first study to our knowledge to compare the histologic and immunohistochemical features of ALTR in two different classes of implants.

We have shown convincing histological evidence that similar common morphologic features exist in ALTR with an early phase of cellular activation and proliferation seen in neo-synovial reaction to other particulate implant materials (e.g. polyethylene) followed by a distinctive sequence of cellular and tissue reactions leading to formation of a variable amount of soft tissue necrosis/

Table 6 Observed histologic subtypes in the Dual-Modular Neck and the Metal-on-Metal (MoM) total hip arthroplasty (THA) groups

Observed subtypes	Dual-Modular Neck THA (N = 54 hips)	MoM THA (N = 18 hips)
Macrophagic	0 (0%)	1 (5.2%)
Macrophagic with Mixed Lymphocytic Infiltrate		
w/ Germinal Centers	15 (27.2%)	2 (11.1%)
w/o Germinal Centers	30 (54.5%)	14 (77.8%)
Granulomatous	9 (16.4%)	1 (5.2%)

All values listed as number (percentage of cases) representing each histologic subtype.
Histologic Subtypes of Adverse Local Tissue Reaction.

infarction. Corroborating evidence is provided by the metachronous development of the reaction in various areas of the periprosthetic tissue, contiguous areas of superficial necrosis, preserved neo-synovial architecture, and absence of necrosis in the bursal tissue until dehiscence of the fluid contained within the pseudocapsule. The time to revision in the DMN group was significantly shorter than the MoM THA, and this suggests different progression rates of ALTR with different implant designs. Progression of ALTR may depend on length of device implantation, toxicity/immunogenicity of corrosion particles, implant design and alignment, patient comorbidities, and host immune reactivity. The modality of failure of the DMN and MoM THA implants analyzed in this study have been attributed in previous publications to the formation of corrosion products at the metallic interacting surfaces and not to technical mistakes or poor design resulting in mechanical failure of the implants [5,9,11]. Gill et al. also found that corrosion at the modular neck-stem junction resulted in early revision relative to the same monoblock stem and bearing components [9]. Additionally, Cooper et al. have shown a similar time to failure of the DMN implant used in our study, further corroborating our results were not due to technical error [11]. A possibility of bias in time to revision might exist because the DMN group had a publicized recall of the implant, however, all patients revised in both cohorts were indicated for revision due to elevated metal ion levels, symptomatic hip pain, MRI findings of moderate to severe adverse tissue reaction, and/ or positive needle biopsies. Our observations are similar to previous studies that have illustrated the distinct histological aspects of the reaction, predominantly in MoM hip resurfacing implants or in mixed resurfacing and THA implants [10,13-19]. Previous publications examining ALTR have used the proposed ALVAL score by Campbell et al. as a grading system of the reaction [16,18,25]. If our interpretation of the natural history of the reaction is correct, the score would be an indication of developmental stage of the adverse reaction rather than a grading system of its biological severity, and therefore of limited clinical value in predicting the course or

the biological outcome of the reaction for each specific type of implant.

Different histologic subtypes were observed in ALTR in our study. A subset of patients in the MoM THA group had a macrophagic pattern of failure with minimal lymphocytic response and absent or minimal necrosis. These patients may have impingement related failure, suggested by black metallic particles in their soft tissue and/ or an immunoprofile that is less responsive to wear debris. A second subgroup of patients had a mixed macrophagic and lymphocytic response with a variable number of plasma cells, eosinophils, and mast cells. This has been described frequently in ALTR from previous studies and represented the most common pattern we observed [13-18]. A third subgroup displayed a granulomatous pattern with or without inflammatory infiltrate or necrosis, and this patient subgroup may have unique immunologic responses to wear debris. We did not observe any cases with an exclusively lymphocytic pattern without presence of particle-laden macrophages, as described by Berstock et al. [37]. This difference may be due to the extensive sampling performed of periprosthetic tissue in our study. The association of these different histologic patterns and clinical outcomes needs to be investigated in future studies.

We demonstrated an association between the presence of extra-cellular and intra-cellular corrosion products in the periprosthetic tissue with the presence of interstitial and perivascular lymphocytic infiltrate. This association suggests that corrosion particle laden macrophages are instrumental in the formation of the lymphocytic infiltrate, although free particulate material can also significantly contribute to the response. Corroborative evidence of our interpretation was the presence of benign lymphocytic aggregates in the bone marrow associated with particle-laden macrophages as previously reported in hip resurfacing implants [15,40]. The appearance of corrosion materials was different between the two implant designs, which also were associated with differing levels of serum cobalt and chromium ions. The MoM THA has two possible sources of corrosion materials or metallic debris: the metal-on-metal articular surface and the head-neck taper junction. The dual modular neck implant also has two possible sources of corrosion: the head-neck taper junction and the neck-stem taper junction, although the predominant one appears to be the latter [11]. These different surface possibilities likely explain the variable corrosion material appearance and distribution. Xia et al. used electron microscopy and EDX to assess macrophage content in ALVAL due to failure of a MoM bearing surface and their results showed nanometer-sized inclusions within the phagosomes with significant chromium content by EDX [41]. We hypothesize that the numerous, predominantly globular small intracellular inclusions seen on light microscopy represent corrosion products generated at the bearing surface, which are not present in the dual modular neck implant. This observation is confirmed by the presence of the same inclusions in resurfacing implants with the same bearing surface (data not shown). In contrast to intracellular corrosion material, both implant types had large extracellular corrosion aggregates of similar morphology. Our data indicate these materials represent corrosion products from the taper junctions at the head-neck and neck-stem, which is consistent with previous studies [5,11,35]. Analysis of material produced from head-neck taper corrosion suggested that chromium orthophosphate was the most common corrosion material produced at modular junctions, and this material could disseminate into the surrounding soft tissue [5,11,35]. These wear products differ in size and shape from the intracellular products that are seen from the bearing surface, possibly explaining biological or clinical differences between different implant types [42]. Moreover, the stratified appearance of the aggregates at light microscopy possibly suggests mixing of fluid proteins and secondary particles released from the exfoliated macrophages forming products of unknown and untested cytotoxicity. Early involvement of the hematopoietic bone marrow by macrophages and large aggregates of particles can also influence the adverse reaction, and this may have future biological significance.

The ALTR reaction seen in the DMN implant is unlikely to be influenced by polyethylene debris. There have been extensive publications in the literature about wear rates of highly cross-linked polyethylene in vivo, and for the X3, femoral head penetration rates remain low at two years (head penetration <0.06 mm) [43]. Moreover, between years 1 and 5, wear rates in vivo were less than 0.001 mm/ year [44]. This data suggests that polyethylene wear is unlikely to contribute to the observed reaction to ALTR seen in our study in the DMN group. This is further corroborated by the fact that only 1 of 54 cases examined in our study had polyethylene debris in their periprosthetic tissue at light microscopy, suggesting that polyethylene debris is unlikely to play a major role in ALTR seen in our study.

Immunohistochemistry results showed a predominant T lymphocytic response with a variable B cell component with the formation in some cases of perivascular germinal centers and tall endothelial cell venules as previously reported [13-17,19]. The analysis of the T cell population pointed towards a mixed pattern with predominant GATA3 positivity (Th2 lymphocytes) but also substantial T-bet and FOXP3 expressing lymphocytes, representing Th1 and Treg subgroups respectively. These findings were associated with the presence of a population of macrophages strongly positive for CD163, a marker of M2 macrophages, a subset frequently correlated with Th2 cytokines [45]. The frequent finding of a variable number of CD117 positive mast cells is also a new important finding with implications in reaction initiation/progression due to their interactions between T and B cell lymphocytes and eosinophils, and their potential to produce M2 inducing cytokines such as IL-4 [46]. Reaction initiation and severity may be explained by the release of chemokines from macrophages under oxidative stress and/or direct lymphocyte cytotoxicity [47-50]. Similar lymphocyte distributions were observed in the cases of osteoarthritis at time zero, and the possibility of a non-specific common pathway in different inflammatory conditions of the synovial membrane not representative of the initial response of the adverse reaction must be considered and confirmatory studies with testing of other specific antibodies are needed. It is also possible that the lymphocyte distributions seen in our study reflect an innate immunologic profile of the synovium with subsequent adaptive modulation, and analysis of pathologic gene expression patterns could be helpful to elucidate the role of these lymphocytic subpopulations in initiation and progression of ALTR [51]. Collectively, the immunohistochemistry studies indicate a complex adaptive immune response potentially involving several cell types. Future molecular analysis will help define the signaling pathways that orchestrate the tissue necrosis and other pathologies underlying ALTR.

The main limitation of this study is the attempt to reconstruct the natural history of the reaction based on one cross sectional observation at the time of implant revision. We compensated for this limitation by extensive topographical sampling of the periprosthetic soft tissue, but we acknowledge that continued longitudinal observation would be needed to confirm our findings.

Conclusion

In conclusion, a common spectrum of neo-synovial proliferation and subsequent necrosis are observed in both implant classes. These findings can represent temporal progression of the reaction, which could have implant-based and patient-based characteristics. The Campbell-ALVAL score would represent an index of the staging of this temporal progression and not of the grading of the severity of ALTR. Cellular composition showed subtle differences in macrophagic and lymphocytic distributions in the two implant classes, suggesting biological differences may exist between different implant classes. The prominence of corrosion products is a consistent feature of ALTR in both implant types; however, their morphologies differ based on implant design. Immunohistochemistry showed a complex adaptive immune response, and future studies on molecular signaling pathways in ALTR are needed. The immunogenicity and toxicity of the new particulate material formed at the implant interacting surfaces and their association with hematopoietic marrow cells are still unknown, especially in patients with pre-existing immunologic disease. Short- and long-term follow-up of all patients affected by ALTR is needed to monitor for local and systemic effects.

Abbreviations
ALTR: Adverse local tissue reaction; DMN: Dual-modular neck implant; MoM: Metal-on-metal implant; THA: Total hip arthroplasty; ALVAL: Aseptic lymphocyte dominated vasculitis-associated lesions.

Competing interests
There are no competing financial or non-financial interests in direct relation to this manuscript for any authors. Author S Jerabek is a consultant for Mako Surgical Corporation.

Authors' contributions
GP conceived of the study, collected and analyzed synovial tissue, and drafted the manuscript. BR assisted with histologic and immunohistochemistry analysis and drafted the manuscript. SAJ analyzed the clinical data. GM performed immunohistochemistry and assisted with study design. GW and DM collected synovial tissue and assisted with manuscript preparation. SRG participated in study design and interpretation of data. PEP participated in study design and coordination. All authors read and approved the final manuscript.

Acknowledgements
We would like to acknowledge the surgeons of the Adult Reconstruction and Joint Replacement Service at the Hospital for Special Surgery for providing periprosthetic tissue for this study; Irina Shuleshko and Yana Bronfman for technical assistance in histology preparation; Licia Montagna, Claudia Parolini, and Paola Piccoli at University of Verona for immunohistochemistry staining; and Philip Rusli for technical assistance for preparation of the manuscript.

Author details
[1]Department of Pathology, Hospital for Special Surgery, 535 East 70th Street, New York, NY 10021, USA. [2]Department of Orthopedic Surgery, Hospital for Special Surgery, New York, NY, USA. [3]Department of Pathology and Diagnostics, University of Verona, Verona and Pederzoli Hospital, Peschiera, Italy. [4]Division of Research, Hospital for Special Surgery, New York, NY, USA.

References
1. Amstutz HC, Grigoris P: **Metal on metal bearings in hip arthroplasty.** *Clin Orthop Relat Res* 1996, **329**(Suppl):S11–S34.
2. Srinivasan A, Jung E, Levine BR: **Modularity of the femoral component in total hip arthroplasty.** *J Am Acad Orthop Surg* 2012, **20**:214–222.
3. Cohen D: **How safe are metal-on-metal hip implants?** *BMJ* 2012, **344**: e1410.
4. Kop AM, Swarts E: **Corrosion of a hip stem with a modular neck taper junction: a retrieval study of 16 cases.** *J Arthroplasty* 2009, **24**:1019–1023.
5. Huber M, Reinisch G, Trettenhahn G, Zweymüller K, Lintner F: **Presence of corrosion products and hypersensitivity-associated reactions in periprosthetic tissue after aseptic loosening of total hip replacements with metal bearing surfaces.** *Acta Biomater* 2009, **5**:172–180.
6. Bosker BH, Ettema HB, Boomsma MF, Kollen BJ, Maas M, Verheyen CC: **High incidence of pseudotumour formation after large-diameter metal-on-metal total hip replacement: a prospective cohort study.** *J Bone Joint Surg Br* 2012, **94**:755–761.
7. Chana R, Esposito C, Campbell PA, Walter WK, Walter WL: **Mixing and matching causing taper wear: corrosion associated with pseudotumour formation.** *J Bone Joint Surg Br* 2012, **94**:281–286.
8. Fabi D, Levine B, Paprosky W, Della Valle C, Sporer S, Klein G, Levine H, Hartzband M: **Metal-on-metal total hip arthroplasty: causes and high incidence of early failure.** *Orthopedics* 2012, **35**:e1009–e1016.
9. Gill IP, Webb J, Sloan K, Beaver RJ: **Corrosion at the neck-stem junction as a cause of metal ion release and pseudotumour formation.** *J Bone Joint Surg Br* 2012, **94**:895–900.
10. Meyer H, Mueller T, Goldau G, Chamaon K, Ruetschi M, Lohmann CH: **Corrosion at the cone/taper interface leads to failure of large-diameter metal-on-metal total hip arthroplasties.** *Clin Orthop Relat Res* 2012, **470**:3101–3108.
11. Cooper HJ, Urban RM, Wixson RL, Meneghini RM, Jacobs JJ: **Adverse local tissue reaction arising from corrosion at the femoral neck-body junction in a dual-taper stem with a cobalt-chromium modular neck.** *J Bone Joint Surg Am* 2013, **95**:865–872.
12. Werner SD, Bono JV, Nandi S, Ward DM, Talmo CT: **Adverse tissue reactions in modular exchangeable neck implants: a report of two cases.** *J Arthroplasty* 2013, **28**:543.e13–5.
13. Davies AP, Willert HG, Campbell PA, Learmonth ID, Case CP: **An unusual lymphocytic perivascular infiltration in tissues around contemporary metal-on-metal joint replacements.** *J Bone Joint Surg Am* 2005, **87**:18–27.
14. Willert HG, Buchhorn GH, Fayyazi A, Flury R, Windler M, Köster G, Lohmann CH: **Metal-on-metal bearings and hypersensitivity in patients with artificial hip joints. A clinical and histomorphological study.** *J Bone Joint Surg Am* 2005, **87**:28–36.
15. Mahendra G, Pandit H, Kliskey K, Murray D, Gill HS, Athanasou N: **Necrotic and vinflammatory changes in metal-on-metal resurfacing hip arthroplasties.** *Acta Orthop* 2009, **80**:653–659.
16. Campbell P, Ebramzadeh E, Nelson S, Takamura K, De Smet K, Amstutz HC: **Histological features of pseudotumor-like tissues from metal-on-metal hips.** *Clin Orthop Relat Res* 2010, **468**:2321–2327.
17. Natu S, Sidaginamale RP, Gandhi J, Langton DJ, Nargol AV: **Adverse reactions to metal debris: histopathological features of periprosthetic soft tissue reactions seen in association with failed metal on metal hip arthroplasties.** *J Clin Pathol* 2012, **65**:409–418.
18. Grammatopoulos G, Pandit H, Kamali A, Maggiani F, Glyn-Jones S, Gill HS, Murray DW, Athanasou N: **The correlation of wear with histological features after failed hip resurfacing arthroplasty.** *J Bone Joint Surg Am* 2013, **95**:e81.
19. Mittal S, Revell M, Barone F, Hardie DL, Matharu GS, Davenport AJ, Martin RA, Grant M, Mosselmans F, Pynsent P, Sumathi VP, Addison O, Revell PA, Buckley CD: **Lymphoid aggregates that resemble tertiary lymphoid organs define a specific pathological subset in metal-on-metal hip replacements.** *PLoS One* 2013, **8**:e63470.
20. Gallo J, Vaculova J, Goodman SB, Konttinen YT, Thyssen JP: **Contributions of human tissue analysis to understanding the mechanisms of loosening and osteolysis in total hip replacement.** *Acta Biomater* 2014, **10**:2354–2366.
21. Cooper HJ, Della Valle CJ, Berger RA, Tetreault M, Paprosky WG, Sporer SM, Jacobs JJ: **Corrosion at the head-neck taper as a cause for adverse local tissue reactions after total hip arthroplasty.** *J Bone Joint Surg Am* 2012, **94**:1655–1661.
22. Fricka KB, Ho H, Peace WJ, Engh CA Jr: **Metal-on-metal local tissue reaction is associated with corrosion of the head taper junction.** *J Arthroplasty* 2012, **27**(8 Suppl):26–31.e1.
23. Dyrkacz RM, Brandt JM, Ojo OA, Turgeon TR, Wyss UP: **The influence of head size on corrosion and fretting behaviour at the head-neck interface of artificial hip joints.** *J Arthroplasty* 2013, **28**:1036–1040.
24. Hayter CL, Gold SL, Koff MF, Perino G, Nawabi DH, Miller TT, Potter HG: **MRI findings in painful metal-on-metal hip arthroplasty.** *AJR Am J Roentgenol* 2012, **199**:884–893.
25. Nawabi DH, Hayter CL, Su EP, Koff MF, Perino G, Gold SL, Koch KM, Potter HG: **Magnetic resonance imaging findings in symptomatic versus**

asymptomatic subjects following metal-on-metal hip resurfacing arthroplasty. *J Bone Joint Surg Am* 2013, 95:895–902.

26. Nawabi DH, Gold S, Lyman S, Fields K, Padgett DE, Potter HG: **MRI Predicts ALVAL and tissue damage in metal-on-metal hip arthroplasty.** *Clin Orthop Relat Res* 2014, 472:471–481.

27. Nawabi DH, Nassif NA, Do HT, Stoner K, Elpers M, Su EP, Wright T, Potter HG, Padgett DE: **What causes unexplained pain in patients with metal-on metal hip devices? A retrieval, histologic, and imaging analysis.** *Clin Orthop Relat Res* 2014, 472:543–554.

28. Willert HG, Semlisch M: **Reactions of the articular capsule to wear products of artificial joint prostheses.** *J Biomed Mater Res* 1977, 11:157–164.

29. Holness CL, Simmons DL: **Molecular cloning of CD68, a human macrophage marker related to lysosomal glycoproteins.** *Blood* 1993, 81:1607–1613.

30. Wang FQ, Chen G, Zhu JY, Zhang W, Ren JG, Liu H, Sun ZJ, Jia J, Zhao YF: **M2-polarised macrophages in infantile haemangiomas: correlation with promoted angiogenesis.** *J Clin Pathol* 2013, 66:1058–1064.

31. Zheng W, Flavell RA: **The transcription factor GATA-3 is necessary and sufficient for Th2 cytokine gene expression in CD4 T cells.** *Cell* 1997, 89:587–596.

32. Szabo SJ, Kim ST, Costa GL, Zhang X, Fathman CG, Glimcher LH: **A novel transcription factor, T-bet, directs Th1 lineage commitment.** *Cell* 2000, 100:655–669.

33. Hori S, Nomura T, Sakaguchi S: **Control of regulatory T cell development by the transcription factor Foxp3.** *Science* 2003, 299:1057–1061.

34. Iemura A, Tsai M, Ando A, Wershil BK, Galli SJ: **The c-kit ligand, stem cell factor, promotes mast cell survival by suppressing apoptosis.** *Am J Pathol* 1994, 144:321–328.

35. Jacobs JJ, Urban RM, Gilbert JL, Skipor AK, Black J, Jasty M, Galante JO: **Local and distant products from modularity.** *Clin Orthop Relat Res* 1995, 319:94–105.

36. Jacobs JJ, Gilbert JL, Urban RM: **Corrosion of metal orthopaedic implants.** *J Bone Joint Surg Am* 1998, 80:268–282.

37. Berstock JR, Baker RP, Bannister GC, Case CP: **Histology of failed metal-on metal hip arthroplasty; three distinct sub-types.** *Hip Int* 2014, 5:0.

38. Langton DJ, Joyce TJ, Jameson SS, Lord J, Van Orsouw M, Holland JP, Nargol AV, De Smet KA: **Adverse reaction to metal debris following hip resurfacing: the influence of component type, orientation and volumetric wear.** *J Bone Joint Surg Br* 2011, 93:164–171.

39. Lindgren JU, Brismar BH, Wikstrom AC: **Adverse reaction to metal release from a modular metal-on-polyethylene hip prosthesis.** *J Bone Joint Surg Br* 2011, 93:1427–1430.

40. Hinsch A, Vettorazzi E, Morlock MM, Rüther W, Amling M, Zustin J: **Sex differences in the morphological failure patterns following hip resurfacing arthroplasty.** *BMC Med* 2011, 9:113.

41. Xia Z, Kwon YM, Mehmood S, Downing C, Jurkschat K, Murray DW: **Characterization of metal-wear nanoparticles in pseudotumor following metal-on-metal hip resurfacing.** *Nanomedicine* 2011, 7:674–681.

42. Caicedo MS, Samelko L, McAllister K, Jacobs JJ, Hallab NJ: **Increasing both CoCrMo-alloy particle size and surface irregularity induces increased macrophage inflammasome activation in vitro potentially through lysosomal destabilization mechanisms.** *J Orthop Res* 2013, 31:1633–1642.

43. Campbell DG, Field JR, Callary SA: **Second-generation highly cross-linked X3™ polyethylene wear: a preliminary radiostereometric analysis study.** *Clin Orthop Relat Res* 2010, 468:2704–2709.

44. Callary SA, Field JR, Campbell DG: **Low wear of a second-generation highly crosslinked polyethylene liner: a 5-year radiostereometric analysis study.** *Clin Orthop Relat Res* 2013, 471:3596–3600.

45. Mills CD: **M1 and M2 macrophages: oracles of health and disease.** *Crit Rev Immunol* 2012, 32:463–488.

46. Amin K: **The role of mast cells in allergic inflammation.** *Respir Med* 2012, 106:9–14.

47. Caicedo MS, Desai R, McAllister K, Reddy A, Jacobs JJ, Hallab NJ: **Soluble and particulate Co Cr-Mo alloy implant metals activate the inflammasome danger signaling pathway in human macrophages: a novel mechanism for implant debris reactivity.** *J Orthop Res* 2009, 27:847–854.

48. Cobelli N, Scharf B, Crisi GM, Hardin J, Santambrogio L: **Mediators of the inflammatory response to joint replacement devices.** *Nat Rev Rheumatol* 2011, 7:600–608.

49. Vanlangenakker N, Vanden Berghe T, Vandenabeele P: **Many stimuli pull the necrotic trigger, an overview.** *Cell Death Differ* 2012, 19:75–86.

50. Samelko L, Caicedo MS, Lim SJ, Della-Valle C, Jacobs J, Hallab NJ: **Cobalt-alloy implant debris induce HIF-1α hypoxia associated responses: a mechanism for metal-specific orthopedic implant failure.** *PLoS One* 2013, 8:e67127.

51. Fujishiro T, Moojen DJ, Kobayashi N, Dhert WJ, Bauer TW: **Perivascular and diffuse lymphocytic inflammation are not specific for failed metal-on metal hip implants.** *Clin Orthop Relat Res* 2011, 469:1127–1133.

15

A retrospective analysis of breast cancer subtype based on ER/PR and HER2 status in Ghanaian patients at the Korle Bu Teaching Hospital, Ghana

Bernard Seshie[1], Nii Armah Adu-Aryee[2], Florence Dedey[2], Benedict Calys-Tagoe[3] and Joe-Nat Clegg-Lamptey[2*]

Abstract

Background: Breast cancer is a heterogeneous disease composed of multiple subgroups with different molecular alterations, cellular composition, clinical behaviour, and response to treatment. This study evaluates the occurrence of the various subtypes and their clinical and pathological behaviour in the Ghanaian breast cancer population at the Korle Bu Teaching Hospital (KBTH).

Methods: Retrospective review of case notes of patients who had completed treatment for breast cancer at the KBTH within the last 5 years was conducted between April 2011 and March 2012. Subtypes were determined by immunohistochemistry classification based on expression of estrogen receptor (ER), progesterone receptor (PR), and human epidermal growth factor receptor-2 (HER-2).

Result: A total of 165 cases contributed to this study. The mean age at diagnosis was 52.5 ± 12.1 years. Tumour size ranged from 0.8 cm to 15 cm with a mean of 4.9 ± 2.8 cm and median of 4 cm. Tumour grade was Grade I 8.3 %, Grade II 60.8 % and Grade III 30.8 %. ER, PR and HER2/neu receptor positivity was 32.1, 25.6 and 25.5 % respectively. Almost half (49.4 %) of the study population had triple negative tumours. Luminal A, luminal B and non-luminal HER2 were 25.6, 12.2, and 12.8 % respectively. No statistically significant association was seen between subtype and tumour size, tumour grade, lymph node status and age at diagnosis.

Conclusion: Triple negative tumour is the most occurring subtype in the Ghanaian breast cancer population treated at the Korle Bu Teaching Hospital. Lack of association seen between subtypes and their clinical and pathological behaviour could be due to small sample size.

Keywords: Breast cancer, Subtype, ER, PR, HER2

Background

Breast cancer is still the most common cancer in women comprising 16 % of all female cancers worldwide [1]. With increasing improvement in treatment modalities like hormonal and chemotherapy, however, mortality has declined [2]. But this decline is faster in white Americans compared to black Americans in the United States of America, although the incidence of breast cancer is lower in the latter [3]. The poorer prognosis in blacks has been attributed to a number of factors, including the observation that blacks appear to be at higher risk of breast cancer at an early age, and are diagnosed with more aggressive and advanced tumours [4, 5]. In Ghana, where more than 50 % of patients present with locally advanced or metastatic disease, 5-year survival was reported as only 25.3 % in 2001 [6].

It is now clear that breast cancer is a heterogeneous disease of multiple subgroups with different molecular alterations, cellular composition, clinical behaviour, and response to treatment [7–9]. Hence, standard clinical prognostic features such as age, tumour size, nodal status, grade, and hormone receptor status may be inaccurate.

* Correspondence: clegglamptey@chs.edu.gh
[2]Department of Surgery, School of Medicine and Dentistry, University of Ghana, Accra, Ghana
Full list of author information is available at the end of the article

Consequently, many patients are perhaps given treatment they may not need and benefit from. On the other hand, the true risk in some patients is underestimated and some may be given false assurances of favourable prognosis [10].

Several studies have attested to the higher prevalence of triple negative tumours with poorer prognosis in breast cancer patients of African origin [5, 11], although a study from Nigeria reported no difference in the pattern of hormone receptors in the African breast cancer population compared to other populations [12].

This study was undertaken to determine the occurrence of the various subtypes of breast cancer in Ghanaian patients seeking treatment at the Korle Bu Teaching Hospital and to determine the clinical and pathological behaviour of the different subtypes (grade, tumour size, lymph node burden and age at diagnosis).

Methods

Data for this study was from an ongoing study on upper limb morbidity following treatment of breast cancer in Ghana, which has been approved by the Ethical and Protocol Review Committee, University of Ghana School of Medicine and Dentistry.

Study population

Korle Bu Teaching Hospital (KBTH) is the largest teaching hospital in Ghana, the leading tertiary hospital and the major referral centre in the country. It also serves as the teaching hospital of the University of Ghana School of Medicine and Dentistry.

Breast Cancer patients who had received and completed treatment for breast cancer at the Korle Bu Teaching Hospital (KBTH) within the last 5 years and were being seen for out-patient review constituted the study population. Data was thus collected between April 2011 and March 2012. During the period 363 consecutive patients who met the above criteria were seen and their case notes reviewed. Immunohistochemistry (IHC) for estrogen receptor (ER), progesterone receptor (PR), and HER-2/neu, which is a prerequisite for this study, was available for 165. They thus constituted the subset for this study. Demographic information (hand dominance and educational level), breast cancer clinico-pathological features (age at diagnosis, tumour size, tumour grade, lymph node status, hormonal receptors status) and treatment modality (type of surgery, chemotherapy) were extracted from the case notes.

Pathology reports from which ER, PR and HER-2/neu, were obtained came from Korle-Bu Teaching Hospital. IHC was performed on formalin-fixed paraffin embedded tissue sections. The ER and PR tests were scored based on an aggregate score of percentage of tumour stained and staining intensity. Aggregate score of more than 2 were considered positive; that is, a minimum of 1–10 % stained associated with minimum intensity. HER-2/neu was considered positive if an IHC 3+ result was found. Flourescence in situ hybridization (FISH) was not available in the institution.

For this study we used Immunohistochemistry (IHC) classification that categorizes tumours according to the expression of estrogen receptor (ER), progesterone receptor (PR), and HER-2/neu. Expression of basal cytokeratin 5/6 and EGFR were not determined in these cases. Hence the triple negative tumours included both core basal phenotype, equivalent to the basal-like by gene expression profiling, and five negative phenotype. Below is the categorization used:

Luminal A (ER/PR+, HER2-)
- ER+/PR+/HER2-; ER-/PR+/HER2-; or ER+/PR-/HER2-

Luminal B (ER/PR+, HER2+)
- ER+/PR+/HER2+; ER-/PR+/HER2+; or ER+/PR-/HER2+

Non-luminal HER2 (ER-/PR-/HER2+)
- ER-/PR-/HER2+

Triple Negative (ER-/PR-/HER2-)
- ER-/PR-/HER2-

Histological grading was by the Bloom-Richardson grading system that combined scores for nuclear grade, tubule formation and mitotic rate [13].

Statistical analysis

SPSS 16.0 was used for the descriptive data analysis. To test for association between subtype and tumour grade, and subtype and lymph node burden contingency table was used and Chi Square test done. One-way ANOVA was conducted to compare the differences in tumour size and age at diagnosis between breast cancer subtypes.

Results

A total of 165 cases contributed to this study. The mean age at diagnosis was 52.5 ± 12.1 years. The youngest patient in the study group was 24 years and the oldest person was 77 years at the time of diagnosis. Figure 1 shows the age distribution at the time of diagnosis. The educational level of the study population is as shown in Fig. 2.

In 50.9 % of the study population the tumour was located in the left breast with the remaining 49.1 % in the right breast. Over 90 % of the patients were right handed. There was however, no correlation between hand dominance and tumour site (Spearman's correlation value of 0.034, p-value of 0.666).

Tumour size ranged from 0.8 cm to 15 cm with a mean of 4.9 ± 2.8 cm and median of 4. Eight tumours were ≥ 10 cm. Tumour size (T in TNM classification)

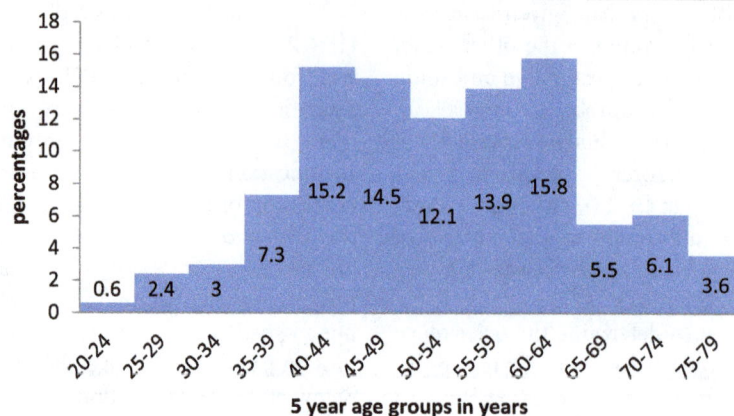

Fig. 1 Age distribution of study patient

values were available for 155 cases. T1 (maximum diameter 2 cm or less) tumour was present in 17/155 (11 %) and T2 (size more than 2 cm but not more than 5 cm), T3 (bigger than 5 cm) and T4 (spread to chest wall, or skin—including inflammatory cancer) tumours were 71 (45.8 %), 42 (27.1 %), and 25 (15.2 %) respectively.

The majority of tumours were Grade 2. The distribution of tumour grade is shown in Fig. 3.

Mastectomy was done in 97.6 % (161/165) of cases. Only 4 cases (2.4 %) had breast conservation surgery (BCS). Apart from 2 patients who had sentinel node biopsy, all the other patients had axillary clearance. Less than 10 lymph nodes were removed in 52.2 % of cases. Mean lymph node (LN) removal was 9.4 ± 4.3 and mean LN involvement was 3.3 ± 3.6. Regional LN involvement (TNM) in 137 patients in which data was available was N0 47 (34.3 %), N1 35 (25.5 %), N2 46 (33.6 %) and N3 9 (6.6 %).

ER, PR and HER 2 neu receptor positivity was 32.1 % (53/165), 25.6 % (42/164) and 25.5 % (40/157) respectively. The distribution of the receptor status by tumour size, tumour grade and LN positivity is shown in Table 1.

Data for breast cancer subtype was available for 156 cases. Almost half (49.4 %) of the study population had triple negative tumours. The distribution of various subtypes is as shown in Fig. 4.

The distribution of the subtype by tumour size, tumour grade and LN positivity is shown in Table 2. Luminal A subtype constituted 53.3 % of T1 tumours, whereas triple negative subtype represented 50 % of T2 tumours, 57.1 % of T3 tumours and 50 % of T4 tumours. However, the difference in tumour size among the subtypes was not significant ($F_{3, 113} = 1.26$, $p = 0.262$). Regarding tumour grade, 45.5 % of Grade 2 tumours and 52.8 % of Grade 3 tumours were triple negative subtype. But there was no statistically significant association between tumour grade and subtype (p-value = 0.515). Although 51.1 % of N2 and 66.7 % of N3 lymph node status were triple negative subtype, no significant association was seen statistically (p-value = 0.547). The same applied to age at diagnosis ($F_{3, 152} = .507$, $p = 0.678$).

In the study population, 43.1 % received between 2 to 6 cycles of neoadjuvant chemotherapy. The commonest combination therapy used as neoadjuvant and adjuvant therapy was Cyclophosphamide—Doxorubicin—5 Fluorouracil (CAF) in 85.5 % of cases. 5-Fluorouracil—Epirubicin—Cyclophosphamide (FEC) 6.2 %, Cyclophosphamide—Methotrexate -5-Fluorouracil (CMF) 6.2 %, and Paclitaxel in only 1.4 %.

Discussion

In this study of patients treated for breast cancer we found predominance of hormone receptor negative tumours (49.4 %). This is consistent with a study from Kumasi-Ghana between July 2004 and June 2009, which reported 42.5 % triple negative tumours in 54 breast cancer patients [14]. An earlier from the same centre that compared Ghanaian breast cancer patients with black American and white American reported a higher percentage of hormone negative tumours of 82.2 % in Ghanaian women compared

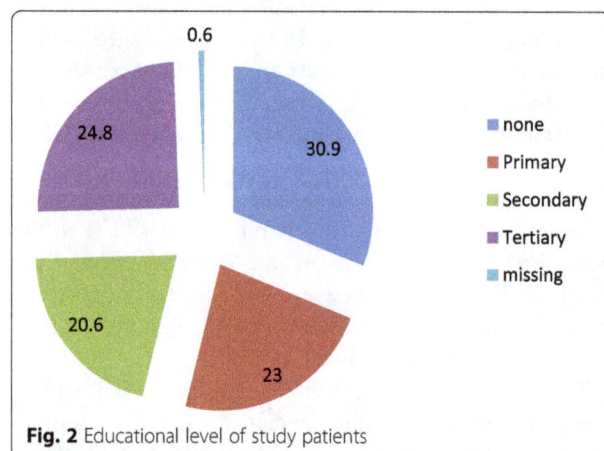

Fig. 2 Educational level of study patients

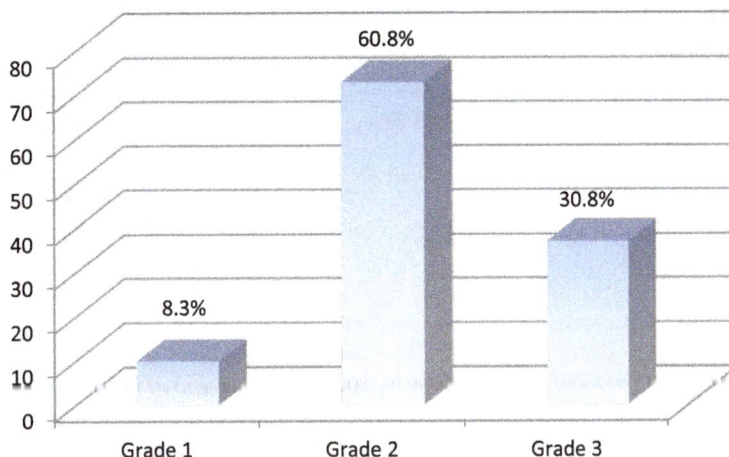

Fig. 3 Histological grade of tumours

to 26.4 and 16.0 % in black American and white American women respectively [11].

DNA microarray analysis of gene expression has identified five subtypes with different gene expression characteristics and differences in behaviour [15]. The usefulness of gene expression pattern rests in its value as a prognostic maker [16]. Although considered as gold standard it has not been widely used due to expense and difficulty using paraffin-embedded material. Hence, the use of immunohistochemisty (IHC) which is simple, workable, and capable of classifying tumours

into subtypes which are surrogates to gene expression pattern [17].

IHC for hormone receptor status, human epidermal growth factor receptor-2 (HER2) status, and at least one basal marker (cytokeratin [CK]5/6 or epidermal growth factor receptor [EGFR]) enable the division of tumours into Luminal 1, Luminal 2, Non-luminal HER2 positive tumours, and triple negative tumours (Fig. 5) and are associated with different behaviour [7].

Using IHC classification based on expression of ER, PR, and HER-2 receptors tumours were grouped in Luminal

Table 1 Distribution of receptor status by tumour size, grade and LN involvement

Tumour size	Receptor status								
	ER+	ER-	Total	PR+	PR-	Total	Her2+	Her2-	Total
T1	9 (17.6)	8 (7.7)	17 (11.0)	7 (17.5)	9 (7.9)	16 (10.4)	4 (10.8)	12 (10.8)	16 (10.0)
T2	24 (47.1)	47 (45.2)	71 (45.8)	21 (52.3)	50 (43.9)	71 (46.1)	17 (46.9)	49 (44.1)	66 (44.6)
T3	12 (20.6)	30 (28.8)	42 (27.1)	6 (15.0)	36 (31.6)	42 (27.3)	9 (24.3)	33 (29.7)	42 (28.4)
T4	6 (11.8)	19 (18.3)	25 (6.1)	6 (15.0)	19 (16.7)	25 (16.2)	7 (18.9)	17 (15.3)	24 (16.2)
Total	51	104	155	40	114	154	37	111	148
Tumour grade									
1	5 (50)	5 (50)	10	4 (40)	6 (60)	10	3 (33.3)	6 (66.7)	9
2	24 (32.9)	49 (67.1)	73	23 (31.9)	49 (68.1)	72	21 (30.4)	48 (69.6)	69
3	8 (21.6)	29 (78.4)	37	5 (13.5)	32 (86.5)	37	8 (22.2)	28 (77.8)	36
Total	37	83	120	32	87	119	32	82	114
Lymph node positivity									
N0	12 (25.5)	35 (74.5)	47	8 (17.0)	39 (83.0)	47	11 (25.0)	33 (75.0)	44
N1	13 (32.1)	22 (62.9)	35	12 (34.3)	23 (65.7)	35	8 (25.0)	24 (75.0)	32
N2	16 (34.8)	30 (65.2)	46	10 (22.2)	35 (77.8)	45	12 (26.1)	34 (73.9)	46
N3	2 (22.2)	7 (77.8)	9	0 (0)	9 (100)	9	3 (33.3)	6 (66.7)	9
Total	43	94	137	30	106	136	34	97	131

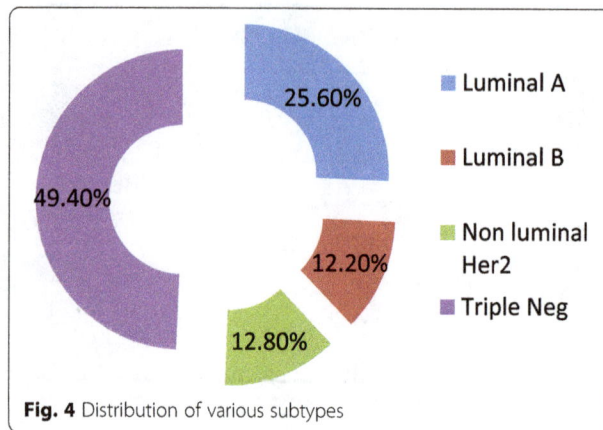

Fig. 4 Distribution of various subtypes

A, Luminal B, Non-luminal HER-2 and triple negative tumours. We observed a high prevalence of triple negative subtype. Indeed, almost half of the cases were triple negative. This is consistent with some studies from Nigeria and Senegal in which majority of tumours were basal-like 27 % or unclassified 28 % subtype (surrogate for triple negative) [18]. However, this is in contrast to another study from Nigeria in which majority of tumours were Luminal A (77.6 %) [12]. Luminal A, although the second most frequently occurring subtype in our study, was present in only 25.60 % of cases. One limitation to our study was the non availability of retrospective data on basal markers (cytokeratin [CK]5/6 or epidermal growth factor receptor [EGFR]) as they are not routinely done in

our centre. This would have enabled us stratify the triple negative tumours into 5 negative phenotype (non-basal triple negative) and core basal phenotype which many studies had shown to have different behaviour with the latter being more aggressive [5, 8, 17, 19, 20].

In addition, BRCA 1 and 2 mutations have not been determined in our study population. Hence, we are unable to evaluate their contribution to the high prevalence of triple negative tumours in this study. However, several studies have documented high proportion of triple negative breast cancer in carriers of these germ-line mutations, especial BRCA 1 [21–25]. Future research is needed in this area because of its implications for treatment. Triple negative breast cancer patients with BRCA 1 or BRCA like tumours can benefit from treatment with PARP inhibitors [26].

In this study triple negative tumours appeared to be associated with high mean tumour size and higher proportion of T2, T3 and T4 tumours compared to other subtypes. Indeed, 53.3 % of T1 tumours were luminal A subtype whereas over 50 % T2 to T4 tumours were Triple negative tumours. They also constitute greater proportion of Grade 2 and Grade 3 tumours and N2 and N3 tumours. These are consistent with other studies that have shown that triple negative breast cancer has very unfavourable and aggressive clinicopathological features [5, 11]. However, we failed to find significant statistical association.

Our findings have implication for treatment of breast cancer in Ghana. In the past, patient with breast cancer were treated blindly with tamoxifen. However, approximately 50 % of our patients may not be suitable for hormonal or targeted therapy because they are either negative for ER/PR or do not over express HER2. Hence, they will not benefit from the advantages of these modalities of treatment [27–30]. Currently chemotherapy remains the only systemic treatment for this category of patients. Fortunately, core basal phenotype which is a subset of triple negative breast cancer has the greatest short-term effect from cytotoxics compared to all other subtypes. But this cannot be said about the 5 negative phenotype [31]. Several studies using post treatment American Joint Committee on Cancer tumour-node-metastasis staging for invasive carcinoma have documented higher complete pathological response in the core basal phenotype of triple negative breast cancer compared to all other subtypes [5, 31]. However, they still have poorer prognosis due to higher likelihood of relapse in those with residual disease [9, 31].

Several of these studies demonstrated the importance of neo-adjuvant chemotherapy in triple negative breast cancer patients. This is not for the sole purpose of tumour reduction to facilitate surgery, but also to assess response to cytotoxic drugs and predict the likelihood of

Table 2 Distribution of subtype by tumour size, grade and LN involvement

Subtype					
Tumour size	Luminal A	Luminal B	Non luminal Her2	Triple Neg	Total
T1	8 (53.3)	2 (13.3)	2 (13.3)	3 (20.0)	15 (100)
T2	17 (25.8)	10 (15.2)	6 (9.1)	33 (50.0)	66 (100)
T3	9 (21.4)	4 (9.5)	5 (11.9)	24 (57.1)	42 (100)
T4	5 (20.8)	2 (8.3)	5 (20.8)	12 (50.0)	24 (100)
Total	39	18	18	72	147
Tumour grade					
1	3 (33.3)	2 (22.2)	1 (11.1)	3 (33.3)	9
2	17 (25.0)	10 (14.7)	10 (14.7)	31 (45.5)	68
3	9 (25.0)	1 (2.8)	7 (19.4)	19 (52.8)	36
Total	29	13	18	53	113
Lymph node positivity					
N0	10 (22.7)	4 (9.1)	7 (15.9)	23 (52.3)	44
N1	12 (37.5)	4 (12.5)	4 (12.5)	12 (37.5)	32
N2	10 (22.2)	7 (15.6)	5 (11.1)	23 (51.1)	45
N3	0(0)	2 (22.2)	1 (11.1)	6 (66.7)	9
Total	32	17	17	64	130

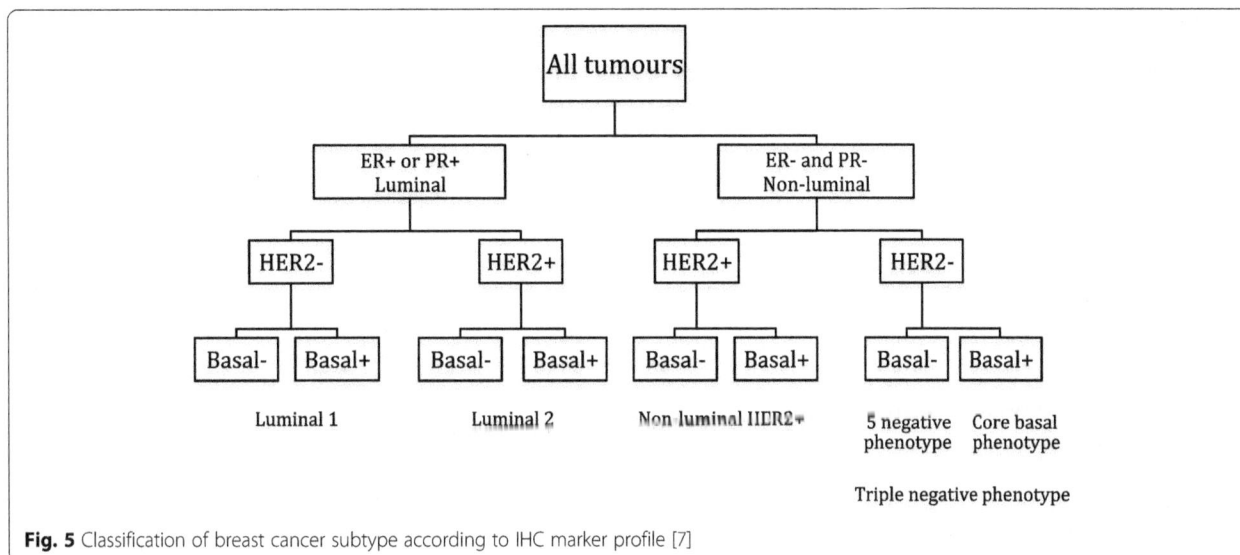

Fig. 5 Classification of breast cancer subtype according to IHC marker profile [7]

relapse in patients with residual disease. But in our study only 43.1 % received between 2 to 6 cycles of neo-adjuvant chemotherapy. In our study 85.5 % of patient received CAF either as neo-adjuvant, adjuvant or both despite almost half of the patients being triple negative. However, studies have shown that basal-like and HER2+ subtypes are more sensitive to neo-adjuvant chemotherapy with paclitaxel- and doxorubicin-containing regimes compared to the luminal subtype [9]. Also for the triple negative tumours (especially BRCA—mutated disease), platinum based chemotherapy and PARP inhibitors may hold some promise [32, 33]. The neoadjuvant/adjuvant treatment of the patients in our study therefore appears to be suboptimal.

For surgical treatment, 97.6 % of the patients had mastectomy, a rather high rate compared to what is reported in Europe, North America and Japan (between 27.5 to 64 % [34–37]. Breast conserving surgery was only done in 2.4 % of our patients, a rather low rate as compared to rates of 54 % to over 70 % elsewhere [35–39]. As many as 66 % of the patients in this study presented with a T1 or 2 tumours while almost 60 % had N0 or 1 lymph node staging. Breast conservation surgery may have been suitable for many of these patients. However, almost half of the patients had triple negative subtype and about 91 % had grade 2 and 3 tumours. These factors, as well as increasing tumour size, have been found to be independent predictors of mastectomy but are not contraindications to BCS [34, 36, 38, 40],. Although there is no optimal mastectomy rate [41], evidence suggests that our patients may be presenting late and refusing treatment for breast cancer partly because of the fear of mastectomy. Indeed, in a previous study at the KBTH, fear of mastectomy was the reason for delayed

presentation and absconding before and during treatment in 24.2 and 57.2 % of patients respectively [42]. Hence, more breast conservation should be encouraged where indicated.

The limitation of this study was the small sample size. We were thus unable to demonstrate statistically any association between the subtypes and clinical and pathological behaviour. We did not also have information about the menopausal status of the participants to determine the proportions of the various subtypes that were premenopausal.

Conclusion

Triple negative tumour is the most commonly occurring subtype in the Ghanaian breast cancer population treated at the Korle Bu Teaching Hospital. Hence, blind hormonal therapy is not justifiable. Lack of significant association between subtypes and their clinical and pathological behaviour could be due to the small sample size. We recommend the inclusion of basal makers in the IHC panel on routine basis.

Abbreviations
KBTH: Korle Bu Teaching Hospital; ER: Estrogen receptor; PR: Progesterone receptor; HER2: Human epidermal receptor 2; IHC: Immunohistochemistry; EGFR: Epidermal growth factor receptor; ESBC: Early stage breast cancer; BCS: Breast conservation surgery; CK: Cytokeratin; CAF: Cyclophosphamide-Doxorubicin-5 Fluorouracil; FEC: 5Fluorouracil-Epirubicin-Cyclophosphamide; CMF: Cyclophosphamide- Methotrexate-5 Fluorouracil; LN: Lymph node.

Competing interests
The authors declare that they have no competing interests.

Authors' contribution
BS, NAA, BCT, FD and JNCL conceptualized the study. BS collected data and all authors analysed the data. BS drafted the manuscript and NAA, BCT, FD and JNCL reviewed and revised the manuscript. All authors read and approved the final manuscript.

Acknowledgements

We thank the following for their roles in the acquisition of the data:
Desmond Ampaw-Asiedu
Doris Kpogo
Janet Adade

Author details

[1]Department of Surgery, Tema General Hospital, Tema, Ghana. [2]Department of Surgery, School of Medicine and Dentistry, University of Ghana, Accra, Ghana. [3]Department of Community Health, School of Public Health, University of Ghana, Accra, Ghana.

References

1. WHO. The Global Burden of Disease: 2004 Update. 2008.
2. Jatoi I, Chen BE, Anderson WF, Rosenberg PS. Breast Cancer Mortality Trends in the United States According to Estrogen Receptor Status and Age at Diagnosis. J Clin Oncol. 2007;25(13):1683–90.
3. Ries LA, Eisner MP, Kosary CL. Cancer Statistics review 1975-2000. In: National Cancer Institute. 2003.
4. Newman LA. Breast Cancer in African American women. Oncologist. 2005;10:1–14.
5. Carey LA, Perou CM, Livasy CA, Dressler LG, Cowan D, Conway K, et al. Race, Breast Cancer Subtypes, and Survival in the Carolina Breast Cancer Study. JAMA. 2006;295:2492–502.
6. Baako BN, Badoe EA. Treatment of Breast Cancer in Accra: 5 year Survival. Ghana Med J. 2001;35:90–5.
7. Blows FM, Driver KE, Schmidt MK, Broeks A, van Leeuwen FE, et al. (2010) Subtyping of Breast Cancer by Immunohistochemistry to Investigate a Relationship between Subtype and Short and Long Term Survival: A Collaborative Analysis of Data for 10,159 Cases from 12 Studies. PLoS Med 7(5): e1000279. doi:10.1371/journal.pmed.1000279.
8. de Ruijter TC, Veeck J, de Hoon JPJ, van Engeland M, Tjan-Heijnen VC. Characteristics of triple-negative breast cancer. J Cancer Res Clin Oncol. 2011;137:183–92.
9. Rouzier R, Perou CM, Fraser Symmans W, Ibrahim N, Cristofanilli M, Anderson K, et al. Breast Cancer Molecular Subtypes Respond Differently to Preoperative Chemotherapy. Clin Cancer Res. 2005;11:5678–85.
10. Bergh J, Holmquist M. Who should not receive adjuvant chemotherapy? International databases. J Natl Cancer Inst Monogr. 2001;30:103–8.
11. Stark A, Kleer CG, Martin I, Awuah B, Nsiah-Asare A, Takyi V, et al. African Ancestry and Higher Prevalence of Triple-Negative Breast Cancer. Cancer. 2010;116:4926–32.
12. Adebamowo AC, Famooto A, Ogundiran OT, Aniagwu T, Nkwodimmah C, Akang EE. Immunohistochemical and molecular subtypes of breast cancer in Nigeria. Breast Cancer Res Treat. 2008;110:183–8.
13. Bloom HJ, Richardson WW. Histological grading and prognosis in breast cancer; a study of 1409 cases of which 359 have been followed for 15 years. Br J Cancer. 1957;11(3):359–77.
14. Ohene-Yeboah M, Adjei E. Breast cancer in Kumasi, Ghana. Ghana Med J. 2012;46(1):8–13.
15. Perou CM, Sùrlie T, Eisen MB, van de Rijn M, Jeffrey SS, Rees CA, et al. Molecular portraits of human breast tumours. Nature. 2000;406.
16. Sørliea T, Perou CM, Tibshiranie R, Aas T, Geisler S, Johnsen H, et al. Gene expression patterns of breast carcinomas distinguish tumor subclasses with clinical implications. Proc Natl Acad Sci U S A. 2001;98(199):10869–74.
17. Nielsen TO, Hsu FD, Jensen K, Cheng M, Karaca G, Hu Z, et al. Immunohistochemical and Clinical Characterization of the Basal-Like Subtype of Invasive Breast Carcinoma. Clin Cancer Res. 2004;10:5367–74.
18. Huo D, Ikpatt F, Khramtsov A, Dangou J-M, Nanda R, Dignam J, et al. Population Differences in Breast Cancer: Survey in Indigenous African Women Reveals Over-Representation of Triple-Negative Breast Cancer. J Clin Oncol. 2009;27:4515–21.
19. Pang J, Toy KA, Griffith KA, Awuah B, Quayson S, Newman LA, et al. Invasive breast carcinomas in Ghana: high frequency of high grade, basal-like histology and high EZH2 expression. Breast Cancer Res Treat. 2012;135(1):59–66.
20. Yang XR, Sherman ME, Rimm DL, Lissowska J, Brinton LA, Peplonska B, et al. Differences in Risk Factors for Breast Cancer Molecular Subtypes in a Population-Based Study. Cancer Epidemiol Biomarkers Prev. 2007;16:439–43.
21. Lakhani SR, Van De Vijver MJ, Jacquemier J, Anderson TJ, Osin PP, McGuffog L, et al. The pathology of familial breast cancer: predictive value of immunohistochemical markers estrogen receptor, progesterone receptor, HER-2, and p53 in patients with mutations in BRCA1 and BRCA2. J Clin Oncol. 2002;20(9):2310–8.
22. Foulkes WD, Stefansson IM, Chappuis PO, Begin LR, Goffin JR, Wong N, et al. Germline BRCA1 mutations and a basal epithelial phenotype in breast cancer. J Natl Cancer Inst. 2003;95(19):1482–5.
23. Fostira F, Tsitlaidou M, Papadimitriou C, Pertesi M, Timotheadou E, Stavropoulou AV, et al. Prevalence of BRCA1 mutations among 403 women with triple-negative breast cancer: implications for genetic screening selection criteria: a Hellenic Cooperative Oncology Group Study. Breast Cancer Res Treat. 2012;134(1):353–62.
24. Young SR, Pilarski RT, Donenberg T, Shapiro C, Hammond LS, Miller J, et al. The prevalence of BRCA1 mutations among young women with triple-negative breast cancer. BMC Cancer. 2009;9:86.
25. Villarreal-Garza C, Weitzel JN, Llacuachaqui M, Sifuentes E, Magallanes-Hoyos MC, Gallardo L, et al. The prevalence of BRCA1 and BRCA2 mutations among young Mexican women with triple-negative breast cancer. Breast Cancer Res Treat. 2015;150(2):389–94.
26. McCabe N, Turner NC, Lord CJ, Kluzek K, Bialkowska A, Swift S, et al. Deficiency in the repair of DNA damage by homologous recombination and sensitivity to poly(ADP-ribose) polymerase inhibition. Cancer Res. 2006;66(16):8109–15.
27. Early Breast Cancer Trialists' Collaborative Group (EBCTCG). Effects of chemotherapy and hormonal therapy for early breast cancer on recurrence and 15-year survival: an overview of the randomised trials. Lancet. 2005;365(9472):1687–717.
28. Samphao S, Eremin JM, El-Sheemy M, Eremin O. Treatment of established breast cancer in post-menopausal women: role of aromatase inhibitors. Surgeon. 2009;7(1):42–55.
29. Romond EH, Perez EA, Bryant J, Suman VJ, Geyer Jr CE, Davidson NE, et al. Trastuzumab plus adjuvant chemotherapy for operable HER2-positive breast cancer. N Engl J Med. 2005;353(16):1673–84.
30. Pienkowski T, Zielinski CC. Trastuzumab treatment in patients with breast cancer and metastatic CNS disease. Ann Oncol. 2010;21(5):917–24.
31. Carey LA, Claire DE, Sawyer L, Gatti L, Moore DT, Collichio F, et al. The Triple Negative Paradox: Primary Tumor Chemosensitivity of Breast Cancer Subtypes. Clin Cancer Res. 2007;13:2329–34.
32. Silver DP, Richardson AL, Eklund AC, Wang ZC, Szallasi Z, Li Q, et al. Efficacy of Neoadjuvant Cisplatin in Triple-Negative Breast Cancer. J Clin Oncol. 2010;28(7):1145–53.
33. Rottenberg S, Jaspers JE, Kersbergen A, van der Burg E, Nygren AO, Zander SA, et al. High sensitivity of BRCA1-deficient mammary tumors to the PARP inhibitor AZD2281 alone and in combination with platinum drugs. Proc Natl Acad Sci U S A. 2008;105(44):17079–84.
34. Feigelson HS, James TA, Single RM, Onitilo AA, Aiello Bowles EJ, Barney T, et al. Factors associated with the frequency of initial total mastectomy: results of a multi-institutional study. J Am Coll Surg. 2013;216(5):966–75.
35. Hanagiri T, Nagata Y, Monji S, Shinohara S, Takenaka M, Shigematsu Y, et al. Temporal trends in the surgical outcomes of patients with breast cancer. World J Surg Oncol. 2012;10:108.
36. McGuire KP, Santillan AA, Kaur P, Meade T, Parbhoo J, Mathias M, et al. Are mastectomies on the rise? A 13-year trend analysis of the selection of mastectomy versus breast conservation therapy in 5865 patients. Ann Surg Oncol. 2009;16(10):2682–90.
37. Damle S, Teal CB, Lenert JJ, Marshall EC, Pan Q, McSwain AP. Mastectomy and contralateral prophylactic mastectomy rates: an institutional review. Ann Surg Oncol. 2011;18(5):1356–63.
38. Garcia-Etienne CA, Tomatis M, Heil J, Friedrichs K, Kreienberg R, Denk A, et al. Mastectomy trends for early-stage breast cancer: a report from the EUSOMA multi-institutional European database. Eur J Cancer. 2012;48(13):1947–56.
39. Dragun AE, Huang B, Tucker TC, Spanos WJ. Increasing mastectomy rates among all age groups for early stage breast cancer: a 10-year study of surgical choice. Breast J. 2012;18(4):318–25.
40. Mahmood U, Hanlon AL, Koshy M, Buras R, Chumsri S, Tkaczuk KH, et al. Increasing national mastectomy rates for the treatment of early stage breast cancer. Ann Surg Oncol. 2013;20(5):1436–43.

16

Estrogen receptor alpha and androgen receptor are commonly expressed in well-differentiated liposarcoma

Davis R Ingram[1], Lloye M Dillon[2], Dina Chelouche Lev[1], Alexander Lazar[3], Elizabeth G Demicco[5], Burton L Eisenberg[4] and Todd W Miller[2]*

Abstract

Background: Liposarcoma (LS) is the second-most common type of soft-tissue sarcoma. Despite advances in knowledge and treatment of this disease, there remains a need for more effective LS therapy. Steroid hormone receptors regulate metabolism in adipocytes. Estrogen receptor alpha (ER), progesterone receptor (PR), and androgen receptor (AR) have been implicated in the pathophysiology of other cancer types. We sought to comprehensively determine temporal expression patterns of these receptors in LS.

Methods: We analyzed 561 histologically subtyped LS specimens from 354 patients for expression of ER, PR, and AR by immunohistochemistry (IHC) using diagnostic-grade reagents and protocols. The fractions of positively stained tumor cells were scored within each specimen. IHC scores were compared across LS subtypes using the Kruskal-Wallis test, and subtypes were compared using Dunn's post-hoc test. Ages of patients with receptor-positive vs. -negative LS were compared by t-test. Genders and races were compared for hormone receptor positivity using Fisher's exact test and Chi-square analysis, respectively. Recurrence-free survival was compared between receptor-positive and negative patients by log-rank test. p< 0.05 was considered significant.

Results: ER and AR were frequently expressed in LS, while few tumors expressed PR. Most of the ER + and AR + samples were of the well-differentiated LS subtype. A smaller fraction of de-differentiated LS expressed ER or AR, but expression was common within well-differentiated regions of tumors histologically classified as de-differentiated LS. In LS specimens from patients who underwent multiple surgeries over time, receptor expression frequently changed over time, which may be attributable in part to intratumor heterogeneity, varying degrees of de-differentiation, and biopsy bias. ER and AR were frequently co-expressed. Receptor status was not significantly associated with gender or race, but AR and PR expression were associated with earlier age at diagnosis. Receptor expression was not associated with altered recurrence-free survival.

Conclusions: ER and AR are commonly expressed in LS, particularly in well-differentiated tumors. These data warrant further functional study to determine receptor function in LS, and the potential efficacy of anti-hormone therapies for the treatment of patients with LS.

* Correspondence: todd.w.miller@dartmouth.edu
[2]Departments of Pharmacology & Toxicology, Norris Cotton Cancer Center, Geisel School of Medicine at Dartmouth, Dartmouth-Hitchcock Medical Center, One Medical Center Drive, HB-7936, Lebanon, NH 03756, USA
Full list of author information is available at the end of the article

138 New Frontiers in Clinical Pathology

Background

Approximately 11,280 patients are diagnosed with one of many types of soft tissue sarcoma each year in the U.S. [1]. Liposarcomas (LS) constitute approximately 24% of extremity and 45% of retroperitoneal soft tissue sarcomas [2], ranking as the second-most common type of soft-tissue sarcoma. LS occurs in three major biologic subgroups: 1) well- or de-differentiated LS (WDLS, DDLS, most common subgroup), 2) myxoid LS (MLS), and 3) pleomorphic LS (PLS). WDLS and MLS are typically low-grade tumors, DDLS are often intermediate grade with intermediate risk for metastasis, and PLS are high-grade and clinically aggressive. It is thought that DDLS starts as WDLS, and tumor cells progressively accumulate genetic lesions as they transition to a less differentiated, non-lipogenic state. Progression to DDLS is associated with more aggressive local disease, increased metastatic potential (10-20%), and increased mortality (50-75%) [3-6]. LS is typically treated by surgical resection, and high-grade lesions are sometimes treated with adjuvant radiation therapy. DNA-damaging chemotherapy is usually not effective against LS. In addition, tumor recurrence is common, particularly with retroperitoneal LS. Therefore, there exists a need for improved LS therapy.

LS likely originates from a lipogenic precursor cell(s). Since lipogenic metabolism is heavily influenced by steroid hormones [7], and adipocytes express nuclear hormone receptors and steroidogenic enzymes such as aromatase [8,9], we postulated that LS cells may similarly express such receptors. Prior studies in limited numbers of patients reported expression of steroid hormone receptors in a fraction of LS cases [10-17]. To expand upon and clarify these findings, we analyzed 561 LS specimens acquired from 353 patients in the largest LS cohort reported to-date to determine the frequencies of expression of estrogen receptor alpha (ER), progesterone receptor (PR), and androgen receptor (AR). Frequent expression of these hormone receptors may prompt clinical testing of anti-hormone strategies, such as those used to treat patients with cancers of the breast (anti-estrogens) or prostate (anti-androgens), or to control pregnancy (anti-progestins), in order to assess the contribution of these receptors to LS growth. These drugs may ultimately prove useful for the treatment of patients with LS.

Methods

Patients and tissues

LS specimens were obtained at Dartmouth-Hitchcock Medical Center and M.D. Anderson Cancer Center between 1986 and 2012 under protocols approved by the Institutional Review Boards of Dartmouth-Hitchcock Medical Center and M.D. Anderson Cancer Center, respectively. Patients provided written informed consent. Tissues were formalin-fixed and paraffin-embedded.

Core samples were used to construct tissue microarrays (TMAs). Clinical records indicated that these TMAs included 379 tumors from 353 patients, where tumors were classified as DDLS ($n=122$), WDLS ($n=146$), MLS ($n=79$), or PLS ($n=32$). WDLS and DDLS are thought to represent different stages of disease progression that can co-exist in the same tumor. Hence, some cores taken from DDLS cases were histologically classified as "WDLS." In total, we analyzed 561 core samples, which were classified as 294 WDLS, 123 DDLS, 112 MLS, and 32 PLS based on histological criteria.

Table 1 Baseline characteristics

Characteristic	n patients
Age at registration	
<30 years	9
30–50 years	106
50.1-70 years	180
>70 years	51
Unreported	7
Gender	
Male	215
Female	138
Race	
White	264
Black	12
Hispanic	38
Asian	7
Unreported	32
Primary tumor type	
Well-differentiated	136
De-differentiated	107
Myxoid	78
Pleomorphic	32
Primary tumor size	
<5 cm	15
5–9.9 cm	55
≥10 cm	221
Undetermined	62
Chemotherapy	
Yes	98
No	236
Unreported	19
Radiation therapy	
Yes	93
No	239
Unreported	21

Immunohistochemistry

Commercially available antibodies against ER alpha (6 F11 monoclonal, dil. 1:35; Leica Biosystems), PR (PgR 1294 monoclonal, dil. 1:200; Dako; recognizes both A and B isoforms), and AR (AR441 monoclonal, dil. 1:30; Dako; recognizes both A and B isoforms) were used for immunohistochemistry (IHC). These antibodies are routinely used for *in vitro* diagnostics in clinical laboratories. A Leica BOND-MAX automated stainer was used with a polymer/HRP detection system. After deparaffinization, 5-μm TMA sections were treated with citrate buffer at 100°C for 25–30 minutes. Slides were probed with primary antibody for 15 minutes, washed, and probed with HRP-polymer anti-mouse IgG for 8 minutes. Signal was detected using 3,3-diaminobenzidine, followed by hematoxylin counterstaining. ER+/PR + breast tumor tissue was used as a positive control for ER and PR IHC. AR + prostate cancer tissue was used as a positive control for AR IHC. Spleen biopsies were included in the TMAs and used as negative control tissues. Tissues were scored based on the estimated percent of positively stained cancer cell nuclei.

Statistics

IHC scores were compared across LS subtypes using the Kruskal-Wallis non-parametric test, and subtypes were compared in a one-by-one fashion using Dunn's post-hoc test. Ages of patients with hormone receptor-positive vs. -negative WDLS/DDLS were compared by *t*-test. Genders and races were compared for hormone receptor positivity using Fisher's exact test and Chi-square analysis, respectively. $p \leq 0.05$ was considered significant.

Results

Frequent expression of ER and AR in WDLS and DDLS

IHC staining of 561 specimens obtained from 379 LS tumors from 353 patients (characteristics listed in Table 1) revealed nuclear ER and AR expression in a significant number of cases (Figure 1). PR staining was less frequently observed. Using the stringent threshold of 10% positively-stained nuclei, we observed the following: 43.1% of WDLS, 17.5% of DDLS, 0% of PLS, and 5.2% of MLS were scored as ER+; 9.8% of WDLS, 7.6% of DDLS, 0% of PLS, and 5% of MLS were scored as PR+; 58.1% of WDLS, 24.1% of DDLS, 6.2% of PLS, and 9.1% of MLS were scored as AR + (Figure 2A). Using the threshold of 1% positively-stained nuclei used in the histological classification of breast cancer, we observed the following: 52.8% of WDLS, 22.5% of DDLS, 3.3% of PLS, and 10.4% of MLS were scored as ER+; 16.5% of WDLS, 10.2% of DDLS, 0% of PLS, and 9% of MLS were scored as PR+; 70% of WDLS, 36.2% of DDLS, 15.6% of PLS, and 19.2% of MLS were scored as AR + .

Since a significant number of specimens expressed ER or AR, we compared IHC scores between histologic subtypes. We detected a statistically significantly higher frequency of ER and AR expression in WDLS compared to each other subtype (Figure 2B, all $p < 0.001$). While some DDLS specimens expressed ER and AR, this subtype was not significantly different from PLS or MLS. PR was

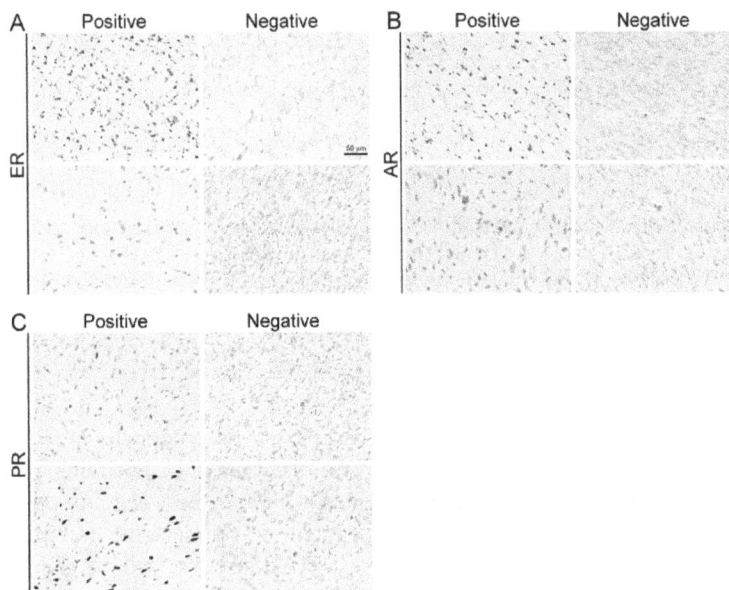

Figure 1 Steroid hormone receptor expression in LS. Sections of LS were stained using antibodies against **A)** ER, **B)** AR, or **C)** PR. Shown are two representative microscopic fields that were scored as receptor-positive or -negative. Scale bar in **(A)** is 50 μm.

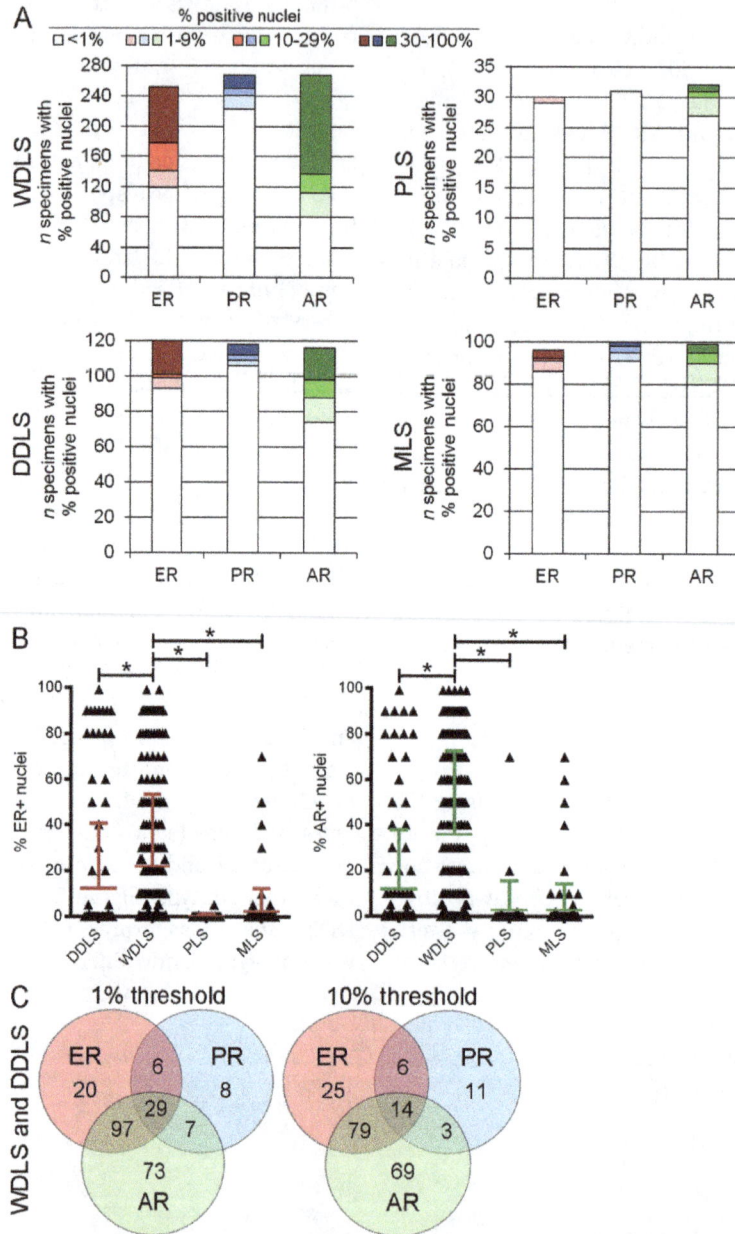

Figure 2 Steroid hormone receptor expression is most common in WDLS. A) LS specimens were scored for% positively-stained nuclei for ER, PR, and AR, then classified by histological subtype and binned according to score as indicated. **B)** ER and AR scores were compared between specimen subtypes. Colored bars indicate mean + SD. *$p < 0.0001$ by Dunn's post-hoc test. **C)** Venn diagrams illustrating the number of WDLS and DDLS specimens with co-expression of hormone receptors using a threshold of 1% or 10% positively-stained nuclei.

not significantly differentially expressed across histologic subtypes.

We then used Venn diagrams to determine the frequency of receptor co-expression within the combined WDLS and DDLS subtypes. Among 347 WDLS/DDLS specimens for which ER and AR IHC were evaluable, ER and AR were co-expressed in 28% and 22.8% of specimens at the 10% and 1% thresholds, respectively (Figure 2C).

Intratumor heterogeneity in ER and AR expression

We observed that hormone receptor expression sometimes differed between tumors acquired from the same patient who underwent multiple surgeries over time. We therefore systematically evaluated hormone receptor expression levels over time in 53 patients who underwent ≥2 surgeries to remove WDLS and/or DDLS (Figure 3). This analysis revealed that many tumors show changes in

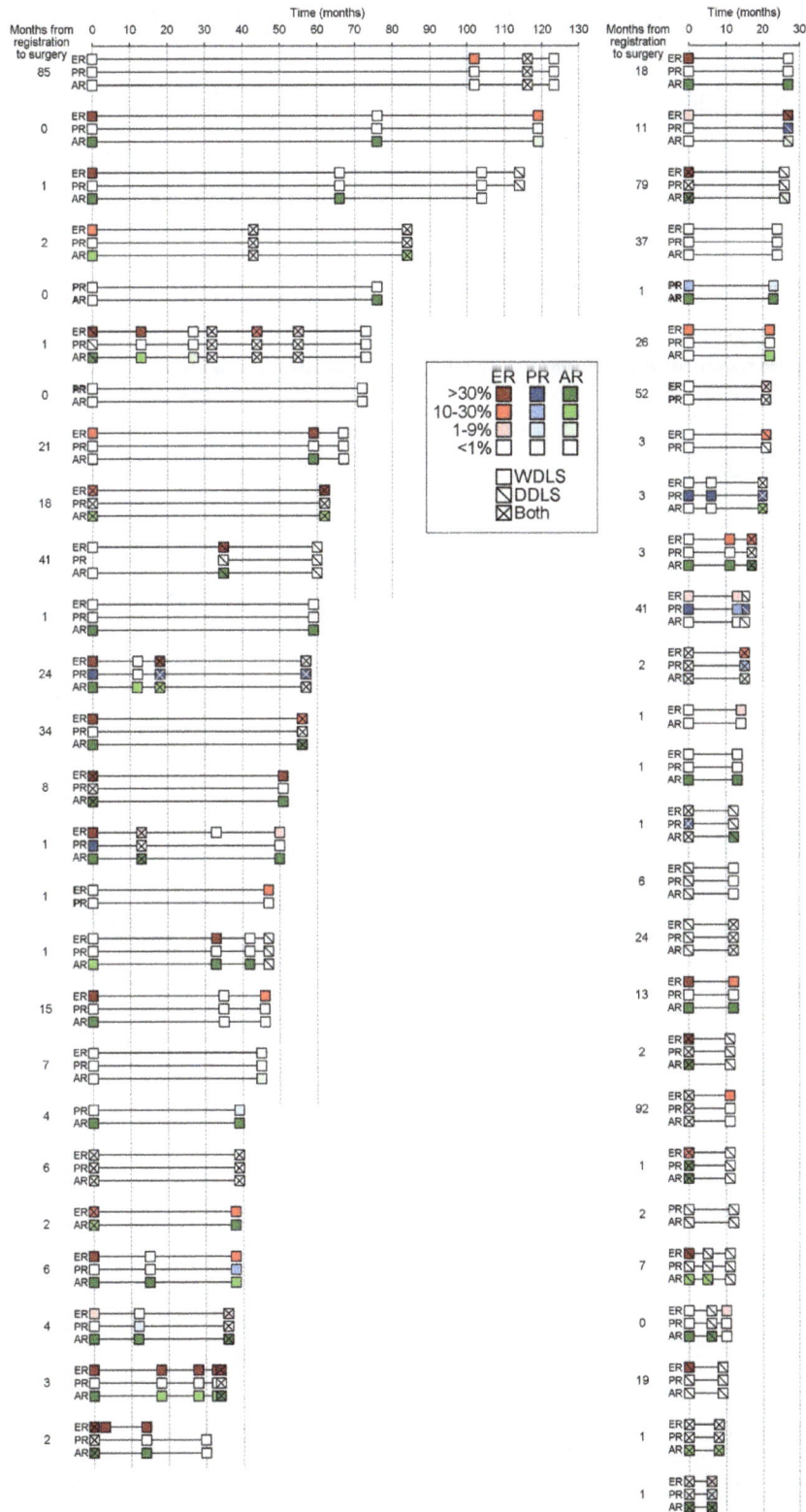

Figure 3 Changes in tumor hormone receptor status over time. Fifty-three patients with WDLS and/or DDLS for whom specimens were obtained from ≥2 surgeries ≥6 months apart were evaluated. In cases where multiple specimens were obtained from the same tumor at the same time point, the% positively-stained nuclei were averaged across specimens. The% positively-stained nuclei and histological classification of each tumor are noted by color intensity and hash marks as indicated in legend.

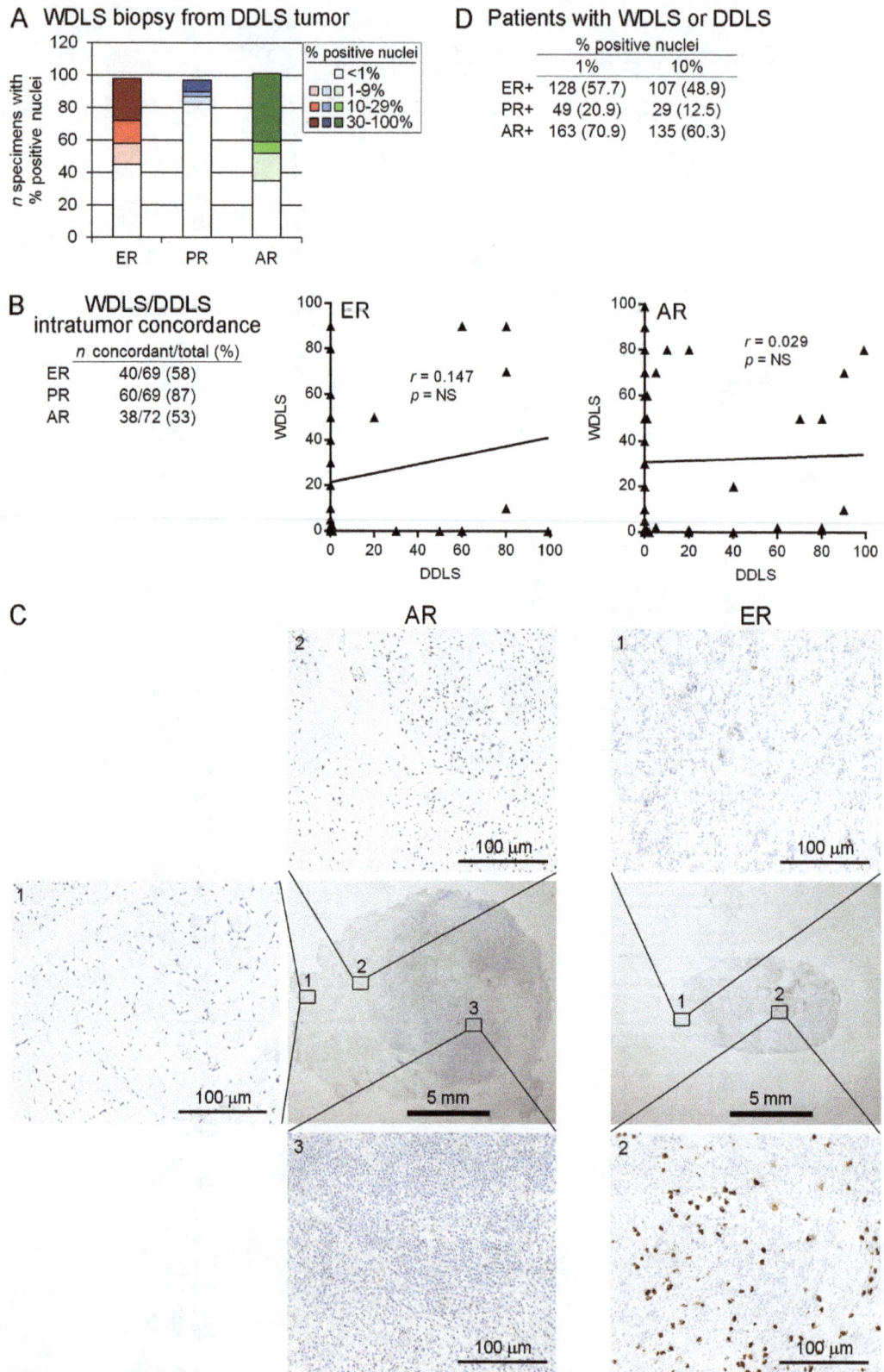

Figure 4 (See legend on next page.)

(See figure on previous page.)
Figure 4 Intratumor heterogeneity in degree of differentiation contributes to heterogeneity in hormone receptor expression.
A) Frequencies of hormone receptor expression among WDLS specimens obtained from tumors classified as DDLS. **B)** Tumors for which 2 specimens were obtained from different regions at the same time point were evaluated for concordance in hormone receptor expression using a threshold of 10% for positivity. Scatterplots show% positive nuclei for ER and AR in tumors for which one DDLS specimen and one WDLS specimen were available. **C)** Representative liposarcoma specimens showing regions of receptor-positivity and -negativity. **D)** Hormone receptor status for patients with WDLS/DDLS as determined using any LS specimen obtained from any surgery.

hormone receptor expression over time, which may be attributable in part to intratumor heterogeneity, varying degrees of de-differentiation, and biopsy bias.

DDLS represents a form of tumor progression in WDLS, and both histologies may co-exist within the same tumor. We evaluated DDLS tumors with synchronous foci of WDLS and DDLS histologies for hormone receptor expression. At a threshold of 10% positively-stained nuclei, 40.8%, 10.3%, and 48.5% of WDLS foci were ER+, PR+, and AR+, respectively. At a 1% threshold, 54.1%, 15.5%, and 65.3% of WDLS foci were ER+, PR+, and AR+, respectively (Figure 4A). Therefore, ER and AR expression are common in WDLS foci within otherwise DDLS tumors.

We then determined the rate of concordance for hormone receptor expression between 2 specimens obtained from different regions of the same WDLS/DDLS tumor; 75 tumors were available for this analysis. Using a threshold of 10% positively-stained nuclei, this analysis revealed rates of 58% and 53% concordance for ER and AR, respectively (Figure 4B). Ninety-two percent (69/75) of these tumors had specimens histologically classified as WDLS and DDLS (one of each). Among the ER-discordant tumors, 82.8% (24/29) showed an ER + WDLS specimen and an ER- DDLS specimen (Figure 4B). Among the AR-discordant tumors, 73.7% (28/38) showed an AR + WDLS specimen and an AR- DDLS specimen. These data suggest

that the high degree of intratumor discordance in ER and AR expression (demonstrated with representative specimens in Figure 4C) is partially attributable to the degree of de-differentiation.

Given that tumor hormone receptor status changed over time (Figure 3), we evaluated associations between patient characteristics and hormone receptor expression using hormone receptor status (threshold of 10% positively-stained nuclei) determined from A) a specimen obtained from the first surgery performed at M.D. Anderson Cancer Center, or B) hormone receptor positivity from a specimen obtained from any WDLS/DDLS surgical specimen (i.e., patient had a receptor-positive specimen at any time point; frequencies shown in Figure 4D). The latter criterion indicated that 48.9% and 60.3% of patients had ER + or AR + WDLS/DDLS at some point during the course of their disease. Hormone receptor status was not significantly associated with gender, race, or tumor size. There was a significant association linking AR expression with earlier age at WDLS/DDLS diagnosis, and a trend linking PR expression with earlier age at diagnosis (Tables 2 and 3). However, the mean ages of onset were similar between receptor-positive and -negative groups. ER and AR expression were not associated with recurrence-free survival in patients with WDLS and/or DDLS using either criterion.

Table 2 Receptor positivity at any time point

| | | n | Age (years) | t-test p | Gender | | Fisher's p |
					Male	Female	
ER	Negative	117	60.6 ± 11.8		74	43	
	Positive	102	59.6 ± 11.1	NS	57	45	NS
	Undetermined	24			13	11	
	Total	243			144	99	
PR	Negative	203	60.4 ± 11.3		121	82	
	Positive	28	56.4 ± 13.2	0.08	14	14	NS
	Undetermined	12			9	3	
	Total	243			144	99	
AR	Negative	90	61.3 ± 11.8		52	38	
	Positive	134	58.6 ± 11.4	0.09	83	51	NS
	Undetermined	19			9	10	
	Total	243			144	99	

Table 3 Receptor positivity at time of first surgery

		n	Age (years)	t-test p	Male	Female	Fisher's p
					\multicolumn{2}{c}{Gender}	
ER	Negative	124	60.9 ± 11.3		80	44	
	Positive	90	59.1 ± 11.6	NS	50	40	NS
	Undetermined	29			14	15	
	Total	243			144	99	
PR	Negative	202	60.4 ± 11.3		122	80	
	Positive	23	55.5 ± 13.7	0.06	11	12	NS
	Undetermined	18			11	7	
	Total	243			144	99	
AR	Negative	100	61.6 ± 11.6		58	42	
	Positive	122	58.0 ± 11.5	0.02	76	46	NS
	Undetermined	21			10	11	
	Total	243			144	99	

Discussion

Given that WDLS have a significantly higher frequency of ER-positivity and AR-positivity than DDLS, and that WDLS foci within DDLS tumors are often ER + and/or AR+, hormone receptor expression is likely associated with a more differentiated LS phenotype. WDLS is often locally aggressive and non-metastasizing, is treated with surgical resection, and occurs repeatedly particularly in the retroperitoneum or mediastinum. WDLS causes morbidity through uncontrolled local effects on vital organs, or through de-differentiation and metastasis. Therefore, therapeutics to control WDLS and prevent de-differentiation may be clinically valuable.

If ER and AR are functionally important for WDLS/DDLS cell proliferation or viability, as is observed in other cancer types such as breast and prostate, anti-hormone therapies may prevent LS progression. However, we caution that hormone receptor expression does not necessarily indicate receptor dependence. AR is expressed in 70-90% of breast cancers [18], but clinical testing of anti-androgen therapy in unselected patients with breast cancer met with little success [19]. AR may be functionally important in certain breast cancer subtypes [20,21], and clinical testing of anti-androgen therapy in patients with such subtypes is ongoing. Furthermore, ER + breast tumors frequently co-express PR. Since PR is encoded by an ER-regulated gene, PR co-expression is typically indicative of ER function. Surprisingly, most ER + LS specimens are PR-, raising the possibility that ER is non-functional. Alternatively, ER may regulate a different set of genes in LS cells, and/or PR levels may be modulated by another mechanism (such as phosphorylation by mitogen-activated protein kinase (MAPK), which promotes degradation [22]).

In vitro evidence to support hormone receptor dependence in LS models would help elucidate receptor function, but few WDLS cell lines exist, and it is arguable whether such cell lines accurately model the disease(s). Transgenic mice that overexpress *IL22* in adipocytes develop WDLS when fed a high-fat diet [23]. If such murine LS tumors are hormone receptor-positive, this may present a useful model to elucidate receptor functionality in LS. There have been no proof-of-principle clinical trials to evaluate the effects of anti-hormone therapies in LS based on pre-treatment tumor hormone receptor status. Another option to explore the role(s) of hormone receptors in LS would be a pilot presurgical clinical study, where patients who have undergone a diagnostic tumor biopsy would be treated with anti-hormone therapy for 2–3 weeks prior to surgical tumor resection. The diagnostic (pre-treatment) biopsy tissue is then compared to the surgical (post-treatment) specimen to determine whether levels of hormone receptor-driven or cell cycle-related genes and proteins have changed. This strategy may be useful to identify LS patients who will (or will not) benefit from adjuvant endocrine therapy [24].

Conclusions

In summary, we demonstrate that a significant fraction of WDLS and DDLS express ER and/or AR. The hormone receptor scoring method used herein is not finely calibrated, which may affect assay sensitivity; however, a less sensitive scoring method may be more likely to detect only cases with more robust (and, likely, more biological important) expression of these receptors. While there appears to be intratumor heterogeneity in hormone receptor expression, both between well- and de-differentiated areas of the same tumor, and over time within a patient's tumor (which may be partially attributable to biopsy bias), endocrine therapeutics may be useful to control hormone receptor-driven LS cells and mitigate disease progression.

Abbreviations
ER: Estrogen receptor alpha; PR: Progesterone receptor; AR: Androgen receptor; LS: Liposarcoma; WDLS: Well-differentiated liposarcoma; DDLS: De-differentiated liposarcoma; MLS: Myxoid liposarcoma; PLS: Pleomorphic liposarcoma.

Competing interests
The authors declare that they have no competing interests.

Authors' contributions
TWM and DCL designed the study. DR, DCL, AL, EGD, and TWM procured tissue samples, generated the tissue microarray, and performed IHC staining. TWM, LD, and BLG scored IHC staining and analyzed data. TWM wrote the manuscript. All authors read, provided input on, and approved the final manuscript.

Acknowledgements
We thank the Norris Cotton Cancer Center Pathology Translational Research and Microscopy Shared Resources.

Funding
This work was supported by the National Institutes of Health R00CA142899 (T.W.M.). We thank the Lobo, Margolis, and Jackson families for their continued support of liposarcoma research.

Author details
[1]Departments of Surgical Oncology, M.D. Anderson Cancer Center, University of Texas, 1515 Holcombe Blvd, Houston, TX, USA. [2]Departments of Pharmacology & Toxicology, Norris Cotton Cancer Center, Geisel School of Medicine at Dartmouth, Dartmouth-Hitchcock Medical Center, One Medical Center Drive, HB-7936, Lebanon, NH 03756, USA. [3]Departments of Surgical Pathology, M.D. Anderson Cancer Center, University of Texas, 1515 Holcombe Blvd, Houston, TX, USA. [4]Departments of Surgery, Norris Cotton Cancer Center, Geisel School of Medicine at Dartmouth, Dartmouth-Hitchcock Medical Center, One Medical Center Dr, Lebanon, NH, USA. [5]Department of Pathology, Mount Sinai Medical Center, One Gustave L. Levy Pl, New York, NY, USA.

References
1. American_Cancer_Society: **Breast Cancer Facts & Figures 2011–2012.** In *Book Breast Cancer Facts & Figures 2011–2012.* Atlanta, GA: American Cancer Society, Inc.
2. Crago AM, Singer S: **Clinical and molecular approaches to well differentiated and dedifferentiated liposarcoma.** *Curr Opin Oncol* 2011, **23:**373–378.
3. Dalal KM, Kattan MW, Antonescu CR, Brennan MF, Singer S: **Subtype specific prognostic nomogram for patients with primary liposarcoma of the retroperitoneum, extremity, or trunk.** *Ann Surg* 2006, **244:**381–391.
4. Henricks WH, Chu YC, Goldblum JR, Weiss SW: **Dedifferentiated liposarcoma: a clinicopathological analysis of 155 cases with a proposal for an expanded definition of dedifferentiation.** *Am J Surg Pathol* 1997, **21:**271–281.
5. McCormick D, Mentzel T, Beham A, Fletcher CD: **Dedifferentiated liposarcoma. Clinicopathologic analysis of 32 cases suggesting a better prognostic subgroup among pleomorphic sarcomas.** *Am J Surg Pathol* 1994, **18:**1213–1223.
6. Hasegawa T, Seki K, Hasegawa F, Matsuno Y, Shimodo T, Hirose T, Sano T, Hirohashi S: **Dedifferentiated liposarcoma of retroperitoneum and mesentery: varied growth patterns and histological grades–a clinicopathologic study of 32 cases.** *Hum Pathol* 2000, **31:**717–727.
7. Kallio A, Guo T, Lamminen E, Seppanen J, Kangas L, Vaananen HK, Harkonen P: **Estrogen and the selective estrogen receptor modulator (SERM) protection against cell death in estrogen receptor alpha and beta expressing U2OS cells.** *Mol Cell Endocrinol* 2008, **289:**38–48.
8. Bulun SE, Chen D, Moy I, Brooks DC, Zhao H: **Aromatase, breast cancer and obesity: a complex interaction.** *Trends Endocrinol Metab* 2012, **23:**83–89.
9. Shin JH, Hur JY, Seo HS, Jeong YA, Lee JK, Oh MJ, Kim T, Saw HS, Kim SH: **The ratio of estrogen receptor alpha to estrogen receptor beta in adipose tissue is associated with leptin production and obesity.** *Steroids* 2007, **72:**592–599.
10. Chaudhuri PK, Walker MJ, Beattie CW, Das Gupta TK: **Presence of steroid receptors in human soft tissue sarcomas of diverse histological origin.** *Cancer Res* 1980, **40:**861–865.
11. Chaudhuri PK, Walker MJ, Beattie CW, Das Gupta TK: **Distribution of steroid hormone receptors in human soft tissue sarcomas.** *Surgery* 1981, **90:**149–153.
12. Chaudhuri PK, Walker MJ, Beattie CW, Das Gupta TK: **The steroid hormone receptors in tumors of adipose tissue.** *J Surg Oncol* 1985, **28:**87–89.
13. Weiss SW, Langloss JM, Shmookler BM, Malawer MM, D'Avis J, Enzinger FM, Stanton R: **Estrogen receptor protein in bone and soft tissue tumors.** *Lab Invest* 1986, **54:**689–694.
14. Suda A, Sato T, Watanabe Y, Yamakawa M, Imai Y: **Immunohistochemical study of steroid hormones and an estrogen binding assay in malignant soft tissue tumors.** *Nihon Seikeigeka Gakkai zasshi* 1990, **64:**814–823.
15. Li XQ, Hisaoka M, Hashimoto H: **Expression of estrogen receptors alpha and beta in soft tissue sarcomas: Immunohistochemical and molecular analysis.** *Pathol Int* 2003, **53:**671–679.
16. Valkov A, Sorbye S, Kilvaer TK, Donnem T, Smeland E, Bremnes RM, Busund LT: **Estrogen receptor and progesterone receptor are prognostic factors in soft tissue sarcomas.** *Int J Oncol* 2011, **38:**1031–1040.
17. Sorbye SW, Kilvaer TK, Valkov A, Donnem T, Smeland E, Al-Shibli K, Bremnes RM, Busund LT: **Prognostic impact of Skp2, ER and PGR in male and female patients with soft tissue sarcomas.** *BMC Clin Pathol* 2013, **13:**9.
18. Gonzalez LO, Corte MD, Vazquez J, Junquera S, Sanchez R, Alvarez AC, Rodriguez JC, Lamelas ML, Vizoso FJ: **Androgen receptor expresion in breast cancer: relationship with clinicopathological characteristics of the tumors, prognosis, and expression of metalloproteases and their inhibitors.** *BMC Cancer* 2008, **8:**149.
19. Millward MJ, Cantwell BM, Dowsett M, Carmichael J, Harris AL: **Phase II clinical and endocrine study of Anandron (RU-23908) in advanced post-menopausal breast cancer.** *Br J Cancer* 1991, **63:**763–764.
20. Lehmann BD, Bauer JA, Chen X, Sanders ME, Chakravarthy AB, Shyr Y, Pietenpol JA: **Identification of human triple-negative breast cancer subtypes and preclinical models for selection of targeted therapies.** *J Clin Invest* 2011, **121:**2750–2767.
21. Ni M, Chen Y, Lim E, Wimberly H, Bailey ST, Imai Y, Rimm DL, Liu XS, Brown M: **Targeting androgen receptor in estrogen receptor-negative breast cancer.** *Cancer Cell* 2011, **20:**119–131.
22. Lange CA, Shen T, Horwitz KB: **Phosphorylation of human progesterone receptors at serine-294 by mitogen-activated protein kinase signals their degradation by the 26S proteasome.** *Proc Natl Acad Sci U S A* 2000, **97:**1032–1037.
23. Wang Z, Yang L, Jiang Y, Ling ZQ, Li Z, Cheng Y, Huang H, Wang L, Pan Y, Wang Z, Yan X, Chen Y: **High fat diet induces formation of spontaneous liposarcoma in mouse adipose tissue with overexpression of interleukin 22.** *PLoS One* 2011, **6:**e23737.
24. Dowsett M, Smith I, Robertson J, Robison L, Pinhel I, Johnson L, Salter J, Dunbier A, Anderson H, Ghazoui Z, Skene T, Evans A, A'Hern R, Iskender A, Wilcox M, Bliss J: **Endocrine therapy, new biologicals, and new study designs for presurgical studies in breast cancer.** *J Natl Cancer Inst Monogr* 2011, **2011:**120–123.

17

5-type HPV mRNA versus 14-type HPV DNA test: test performance, over-diagnosis and overtreatment in triage of women with minor cervical lesions

Bjørn Westre[1], Anita Giske[1], Hilde Guttormsen[1], Sveinung Wergeland Sørbye[2*] and Finn Egil Skjeldestad[3]

Abstract

Background: Repeat cytology and HPV testing is used in triage of women with minor cytological lesions. The objective of this study was to evaluate 14-type HPV DNA and 5-type HPV mRNA testing in delayed triage of women with ASC-US/LSIL.

Methods: We compared a DNA test (Roche Cobas 4800) and an 5-type mRNA test (PreTect HPV-Proofer). In total 564 women were included in the study.

Results: The sensitivity among solved cases for CIN3+ were 100 % (15/15) for both tests. The sensitivity for CIN2+ of the HPV DNA test was 100 % (38/38) relative to 79 % (30/38) for the 5-type HPV mRNA test. The corresponding estimates of specificity for CIN2+ among solved cases were 84 % (393/466; 95 % CI: 81–88) and 91 % (451/498; 95 % CI: 88–93). The positive predictive values for CIN3+ were 13.5 % (15/111) for DNA+ and 19.5 % (15/77) for 5-type mRNA+. Significantly more women screened with 5-type mRNA than DNA returned to screening (81 % vs 71 %, $p < 0.01$). Subsequently, significantly fewer women were referred for colposcopy/biopsies/treatment (19 % (105/564) vs 29 % (165/564), $p < 0.01$).

Conclusions: 5-type HPV mRNA is more specific than 14-type HPV DNA in delayed triage of women with ASC-US/LSIL. The referral rate for colposcopy was 57 % higher for DNA+ relative to mRNA+ cases (165 vs 105), with the same detection rate of CIN3+, but the 5-type mRNA test had lower sensitivity for CIN2+. It is important to consider the trade-off between sensitivity and specificity of the diagnostic test when designing screening algorithms.

Keywords: HPV, DNA, mRNA, Screening, Triage, CIN, CIN2, CIN3, Cervical cancer

Background

Cervical cancer is the third most common cancer in women worldwide [1]. Persistent infection of human papillomavirus (HPV) causes virtually all cases of cervical cancer [2]. In Europe most cervical cancer cases are caused by HPV types 16, 18, 31, 33, and 45 [1, 3]. Cervical cancer can be prevented by early detection and treatment of precancerous lesions [4]. Women with minor cytological cervical lesions have an increased risk of having, or developing, high-grade dysplasia compared

to women with normal cytology. However, most minor cytological lesions regress spontaneously, and therefore careful triage is crucial in order to avoid unnecessary referrals and overtreatment [5]. In Norway, HPV test is used in delayed triage of women with atypical squamous cells of undetermined significance (ASC-US) or low-grade squamous intraepithelial lesions (LSIL) [6]. If the HPV test is positive, the woman is referred to colposcopy.

The HPV E6/E7 mRNA test PreTect HPV-Proofer which detects HPV E6/E7 mRNA from the five most prevalent types causing cervical cancer has been shown to have a higher clinical specificity and positive predictive value (PPV) than HPV DNA tests [7–14]. A high specificity and a low positivity rate of a triage test indicates a low

* Correspondence: sveinung.sorbye@unn.no
[2]Department of Clinical Pathology, University Hospital of North Norway, 9038 Tromsø, Norway
Full list of author information is available at the end of the article

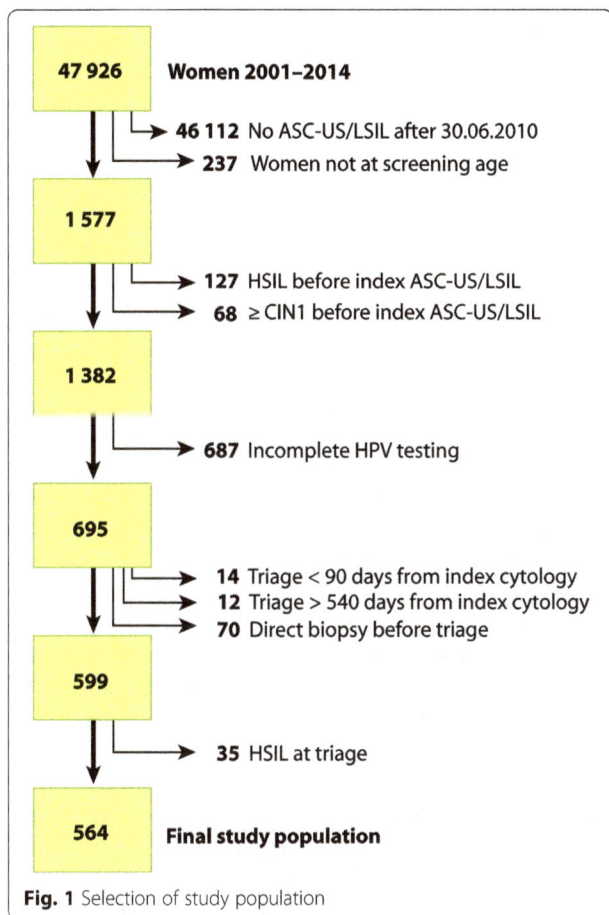

Fig. 1 Selection of study population

referral rate for colposcopy [8]. In this study we performed a direct comparison of a 5-type HPV mRNA and a 14-type HPV DNA test in delayed triage of ASC-US/LSIL related to referral rates for colposcopy, biopsy rates, and histological outcomes.

Methods

Organized cervical cancer screening was introduced in Norway in 1995 with the recommendation that all women 25 to 69 years have a Pap smear collected every third year [15]. During the study period the Norwegian cervical cancer program recommended delayed triage with repeat cytology and HPV testing 6–12 months after the index diagnosis of ASC-US/LSIL. Women with high-grade squamous intraepithelial lesions (HSIL) or repeated ASC-US/LSIL with a positive HPV test were referred to colposcopy/biopsy immediately after triage. Women with a normal smear and a positive HPV test were recommended a repeat HPV test within 12 months, whereas women with an ASC-US/LSIL/normal smear with a negative HPV test were returned to the screening program at a three-year interval [9].

This study compared test performance of the HPV mRNA test PreTect HPV-Proofer (PreTect AS, Norway), which detects E6/E7 mRNA of 5 HPV types, and the HPV DNA test Cobas 4800 (Roche Molecular Diagnostics), which detects 14 HPV types. We followed the manufacturer's instructions in preparation of aliquots and detection of mRNA, while we analyzed HPV DNA in accordance with national guidelines [10]. The conventional cytology

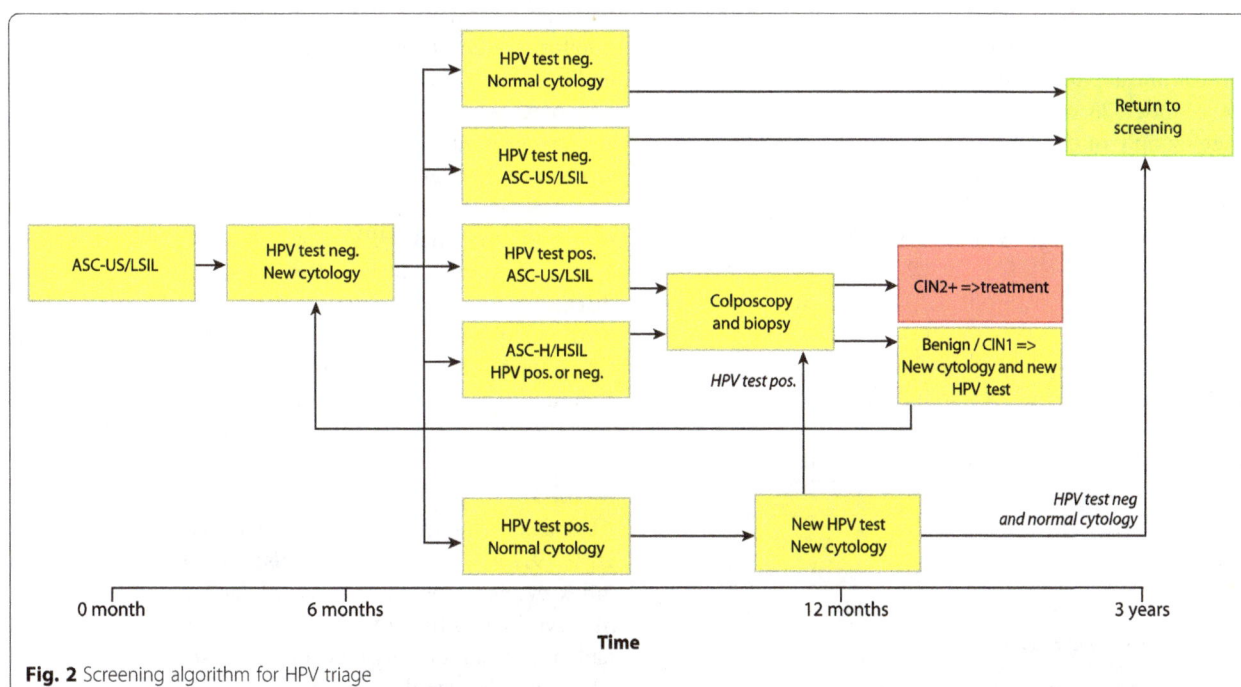

Fig. 2 Screening algorithm for HPV triage

Table 1 Outcome of triage by HPV test (*n* = 564)

	DNA		5-type-mRNA	
	N = 564	% (95 % CI)	*N* = 564	% (95 % CI)
Back to screening	399	70.7 (66.9–74.5)	459	81.4 (78.2–84.6)*
Met for biopsy	105	18.6 (15.4–21.8)	77	13.7 (10.9–16.5)
Scheduled, not met for biopsy	36	6.4 (4.4–8.4)	15	2.7 (1.4–4.0)*
Incomplete follow-up	24	4.3 (2.6–6.0)	13	2.3 (1.1–3.5)

*$p < 0.05$
Triage repeat cytology and HPV test 3–18 months after index ASC-US/LSIL cytology
DNA HPV DNA test (Cobas 4800)
5-type-mRNA HPV mRNA test (PreTect HPV-Proofer)

(Pap smear) consists of sampling cells from the cervical area. The sample is obtained using a brush, and the cells are placed directly onto a glass slide and spray fixed. Then the same brush is placed into a liquid medium (ThinPrep, Cytyc Corporation, Marlborough, USA) for HPV testing. In Norway, many hospitals have switched from conventional Pap smears to liquid-based cytology (LBC), but Ålesund Hospital still uses conventional Pap smears.

The Department of Pathology, Ålesund Hospital, located on the western coast of Norway, serves a background population of approximately 50 000 women at screening age 25–69 years and assesses 12 000 cervical smears annually. Since 1999 the department has used the clinical database SymPathy for administration of cytological and histological specimens. From January 1, 2001, through September 15, 2014, we identified 47 926 women with 160 466 valid smears, among which 1 577 women had a diagnosis of ASC-US/LSIL after June 30, 2010. Our study commenced on January 4, 2012, when the department introduced the HPV DNA test. After excluding women with a history of HSIL, or biopsy with cervical intraepitelial neoplasi grade 1 or worse (CIN1+), those under 25 or over 69 years of age, and cases with none or only one HPV test, 695 women were eligible for study participation (Fig. 1).

The Norwegian cervical cancer screening program recommended triage 6 to 12 months after the index ASC-US/LSIL [6, 9] (Fig. 2). We expanded the triage follow-up window from 90 to 540 days after the index

smear. Therefore women having triage <90 days (*n* = 14) or >540 days (*n* = 12) after index smear, and women having direct biopsy (reflex testing) before or at triage (*n* = 70), and women who had HSIL at triage (*n* = 35) were excluded, leaving 564 women for final analyses. Either a positive HPV DNA or a positive HPV mRNA test triggered colposcopy.

We defined solved cases as subjects who returned to the screening program from either a valid smear/negative HPV test, or having had a biopsy, which determined future follow-up/treatment. Corresponding dates were "outcome" dates for solved cases, while we censored cases not met for biopsy or incomplete follow-up at last day of study, September 15, 2014. Abnormal cervical cytology was classified using the Bethesda system. Cervical biopsies were reported using WHO histological classification of tumors of the uterine cervix (http://screening.iarc.fr/colpochap.php?-chap=2). All biopsies were reviewed by one experienced pathologist (BW). Biopsies with uncertain cellular changes were immunostained with p16 (INK4a) (Roche mtm laboratories AG). If there was a discrepancy between biopsy and treatment histology, the most severe histology was endpoint.

The sensitivity of the HPV tests is defined as the proportion of high-grade dysplasia (CIN2+) detected by the two different HPV tests. In the calculations of specificity, it is assumed that HPV negative samples without detected dysplasia during the follow-up period were disease-free.

All analyses were done in SPSS, version 22.0, with Chi-square test for categorical variables, *t*-test for continuous variables, and survival analyses for clinically solved cases. Significance level was set to $p < 0.05$.

Table 2 Most severe histology from biopsy/cone specimen by HPV test

Histology	HPV DNA		5-type-mRNA	
	N = 105	% (95 % CI)	*N* = 77	% (95 % CI)
Normal/CIN1	67	63.8 (54.6–73.0)	47	61.0 (50.1–71.9)
CIN2	23	21.9 (14.0–29.8)	15	19.5 (10.7–28.3)
CIN3+	15	14.3 (7.6–21.0)	15	19.5 (10.7–28.3)

CIN cervical intraepitelial neoplasi
HPV DNA HPV DNA test (Cobas 4800)
5-type-mRNA HPV mRNA test (PreTect HPV-Proofer)

Results

At index cytology 84 % (473/564) were ASC-US and 16 % (91/564) LSIL. At the most recent screen prior to index cytology 79 % (444/564) of the women had a normal cytology within the screening interval, 4 % (24/564) had a normal cytology beyond the screening interval, whereas index cytology represented the first smear, ever,

Table 3 Test performance of HPV DNA test (N = 504) and 5-type-mRNA test (N = 536) in solved cases

Triage status	CIN2+	CIN1-	Total
HPV DNA positive	38	73	111[a]
HPV DNA negative	0	393	393
Total	38	466	504
Triage status	CIN2+	CIN1-	Total
HPV mRNA positive	30	47	77
HPV mRNA negative	8	451	459
Total	38	498	536

CIN2+ CIN2, CIN3, ACIS, and cervical cancer

CIN1- Normal and CIN1

[a]Of the 111 women with a positive HPV DNA test, six women had normal cytology and a negative HPV DNA test at second follow-up and returned to screening at 3-year interval

for 17 % (96/564) of the women. The mean age was 39 years (SD 10.5 years) and nearly 40 % (217/564) of the women were 25–34 years of age.

Mainly from triage, but also after follow-up of a normal cytology with a positive HPV test at triage, the 5-type mRNA test scheduled significantly more women back to screening, 81 % (459/564), than the DNA test, 71 % (399/564) (p < 0.01). There was no difference in incomplete follow-ups by screening test, HPV DNA test 4 % (24/564)/mRNA test 2 % (13/564) (p = 0.09). Accordingly, the DNA test targeted significantly more women for biopsy, 25 % (141/564) than the 5-type mRNA test, 16 % (92/564) (p < 0.01) (Table 1). In total 141 women were recommended colposcopy by the DNA test, and 105 (74 %) met for biopsy. Out of the 92 women scheduled for biopsy by the 5-type mRNA test, 77 (84 %) made a visit (p = 0.12).

There was no difference in histology outcome by screening test among women who had biopsy and/or treatment. Both tests identified 14 women with CIN3 and one woman with squamous cell carcinoma (Table 2). The positive predictive value (PPV) for CIN2+ was 34 % (38/111) for HPV DNA and 39 % (30/77) for the 5-type mRNA test. The PPVs for CIN3+ were 13.5 % (15/111) and 19.5 % (15/77) for the DNA and the 5-type mRNA test (Table 3). The increased referral rate to biopsy among DNA-tested women relative to mRNA-tested women resulted in 10 more cases of normal histology, 10 more cases of CIN1, and eight more cases of CIN2 (Table 4).

At triage, 65 % (366/564) were negative in both tests (DNA-/mRNA-), while 29 % (165/564) and 19 % (105/564) were positive with the DNA or 5-type mRNA test, respectively. In total, 98 women were double positive (DNA+/mRNA+). Among the 73 HPV DNA positive and 5-type mRNA negative women (DNA+/mRNA-), 69 were positive for HPV types other than 16 and 18, two for HPV16, and two for HPV18. Among women with a negative HPV DNA test, seven tests were positive with the 5-type mRNA test (DNA-/mRNA+), four HPV16 and three HPV other than 16 and 18. Among the 53 women testing positive for HPV16 (DNA+ and/or mRNA+), 44 tested positive in both tests (DNA+/mRNA+), 48 tested positive for HPV DNA, and 49 for 5-type mRNA. Similar results for HPV18, 11 women out of 14 were double positive (DNA+/mRNA+), 13 tested positive for HPV DNA, while 12 tested positive for 5-type mRNA. The largest difference was for HPV other types than HPV16 and HPV18. Only 39 out of 116 tested positive in both tests (DNA+/mRNA+), 110 tested positive for DNA, and 44 tested positive for 5-type mRNA.

Table 4 HPV positivity, genotype, and HPV test by stage of triage and histology

	HPV DNA					5-type-mRNA				
		HPVNeg.	HPV 16	HPV 18	HPV other		HPVNeg.	HPV 16	HPV 18	HPV other
Stages of triage	N	%	%	%	%	N	%	%	%	%
At triage[a]	564	69.7	8.5	2.3	19.5	564	81.4	8.7	2.1	7.8
Recommended biopsy[b]	141		28.4	8.5	63.1	92		45.7	10.9	43.5
Had biopsy[c]	105		36.2	7.6	56.2	77		51.9	9.1	39.0
By histology	N	%	%	%	%	N	%	%	%	%
Normal/CIN1	67		26.9	7.5	65.7	47		44.7	8.5	46.8
CIN2	23		39.1	13.0	47.8	15		53.3	20.0	26.7
CIN3	14		71.4	0.0	28.6	14		71.4	0.0	28.6
Sq. cell carcinoma	1		0.0	0.0	100	1		0.0	0.0	100

HPV DNA other HPV type 31, 33, 35, 39, 45, 51, 52, 56, 58, 59, 66, and 68

5-type-mRNA other HPV type 31, 33, and 45

CIN cervical intraepitelial neoplasi

[a]The Norwegian cervical cancer screening program recommended triage 6 to 12 months after the index ASC-US/LSIL

[b]Women with either a positive HPV DNA or a positive HPV mRNA test are recommended biopsy

[c]In total 141 women were recommended colposcopy by the DNA test, and 105 (74 %) met for biopsy. Out of the 92 women scheduled for biopsy by the 5-type mRNA test, 77 (84 %) made a visit (p = 0.12)

Table 4 summarizes HPV positivity, genotype, stage of triage and histology by HPV test. The DNA test detected 23 cases of CIN2, relative to 15 with the 5-type mRNA test. There was concordance between tests in eight cases of HPV16, three cases of HPV18, and three cases of HPV other than 16 and 18. One CIN2 case testing HPV16 in the DNA test tested HPV other than 16 and 18 in the 5-type mRNA test. The eight additional cases of CIN2 detected by the DNA test were all negative for HPV 16/18 and positive for other than 16 and 18: three in the age group 25–34 years and five in the 35–69 group. All cases with CIN3 ($n = 14$) were concordant for HPV type in both tests ($n = 10$ for HPV16, $n = 4$ for HPV other than 16 or 18).

In total 89 % (504/564) of the DNA cases were solved across the time frame of the study, relative to 95 % (536/564) of the 5-type mRNA-tested cases ($p < 0.01$). The cumulative proportions of cases solved within 12 and 36 months were significantly higher for 5-type mRNA-tested subjects, 92 % (95 % CI: 90–94) and 96 % (95 % CI: 94–98), than DNA-tested subjects, 85 % (95 % CI: 82–88) and 90 % (95 % CI: 87–93)).

The sensitivity among solved cases for CIN2+ of the HPV DNA test was 100 % (38/38) relative to 79 % (30/38, 95 % CI: 67–92) for the 5-type mRNA test. The corresponding estimates of specificity among solved cases were 84 % (393/466, 95 % CI: 81–88), and 91 % (451/498, 95 % CI: 88–93) (Table 3) ($p < 0.01$). In Tables 5, 6, 7 and 8 we provide data on triage cytology (ASC-US or LSIL) by HPV test for CIN2+ and CIN3 +.

Discussion

Our study shows that the 5-type HPV mRNA test had significantly lower positivity rate (19 %) than the 14-type HPV DNA test (29 %), which led to a significantly higher referral rate to colposcopy for the HPV DNA test. Both tests diagnosed equal numbers of women with CIN3+, whereas the DNA test detected eight more cases of

Table 6 Test performance of HPV DNA test and 5-type HPV mRNA test in repeated ASC-US in solved cases versus CIN3+

Triage status	CIN3+	CIN2-	Total
HPV DNA positive	9	78	87
HPV DNA negative	0	28	28
Total	9	106	115

Triage status	CIN3+	CIN2-	Total
HPV mRNA positive	9	54	63
HPV mRNA negative	0	50	50
Total	9	104	113

CIN2+ CIN2, CIN3, ACIS, and cervical cancer
CIN1- Normal and CIN1

CIN2. All these CIN2 cases were of HPV types other than 16/18 in both tests, and they were negative for HPV mRNA 31, 33, and 45.

In agreement with other studies, the positivity rate of the HPV DNA test in triage of ASC-US/LSIL is nearly double compared to the 5-type HPV mRNA test (Table 9 [6, 7, 10–12, 16]). We found a 57 % higher referral rate using HPV DNA versus 5-type mRNA while others have reported a double referral rate ratio using HPV DNA compared to 5-type mRNA [6, 7, 10].

Most studies report a higher sensitivity for CIN2+ and CIN3+ using the HPV DNA test or 14-type HPV mRNA test (Hologic APTIMA) compared to the 5-type HPV mRNA test, whereas the specificity is significantly higher for 5-type HPV mRNA compared to HPV DNA (or 14-type HPV mRNA test) [6, 7, 16–18]. The higher specificity reflects the higher positive predictive value (PPV) for the HPV 5-type mRNA test relative to the HPV DNA test (or 14-type HPV mRNA test).

The major difference in test performance between the DNA and the 5-type mRNA test was HPV types other than 16/18, which were in most cases HPV mRNA-negative for 31/33/45. The choice of test is crucial to

Table 5 Test performance of HPV DNA test and 5-type HPV mRNA test in repeated ASC-US in solved cases versus CIN2+

Triage status	CIN2+	CIN1-	Total
HPV DNA positive	25	62	87
HPV DNA negative	0	28	28
Total	25	90	115

Triage status	CIN2+	CIN1-	Total
HPV mRNA positive	18	45	63
HPV mRNA negative	5	45	50
Total	23	90	113

CIN2+ CIN2, CIN3, ACIS, and cervical cancer
CIN1- Normal and CIN1

Table 7 Test performance of HPV DNA test and 5-type HPV mRNA test in repeated LSIL in solved cases versus CIN2+

Triage status	CIN2+	CIN1-	Total
HPV DNA positive	13	31	44
HPV DNA negative	0	5	5
Total	13	36	49

Triage status	CIN2+	CIN1-	Total
HPV mRNA positive	12	17	29
HPV mRNA negative	1	19	20
Total	13	46	49

CIN2+ CIN2, CIN3, ACIS, and cervical cancer
CIN1- Normal and CIN1

Table 8 Test performance of HPV DNA test and 5-type HPV mRNA test in repeated LSIL in solved cases versus CIN3+

Triage status	CIN3+	CIN2-	Total
HPV DNA positive	6	38	44
HPV DNA negative	0	5	5
Total	6	43	49
Triage status	CIN3+	CIN2-	Total
HPV mRNA positive	6	23	29
HPV mRNA negative	0	20	20
Total	6	43	49

CIN2+ CIN2, CIN3, ACIS, and cervical cancer
CIN1- Normal and CIN1

avoid over-diagnosis in triage of women with minor cytological lesions. Our data indicates that the difference in sensitivity/loss of CIN2 may be attributed to HPV types with a low oncogenic potential with slow progression into cancer. The next screening round will capture these women for follow-up/treatment if there is any progression. A triage HPV test with high specificity, targeting the HPV types with the highest potential for progression to cervical cancer, will reduce over-diagnosis and overtreatment, as observed in this study. Over-diagnosis is a cost-driver in unnecessary conizations and may lead to an increased risk of premature births and late abortions in subsequent pregnancies [19, 20] in this young population.

In our study the 5-type HPV mRNA test detected the same number of CIN3+, with a significant lower positivity rate and significant lower referral rate to colposcopy than the HPV DNA test. The risk of cervical cancer in women with ASC-US/LSIL is low and even lower if the HPV mRNA test is negative [6, 16, 21]. In Europe, HPV16 predominates in both CIN3 and cervical cancer. Other HPV types have a slower progression into cancer [22]. In countries with an organized cervical cancer screening program the risk of development of cervical cancer is higher for HPV types 16, 18, 31, 33 and 45 than for other HPV types [23]. These observations support the use of a specific HPV mRNA test detecting the five main HPV types in triage of women with minor cytological lesions.

In a meta-analysis of the accuracy of 5-type HPV mRNA tests, the pooled sensitivity for CIN2+ of the 10 included studies was 75 % and 76 % for the triage of ASC-US and LSIL, respectively [14]. It is well known that many cervical lesions with moderate or severe dysplasia will regress spontaneously. Only 5 % of women with CIN2 will develop cervical cancer without treatment [24]. Only 31 % of colposcopically visible lesions with CIN3 will progress to invasive cancer within 30 years [25]. About 40 % of CIN2 will regress within two years, and the regression rate of CIN2 caused by other HPV types than HPV type 16 is even higher [26]. It is probable that the 5-type HPV mRNA test in triage of women with minor cervical lesions identifies the majority of the lesions that are destined to progress to cancer [27, 28]. When women with ASC-US/LSIL and a negative 5-type mRNA test are returned to screening in three years, we can reduce overtreatment of women with CIN1-2 caused by HPV types with a low risk of progression [22, 23, 26, 29].

Table 9 Test-performance of the 5-type mRNA test and 13–14 types DNA tests in delayed triage and reflex testing of women with minor cytological lesions and CIN3+ as outcome

Ref.	Data collection	Year publ.	Country	Study design	Timing HPV test	Length f-up (mo)	Diagnosis	HPV test	N	N HPV positive	N Met for biopsy	CIN3+ Sens.	Spes.	PPV	NPV
6	July 2005–Dec. 2009	2013	Norway	Case-series	Delayed triage	≤36	Repeat ASCUS/LSIL	HC II	2150	1504	1 184	NR			
								5 mRNA	1543	510	435				
7	Jan. 2004–Dec. 2006	2011	Italy	Head-to-head	Reflex testing	≤2	ASCUS/LSIL	HC II	795	614	377	NR			
								5 mRNA	755	204	132				
10	Jan. 2012–Sept. 2012	2014	Norway[a]	Head-to-head	Delayed triage	≤33	Repeat ASCUS/LSIL	COBAS	281	92	65	100	77.8	6.2	100
								5 mRNA	281	37	26	75.0	91.6	11.5	99.6
11	Aug. 2005–Jan. 2007	2008	UK	Head-to-head	Reflex testing	Same day	≤ mild dyskaryosis	HC II	567	NR	NRe	100	26.0	11.1	100
								5 mRNA	558			89.4	72.8	23.2	NR
12	Sept. 2007–Oct. 2009	2012	UK	Head-to-head	Reflex Testing	Same day	≤ mild dyskaryosis	HC II	670	526	NRe	100	NR	9.2	100
								5 mRNA	641	272		80.9		16.6	NR
16	NR	2010	Canada	Head-to-head	Reflex testing	≤6	ASCUS/LSIL	HC II	781	619	NRe	NR			
								5 mRNA	781	328					
A	Jan. 2012–Sep. 2013		Norway[a]	Head-to-head	Delayed testing	≤33	Repeat ASCUS/LSIL	COBAS	564	171	105	100	80.0	13.9	100
								5 mRNA	564	105	77	100	85.2	16.3	100

A Present study
Sens Sensitivity; Spes. Specificity; PPV positive predictive value; NPV negative predictive value; NR Not reported; NRe Not relevant. All women had colposcopy regardless of HPV result
[a]Only solved cases are included in test-performance analysis

The experience in the Department of Pathology, Ålesund Hospital, is that the 5-type HPV mRNA test has a high specificity and a high positive predictive value. This makes it useful for triage of women with minor cervical lesions.

Conclusions

5-type HPV mRNA is more specific than HPV DNA in triage of women with repeated ASC-US/LSIL. The referral rate for colposcopy after repeated ASC-US/LSIL was 57 % higher for DNA+ relative to mRNA+ cases, with the same detection rate of CIN3+. It is important to consider the trade-off between sensitivity and specificity of the diagnostic test when designing screening algorithms.

Abbreviations
ASC-H, atypical squamous cells – cannot exclude HSIL; ASC-US, atypical squamous cells of undetermined significance; CIN, cervical intraepithelial neoplasia, also known as cervical dysplasia; CIN1, CIN2, CIN3, cervical intraepithelial neoplasia grade 1, 2 or 3, also known as low grade, moderate or severe cervical dysplasia; CIN2+, CIN2, CIN3, adenocarcinoma in situ (ACIS) or cervical cancer DNA: Deoxyribonucleic acid; HPV, human papillomavirus; HPV DNA test, cobas 4800 detects DNA from 14 high-risk HPV types (16, 18, 31, 33, 35, 39, 45, 51, 52, 56, 58, 59, 66 and 68) at clinically relevant infection levels; HPV mRNA test, PreTect HPV-Proofer detects E6/E7 mRNA of 5 HPV types (16, 18, 31, 33 and 45); HSIL, High grade squamous intraepithelial lesion; LBC, liquid-based cytology; LSIL, low grade squamous intraepithelial lesion; mRNA, messenger RNA; NPV, negative predictive value; Pap smear, the Papanicolaou test, also known as Pap test, cervical smear or cervical cytology; PPV, positive predictive value; RNA, ribonucleic acid; WHO, the World Health Organization

Acknowledgements
Not applicable.

Funding
This research was supported by a grant from the Helse Møre og Romsdal Trust. The funders had no role in study design, data collection and analysis, decision to publish, or preparation of the manuscript.

Authors' contributions
BW, SWS and FES participated in the design of the study. AG and HG screened all the PAP-smears and performed HPV mRNA testing. BW reviewed all the histological diagnosis. SWS and FES performed the statistical analysis. All authors read and approved the final manuscript.

Authors' information
Not applicable.

Competing interests
The authors declare that they have no competing interests.

Author details
[1]Department of Pathology, Ålesund Hospital, Møre and Romsdal Health Trust, Ålesund, Norway. [2]Department of Clinical Pathology, University Hospital of North Norway, 9038 Tromsø, Norway. [3]Research Group Epidemiology of Chronic Diseases, Department of Community Medicine, UiT The Arctic University of Norway, Tromsø, Norway.

References
1. Arbyn M, Castellsague X, de Sanjose S, Bruni L, Saraiya M, Bray F, et al. Worldwide burden of cervical cancer in 2008. Ann Oncol. 2011;12:2675–86.
2. Ramakrishnan S, Partricia S, Mathan G. Overview of high-risk HPV's 16 and 18 infected cervical cancer: pathogenesis to prevention. Biomed Pharmacother. 2015;70:103–10.
3. de Sanjose S, Quint WG, Alemany L, Geraets DT, Klaustermeier JE, Lloveras B, et al. Human papillomavirus genotype attribution in invasive cervical cancer: a retrospective cross-sectional worldwide study. Lancet Oncol. 2010;11:1048–56.
4. Saslow D, Solomon D, Lawson HW, Killackey M, Kulasingam SL, Cain J, et al. American Cancer Society, American Society for Colposcopy and Cervical Pathology, and American Society for Clinical Pathology screening guidelines for the prevention and early detection of cervical cancer. Am J Clin Pathol. 2012;137:516–42.
5. Arbyn M, Martin-Hirsch P, Buntinx F, Van Ranst M, Paraskevaidis E, Dillner J. Triage of women with equivocal or low-grade cervical cytology results: a meta-analysis of the HPV test positivity rate. J Cell Mol Med. 2009;13:648–59.
6. Nygard M, Roysland K, Campbell S, Dillner J. Comparative effectiveness study on human papillomavirus detection methods used in the cervical cancer screening programme. BMJ Open. 2014;4:e003460.
7. Benevolo M, Vocaturo A, Caraceni D, French D, Rosini S, Zappacosta R, Terrenato I, Ciccocioppo L, Frega A, Giorgi Rossi P. Sensitivity, specificity, and clinical value of human papillomavirus (HPV) E6/E7 mRNA assay as a triage test for cervical cytology and HPV DNA test. J Clin Microbiol. 2011;49(7):2643–50. doi:10.1128/JCM.02570-10.
8. Koliopoulos G, Chrelias C, Pappas A, Makridima S, Kountouris E, Alepaki M, Spathis A, Stathopoulou V, Panayiotides I, Panagopoulos P, Karakitsos P, Kassanos D. The diagnostic accuracy of two methods for E6&7 mRNA detection in women with minor cytological abnormalities. Acta Obstet Gynecol Scand. 2012;91(7):794–801. doi:10.1111/j.1600-0412.2012.01414.x.
9. Sorbye SW, Fismen S, Gutteberg T, Mortensen ES. Triage of women with minor cervical lesions: data suggesting a "test and treat" approach for HPV E6/E7 mRNA testing. PLoS One. 2010;5:e12724.
10. Sorbye SW, Fismen S, Gutteberg TJ, Mortensen ES, Skjeldestad FE. HPV mRNA is more specific than HPV DNA in triage of women with minor cervical lesions. PLoS One. 2014;9:e112934.
11. Szarewski A, Ambroisine L, Cadman L, Austin J, Ho L, Terry G, et al. Comparison of predictors for high-grade cervical intraepithelial neoplasia in women with abnormal smears. Cancer Epidemiol Biomarkers Prev. 2008;17:3033–42.
12. Szarewski A, Mesher D, Cadman L, Austin J, Ashdown-Barr L, Ho L, et al. Comparison of seven tests for high-grade cervical intraepithelial neoplasia in women with abnormal smears: the Predictors 2 study. J Clin Microbiol. 2012;50:1867–73.
13. Trope A, Sjoborg K, Eskild A, Cuschieri K, Eriksen T, Thoresen S, et al. Performance of human papillomavirus DNA and mRNA testing strategies for women with and without cervical neoplasia. J Clin Microbiol. 2009;47:2458–64.
14. Verdoodt F, Szarewski A, Halfon P, Cuschieri K, Arbyn M. Triage of women with minor abnormal cervical cytology: meta-analysis of the accuracy of an assay targeting messenger ribonucleic acid of 5 high-risk human papillomavirus types. Cancer Cytopathol. 2013;121:675–87.
15. Nygård JF, Skare GB, Thoresen SO. The cervical cancer screening programme in Norway, 1992–2000: changes in Pap smear coverage and incidence of cervical cancer. J Med Screen. 2002;9:86–91.
16. Ratnam S, Coutlee F, Fontaine D, Bentley J, Escott N, Ghatage P, et al. Clinical performance of the PreTect HPV-Proofer E6/E7 mRNA assay in comparison with that of the Hybrid Capture 2 test for identification of women at risk of cervical cancer. J Clin Microbiol. 2010;48:2779–85.
17. Arbyn M, Ronco G, Anttila A, Meijer CJ, Poljak M, Ogilvie G, et al. Evidence regarding human papillomavirus testing in secondary prevention of cervical cancer. Vaccine. 2012;30 Suppl 5:F88–99.
18. Arbyn M, Roelens J, Cuschieri K, Cuzick J, Szarewski A, Ratnam S, et al. The APTIMA HPV assay versus the Hybrid Capture 2 test in triage of women with ASC-US or LSIL cervical cytology: a meta-analysis of the diagnostic accuracy. Int J Cancer. 2013;132:101–8.
19. Arbyn M, Kyrgiou M, Simoens C, Raifu AO, Koliopoulos G, Martin-Hirsch P, et al. Perinatal mortality and other severe adverse pregnancy outcomes associated with treatment of cervical intraepithelial neoplasia: meta-analysis. BMJ. 2008;337:a1284. doi:10.1136/bmj.a1284.:a1284.
20. Bruinsma FJ, Quinn MA. The risk of preterm birth following treatment for precancerous changes in the cervix: a systematic review and meta-analysis. BJOG. 2011;118:1031–41.

21. Sorbye SW, Fismen S, Gutteberg TJ, Mortensen ES. HPV mRNA test in women with minor cervical lesions: experience of the University Hospital of North Norway. J Virol Methods. 2010;169:219–22.

22. Tjalma WA, Fiander A, Reich O, Powell N, Nowakowski AM, Kirschner B, et al. Differences in human papillomavirus type distribution in high-grade cervical intraepithelial neoplasia and invasive cervical cancer in Europe. Int J Cancer. 2013;132:854–67.

23. Powell NG, Hibbitts SJ, Boyde AM, Newcombe RG, Tristram AJ, Fiander AN. The risk of cervical cancer associated with specific types of human papillomavirus: a case–control study in a UK population. Int J Cancer. 2011;128:1676–82.

24. Ostor AG. Natural history of cervical intraepithelial neoplasia: a critical review. Int J Gynecol Pathol. 1993;12:186–92.

25. McCredie MR, Sharples KJ, Paul C, Baranyai J, Medley G, Jones RW, et al. Natural history of cervical neoplasia and risk of invasive cancer in women with cervical intraepithelial neoplasia 3: a retrospective cohort study. Lancet Oncol. 2008;9:425–34.

26. Castle PE, Schiffman M, Wheeler CM, Solomon D. Evidence for frequent regression of cervical intraepithelial neoplasia-grade 2. Obstet Gynecol. 2009;113:18–25.

27. Basu P, Roychowdhury S, Bafna UD, Chaudhury S, Kothari S, Sekhon R, et al. Human papillomavirus genotype distribution in cervical cancer in India: results from a multi-center study. Asian Pac J Cancer Prev. 2009;10:27–34.

28. Kraus I, Molden T, Holm R, Lie AK, Karlsen F, Kristensen GB, et al. Presence of E6 and E7 mRNA from human papillomavirus types 16, 18, 31, 33, and 45 in the majority of cervical carcinomas. J Clin Microbiol. 2006;44:1310–7.

29. Zappacosta R, Gatta DM, Marinucci P, Capanna S, Lattanzio G, Caraceni D, et al. Role of E6/E7 mRNA test in the diagnostic algorithm of HPV-positive patients showing ASCUS and LSIL: clinical and economic implications in a publicly financed healthcare system. Expert Rev Mol Diagn. 2015;15:1–14.

18

Elevation of small, dense low density lipoprotein cholesterol—a possible antecedent of atherogenic lipoprotein phenotype in type 2 diabetes patients in Jos, North-Central Nigeria

Kenneth O. Inaku[1][*] [iD], Obasola O. Ogunkeye[2], Fayeofori M. Abbiyesuku[3], Evelyn K. Chuhwak[4], Christian O. Isichei[2], Lucius C. Imoh[5], Noel O. Amadu[5] and Alexander O. Abu[5]

Abstract

Background: The global prevalence of type 2 diabetes is increasing. Dyslipidaemia is a known complication of diabetes mellitus manifesting frequently as cardiovascular diseases and stoke. Elevation of small, dense low density lipoprotein has been recognised as a component of the atherogenic lipoprotein phenotype associated with cardiovascular complications. We speculate that the elevation of this lipoprotein particle may be the antecedent of the atherogenic lipoprotein phenotype. This study therefore aims to determine the pattern of dyslipidaemia among diabetes mellitus patients in Jos, North-Central Nigeria.

Methods: One hundred and seventy-six patients with type 2 diabetes and 154 age-matched controls were studied. The patients with diabetes were regular clinic attenders and had stable glycaemic control. None were on lipid-lowering therapy. Anthropometric indices, blood pressure, and lipids (including total cholesterol, high density lipoprotein cholesterol, and triglyceride) were measured by chemical methods using the Hitachi 902 analyzer. Low density lipoprotein cholesterol was calculated using the Friedewald's equation. Small, dense low density lipoprotein cholesterol, −sdLDL-C was measured using the precipitation method by Hirano et al. Means of the different groups were compared using EPI Info and a P-value of <0.05 was accepted as significant difference.

Results: Total cholesterol, low density lipoprotein cholesterol, triglyceride and small, dense lipoprotein cholesterol were all significantly higher in diabetes patients than controls except high density lipoprotein cholesterol. The percentage of LDL-C as sdLDL-C among the diabetes versus control group was 45% ± 17.79 v 32.0% ± 15.93. Serum sdLDL-C concentration was determined to be 1.45 ± 0.64 among diabetes patients and 0.8 ± 0.54 among control subjects. 75% of diabetes patients had hypertension and were taking blood pressure lowering medications.

Conclusion: The classical atherogenic lipoprotein phenotype was not demonstrated among subjects with type 2 diabetes mellitus in this study, but the elevation of serum small dense low density lipoprotein cholesterol in patients with sustained hypertension suggests the establishment of atherogenic complications among our diabetes patients.

Keywords: Type 2 diabetes mellitus, Dyslipidaemia, Small, dense LDL-C, Atherogenesis, High density lipoprotein

* Correspondence: keninaku@yahoo.com; keninaku@unical.edu.ng
[1]Department of Chemical Pathology, Faculty of Medicine, College of Medical Sciences, University of Calabar, Calabar, Cross River State, Nigeria
Full list of author information is available at the end of the article

Background

Type 2 diabetes is an increasingly common chronic illness with an accompanying risk of cardiovascular complications [1]. In 2015, an estimated 415 million people worldwide were said to be living with diabetes representing 8.8% of the global adult population. By 2040, that number is expected to rise to 642 million [2]. With some 75% of people with diabetes living in low and middle income countries, diabetes is no longer a disease of the Western countries. Nigeria has a national prevalence of about 1.9% [2] although this may fall below the true prevalence of the disease in Nigeria due to the poor health care services especially in rural areas where majority of ailments go undiagnosed.

Diabetes mellitus is frequently associated with serious health complications and premature deaths. Globally, it is estimated to account for 50 million deaths annually at a frequency of 1 death every 6 s [2]. Approximately 80% of all diabetes associated mortality and hospitalisations can be attributed to cardiovascular complications [3]. Dyslipidaemia in type 2 diabetes may exist alone or in association with metabolic syndrome, and this association increases cardiovascular risk [4]. The typical pattern of diabetic dyslipidaemia consists of elevated very low density lipoprotein (VLDL) triglycerides, low high density lipoprotein cholesterol (HDL-C) and a predominance of small, dense low density lipoprotein cholesterol (sdLDL-C) [5]. This diabetic dyslipidaemia was first described in 1990 by Austin et al. as a risk conferring lipoprotein profile termed "atherogenic dyslipidaemia" or "the atherogenic lipoprotein phenotype" (ALP) [6]. The increase in the number of atherogenic particles reflected by high apolipoprotein B (apoB) concentrations may contribute to an increased cardiovascular disease (CVD) mortality in people with diabetes (phenotype B) [4, 7]. This is in contrast to phenotype A pattern, in which large, more buoyant LDL predominates.

LDL-C remains the target for diagnosing and monitoring dyslipidaemia in type 2 diabetes [8]. The bulk of research on dyslipidaemias in Nigeria, both in the general population and specifically among type 2 diabetes patients, has concentrated on measuring traditional lipid indices such as total cholesterol (TC), LDL-C, HDL-C and triglyceride (TG) [9]. We are unaware of studies in Nigeria that have estimated LDL-C subfractions in diabetes versus controls. Since lipids can be affected by diet, environment and lifestyle, there is a need to investigate the metabolism of sdLDL-C as a component of dyslipidaemia among people with diabetes living in Jos, Nigeria. We hypothesise that the level of sdLDL-C will be higher in diabetes subjects than controls.

Methods

Study area

The protocol for this study was approved by the Ethics Committee of the Jos University Teaching Hospital (JUTH). The study area was Jos and Bukuru metropolis in the Plateau State of Nigeria. The population is made up of civil servants, students and traders.

Study design and population

This is a descriptive, cross-sectional study. Subjects aged 35-65 years were recruited from type 2 diabetes patients attending both the Medical outpatient department (MOPD) and the General Outpatient department (GOPD) of the Jos University teaching hospital (JUTH) from June to September 2012. They were selected by the attending physician after being confirmed to be regular attendees in clinics for at least 3 consecutive visits, taking prescribed medications and never having been on lipid lowering medications. No patient was enrolled twice. Controls were individuals without diabetes or hypertension drawn from hospital staff, patients' relatives and members of the general public who had no symptoms suggestive of diabetes mellitus or hypertension. They were examined to confirm their status. All participants gave written informed consent before enrolling in the study.

Each participant was administered a questionnaire. The questionnaire was completed by the individuals if they could read and write English language and otherwise by the researcher or his trained assistant. Demographic and anthropometric indices such as age, sex, weight and height, blood pressure were recorded. Blood pressure was recorded while patient was sitting using a table mercury column sphygmomanometer after about 5-10 min of rest. Hypertension was defined by systolic or diastolic blood pressure above 139/89 mmHg on more than one occasion or taking blood pressure lowering medications. Body mass index was calculated from the formula: weight (kg)/height (m^2). A history of past or present use of lipid-lowering medications was also noted.

Exclusion criteria

1) individuals on known lipid-lowering drugs; 2) subjects with a triglyceride level above 4.5 mmol/L; 3) pregnant women; 4) individuals with acute or chronic illness (except type 2 diabetes and hypertension); 5) anyone who did not give written informed consent; 6) any subject on admission to hospital irrespective of type or nature of illness. 6) Hypertensive controls without diabetes.

Sample collection and analysis

Blood sampling

About 5 ml of venous blood was collected into a plain bottle from each subject following an overnight fast of at least 10 h. The blood was allowed to clot and retract at room temperature before centrifuging at 3500 rpm for 5 min. Serum was separated and stored at -20 °C and used for the assays within 7 days of sampling. Refrigerator temperature recording was done twice daily to ensure adequate preservation of the samples. This is a part of the daily routine in the AIDS Prevention in Nigeria (APIN) Laboratory. Blood samples were analysed for total cholesterol (TC), high density lipoprotein cholesterol (HDL-C), and triglyceride (TG) by automated colorimetric enzymatic analysis using Cobas (Roche Diagnostics GmbH, Sandhofer Strasse 116, Mannheim, Germany) commercial kits on the Roche/Hitachi 902 automatic analyser (Hitachi High-Technology Corporation, Minato-ku, Tokyo 105-8717, Japan). Low density lipoprotein cholesterol was calculated using Friedewald's formula [10] provided the TG level was <4.5 mmol/L. Small, dense low density lipoprotein cholesterol (sdLDL-C) was isolated using the precipitation method of Hirano et al. [11]. The precipitation reagent (0.1 ml) contained 150 U/ml of heparin-sodium salt (Sigma) and 90 mmol/l of $MgCl_2$ (Sigma), and was added to 0.1 ml of plasma, mixed, and incubated for 10 min at 37 °C. The samples were then placed in an ice bath for 15 min, and then the precipitate was collected by centrifugation at 15000 rpm for 15 min at 4 °C. Aliquots of the supernatant were then used to measure the cholesterol concentration by the same kit method used for total cholesterol. The within- and between-run coefficient of variations (CVs) for cholesterol measurements was 0.48% and 4.72% and for TG measurements it was 0.45% and 9.9% respectively. We calculated large buoyant LDL-C as LDL-C – sdLDL-C, and we also calculated the percentage of LDL-C as sdLDL-C as sdLDL-C/LDL-C × 100.

Data analysis

Data was entered into Microsoft Excel and imported into Epi Info™ version 7 [12] for analysis. Socio-demographic characteristics of the diabetes and control groups were analyzed for differences, using unpaired Student's t-tests. Mean (SD) or 95% confidence interval (CI) of the mean was computed for all lipid variables. A comparison of means across groups where there are more than 2 groups as in Table 7 was made using analysis of variance (ANOVA). P-values <0.05 were considered to be statistically significant for all tests.

Results

The study cohort consisted of 176 patients with type 2 diabetes and 154 controls aged 35-65 years. Among the patients with diabetes, there were 60 men (34%) and 116 women (65%), while in the controls there were 69 men (45%) and 85 women (55%). The duration of diabetes ranged from 1 to 22 years, with a mean of 6.48 ± 4.8 years. Among these, 141 (80%) have had diabetes for at least

10 years while 35 (20%) have been diagnosed over 10 years prior to the time of this study. The age and weight between the diabetes and control groups were not statistically significantly different since they were age matched. However, the diabetes group had a statistically significantly higher body mass index (BMI), systolic and diastolic blood pressure than the controls (Table 1). One hundred and thirty-two (75%) of the patients with diabetes had hypertension and were being treated with blood pressure lowering medications. The duration of hypertension ranged from 1 to 31 years with an average of 7.40 ± 7.81. Nine (0.05%) of the diabetes subjects reported a past history of cardiovascular event ranging from transient ischemic attack (TIA) to stroke. There was no report of a history of myocardial infarction among the subjects. Diabetes was being managed with metformin as first line with sulphonylureas or thiazolidiandiones such as chlropropamide and pioglitazone respectively as adjunct. Five (0.03%) patients were treated with insulin in combination with metformin and 2 (0.01%) patients were being managed with insulin only. Two patients did not need medications to control their blood glucose level and were on diet modification only. None of the diabetes subjects was taking lipid lowering medications at least 6 month prior to, and during the study period.

We compared lipid parameters between patients with diabetes and controls (Table 2). Mean serum concentrations of TC (5.16 ± 1.31 v 4.35 ± 1.02 mmol/l, $P < 0.01$), TG (1.42 ± 0.63 v 1.00 ± 0.56 mmol/L, $P < 0.01$), LDL-C (3.31 ± 1.20 v 2.60 ± 0.91 mmol/L, $P < 0.01$) and small, dense LDL-C (1.45 ± 0.64 v 0.80 ± 0.54 mmol/l, $P < 0.01$) were all higher in patients with diabetes than control. Only HDL-C (1.21 ± 0.36 v 1.26 ± 0.40 mmol/l, $P = 0.19$) and large buoyant LDL-C (1.86 ± 1.09 v1.84 ± 0.93 mmol/l, $P = 0.85$) were not significantly different. The percentage of LDL-C as sdLDL-C among the diabetes patients and controls was 45% and 32%, respectively. All the different lipid and lipoprotein ratios examined were higher among the diabetes patients than the controls except HDL-C/LDL-C, which was higher among controls (0.56 ± 0.36) than the diabetes patients (0.41 ± 0.9 mmol/l).

Table 1 Demographics and some indices of diabetes patients and controls

Characteristics	Diabetics (n = 176)	Controls (n = 154)	P-value
Age (years)	55 ± 8.5	54 ± 7.3	0.89
Weight (Kg)	74 ± 14.9	72 ± 11.7	0.14
BMI (Kg/m²)	28.5 ± 5.0	26.7 ± 4.6	< 0.01
Systolic BP (mmHg)	138 ± 29.0	121 ± 17.9	< 0.01
Diastolic BP (mmHg)	87 ± 15.8	80 ± 10.3	< 0.01

Values are expressed as mean ± SD. Unpaired Student's t-tests, P < 0.05 = significant

Table 2 Serum lipid concentration in diabetes patients and controls

Variable	Diabetics (*n* = 176) Mean ± SD	Controls (*n* = 154) Mean ± SD	*P*-value
Total Cholesterol (mmol/L)	5.16 ± 1.31	4.35 ± 1.02	< 0.01
Triglycerides (mmol/L)	1.42 ± 0.63	1.00 ± 0.56	< 0.01
HDL-C (mmol/L)	1.21 ± 0.36	1.26 ± 0.40	0.19
LDL-C (mmol/L)	3.31 ± 1.20	2.60 ± 0.91	< 0.01
sdLDL-C (mmol/L)	1.45 ± 0.64	0.80 ± 0.54	< 0.01
lbLDL-C (mmol/L)	1.86 ± 1.09	1.84 ± 0.93	0.85
% LDL-C as sdLDL-C	45.0 ± 17.79	32.0 ± 15.93	< 0.01
TC/HDL-C	4.63 ± 2.40	3.69 ± 1.19	< 0.01
HDL-C/LDL/C	0.41 ± 0.19	0.56 ± 0.36	< 0.01
LDL-C/HDL-C	3.05 ± 2.22	2.29 ± 1.04	< 0.01

Values are expressed as mean ± SD, Unpaired Student's t-tests, P < 0.05 = significant

Table 3 compares the mean lipid parameters in the diabetes group between men and women. The total cholesterol, HDL-C, LDL-C and sdLDL-C and lbLDL-C were all statistically significantly higher in women than men with diabetes. The TG value is the same in women as in men with diabetes. Men with diabetes are more likely to have up to 47% (95% CI 42.84–52.16) of their LDL-C as small dense LDL-C. The difference in the percentage of LDL-C as sdLDL-C in women and men (44.83% v 47.50%, *P* = 0.37) did not reach statistical significance.

Table 4 compares serum lipid concentrations between male and female controls. The mean total cholesterol among men was 4.38 mmol/l (95% CI 4.12–4.63), and 4.32 mmol/l (95% CI 4.11–4.53) in women. The difference was not statistically significant (*P* < 0.75). Triglyceride were higher in men (1.11 mmol/l, 95% CI 0.97–1.25) than in women (0.92 mmol/l, 95% CI 0.81–1.02) and the difference was statistically significant (*P* = 0.03). The mean HDL-C was not different in women (1.32 mmol/l, 95% CI 1.22–1.42) than men (1.20 mmol/l, 95% CI 1.12–1.27, *P* = 0.05). LDL-C was the same (*P* = 0.51) in men (2.7 mmol/l, 95% CI 2.50–2.90) as in women (2.60 mmol/l, 95% CI 2.40–2.80). This was also the case with sdLDL-C, which was the same (*P* = 0.39) in women (0.83 mmol/l, 95% CI 0.70-0.96) as in men (0.76 mmol/l, 95% CI 0.56-0.86). The percentage of LDL-C as sdLDL in women was the same (*P* = 0.56) at 33.89% (95%CI 28.86–38.93) as in men at 31.46% (95% CI 24.97–37.96).

The serum lipid concentrations were compared among men with diabetes and men without diabetes (Table 5). TC, HDL-C, LDL-C, and lbLDL-C were not statistically significantly different between the two groups. TG, sdLDL-C and percentage of LDL-C as sdLDL reached statistical significant difference between the groups. Men with diabetes are likely to have as much as 47.50% (95% CI 42.84%–52.16%) of LDL existing as sdLDL-C.

Table 6 represents a comparison between the different lipid parameters measured in women who have diabetes and those without diabetes. Except for HDL-C and lbLDL-C, the rest of the lipids and lipoproteins measured should statistically significant difference between the two

Table 4 Serum lipid concentrations in men and women controls

Variable	Men (*n* = 69)	Women (*n* = 85)	*P*-value
Total cholesterol (mmol/l)	4.38 (4.12–4.63)	4.32 (4.11–4.53)	0.75
Triglycerides (mmol/l)	1.11 (0.97–1.25)	0.92 (0.81–1.02)	0.03
HDL–C (mmol/l)	1.20 (1.12–1.27)	1.32 (1.22–1.42)	0.05
LDL–C (mmol/l)	2.70 (2.50–2.90)	2.60 (2.40–2.80)	0.51
sdLDL–C (mmol/l)	0.76 (0.65–0.86)	0.83 (0.70–0.96)	0.39
lbLDL–C (mmol/l)	1.94 (1.72–2.16)	1.77 (1.57–1.96)	0.25
%LDL as sdLDL	31.46 (24.97–37.96)	33.89 (28.86–38.93)	0.56

Values are expressed as mean (95% confidence interval), Unpaired student's t-test, P < 0.05 = significant

Table 3 Serum lipid concentration in diabetic men and women

Variable	Men (*n* = 60)	Women (*n* = 116)	*P*-value
Total Cholesterol (mmol/l)	4.75 (4.45–5.05)	5.37 (5.13–5.16)	< 0.01
Triglycerides (mmol/l)	1.39 (1.23–1.54)	1.43 (1.32–1.55)	0.68
HDL–C (mmol/l)	1.11 (1.04–1.19)	1.26 (0.99–1.33)	0.01
LDL–C (mmol/l)	3.02 (2.76–3.28)	3.46 (3.23–3.69)	0.01
sdLDL–C (mmol/l)	1.38 (1.23–1.53)	1.48 (1.36–1.60)	0.32
lbLDL–C (mmol/l)	1.64 (1.41–1.87)	1.98 (1.77–2.19)	0.03
%LDL as sdLDL	47.50 (42.84–52.16)	44.83 (41.39–48.27)	0.37

Values are expressed as mean (95% Confidence interval of the mean); Unpaired Student's t-tests, P < 0.05 = significant

Table 5 Serum lipid concentrations in men with diabetes compared with men without diabetes

Variable	Diabetes (*n* = 60)	Controls (*n* = 69)	*P*-value
Total cholesterol (mmol/l)	4.75 (4.45-5.05)	4.38 (4.12-4.63)	0.068
Triglycerides (mmol/l)	1.39 (1.23-1.56)	1.11 (1.09-1.25)	0.012
HDL–C (mmol/l)	1.11 (1.04-1.19)	1.20 (1.12-1.27)	0.116
LDL–C (mmol/l)	3.02 (2.76-3.28)	2.70 (2.50-2.90)	0.759
sdLDL–C (mmol/l)	1.38 (1.23-1.53)	0.76 (0.65-0.86)	< 0.001
lbLDL–C (mmol/l)	1.64 (1.41-1.89)	1.94 (1.72-2.16)	0.069
%LDL as sdLDL	47.50 (42.84-52.16)	31.46 (24.97-37.96)	0.001

Values are expressed as mean (95% confidence interval), Unpaired student's t-test, P < 0.05 = significant

Table 6 Serum lipid concentrations in women with diabetes compared with women without diabetes

Variable	Diabetes (n = 116)	Controls (n = 85)	P-value
Total cholesterol (mmol/l)	5.37 (5.13–5.61)	4.32 (4.11–4.53)	< 0.001
Triglycerides (mmol/l)	1.43 (1.32–1.55)	0.92 (0.81–1.02)	< 0.001
HDL–C (mmol/l)	1.26 (1.19–1.33)	1.32 (1.22–1.42)	0.317
LDL–C (mmol/l)	3.46 (3.23–3.69)	2.60 (2.40–2.80)	< 0.001
sdLDL–C (mmol/l)	1.48 (1.36–1.60)	0.83 (0.70–0.96)	< 0.001
lbLDL–C (mmol/l)	1.98 (1.77–2.19)	1.77 (1.57–1.96)	0.136
%LDL as sdLDL	44.83 (41.39–48.27)	33.89 (28.86–38.93)	< 0.001

Values are expressed as mean (95% confidence interval), Unpaired student's t-test, $P < 0.05$ = significant

groups with all the parameters including TC, TG, LDL-C, sdLDL-C and percentage LDL as sdLDL observed to be higher among diabetes subjects. Women with diabetes are more likely to have as much as 44.83% of their LDL-C existing as sdLDL-C.

The diabetic group was divided into 3 subgroups based on their age—Table 7. Subgroup 1 was 35 to 45 years old and amounted to 26(14.8%) in number. Subgroup 2 included those who were 46–60 years old. They were 98 in number and made up 55.7% of the total diabetics. The third subgroup was >60 years, 52 in number and accounted for 29.5% of the total diabetes patients. There was no statistically significant difference in any of the lipid parameters considered across the 3 age groups.

Discussion

Our data has shown that dyslipidaemia is a problem among type 2 diabetes patients as has been well reported in other similar studies [13–15]. Although there was increase in almost all lipid parameters measured in this study among diabetes patients than controls, the mean TC, TG, LDL-C, and HDL-C in diabetes patients did not meet definitions for dyslipidaemia using criteria such as the National Cholesterol Education Program/Adult

Treatment Panel III (NCEP ATP III)] [16]. This observation is in agreement with some previous studies in Nigeria that showed that black Africans have a low prevalence of dyslipidaemia [17]. The high fibre, unrefined carbohydrate diet with low saturated fat commoner among Nigerians may account for this picture. Some researchers have found that diets high in carbohydrates, glycaemic index or both have an adverse relationship to total cholesterol, LDL-C and HDL-C levels with a moderate increase in the overall TC:HDL-C ratio [18]. The implication is that the apparent beneficial effect of a low cholesterol level may not persist in the long run. However, this observation was made in a highly motivated population and the composition of carbohydrates in their diet may be more refined carbohydrates in comparison to the average Nigerian diet. Notably, the TC:HDL-C ratio in our study was found to be lower than what was reported in other studies that involved Whites with no risk factors for CHD [18, 19].

Suppressed HDL-C has been reported as a component of diabetic dyslipidaemia [20, 21] and an important indicator for an elevated risk of CAD in diabetes even if TC and TG were strictly normal [22]. This study did not however demonstrate a reduction of HDL-C in the diabetes patients. Some researchers have suggested that protective HDL-C was significantly higher in tropical Africa including diabetes patients in Nigeria [14, 23]. The apparently high HDL-C among diabetes patients in this study and others is in keeping with the relatively low-incidence of acute myocardial infarction (AMI) in our environment [23–25]. No participant in this study reported a past episode of AMI. Epidemiological and other studies have consistently confirmed the inverse relationship between HDL-C and CAD [3, 26, 27]. The beneficial effects of HDL are primarily link to their role in reverse cholesterol transport mechanism, i.e., the cholesterol in HDL is being transported back to the liver for excretion out of the body. HDL is also believed to be involved in beneficial mechanisms such as inhibition of lipid peroxidation, cellular adhesion and/or platelet activation resulting in low levels of dyslipidaemia.

Table 7 Comparison of mean lipid parameters among diabetes patients according to age groups

Variable/Age (years)	Subgroup 1 < 46 (n = 26)	Subgroup 2 46-60 (n = 98)	Subgroup 3 > 60 (n = 52)	F-value	p-value
TC (mmol/L)	4.7 ± 0.9	5.36 ± 1.4	5.01 ± 1.3	3.058	0.050
TG (mmol/L)	1.29 ± 0.6	1.45 ± 0.7	1.43 ± 0.6	0.697	0.499
HDL-C (mmol/L)	1.19 ± 0.2	1.23 ± 0.4	1.18 ± 0.3	0.358	0.700
LDL-C (mmol/L)	2.98 ± 0.9	3.45 ± 1.3	3.21 ± 1.1	1.862	0.158
sdLDL-C (mmol/L)	1.25 ± 0.4	1.46 ± 0.6	1.50 ± 0.7	1.432	0.242
lLDL-C (mmol/L)	1.72 ± 0.6	1.99 ± 0.6	1.69 ± 0.5	1.544	0.216
%LDL-C as dLDL-C	45.70 ± 15.4	44.02 ± 15.5	48.78 ± 16.9	0.896	0.410

Values are expressed as Mean ± SD, ANOVA, $p < 0.05$ = significant

This is probably the first study that has estimated the level of LDL sub-fractions in diabetics and non-diabetic controls in our setting. The mean sdLDL-C concentration among the controls in this study compares closely with the findings in a healthy adult population in Japan, where the cut-off for increased sdLDL-C was determined to be >0.9 mmol/l and supported by results from the FOS [28]. Although it may not be wise to apply this cut-off to our subject, the mean value of sdLDL-C among our control subjects was determined to be 0.8 ± 0.54 mmol/L. This may not represent the true value in our population due to the apparently small sample size in this study. Future studies involving larger sample sizes are needed to determine this cut off in our populations. Since it has been established that dyslipidaemia, especially involving increase in sdLDL-C is the basis of atherosclerosis and intima-media thickening of blood vessels [29, 30], we suggest that the dyslipidaemia demonstrated in our study subjects probably contributed to the establishment or maintenance of hypertension in the 75% of diabetes subjects found to be hypertensive. This is much higher than an earlier reported incidence of hypertension among diabetes patients who are Nigerians [31] and indicates that the problem may be increasing. It can also be expected that other unmeasured indices of atherogenesis are likely to worsen in these subjects as long as the blood levels of sdLDL-C and TG remain elevated. Small, dense LDL has been shown to be a marker for atherosclerosis owing to its susceptibility to oxidation and ability to binds more readily to arterial wall proteoglycans. Moreover, it has been shown to be an independent predictor of coronary artery disease in healthy men [19].

Patients with AMI have been observed to show a reduction of LDL size quite early in the course of the event. This abnormality appears to precede all other plasma lipoprotein modifications and is persistent throughout the period of admission [32]. In this study, the level of sdLDL was significantly higher among diabetes subjects than controls. This may have been partly responsible for the few (0.05%) reported cases of transient ischemic attack and stroke among our diabetes subjects. There was no reported case of AMI among our study participants. One reason for the low CVD episodes may be the presence of high HDL-C observed among participants of this study, as explained earlier. The second possible explanation is the diet composition and frequent engagement of our study subjects in some moderate physical activities. However, our findings were in harmony with other researchers who reported a very low incidence of AMI (0.2% of annual adult admissions and 0.04% of all adult admissions) over a 10 year period in Benin, Southern Nigeria [33]. A prevalence of 0.9% for ishaemic heart disease (IHD) and 0.004% for AMI of all medical admissions under a 5 year period was reported in Kano, Northern Nigeria [25]. However, a gradual

increase in the number of people presenting with AMI in the University of Benin Teaching Hospital (UBTH) during the study period was also demonstrated [33]. With the recent increase in reported cases of sudden unexplained deaths among Nigerians, there is reason to believe that the present prevalence of CVD will be much higher today. Moreover, the prevalence of sdLDL among healthy non-diabetics in a small Mediterranean Island was determined to be 30 – 35% of total LDL-C in adult men. [34] This study reported 32% of LDL-C as sdLDL-C among non-diabetic men which is almost the same as the Mediterranean study. Among diabetes patients, a slightly higher prevalence of 50% was reported [34] which is higher than the 45% noted in this study.

Improving glycaemic control has been shown to have a favourable effect on lipid and lipoprotein concentrations in type 2 diabetes [35, 36]. However, other researchers have demonstrated that DM subjects with good glycaemic control continued to exhibit a predominance of small, dense LDL particles [37]. This may be due to the presence of hyperinsulinaemia either from insulin resistance or the use of oral hypoglycaemic agents [38]. In this study, diabetes patients were regular clinic attenders and were in good glycaemic control—one criterion considered during patient selection. Since the study was carried out using a one-off measurement of the lipid profile rather than serial measurements, it was not considered necessary to confirm long-term glycaemic control with HbA1c. However, HbA1c measurements would have strengthened our clinical judgment. This is a limitation of this study. Nevertheless, this study has demonstrated that dyslipidaemia is an issue among diabetes patients in our environment. We suggest that early initiation of lipid lowering medications may go a long way to delay or even prevent the development of hypertension and other effects of dyslipidaemia common among type 2 diabetes patients.

Conclusion

The classical atherogenic lipoprotein phenotype was not demonstrated among subjects with type 2 diabetes mellitus in this study. This may explain to some extent the low incidence of CVD among our diabetes patients. However, dyslipidaemia characterised by an elevation of small, dense LDL-C and triglyceride is a big issue among diabetes patient in our environment and is increasing. If the elevation of small dense low density lipoprotein cholesterol is truly the antecedent of the full blown atherogenic lipoprotein phenotype, it is reasonable to suggest that lipid-lowering medication should be helpful in the management of these patients. A clinical trial of early use of lipid-lowering medication on the basis of elevation of small dense low density lipoprotein cholesterol in diabetes subjects would probably be necessary to support our speculation.

Abbreviations

ALP: Atherogenic lipoprotein phenotype; AMI: Acute myocardial infarction; ANOVA: Analysis of variance; APIN: AIDS Prevention in Nigeria; Apo B: Apolipoprotein B; BMI: Body Mass Index; CAD: Coronary artery disease; CHD: Coronary heart disease; CI: Confidence interval; CVD: Cardiovascular disease; DM: Diabetes mellitus; FOS: Framingham offspring study; HDL-C: High density lipoprotein cholesterol; IHD: Ischemic heart disease; JUTH: Jos University Teaching Hospital; lbLDL-C: Large buoyant low density lipoprotein cholesterol; LDL-C: Low density lipoprotein cholesterol; MOPD: Medical out-patient department; NCEP ATP III: National Cholesterol Education Program-Adult Treatment Panel III; SD: Standard deviation; sdLDL-C: small, dense low density lipoprotein cholesterol; TC: Total cholesterol; TG: Triglyceride; TIA: Transient ischemic attack; UBTH: University of Benin Teaching Hospital; VLDL-C: Very low density lipoprotein cholesterol

Acknowledgements

We are especially grateful to Mr. Matt Hodgkinson of AuthorAID for editing the manuscript for publication. Many thanks to AuthorAID for providing the platform that linked us to their experienced mentors. We also thank Professor E E Ekanem who assisted with some of the data analysis. We owe our gratitude to Dr. Lucy Inaku and Dr. Okokon Ita for assisting with collection of data.

Funding

No funds were received for this research from any donor by any of the authors.

Authors' contributions

OOO, KOI, FMA conceived and designed the experiments. KOI, LCI, NOA, AOA performed the experiments. KOI, OOO, LCI analyzed the data. Selection/recruitment of participants was done by EKC, KOI while KOI, OOO, FMA, EKC and COI wrote the paper. All authors read and approved the final manuscript.

Competing interests

The authors declare that they have no competing interests.

Author details

[1]Department of Chemical Pathology, Faculty of Medicine, College of Medical Sciences, University of Calabar, Calabar, Cross River State, Nigeria. [2]Department of Chemical Pathology, Faculty of Medical Sciences, University of Jos, Jos, Plateau State, Nigeria. [3]Department of Chemical Pathology, Faculty of Medicine, University of Ibadan, Ibadan, Oyo State, Nigeria. [4]Department of Internal Medicine, Faculty of Medical Sciences, University of Jos, Jos, Plateau State, Nigeria. [5]Department of Chemical Pathology, University of Jos Teaching Hospital, Jos, Plateau State, Nigeria.

References

1. Hobbs FD. Reducing cardiovascular risk in diabstes: beyond glycaemic and blood glucose control. Internatonal. J Cardiol. 2006;110:137–45.
2. IDF Diabetes Atlas. 7th Edition. Brussels, Belgium: International Diabetes Federation; 2015. https://www.idf.org/e-library/.../diabetes atlas/13-diabetes-atlas-seventh-edition.html. Accessed 16 Feb 2017.
3. Golberg RB. Hyperlipidemia and cardiovascular risk factors in patients with type 2 diabetes. Am J Manag Care. 2000;6(13Suppl):S682–91.
4. Syvanne M, Taskinem M. Lipids and lipoproteins as coronary risk factors in NIDDM. Lancet. 1997;350(Suppl 1):20–3.
5. American Diabetes Association. Management of Dyslipidemia in adults with diabetes. Diabetes Care. 2003;26(Suppl1):S83–6.
6. Austine MA, King MC, Vranizan KM, Krauss RM. Atherogenic lipoprotein phenotype. A proposed genetic marker for coronary heart disease risk. Circulation. 1990;82(2)495 506.
7. Wagner AM, Perez A, Calvo F, Apolipoprotein B. Identifies dyslipidaemic phenotypes associated with cardiovascular risk in normocholesterolaemic type 2 diabetic patients. Diabetes Care. 1999;22:812–7.
8. American Diabetes Association. Standards of medical care in diabetes — 2017. Diabetes Care. 2017;40(Suppl. 1):S75–87.
9. Oguejiofor OC, Onwukkwe CH, Odenigbo CU. Dyslipidaemia in Nigeria: Prevalence and pattern. Ann Afr Med. 2014;11(4):197–202.
10. Friedwald WT, Levy RI, Fredrickson DS. Estimation of the Concentration of Low-density Lipoprotein Cholesterol in Plasma, without Use of the Preparative Ultracentrifuge. Clinical Chemistry. 1972;18(6):499–502.
11. Hirano T, Ito Y, Saegusa H, Yoshino G. A novel and simple method for quantification of small, dense LDL. J Lipd Res. 2003;44:2193–201.
12. Dean AG, Arner TG, Sunki GG, Friedman R, Lantiga M, Sagman S, Zubieta JC et al. Epi info, a database and statis. CDC, Atlanta, GA, USA. 2011;
13. Ogbera AO, Fasamade OA, Chinyere SAA. Characterization of lipid parameters in diabetes mellitus-a Nigerian report. Int Arch Med. 2009;2:19.
14. Okafor CI, Fasimade OA, Oke DA. Pattern of dyslipidaemia among Nigerians with type 2 diabetes mellitus. Nig J Clin Pr. 2008;11:25–31.
15. AbdulAzeez IM, Okesina AB, Adebisi SA, Adunmo GO, AbdulAzeez IF, et al. Correlation between glycaemic control and lipid profile in Nigerian type II diabetic patients. Ann Trop Pathol. 2015;6:67–73.
16. American Medical Associaton. Executive summary of the third report (NCEP) expert panel on detection, evaluation, and treatment of high blood cholesterol in adults (adult treatment panel III). JAMA. 2015;285(19):2486–97.
17. Kesteloot H, Oviasu VO, Obasohan AO, Olomu A, Cobbaert CLW. Serum lipid and apoprotein levels in a Nigerian population sample. Atherosclerosis. 1989;78:33–8.
18. Ma Y, Chiruboga DE, Olendzki BC, Li W, Leung K, Hafner AR, et al. Association between carbohydrate intake and serum lipids. J Am Coll Nutr. 2006;25(2):115–63.
19. Ochene IS, Chiriboga DE, Stanek EJI, Harmatz MG, Nicolosi R, Seperia G, et al. Seasonal variation in serum cholesterol: treatment implications and possible mechanisms. Arch Intern Med. 2004;164:863–70.
20. Taskinen MR. Diabetic dyslipidaemia. Atheroscler Suppl. 2002;3(1):47–51.
21. Hafner SM. Lipoprtein disorders associated with type 2 diabetes mellitus and insulin resistance. Am J if Cardiol. 2002;90(Supplement): 55i–61i.
22. Yoshino G, Hirano T, Kazumi T. Atherogenic lipoproteins and diabetes mellitus. J Diabetes Complicat. 2002;16:29–34.
23. Stanford WL, Onyemelukwe GC. Serum lipids in Nigerians: the effect of diabetes mellitus. Trop Geogr Med. 1981;33:323–8.
24. Falase AO, Oladipo OO, Kanu EO. Relatively low incidence of myocardial infarction in Nigerians. Cardiol Trop. 2001;27:10745–7.
25. Sani MU, Adamu B, Mijinjawu MS, Abdu A, Karaye KM, Maiyaki MB, et al. Ischaemic heart disease in Aminu Kano teaching hospital, Kano, Nigeria: a 5 year review. J Med. 2006;15(2):128–31.
26. Castelli WP. Cholesterol and lipids in the risk of coronary heart disease-the Framingham heart study. Can J Cardiol. 1998;4(supplement A):5A–10A.
27. Hirano T, Ito Y, Koba S, Toyoda M, Ikejiri A, Saegusa H, et al. Clinical significance of small dense low density lipoprotein cholesterol levels determined by the simple precipitation method. Arterioscler Throm Vasc Biol. 2004;24(3):558–563.
28. Masumi AI, Otokozawa S, Aszatalos BF, Ito Y, Nakajima K, White C, et al. Small dense LDL cholesterol and coronary heart disease: results from the Framingham offspring study. Clin Chem. 2010;56:6.
29. Skoglund-Andersson C, Tang R, Bond MG, de Faire U, Hamstein A, Karpe FLDL. Particle size distribution is associated with carotid intima-thickness in healthy 50 year-old men. Atheroscler Throm Vasc Biol. 1999;19:2422–30.
30. Berneis K, Jeanneret C, Muser AR. Low-density lipoprotein size and subclasses are markers of clinically apparent and non-apparent atherosclerosis in type 2 diabetes. Metab Clin Exp. 2005;54(2):227–34.
31. Okeshina AB, Omotobo ABO, Gadzama AA, Ogunrimola EO. Frequency of hypertension in diabetes patients: relationship with metabolic control, body mass index, age and sex. Int Diab Dig. 1996;7:39–40.
32. Rizzo M, Berneis K. Should we measure the LDL peak size? Int J Cardiol. 2006;107:166–70.
33. Joseph VA. Frequency and pattern of acute myocardial infarction in the university of Benin teaching hospital, Nigeria. Niger Med Pract. 2009;55(6): 97–100.

34. Rizzo M, Barbagallo CM, Serverino M. Low density lipoprotein particle size in a population living in a small Mediterranean Island. Eur J Clin Investig. 2003; 33:126–33.

35. Kannel WB, McGee DL. Diabetes and Glucose Tolerance as Risk Factors for Cardiovascular Disease: The Framingham Study. Diabetes Care. 1979;2(2): 120-126.

36. Wagner AM, Oscar J, Rilga M, Bonet R, de Leiva A, et al. Effect of Improving glycaemic control on LDL particle size in type 2 diabetes, Metabolism. 2003; 52(12):1576-1578.

37. Tan C, Chew LS, Chio LF, Tai ES, Lim HS, Lim SC, et al. Cardiovascular risk factors and LDL subfraction profile in type 2 diabetes mellitus with good glycaemic control. Diabetes Res abd Clin Pract. 2001;51:107–14.

38. Brownlee M. The pathobiology of diabetic complications. Diabetes. 2005;54: 1615–25.

19

Peritumoral lymphatic vessel density and invasion detected with immunohistochemical marker D240 is strongly associated with distant metastasis in breast carcinoma

Nur Fatiha Norhisham, Choi Yen Chong and Sabreena Safuan*iD

Abstract

Background: Detection of vascular invasion by hematoxylin and eosin staining is the current pathological assessment practice to diagnose breast carcinoma. However, conventional hematoxylin and eosin staining failed to distinguish between blood vessel invasion and lymphatic vessel invasion. Both are important prognostic criteria however with different outcomes. The aim of this study is to distinguish between blood vessel invasion and lymphatic vessel invasion using conventional assessment and immunohistochemical markers. The prognostic significance of both circulatory invasions in invasive breast carcinoma was also investigated.

Methods: Consecutive sections of breast carcinoma samples from 58 patients were stained with CD34 and D240 to stain blood and lymphatic vessels respectively. Hematoxylin and eosin staining was carried out on another consecutive section as conventional staining.

Results: Although blood vessel density is higher in the sections (median = 10.3 vessels) compared to lymphatic vessel density (median = 0.13), vessel invasion is predominantly lymphatic invasion (69.8 and 55.2% respectively). Interestingly, peritumoral lymphatic vessel density and peritumoral lymphatic invasion was significantly associated with distant metastasis ($p = 0.049$ and $p = 0.05$ respectively). The rate of false positive and false negative interpretation by hematoxylin and eosin was 46.7 and 53.3% respectively.

Conclusions: Lymphatic vessel invasion is a strong prognostic markers of breast carcinoma invasion and the use of immunohistochemical markers increase the rate and accuracy of detection.

Keywords: Lymphatic invasion, D2-40, CD34, Breast carcinoma

Background

Breast carcinoma is one of the leading cancer worldwide with more than 190,000 new cases reported each year in the US [1]. From this figure, the estimated deaths is about 21%. The prognosis of breast cancer is based on the age and menopausal status of the patients, tumor size, histological types and grade, hormone and growth factor receptors and vascular invasion [2].

Currently, vascular invasion is detected microscopically as the presence of tumor cells within the blood or lymphatic vessels using haematoxylin and eosin (H&E) staining [2]. Patients with positive vascular invasion often has poorer prognosis than those with negative invasion. The presence of vascular invasion was also associated with axillary lymph node involvement, systemic relapse and local recurrence [3, 4]. However, conventional assessment of vascular invasion by H&E stained slides was reported to have high rate of false interpretation. Retraction artefacts of the tissue sections tend to be reported as positive invasion while packed tumor cells in a vessel may be

---
* Correspondence: sabreena@usm.my
School of Health Sciences, Universiti Sains Malaysia, 16150 Kubang Kerian, Kelantan, Malaysia

missed, leading to false positive and false negative observation of the tissue respectively. There was a low level of concordence (kappa = 0.3) between two observers in reporting vascular invasion of H&E stained tissue section [5]. In addition, H&E staining failed to distinguish between lymphatic vessel invasion and blood vessel invasion in patients' samples.

D240 is a monoclonal antibody that bind to an O-linked sialoglycoprotein on lymphatic endothelial cells but not on blood endothelial cells. Therefore, D240 antibody has been used as reliable marker to evaluate lymphatic invasion in many research settings [6, 7]. The commercially available D240 antibody binds to a fixation resistant epitope on podoplanin molecules, an integral transmembrane glycoprotein. Ultrastructural analysis revealed the predominat localisation to the luminal surface of lymphatic vessels. CD34 is a common endothelial marker used to detect the presence of blood vessels. This antibody detects a 110 kDa transmembrane glycoprotein expressed on endothelial cells, embryonic fibroblasts and some nervous tissues [8].

The aim of this study is to compare the incidence of lymphatic vessel invasion and blood vessel invasion in breast carcinoma cohort between conventional H&E staining and immunohistochemical staining. The significance of using immunohistochemical markers in relation to adverse clinicopathological criteria is also evaluated.

Methods

Patients and specimens

This study was conducted on 58 consecutive formalin fixed paraffin embedded (FFPE) archival specimens of breast carcinoma obtained from Universiti Sains Malaysia Hospital. Clinical characteristics of the patients and tumors are summarized in Table 1.

Immunohistochemistry

Two consecutive FFPE breast carcinoma sections from each patient were stained with CD34 and D240 to assess blood vessels and lymphatic vessels respectively. Staining optimization was conducted on breast sections before using them in the main cohort. 4 μm thick whole sections from each specimen were deparaffinized in two xylene baths for 5 min each and then rehydrated in a series of descending ethanol concentrations (100, 90, 70, 50 and 30% in water for 1 min at each concentration). Antigen retrieval was carried out in 0.01 mol/L-1 sodium citrate buffer (pH6) in a microwave for 20 min; 10 min at full power (750 W) followed by 10 min at low power (450 W). Endogenous hydrogen peroxidase activity was then blocked in 0.3% hydrogen peroxide in methanol for 10 min. Sections were incubated with the primary antibody diluted in antibody diluent (DAKO, Denmark) (1:100 for CD34 and D2-40) for 1 h at room

temperature. Unbound primary antibody was washed with TBS prior to the addition of HRP-labeled polymer for 30 min. Sections were then washed and immunohistochemical reactions were developed using 3, 3′ diaminobenzidine (Liquid DAB+ Substrate Chromogen System, DAKO, K3468) for 7 min.

Counterstained with haematoxylin was carried out for 3 min and rinsed off under running tap water. Sections were dehydrated in a series of ascending ethanol concentrations (30,50,70, 90 and 100% in water for 1 min at each concentration), fixed in xylene and mounted with DPX. Sections were left to dry overnight before viewing under the microscope. Tonsil sections were used as both positive and negative controls each time staining was conducted. The procedure as above was applied for positive controls. For negative controls, primary antibody was omitted.

Microscopic analysis

All microscopic analysis was carried out using light microscope (Olympus, Japan).

Assessment of microvessel density and lymphatic vessel density

Microvessel density was assessed by counting three hotspots with the highest number of vessels at 100× magnification. The mean value of the hotspots was used in the analysis. For lymphatic vessel density, the positively stained D240 vessels were counted manually across the tissue section. This ensure the accuracy of result as lymphatic vessels are present in much lower density that blood vessel density. For vessel density, both the peritumoral and intratumoral area were counted. Intratumoral was defined as the area within the tumor while peritumoral was defined as the peripheral area at 1 microscopic field of view (×200) from the intratumoral area.

Assessment of vascular invasion

Figure 1 shows the examples of immunohistochemistry staining with D240 antibody. Lymphatic vessel invasion was identified as the presence of tumor cells within a D2-40 stained vessel. As CD34 can also stain a subset of lymphatic vessels, blood vessel invasion was defined when tumour cells were detected in CD34 positive but D240 negative vessels. The frequency of vascular invasion detected by H&E staining was compared with that detected by IHC. False positive cases were recorded when H&E sections were positive for vascular invasion but negative in IHC. False negatives were recorded when vascular invasion was negative in the H&E sections but positive in IHC. 20% of the specimens were randomly chosen and analysed by second scorer blinded to the results to measure concordance between observers.

Table 1 Clinicopathological characteristics of breast carcinoma patients and tumors

Clinical criteria	Frequency, n (%)	Clinical criteria	Frequency, n (%)
Age of diagnosis		Recurrence	
≤40	4 (6.9)	No	56 (96.6)
≥40	54 (93.1)	Yes	2 (3.4)
Ethnicity		Estrogen Receptor	
Malay	54 (93.1)	Positive	32 (55.2)
Chinese	4 (6.9)	Negative	26 (44.8)
Tumor Size (mm)		Progesteron Receptor	
<30	11 (19.0)	Positive	28 (48.3)
30 ≤ × < 60	27 (46.6)	Negative	30 (51.7)
>60	17 (29.3)		
No data	3 (5.1)		
Tumor Grading		Lymph nodes involvement	
Grade I	10 (17.2)	1	19 (32.8)
Grade II	27 (46.6)	2-4	6 (10.3)
Grade III	16 (27.6)	>4	16 (27.6)
Not determined	5 (8.6)	Not involved	17 (29.3)
Distant Metastasis		Lymphovascular Invasion (H&E)	
Yes	15 (25.9)	Positive	26 (44.8)
No	37 (63.8)	Negative	28 (48.3)
Not determined	6 (10.3)	Not determined	4 (6.9)
Mastectomy			
Full	10 (17.2)		
Partial	48 (82.8)		

Statistical analysis

Vessels density was classified into high and low category based on the median value. Vessel invasion was divided into negative and positive groups and used as a basis to determine association between all parameters. The relationship between vascular invasion, vessels density and clinical criteria were assessed using chi square test (Fisher exact if the cell count was less than 5). Multivariate analyses were carried out using binomial logistic regression and multiple regression analysis based on the type of variables. Some tumors were not scored because of missing tissue and lack of peritumoral area. P value of less than 0.05 determined significant relationship. Variations between observers were measured using kappa score. Statistical analysis was carried out using IBM SPSS Statistic 24.

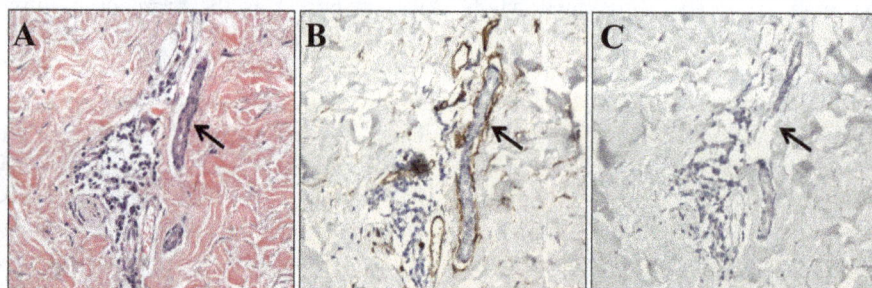

Fig. 1 Example of true positive lymphatic vessel invasion determined in D2-40 stained tissue. H&E stained tissue scored as positive lymphovascular invasion (**a**). At the same field of microscopic field view (200× magnification), lymphatic vessel invasion was clearly observed in D2-40 stained tissue (**b**). In CD34 stained tissue (**c**), blood vessel invasion was scored as negative

Results

Distribution of lymphatic and blood vessels

Microvessel density ranged from 5 to 26 vessels with a median of 10.3 vessels. Peritumoral lymphatic vessel density and intratumoral lymphatic vessel density showed a median of $0.052/mm^2$ and $0.078/mm^2$ respectively.

Frequency of lymphatic and blood vessels invasion

25.7% ($n = 15$) showed no vascular invasion on both intratumoral and peritumoral area. Of the 43 samples with vascular invasion, 69.8% ($n = 30$) showed lymphatic vessel invasion. Of the LVI positive specimens, 33.3% ($n = 10$), 26.7% ($n = 8$) and 40.0% ($n = 12$) were intratumoral invasion, peritumoral invasion and both intratumoral and peritumoral invasion respectively.

In comparison to IHC staining, only 55.2% ($n = 32$) showed invasion positive in H&E stained slides. When compared with all cases, 7 cases were false positive while 8 cases showed false negative results. Figure 1 shows the example of positive D2-40 staining which was scored as vascular invasion negative in H&E section. Figure 2 shows the determination of lymphatic vessel invasion positive which was scored as invasion positive in H&E staining. The kappa scores of invasion using immunohistochemical markers between observers were 0.87 and 0.88 for CD34 and D240 respectively. The kappa score of H&E staining between observers was 0.61.

Association of lymphatic and blood vessel density with clinical criteria

Table 2 shows the association of lymphatic vessel density with clinical criteria. Peritumoral and total lymphatic vessel density was significantly associated with age ($p = 0.020$ and 0.017 respectively) Total lymphatic vessel density was also associated with grade ($p = 0.018$). Interestingly, peritumoral lymphatic vessel density was significantly associated with distant metastasis ($p = 0.049$). Blood vessel density was not associated with all clinical criterias.

However, in multivariate analysis none of these variables retain their significant association (peritumoral lymphatic vessel density: age $p = 0.820$, distant metastasis $p = 0.291$ and total lymphatic vessel density: grade $p = 0.728$; age $p = 0.916$).

Association of lymphatic and blood vessel invasion with clinical criteria

Table 3 shows the association of lymphatic vessel invasion with clinical criteria. Peritumoral lymphatic invasion was significantly associated with age ($p = 0.012$) and distant metastasis ($p = 0.05$). Blood vessel invasion was not significantly associated with all clinical criterias. In multivariate analysis, only age retain the significant association with peritumoral lymphatic vessel invasion ($p = 0.001$).

Discussion

The aim of this study was to compare the incidence of lymphatic invasion and blood invasion in breast carcinoma cohort between conventional H&E staining and immunohistochemical staining. It also aimed to investigate the association of lymphatic/blood vessel density and invasion with adverse clinical criteria.

Previous studies showed that lymphatic invasion and blood vessel invasion cannot be distinguished when H&E staining was used in tissue biopsy [8, 9]. The presence of lymphatic and blood endothelial cells specific markers, D2-40 and CD34, respectively made the identification of these vessels possible. It is important to know which type of invasion occurs in individual patients, which has been shown in this study because blood and lymphatic vessel invasion have different prognostic outcomes. In addition, personalized therapy could be designed to cater the needs of every patients based on their invasion routes. Furthermore, this study demonstrated that the concordance score between observers with the usage of immunohistochemical markers is excellent compared to the lower score when reporting

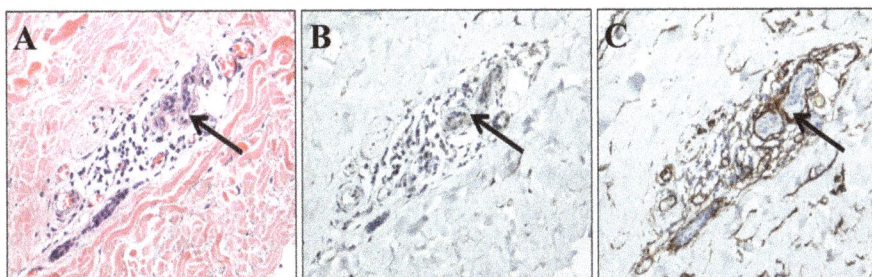

Fig. 2 H&E (**a**), D2-40 (**b**) and CD-34 (**c**) staining of consecutive tissue section. This sample was scored as lymphovascular invasion negative by H&E. However, CD34 staining (**c**) clearly showed the presence of tumor cells within CD34 stained vessel and was scored as blood vessel invasion positive. Lymphatic invasion was scored as negative (**b**). Noted that IHC was able to distinguih between lymphatic and blood vessel invasion. (200× magnification)

Table 2 Association of lymphatic vessel density with clinical criteria

		Total LVD			Intra-tumoral LVD			Peri-tumoural LVD		
		Low	High	p-value	Low	High	p-value	Low	High	p-value
Age	<40	0 (0.0)	4 (13.3)	**0.020**	2 (7.4)	2 (6.9)	0.941	0 (0.0)	4 (13.8)	**0.017**
	≥40	27 (100.0)	26 (86.7)		25 (92.6)	27 (93.1)		28 (100.0)	2 (86.2)	
Tumor size	<30	2 (7.7)	9 (31.0)	0.080	3 (11.1)	8 (28.6)	0.255	3 (11.1)	8 (28.6)	0.255
	30 ≤ x < 60	15 (57.7)	12 (41.4)		15 (55.6)	12 (42.9)		15 (55.6)	12 (42.9)	
	60 ≥	9 (34.6)	8 (27.6)		9 (33.3)	8 (28.6)		9 (33.3)	8 (28.6)	
Grade	I	2 (7.7)	8 (26.7)	**0.018**	1 (3.7)	9 (31.0)	**0.030**	13 (11.1)	7 (24.1)	0.079
	II	13 (50.0)	14 (46.7)		15 (55.6)	12 (41.4)		14 (51.9)	13 (44.8)	
	III	11 (42.3)	5 (16.7)		10 (37.0)	6 (20.7)		10 (37.0)	6 (20.7)	
	No grade	0	3 (10.0)		1 (3.7)	2 (6.9)		0	3 (10.3)	
Distant metastasis	Yes	7 (25.9)	8 (27.6)	0.989	8 (29.6)	7 (23.3)	0.065	7 (25.0)	8 (27.6)	**0.049**
	No	18 (66.7)	19 (65.5)		19 (70.4)	19 (63.3)		21 (75.0)	17 (58.6)	
	Not determine	2 (7.4)	2 (6.9)		0	4 (13.3)		0	4 (13.8)	
Recurrence	No	26 (96.3)	29 (96.7)	0.940	27 (100)	27 (93.1)	0.1	27 (96.4)	28 (96.6)	0.980
	Yes	1 (3.7)	1 (3.3)		0	2 (6.9)		1 (3.6)	1 (3.4)	
ER	Positive	16 (61.5)	16 (55.2)	0.632	16 (61.5)	15 (53.6)	0.554	17 (63.0)	15 (53.6)	0.480
	Negative	10 (38.5)	13 (44.8)		10 (38.5)	13 (46.4)		10 (37.0)	13 (46.4)	
PR	Positive	15 (55.6)	13 (44.8)	0.422	13 (48.1)	14 (50.0)	0.891	16 (57.1)	12 (42.9)	0.284
	Negative	12 (44.4)	16 (55.2)		14 (51.9)	14 (50.0)		12 (42.9)	16 (57.1)	
Lymph nodes involvement	0	8 (29.6)	11 (37.9)	0.374	8 (30.8)	11 (37.9)	0.678	7 (25.0)	12 (42.9)	0.266
	1	3 (11.1)	3 (10.3)		3 (11.5)	3 (10.3)		4 (14.3)	2 (7.1)	
	2 to 4	6 (22.2)	10 (34.5)		6 (23.1)	10 (31.0)		7 (25)	9 (32.1)	
	>4	10 (37.0)	5 (17.2)		9 (34.6)	6 (20.7)		10 (35.7)	5 (17.9)	

*Bold datas refer to statistically significant association (p<0.05)

vascular invasion of H&E stained tissue section [5]. These showed that immunohistochemical markers could be used in clinical setting with patients samples to minimized the rate of error.

In this study, it was shown that although the frequency of blood vessel density was higher compared to lymphatic vessel density, the incidence of lymphatic vessel invasion exceeded that of blood vessel invasion. Clearly, breast carcinoma preferentially used lymphatic vessels as a route of metastasis. Similar data were also reported by previous study showing that lymphatic vessel invasion incidences exceeded of that blood vessel invasions which were 35 and 16% respectively. Mohammed and colleagues also showed significant invasions of the lymphatics (97%) compared to the blood vessels (3%). These results and our results indicated clearly that breast carcinoma preferentially used lymphatic vessels as a route of metastasis. It was not known what drive tumor cells to invade lymphatic vessels when there are higher number of blood vessel in the tumoral area. One explanation is the anatomical structure of the lymphatic vessel itself which would not offer a significant barrier for the entry of tumor cells [10]. The lack of basement membrane and supporting structure in the lymphatic vasculature may ease the intravasation of tumor cells into the lymphatic circulation. In contrary, lymphatic endothelium might also play an active role in tumor cells recruitment. They may secrete chemokines that attracted the tumor cells to the lymphatic capillaries. Chemokines receptor-ligand relationships are important to regulate leukocytes trafficking and this relationship was hypothesized to be exploited by cancer cells to modulate entry into the lymphatic circulation [11, 12].

The presence of intratumoral lymphatic vessel invasion has been debatable as it was thought that lymphatic vessel could not penetrate the high pressure environment inside the tumor mass. With the discovery of new molecular markers and better imaging systems, the presence of intratumoral lymphatics has been reported [13]. In this study, we reported the presence of intratumoral lymphatic vessel invasion however no significant association was observed with any clinical criteria under study. Previous study has demonstrated the association between intratumoral lymphatic invasion with markers of aggressiveness [14] which was

Table 3 Association of lymphatic vessel invasion with clinical criteria

		Intra-tumoral LVI			Peri-tumoral LVI			Total LVI		
		Positive	Negative	p-value	Positive	Negative	p-value	Positive	Negative	p-value
Age	<40	2 (7.1)	2 (7.1)	1.0	4 (14.8)	0 (0)	**0.012**	4 (10.5)	0 (0)	0.065
	≥40	26 (92.9)	26 (92.9)		23 (85.2)	30 (100)		34 (89.5)	19 (100)	
Tumor size	<30	7 (25)	4 (14.8)	0.548	4 (14.8)	7 (25)	0.636	9 (23.7)	2 (11.8)	0.497
	30 ≤ × < 60	12 (42.9)	15 (55.6)		14 (51.9)	13 (46.4)		17 (44.7)	10 (58.8)	
	60 ≥	9 (32.1)	8 (29.6)		9 (33.3)	8 (28.6)		12 (31.6)	5 (29.4)	
Grade	I	3 (10.7)	7 (25.0)	0.387	5 (18.5)	5 (17.2)	0.197	5 (13.2)	5 (27.8)	0.607
	II	14 (50.0)	13 (46.4)		15 (55.6)	12 (41.4)		19 (50)	8 (44.4)	
	III	10 (35.7)	6 (21.4)		7 (25.9)	9 (31.0)		12 (31.6)	4 (22.2)	
	No grade	1 (3.33)	2 (7.1)		0	3 (10.3)		2 (5.3)	1 (5.6)	
Distant metastasis	Yes	9 (32.1)	6 (21.4)	0.432	7 (25.9)	8 (26.7)	**0.05**	11 (28.9)	4 (21.1)	0.607
	No	18 (64.3)	19 (67.9)		20 (74.1)	18 (60.0)		25 (65.8)	13 (68.4)	
	Not determine	1 (3.6)	3 (10.7)		0	4 (13.3)		2 (5.3)	2 (10.5)	
Recurrence	No	26 (92.9)	28 (100)	0.92	27 (100)	28 (93.3)	0.105	36 (94.7)	19 (100)	0.198
	Yes	2 (7.1)	0		0	2 (6.7)		2 (5.3)	0	
ER	Positive	16 (59.3)	15 (55.6)	0.632	15 (57.7)	17 (58.6)	0.944	21 (56.8)	11 (61.1)	0.738
	Negative	11 (40.7)	12 (44.4)		11 (42.3)	2 (41.4)		16 (43.2)	7 (38.9)	
PR	Positive	13 (46.4)	14 (51.9)	0.687	13 (48.1)	15 (51.7)	0.789	17 (44.7)	11 (61.1)	0.251
	Negative	15 (53.6)	13 (48.1)		14 (51.9)	14 (48.3)		21 (55.3)	7 (38.9)	
Lymph nodes involvement	0	10 (37.0)	9 (32.1)	0.983	7 (25.9)	12 (41.4)	0.088	13 (35.1)	6 (31.6)	0.763
	1	3 (11.1)	3 (10.7)		1 (3.7)	5 (17.2)		3 (8.1)	3 (15.8)	
	2 to 4	7 (25.9)	8 (28.6)		11 (40.7)	5 (17.2)		10 (27)	6 (31.6)	
	>4	7 (25.9)	8 (28.6)		8 (29.6)	7 (24.1)		11 (29.7)	4 (21.1)	

*Bold datas refer to statistically significant association (p<0.05)

not observed in this cohort perhaps due to the number of samples used.

The clear association observed between peritumoral lymphatic vessel density and invasion with distant metastasis indicates that peritumoral lymphatic vessels have important role in breast carcinoma metastasis to secondary organs. Distant metastasis is a major factor that lead to poor prognosis of cancer patients. Statistics shows that 90% of cancer-related death occurs as a result of metastasis [15]. The highly significant association between these two variables may indicate that targeted therapy directed to peritumoral density could be designed to reduce metastatic dissemination of cancer cells especially in breast carcinoma patients.

Conclusions

In conclusion, although blood vessel density in breast carcinoma patients is higher compared to lymphatic vessel density, vascular invasion in breast carcinoma is predominantly lymphatic vessel invasion. The fact that peritumoral lymphatic vessel invasion was strongly correlated with distant metastasis shows that it is a strong predictor of breast carcinoma outcome. This study should be repeated in larger cohort with relapse-free survival and overall survival data. We strongly reccommended that IHC markers be used alongside H&E staining to improve the detection rate and false interpretation of tissue samples.

Abbreviations
BVI: Blood vessel invasion; FFPE: Formalin fixed paraffin embedded; H&E: Hematoxylin and eosin; LVI: Lymphatic vessel invasion

Acknowledgements
The authors thank Faezahtul Arbaeyah Hussain for technical support.

Funding
This work was supported by Short Term Research Grant, Universiti Sains Malaysia (grant number: 304/PPSK/61312137).

Authors' contributions
NFN was involved in the acquisition and analysis of data and drafting manuscript. CCY collected the samples and performed staining. SS analysed the data, drafted and revised the manuscript. All authors read and approved the final manuscript.

Competing interests

The authors declare that they have no competing interests.

References

1. Jemal A, Siegel R, Ward E, Hao Y, Xu J, Murray T, Thun MJ. Cancer Statistics, 2008. CA: A Cancer Journal for Clinicians CA: Cancer J Clin. 2008;58:26.

2. Dobi A, et al. Breast cancer under 40 years of age: increasing number and worse prognosis. Pathol Oncol Res. 2011;17(2):425–8.

3. Storr SJ, et al. Objective assessment of blood and lymphatic vessel invasion and association with macrophage infiltration in cutaneous melanoma. Mod Pathol. 2011;25:493–504.

4. Longatto-Filho A, et al. Lymphatic vessel density and epithelial D2-40 immunoreactivity in pre-invasive and invasive lesions of the uterine cervix. 2007. p. 45–51.

5. Mohammed R, et al. Improved methods of detection of lymphovascular invasion demonstrate that it is the predominant method of vascular invasion in breast cancer and has important clinical consequences. Am J Surg Pathol. 2007;31:9.

6. Mohammed RAA, et al. Objective assessment of lymphatic and blood vascular invasion in lymph node-negative breast carcinoma: findings from a large case series with long-term follow-up. J Pathol. 2011;223(3):358–65.

7. Doeden K, et al. Lymphatic invasion in cutaneous melanoma is associated with sentinel lymph node metastasis. J Cutan Pathol. 2009;36(7):772–80.

8. Essner R. Sentinel lymph node biopsy and melanoma biology. 2006. p. 2320s–5s.

9. El-Gohary YM, et al. Prognostic significance of intratumoral and peritumoral lymphatic density and blood vessel density in invasive breast carcinomas. 2008. p. 578–86.

10. Witte M, et al. Structure function relationships in the lymphatic system and implications for cancer biology. Cancer Metastasis Rev. 2006;25(2):159–84.

11. Kawai Y, et al. Chemokine CCL2 facilitates ICAM-1-mediated interactions of cancer cells and lymphatic endothelial cells in sentinel lymph nodes. Cancer Sci. 2009;100(3):419–28.

12. Johnson LA, Jackson DG. Cell traffic and the lymphatic endothelium. Ann N Y Acad Sci. 2008;1131(1):119–33.

13. Ji RC, Eshita Y, Kato S. Investigation of intratumoural and peritumoural lymphatics expressed by podoplanin and LYVE-1 in the hybridoma-induced tumours. Int J Exp Pathol. 2007;88(4):257–70.

14. Straume O, Akslen LA. Lymphatic vessel density and prognosis in cutaneous melanoma. Br J Cancer. 2004;91(6):1224–5.

15. Parkin DM, et al. Fifty years of cancer incidence. Int J Cancer. 2010;127(12):2918–27.

20

Biochemical and histological alterations induced by the smoke of allethrin based mosquito coil on mice model

M. Abdulla Al-Mamun[1,2], M. Ataur Rahman[2], M. Habibur Rahman[2], K.M.F. Hoque[2], Z. Ferdousi[2], Mohammad Nurul Matin[2] and M. Abu Reza[2*]

Abstract

Background: Mosquito coil (MC) emits insecticide upon burning which provides limited protection against lethal mosquito borne diseases. However, apart from killing the insect, toxicities associated with the inhalation of these insecticides poses severe health hazards. However, the use of MC is increasing day by day in third world countries in particular but, yet to receive enough attention of both policy maker and general public. The current study was aimed to assess the MC smoke induced damage of pulmonary and hepatic tissues along with observing the alterations of several blood biochemical parameters in mice model.

Methods: A total of twenty four Swiss albino mice were allowed to inhale the smoke of allethrin based MC at different duration per day for 120 days. By the end of treatment period, blood sample was drawn from each mouse and blood biochemical parameters including alanine transaminase (ALT), aspartate transaminase (AST), blood urea nitrogen(BUN), serum total protein, cholesterol, low density lipoprotein (LDL) and triglyceride (TG) were analyzed. Intact lung and liver were collected for histological analysis using standard protocol.

Results: Biochemical study indicates elevated activity of two hepatic enzymes: ALT (89%), AST (85%), in comparison with the respective control. Increased level of some parameters of lipid profile including cholesterol (36%), LDL (48%) and triglyceride (30%) in smoke inhaled mice is the new finding of this study. On the contrary, the activity of serum total protein and BUN was decreased by 20% and 24%, respectively in inhaled mice. Pulmonary tissue of treated mice shows severe forms of emphysema and hyperplasia, especially in the peripheral region of lung, which is the hallmark of chronic obstructive pulmonary disease (COPD). Histological study of hepatic tissue shows apoptosis mediated damage of hepatocytes along with severe form of necrosis. Infiltration of Inflammatory cells was also observed in both of the organs.

Conclusion: Results from the present studies suggest that chronic exposure of allethrin based MC is responsible factor for severe health complications such as COPD due to the alterations of the key biochemical parameters of blood and histo-organization of lung and liver.

Keywords: Allethrin, Apoptosis, Histology, Liver, Lung, Mice and mosquito coil

---

* Correspondence: rezaru@gmail.com; reza.gen@ru.ac.bd
[2]Protein Science Lab, Department of Genetic Engineering and Biotechnology, University of Rajshahi, Rajshahi 6205, Bangladesh
Full list of author information is available at the end of the article

Background

Mosquito coil is the slow-burning structure made mainly of insecticides along with inert materials such as wood floor, coconut shell powder, starch etc. Upon burning, MC emits smokes, containing single or multiple insecticides, which creates a defending environment and protects the subject from several mosquito borne lethal diseases including malaria, filaria and dengue. Pyrethroids and Pyrethrins are the main active ingredients of MC. Among the several types of pyrethroid, allethrin especially d-transallethrin (belong to the type I pyrethroids) is being used in almost all brands of mosquito coil in South Asian territory. Allethrin is a type of neurotoxin, acting both on the peripheral and central nervous systems by modifying the kinetics of voltage-sensitive sodium channel, resulting in increasing of sodium permeability across the channel and paralysis of insect's organs [1]. On the other hand pyrethroids have well been reported to induce oxidative stress and alter antioxidant level in different organ systems of rodent animal [2, 3].

MC smoke is considered as a potent air pollutant in indoor environment. One MC, upon burning, produces such amount of particulate matter equivalent to that of 75–137 cigarettes [4]. Along with insecticides, MC smoke also contains sub-micrometer particles, volatile, semi-volatile organic compounds and gaseous pollutants such as polyaromatic hydrocarbons [5, 6]. After using the MC in a room, it was observed that the maximum concentration of allethrin (0.0120 ppm) prevails till 30–35 min followed by a gradual decline in 6 h [7]. During overnight burning, subjects at close proximity are exposed to sub-micrometer particles, metal fumes, free radicals and vapors from smoke which ultimately reaches the alveolar region of lung and leading to irritation of the upper respiratory tract [6]. Chronic inhalation of MC smoke has been reported to correlate with asthma and persistent wheeze in human [8] along with focal declination and metaplasia in tracheal epithelium in rodents [5, 9]. Prolong exposure and subsequent entry of allethrin along with other MC derived particulate matters into red blood cells lead to the alteration of blood biochemical parameters including hemoglobin percentages [10, 11]. Exposure of pyrethrin based MC smoke has also been reported to considerable increase in white blood cell (WBC), especially basophil and lymphocyte in rat [12]. This noxious synthetic chemical is proven to be responsible for cellular, tissue and organs injury due to exerting its action on the membrane phospholipids, resulting membrane fluidity and tissue damage [11, 13].

The toxic smoke, emitted from MC is also reported to be responsible for inducing chromosomal aberrations in pulmonary alveolar macrophages and bone marrow [14, 15]. Recently, Madhubabu et al., (2012) have shown that MC smoke induces elevated level of reactive oxygen species (ROS) as well as over-expression of stress responsive gene, p53 [16]. Oxidative stress (DNA damage mediated) induced up-regulation of p53 is considered as the critical and early event of mitochondria mediated apoptosis [17]. Therefore, it could be postulated that MC smoke would induce apoptotic mediated tissue damage in subject with prolong exposure.

Subtropical climate, Poor drainage system and dense population are triggering the mosquito pressure day by day in tropical region including Bangladesh. As a cheap and instant remedy, middle and lower income groups are regularly using MC. Thus, a huge number of people are undesirably exposing to toxic fine particles and free radicals present in the smoke of MC and are subjecting themselves to various health complications regularly [18]. Therefore, this study was aimed to analyze the patterns of damages in the histo-architecture of lung and liver tissues as well as the alteration of biochemical parameters of blood in mice model inhaled with the mosquito coil smoke.

Methods
Chemical and reagents
Picric acid, Ethanol, glacial acetic acid and diethyl-ether (Sigma, USA); ALT, AST and BUN kit (Human, Germany), total protein reaction reagents (Spinreact, Spain), Cholesterol, triglycerides, LDL cholesterol kit (SIEMENS Laboratories Ltd., UK) and all other chemicals used in the experiments were of international standard.

Experimental animal, ethics statement, mosquito coil and inhalation treatment
A total of thirty female Swiss albino mice (25-30 g) were purchased from the department of Pharmacy, Jahangirnagar University, Dhaka, Bangladesh. The animals were kept in the animal house of the department of Biochemistry and Molecular Biology, University of Rajshahi, Bangladesh for acclimatization in the experimental environment.

The protocols used to carry out the current study along with handling and caring of experimental animals were reviewed, assessed and approved by the Institutional Animal, Medical Ethics, Biosafety and Biosecurity Committee (IAMEBBC) for Experimentations on Animal, Human, Microbes and Living Natural Sources (license no: 225/320-IAMEBBC/IBSc), Institute of Biological Sciences, University of Rajshahi, Bangladesh.

Mosquito coil, used in this study was purchased from local super market of Rajshahi by the trade name of Mortein power booster coil from Reckitt Benckiser, Bangladesh Ltd. The active ingredient of this brand was 0.12% w/w d-transallethrin and rest of the composition (99.88% w/w) was inert materials.

Forty days old mice were randomly distributed into control and inhaled group: Control group (six mice) was allowed to receive normal air at separate chamber. The inhaled group was then divided again into four subgroups (each containing six mice): group-1, group-2, group-3 and group-4. Each of these groups was allowed to inhale the smoke of MC at the duration of ½, 1, 2 and 3 h/d, respectively for 120 days. Inhalation treatment was conducted in limited ventilated space, creating a closed door setting mimicking the flat house.

Biochemical study

Blood sample was drawn from caudal vena cava of each mouse by direct punching of syringe (3 mm) into the vain. Collected blood sample was kept for half an hour and then centrifuged at 5000 rpm for 10 min at 4 °C to separate serum as clear supernatant and stored at −20 °C for biochemical analysis.

The activity of ALT and AST was determined by colorimetric method, described previously by Reitman and Frankel [19]. BUN level was estimated by enzymatic colorimetric method [20]. Serum total protein was measured by Biuret method, originally described by Josephson et al. [21]. Total cholesterol was estimated by enzymatic-(hydrolysis and oxidation) colorimetric reaction (CHOD-PAP- method), described originally by Allain et al. [22]. Activity of TG and LDL were determined by enzymatic colorometric reaction (GPA-PAP-Method) [23, 24].

Histological study

Histological study was carried out using the protocol previously described by Carleton et al. [25]. In brief, at the ending of treatment period, animals from each group were anesthetized with diethyl-ether and sacrificed by cervical dislocation. Intact lung and liver tissues were surgically removed quickly and washed with 0.9% normal saline followed by fixing with Bouin's solution for overnight. Tissues were then washed thoroughly under running tap water and subsequently passed through gradually increasing concentrations of alcohol (from 70% to 100%) for

dehydration followed by embedding in paraffin. The paraffin blocks containing tissue were sectioned at 6 μm thickness by rotary microtome (SHIBUYA, optical Co LTD, Tokyo, Japan) and stained with hematoxiline and eosin solution. Finally, the slides were visualized under light microscope (optika, Italy) and photographs were taken by the camera attached to it.

Statistical analysis

Statistical analysis for the assessment of the alterations of biochemical parameters of blood comparing with the respective control (pair comparison) was performed using student's t-test method. Descriptive statistical analysis was performed to estimate mean and standard deviation. Additionally, "p for trend" test was carried out using regression method to evaluate the relationship between the effect and treatment doses as a continuous variable. Data was expressed as mean ± SD ($n = 6$). The significance was set at $P < 0.05$. All analysis was performed using 'STATA' software, version 12.

Results
Biochemical alterations of blood parameters

Toxicological effects of allethrin based MC on different biochemical parameters of blood are presented in Table 1. The blood profiles, representing liver function, show significant changes in smoke inhaled groups in comparison with their respective control. Data indicates that the activity of two key hepatic enzymes i.e. ALT and AST were increased significantly (at $P < 0.05$) by 89% and 85%, respectively in mice exposed to MC smoke for 3 h/d. On the other hand, with the same exposure, the activity of BUN and total protein was decreased by 24% and 20% respectively. Increased levels of cholesterol, LDL and triglyceride were observed in the treated mice, and the values in 3 h/day inhaled mice were higher by 36%, 48% and 30% than the control, respectively. Trends for p value indicates that when the treatments duration were increased, the activity of ALT, AST, cholesterol, LDL and triglyceride were increased as well as BUN and total protein concentration were decreased as a continuous

Table 1 Inhalation effects of the mosquito coil smoke on biochemical parameters of blood

Parameters	Control	Inhalation treatment				Trend for p value
		Group 1 (1/2 h)	Group 2 (1 h)	Group 3 (2 h)	Group 4 (3 h)	
ALT (U/L)	10.20 ± 1.32	11.03 ± 0.92	12.66 ± 2.44*	14.83 ± 2.86*	19.30 ± 2.00*	+0.001
AST (U/L)	41.10 ± 3.26	47.83 ± 4.18*	56.20 ± 4.10*	62.62 ± 5.8*	76. 96 ± 7.46*	+0.001
BUN (mg/dl)	9.66 ± 0.68	8.66 ± 0.75	8.46 ± 0.66	7.93 ± 0.41*	7.33 ± 0.51*	−0.001
Total protein (g/dl)	5.40 ± 0.32	5.13 ± 0.24	5.2 ± 0.23	4.8 ± 0.22*	4.32 ± 0.19*	−0.001
Cholesterol (mg/dl)	99.0 ± 4.68	105.3 ± 6.02	116.6 ± 4.93*	128.4 ± 9.45*	135.6 ± 8.11*	+0.001
LDL (mg/dl)	64.66 ± 3.51	69.43 ± 7.78	75.20 ± 5.0*	88.0 ± 6.88*	95.3 ± 8.16*	+0.001
Triglyceride(mg/dl)	86.8 ± 2.77	93.0 ± 5.36	96.66 ± 4.68*	100.3 ± 6.08*	112.58 ± 7.3*	+0.001

Data represent as averages ± SD ($n = 6$), significance was set at *$P < 0.05$ with respect to the control group variable. Taken together, the biochemical parameters were altered by the inhalation with the mosquito coil smoke in a dose-dependent manner.

Histological changes in pulmonary tissues

Pulmonary tissue of inhaled mice illustrates various degrees of histo-architectural changes in a doses dependent manner in comparison with that of control (Fig. 1). Transverse section of lung of control mice shows normal and compact organization with thin intra-alveolar septa and alveolar sacs (Fig. 1A). However, among of the smoke inhaled groups, mice, inhaled the MC smoke for 1/2 h/d show normal structure only with mild enlargement of air space (Fig. 1B). On the other hand, exposure of the smoke for 3 h/d results in mass infiltration of inflammatory cells (ICI) around the air way and in alveolar septa along with massive enlargement of air space (EAS Fig. 1E-F) by the disruption of

inters alveolar septa and bronchiolar epithelial wall (DBW in Fig. 1E). The ruptured alveoli further join with each other and form large air space especially in the peripheral region of lung (Fig. 1E and F). It implies that air ventilation through the bronchi and bronchiole in treated mice might be considerably reduced due to constricted bronchi (CB in Fig. 1C and F). Besides these, marked form of hyperplasia was also observed by thickening of bronchiolar epithelial wall (TBW) as well as alveolar septa (TAS) in animal inhaled the smoke for 2 h to 3 h/d (Fig. 1D-F). Higher duration inhalation also resulted in pulmonary edema (PE in Fig. 1C-F).

Histological changes in hepatic tissue

Toxicological effects of MC smoke on hepatic tissue in control and smoke inhaled mice are shown in Fig. 2. Microscopic observation of control liver shows regular and compact configuration with well-organized hepatocytes and

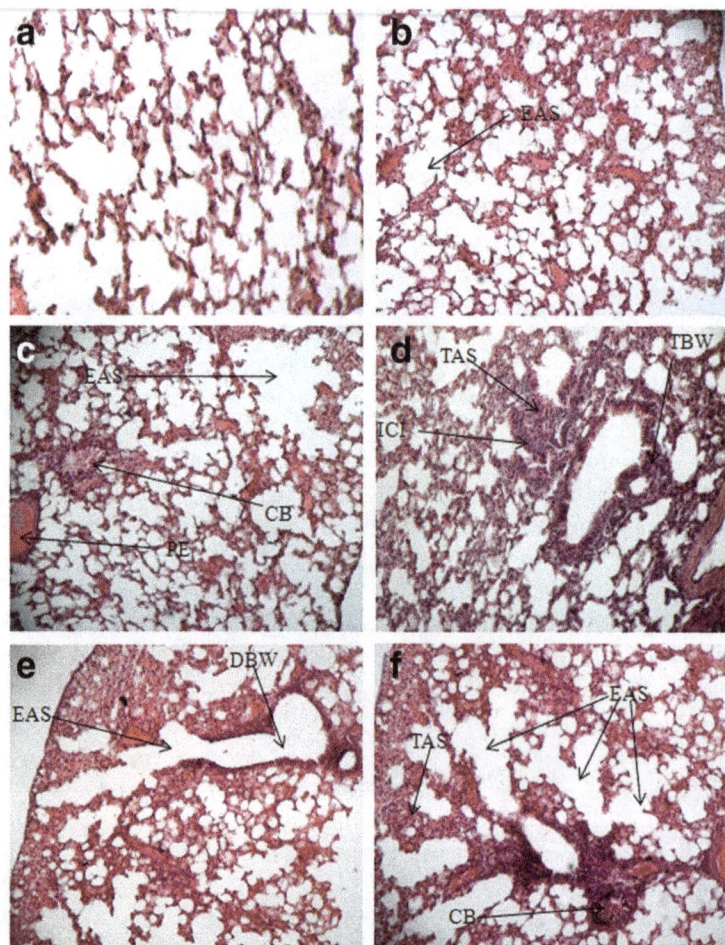

Fig. 1 Histological section of lung tissue of mice inhaled with the mosquito coil smoke in the duration for 120 d/d. (**a**) Control mice; (**b**) ½ h inhalation/d; (**c**) 1 h inhalation/d; (**d**) 2 h inhalation/d and (**e**) & (**f**) 3 h inhalation/d. EAS indicates enlargement of air space, ICI indicates inflammatory cellular infiltration, CB represents constricted bronchi, PE represents pulmonary edema, TAS indicates thickening of alveolar septa, TBW indicates thickening of bronchiolar epithelial wall and DBW indicates disruption of bronchiolar epithelial wall. Sections were stained with hematoxylin and eosin (Original magnification, X400)

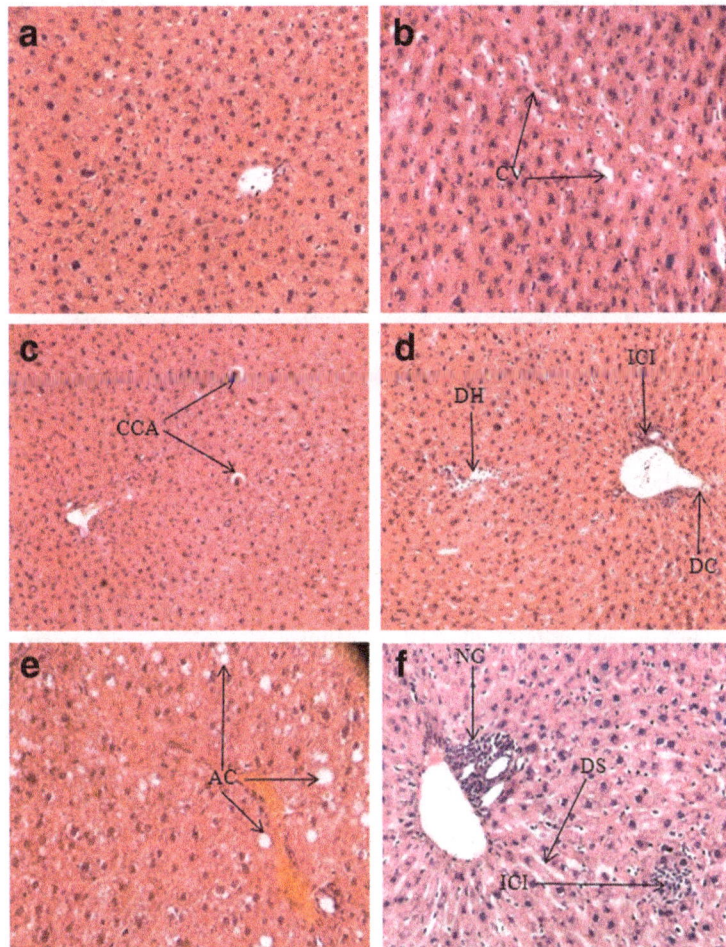

Fig. 2 Histological section of live tissue of mice inhaled with the mosquito coil smoke in the duration for 120 d/d. (**a**) Control mice; (**b**) ½ h inhalation/d; (**c**) 1 h inhalation/d; (**d**) 2 h inhalation/d and (**e**) & (**f**) 3 h inhalation/d. CV indicates cytoplasmic vacuolation, CCA indicates condensation of cytoplasm of ongoing apoptotic cell, DH represents degeneration hepatocytes, ICI represents inflammatory cellular infiltration, DC indicates dilation of central vein, AC indicates apoptotic cells, NC indicates necrosis and DS is for dilation of sinusoid. Sections were stained with hematoxylin and eosin (Original magnification, X400)

central vein (Fig. 2A). While, necrotic (NC) and apoptotic (AC) degeneration of hepatocytes along with infiltration of inflammatory cells (ICI) around the central vein and in the sinusoidal space were found in the liver of mice, exposed to the smoke of MC for 3 h and 2 h/day (fig. 2 D-F). Treated mice with higher duration of inhalation show degenerated hepatocytes (DH), dilation of central vein (DC) and dilation of sinusoid (DS) (Fig. 2D and F). Apoptotic characteristic such as condensation of cytoplasm (CCA) was observed in 1 h inhaled group (Fig. 2C). No significant histological changes but cytoplasmic vacuolation (CV) were found in mice exposed to smoke of MC for 1/2 h (Fig. 2B).

Discussion

MC contains pyrethrin based insecticide but still widely being used in the tropical and subtropical region including Bangladesh as a common approach to protect mosquito from entering into home. MC generally has higher acceptance over liquid vaporizer due to its lower cost and ease of use. Upon burning, MC releases over 60 organic compounds, fine and ultrafine particles and heavy metals [5]. The smoke is composed of two phases: gas and particle phase [26]. During overnight burning, the smoke of particle phase containing carbon particles, heavy metals, aldehydes ultimately reaches peripheral region of lung and leading to progressive cellular injury and destruction of mucus membrane [9].

The present study demonstrates that critical biochemical parameters of blood were altered significantly in MC smoke inhaled animals. The activity of transaminases (ALT and AST) was increased significantly (at $P < 0.05$) in smoke inhaled animals (Table 1). Elevated activity of these hepatic enzymes is strongly correlated with hepatic injury [11]. It is either due to the direct effects of allethrin on the membrane phospholipids of hepatocytes and/or indirect effects caused due to the by-products derived from pyrethroid metabolism. Allethrin is membrane active substance, which acts upon membrane phospholipids and increases membrane fluidity [13] and leading to leak out cellular enzymes in extracellular matrix eventually increasing transaminases activity in blood. Elevated transaminase level has also been reported previously by Karthikeyan et al., (2006) in mice, exposed to mosquito repellent mat vapor [27].

The exposure of MC smoke resulted dose dependent depletion of BUN and total protein activity in all inhaled animals. This finding is also supported by a number of observations which demonstrated that kidney functions were not negatively altered in MC smoke inhaled rat [5, 11]. Similarly, the MC smoke has previously been reported to reduce serum total protein activity both in rodent animal and human subject [27, 28]. Higher protein degradation with subsequent reduction of total protein activity of blood in smoke inhaled subject has also been confirmed by marked increase of plasma free amino acid levels [28].

The elevated activity of some parameters of lipid profile in smoke inhaled mice in current study (Table 1) is not accord with the findings conducted by Narendra et al.,(2008), which demonstrates decreased plasma CHOL and LDL activity in human subjects, who inhaled the smoke of allethrine based MC regularly for long period of time [28]. Elevated LDL activity is considered to be the risk factor for cardiac condition, because it transports cholesterol from the liver to peripheral tissues. However, it is the first study that documented the raised cholesterol level in rodent animal treated with allethin based MC smoke via inhalation.

The oxidative damage, induced by ROS is the hallmark of cellular stress which modulates a number of signaling pathways including carcinogenesis, apoptosis, necrosis and inflammatory pathway. Free radical and volatile organic compounds present in the smoke of MC is considered as the potent contributor of oxidative DNA damage and tissue injury. Under these stress conditions, the histological organization of pulmonary and hepatic tissues becomes affected which led to severe organ injury. Histological study of lung tissue demonstrates extensive destruction of the alveolar septa and bronchial epithelial wall resulting in loss of alveoli as well as capillary surface area. Thus, the current study shows the clear evidence of severe emphysema as a result of long time inhalation of allethrin based MC smoke (Fig. 1E-F). The key event of the development of emphysema is the imbalance between proteases and anti-proteases, which is well established [29]. The ROS, induced by MC smoke, interferes with the antioxidant defense system [16], which would triggers inflammatory response in damage sites [30]. Furthermore, over expression of p53 in MC induced animals [16] is also considered as the potent contributor of pulmonary and hepatic inflammation. Under stress

condition, p53 has been reported to activate pro-inflammatory cytokines at the site of stress induced pulmonary tissue in cigarette smoke inhaled rat [31]. However, the recruited inflammatory cells along with proteolytic enzymes act upon the anti-proteases (collagen and elastin) in alveolar region and inactivate them which in turn results in the destruction of alveolar septa and eventually develop emphysema [29]. Additional evidence has also confirmed the involvement of neutrophil in the degradation of elastin fibers with subsequent development of emphysema [32].

Emphysema in smoke inhaled animals is also accompanied by extensive thickening of alveolar septa and bronchial epithelial wall, which indicate hyperplasia (over tissue growth). Co-existence of emphysema and hyperplasia in pulmonary tissue was also observed in mice expressing TNF-α at elevated level [33]. Therefore, it can be postulated that current pulmonary injury would also due to the up-regulation of TNF-α in some extent. Because, elevated TNF-α level has been reported to deplete the total cellular glutathione (antioxidant enzyme) level in both in vitro and in vivo model [34, 35]. However, over tissue growth (TAS and TBW in Fig. 1D) in the current findings would also be due to extensive proliferation and deposition of two primary connective tissue components i,e. elastin and collagen in emphysematous areas [36]. Accumulation of inflammatory cells probably induces deposition of extracellular matrix in the sub epithelium region and contributes in thickening of bronchial epithelial wall [37]. The structure of epithelial lining of bronchi is converted from pseudo-stratified columnar ciliated epithelium into thickened constricted bronchi (CB in fig-1C and 1B), which might limit air passing through the bronchi to the peripheral region of lung- major clinical feature in patient with COPD [38]. The activation of fibroblasts by inflammatory cells and with subsequent thickening of bronchial epithelial wall and alveolar septa are considered as airway resistance and airway remodeling against ongoing destruction of alveolar septa [37].

The co-existence of necrotic and apoptotic mediated liver damage is the novel finding of this study (AC and NC in Fig. 2E-F). Necrotic characteristics were mainly found in higher duration inhaling groups (3 h and 2 h), probably due to allethrin induced toxicity on cell membranes. Necrotic cells death characteristically affects large fields of tissue (NC in figure- 2F) rather than a single cell and induce to release cytoplasmic contents into the surrounding cellular environment which leads to trigger inflammatory cells to be accumulated (NC in Fig. 2E-F).

Histological observation of hepatic tissue also reveals degeneration of hepatocytes in such a way, affecting single cell or small area of tissue without recruiting inflammatory cells: the critical feature of apoptotic cells (AC in Fig. 2E) [39]. Some hepatocytes of 1 h inhaled mice shows condensation of cytoplasm and chromatin- the key event of apoptosis mediated cell death (CCA in fig-2C). However, it is the first time study that we have observed apoptotic mediated cell death induced by the smoke of allethrin based MC. Oxidative DNA damage with subsequent up-regulation of p53 is the perquisite of mitochondria mediated apoptosis [40]. Several studies earlier reported that ROS induced DNA damage and up-regulation of p53 in MC smoke inhaled rat [15, 16]. Although, the mechanism and cellular features of apoptosis and necrosis are different, but both the phenomenon share a common a biochemical network described or "apoptosis-necrosis continuum" [41]. The interplay between apoptosis and necrosis may take place at the same time in the same tissue depending upon the types and degrees of death stimuli [42], which would also be supportive to the current dose dependent co-existence of apoptosis and necrosis in smoke inhaled tissues.

This study has some limitations relating to the conclusion of the results. Here, we stained the respiratory and hepatic tissue only with hematoxiline-eosin, though other staining technique such as DAPI staining could be done to observe apoptotic cells more precisely. In this study, we could not check the function of respiratory system such as X-ray analysis respiratory system due to lack of proper facilities. In spite of some confines, these findings would help to select proper medication for diseases induced by the mosquito coil smoke, and this study gives the proposal to modify the chemical structure of the insecticide for avoiding unexpected effects on human body.

Conclusion

In this study, we found the biochemical and histological effects of the mosquito coil smoke using mice model. Biochemically, inhalation of the mosquito coil smoke altered dose dependently in all of the blood parameters tested. In histological approach, the progressive destruction of lung tissue and sequential necrotic degeneration of liver tissue were newly characterized as toxicological phenomena of the mosquito coil smoke.

Abbreviations

ALT: Alanine transaminase; AST: Aspartate transaminase; BUN: Blood urea nitrogen; CHOL: Cholesterol; COPD: Chronic obstructive pulmonary diseases; DAPI: 4',6-diamidino-2-phenylindole; dl: deciliter; g: gram; HDL: High density lipoprotein; L: Liter; LDL: Low density lipoproteins; MC: Mosquito coil; ml: milliliter; NC: Necrosis; PARP: Poly (ADP ribose) polymerase; ROS: Reactive oxygen; rpm: rotation per minutes; species; TG: Triglycerides; TNF: Tumor necrosis factor; U: Unit

Acknowledgements
The authors are thankful to Md, Mizanur Rahman, Assistant professor, Department of Global Health Policy, The University of Tokyo, Bunkyo-ku, Tokyo, Japan, for assisting statistical analysis, Professor M. Khalid Hossain, Department of Biochemistry and Molecular Biology, University of Rajshah and Dr. Md. Salah Uddin, Assistant professor, Department of Genetic Engineering and Biotechnology, University of Rajshahi for technical and laboratory support.

Funding
This work was funded internally by the Department of Genetic Engineering and Biotechnology, University of Rajshahi, Bangladesh.

Authors' Contributions.
MAA: Conceived designed and conducted the study as well as wrote the first draft of the manuscript. AR*: Conceived, designed and supervise the study as well as revised the manuscript. NM: NM: Conceived and co-supervise the study as well as revised the manuscript. ZF: Provided statistical and methodological support as well as revised the manuscript. KMF: Provided statistical and methodological support. AR: Conducted the study. HR: Conducted the study. All authors have read and approved the final manuscript.

Competing interests
The authors have declared that they have no competing interests.

Author details
[1]Department of Biotechnology, The University of Tokyo, Bunkyo-ku, Tokyo, Japan. [2]Protein Science Lab, Department of Genetic Engineering and Biotechnology, University of Rajshahi, Rajshahi 6205, Bangladesh.

References
1. Soderlund DM, Bloomquist JR. Neurotoxic actions of pyrethroid insecticides. Annu Rev Entomol. 1989;34:77–96.
2. El-Demerdash FM. Oxidative stress and hepatotoxicity induced by synthetic pyrethroids-organophosphate insecticides mixture in rat. J Environ Sci Health C Environ Carcinog Ecotoxicol Rev. 2011;29:145–58.
3. Mossa AT, Refaie AA, Ramadan A, Bouajila J. Amelioration of Prallethrin-induced oxidative stress and hepatotoxicity in rat by the administration of Origanum majorana essential oil. Biomed Res Int. 2013:1–11.
4. Liu W, Zhang J, Hashim JH, Jalaludin J, Hashim Z, Goldstein BD. Mosquito coil emissions and health implications. Environ Health Perspect. 2003;111:1454–60.
5. Liu WK, Sun SE. Ultrastructural changes of tracheal epithelium and alveolar macrophages of rats exposed to mosquito-coil smoke. Toxicol Lett. 1988;41:145–57.
6. Chang JY, Lin JM. Aliphatic aldehydes and allethrin in mosquito coil smoke. Chemosphere. 1998;36:617–24.
7. Ramesh A, Vijayalakshmi A. Monitoring of allethrin, deltamethrin, esbiothrin, prallethrin and transfluthrin in air during the use of household mosquito repellents. J Environ Monit. 2001;3:191–3.
8. Fagbule D, Ekanem EE. Some environmental risk factors for childhood asthma: a case-control study. Ann Trop Paediatr. 1994;14:15–9.
9. Liu WK, Wong MH. Toxic effects of mosquito coil (a mosquito repellent) smoke on rats. Toxicol Lett. 1987;39:223–39.
10. Narendra M, Bhatracharyulu NC, Padmavathi P, Varadacharyulu NC. Prallethrin induced biochemical changes in erythrocyte membrane and red cell osmotic haemolysis in human volunteers. Chemosphere. 2007;67:1065–71.
11. Idowu ET, Aimufua OJ, Ejovwoke YO, Akinsanya B, Otunbanjo OA. Toxicological effects of prolonged and intense use of mosquito coil emission in rats and its implications on malaria control. Rev Biol Trop. 2013;61:1463–73.
12. Garba SH, Shehu MM, Adelaiye AB. Toxicological effects of inhaled mosquito coil smoke on the rat spleen: a haematological and histological study. J Med Sci. 2007;7:94–9.
13. Moya-Quiles MR, Munoz-Delgado E, Vidal CJ. Effect of the pyrethroid insecticide allethrin on membrane fluidity. Biochem Mol BiolInt. 1995;36:1299–308.
14. Das RK, Sahu K, Dash BC. Induction of chromosome aberrations and micronuclei in pulmonary alveolar macrophages of rats following inhalation of mosquito coil smoke. Mutat Res. 1994;320:285–92.
15. Moorthy MV, Murthy PB. Analysis of sister chromatid exchange, micronucleus and chromosomal aberration frequencies in rodents exposed to mosquito coil smoke by inhalation route. Toxicol Lett. 1994;70:357–62.
16. Madhubabu G, Yenugu S. Effect of continuous inhalation of allethrin-based mosquito coil smoke in the male reproductive tract of rats. InhalToxicol. 2012;24:143–52.

17. Vaseva AV, Moll UM. The mitochondrial p53 pathway. BiochimBiophysActa. 2009;1787:414–20.

18. Roshnee G, Cao GQ, Chen H. Hypersensitivity pneumonitis due to residential mosquito-coil smoke exposure. Chin Med J. 2011;24:1915–8.

19. Reitman Sand Frankel S. A colorimetric method for the determination of serum glutamic oxalacetic and glutamic pyruvic transaminases. Am J ClinPathol. 1957;28:56–63.

20. Fawcett JK, Scott JE. A rapid and precise method for the determination of urea. J ClinPathol. 1960;13:156–9.

21. Josephson B, Gyllensward C. The development of the protein fractions and of cholesterol concentration in the serum of normal infants and children. Scand J Clin Lab Invest. 1957;9:29–38.

22. Allain CC, Poon LS, Chan CS, Richmond W, Fu PC. Enzymatic determination of total serum cholesterol. ClinChem. 1974;20:470–5.

23. Bucolo G, David H. Quantitative determination of serum triglycerides by the use of enzymes. ClinChem. 1973;19:476–82.

24. Okada M, Matsui H, Ito Y, Fujiwara A, Inano K. Low-density lipoprotein cholesterol can be chemically measured: a new superior method. J Lab Clin Med. 1998;132:195–201.

25. Carleton HM, Drury RAB, Wallington EA. Carleton's histological technique. Ulster Med J. 1967;36:1.

26. Lalonde C, Demling R, Brain J, Blanchard J. Smoke inhalation injury in sheep is caused by the particle phase not the gas phase. J Appl Physiol. 1994;77:15–22.

27. Karthikeyan S, Gobianand K, Pradeep K, Mohan CV, Balasubramanian MP. Biochemical changes in serum, lung, heart and spleen tissues of mice exposed to sub-acute toxic inhalation of mosquito repellent mat vapour. J Environ Biol. 2006;27:355–8.

28. Narendra M, Kavitha G, HelahKiranmai A, Raghava Rao N, Varadacharyulu NC. Chronic exposure to pyrethroid-based allethrin and prallethrin mosquito repellents alters plasma biochemical profile. Chemosphere. 2008;73::360–4. 26.

29. Janoff A. Elastases and emphysema. Current assessment of the protease-antiprotease hypothesis. Am Rev Respir Dis. 1985;132:417–33.

30. Johar D, Roth JC, Bay GH, Walker JN, Kroczak TJ, Los M. Inflammatory response, reactive oxygen species, programmed (necrotic-like and apoptotic) cell death and cancer. RoczAkad Med Bialymst. 2004;49:31–9.

31. Tiwari N, Marudamuthu AS, Tsukasaki Y, Ikebe M, Fu J, Shetty S. p53 and PAI-1-mediated induction of C-X-C chemokines and CXCR2: importance in pulmonary inflammation due to cigarette smoke exposure. Am J Physiol Lung Cell Mol Physiol. 2016;00290

32. Shapiro SD. Elastolytic metalloproteinases produced by human mononuclear phagocytes. Potential roles in destructive lung disease. Am J Respir Crit Care Med. 1994;150:160–4.

33. Lundblad LK, Thompson-Figueroa J, Sullivan MJ, Poynter ME, Irvin CG, Leclair T, Bates JH. Tumor necrosis factor-alpha overexpression in lung disease: a single cause behind a complex phenotype. Am J Respir Crit Care Med. 2005;171:1363–70.

34. Glosli H, Tronstad KJ, Wergedal H, Müller F, Svardal A, Aukrust P, Berge RK, Prydz H. Human TNF-alpha in transgenic miceinduces differential changes in redox status and glutathione regulating enzymes. FASEB J. 2002;16:1450–2.

35. Ferro TJ, Hocking DC, Johnson A. Tumor necrosis factor-alpha alters pulmonary vasoreactivity via neutrophil-derived oxidants. Am J Phys. 1993;265:L462–71.

36. Setlakwe EL, Lemos KR, Lavoie-Lamoureux A, Duguay JD, Lavoie JP. Airway collagen and elastic fiber content correlates with lung function in equine heaves. Am J Physiol Lung Cell MolPhysiol. 2014;307:L252–60.

37. Knight D. Epithelium-fibroblast interactions in response to airway inflammation. Immunol Cell Biol. 2001;79:160–4.

38. Hogg JC, Timens W. The pathology of chronic obstructive pulmonary disease. Annu Rev Pathol. 2009;4:435–59.

39. Elmore S. Apoptosis: a review of programmed cell death. Toxicol Pathol. 2007;35:495–516.

40. Wang X. The expanding role of mitochondria in apoptosis. Genes Dev. 2001;15:2922–33.

41. Zeiss CJ. The apoptosis-necrosis continuum: insights from genetically altered mice. Vet Pathol. 2003;40:481–95.

42. Zong WX, Thompson CB. Necrotic death as a cell fate. Genes Dev. 2006;20:1–15.

21

De novo acute lymphoblastic leukemia-like disease of high grade B-cell lymphoma with *MYC* and *BCL2* and/or *BCL6* rearrangements

Akiko Uchida[1], Yasushi Isobe[1*] (iD), Yu Uemura[1], Yuji Nishio[1], Hirotaka Sakai[1], Masayuki Kato[1], Kaori Otsubo[2], Masahiro Hoshikawa[3], Masayuki Takagi[3] and Ikuo Miura[1]

Abstract

Background: B-cell lymphomas harboring the 8q24/*MYC* plus 18q21/*BCL2* translocations are now referred to as high grade B-cell lymphoma with *MYC* and *BCL2* and/or *BCL6* rearrangements (HGBL-MBR). Although HGBL-MBR is frequently found in cases with diffuse large B-cell lymphoma or Burkitt lymphoma-like B-cell lymphoma, acute lymphoblastic leukemia (ALL)-like disease of HGBL-MBR (AL-HGBL-MBR) has been reported incidentally.

Case presentation: A 69-year-old Japanese woman developed remittent fever and increasing systemic bone pain. The bone marrow examination revealed that more than 90% of nuclear cells were blastoid cells, which were positive for CD10, CD19, CD20, and surface IgMκ and negative for terminal deoxynucleotidyl transferase (TdT). Cytogenetic studies confirmed that the patient had de novo AL-HGBL-MBR with the extra copies of *MYC* and loss of chromosome 17p. She showed resistance to chemoimmunotherapy and died seven months after the diagnosis. The literature review identified further 47 de novo AL-HGBL-MBR cases within the last 32 years. The median age was 61 years (range, 27 – 86); the male/female ratio was 2.0. Thirty-eight cases (79%) presented a clinical picture of ALL at diagnosis; 14 (36%) of 39 available cases showed central nervous system involvement. Loss of 17p and translocations at 2p12–13, 3q27, 9p13 were frequently observed as additional cytogenetic abnormalities. Although the median survival of 46 available cases was only five months (range, 0.1–18), rituximab use significantly improved the survival of AL-HGBL-MBR (log-rank test, $P = 0.0294$).

Conclusion: Our patient and most reported de novo AL-HGBL-MBR cases showed resistance to conventional chemoimmunotherapy and disastrous consequences. AL-HGBL-MBL is a rare, but should be considered a distinct clinical condition in HGBL-MBR. Other therapeutic strategies, such as using inhibitors of MYC and BCL2, are needed to overcome the chemoresistance of AL-HGBL-MBR.

Keywords: High grade B-cell lymphoma with *MYC* and *BCL2* and/or *BCL6* rearrangements, Acute lymphoblastic leukemia-like disease, T(14;18)(q32;q21), *MYC*, *BCL2*

* Correspondence: yisobe@marianna-u.ac.jp
[1]Division of Hematology & Oncology, Department of Internal Medicine, St.
Marianna University School of Medicine, 2-16-1 Sugao, Miyamae-ku,
Kawasaki, Kanagawa 216-8511, Japan
Full list of author information is available at the end of the article

Background

Recurrent reciprocal chromosomal translocations have been observed in specific subtypes of B-cell lymphomas [1, 2]. Although the presence of t(8;14)(q24;q32) and t(14;18)(q32;q21) are hallmarks of Burkitt lymphoma (BL) and follicular lymphoma (FL), respectively, these translocations occur at different B-cell differentiation stages [1, 2]. The *IGH-BCL2* fusion resulting from t(14;18) is generated from the failure of VDJ recombination in the bone marrow (BM) at an early B-cell stage, whereas the *IGH-MYC* fusion resulting from t(8;14) almost always occurs as a consequence of the aberrant class-switch recombination in germinal centers (GCs) of lymphoid tissues [1–3].

B-cell lymphomas harboring concurrent translocations of 8q24/*MYC* mainly in combination with 18q21/*BCL2* are called "double-hit" lymphoma and now defined as "high grade B-cell lymphoma with *MYC* and *BCL2* and/ or *BCL6* rearrangements (HGBL-MBR)" according to the current World Health Organization classification (WHO) of lymphoid neoplasms [2, 4]. HGBL-MBR is frequently found in diffuse large B-cell lymphoma (DLBCL) and BL-like B-cell lymphoma cases, which show poor prognosis when treated with standard regimen, R-CHOP (rituximab plus cyclophosphamide, doxorubicin, vincristine, and prednisone), with a median survival of around 12 months [5–7]. Although the WHO classification defines HGBL-MBR as the terminal deoxynucleotidyl transferase (TdT)-negative mature B cell neoplasm in spite of the cell morphology [4], several cases with acute lymphoblastic leukemia (ALL)-like disease of HGBL-MBR (AL-HGBL-MBR) have been reported incidentally [8–33]. AL-HGBL-MBR is clinically characterized as the acute onset disease with the initial manifestation of BM infiltration by blastoid B cells but lacks obvious tumors, suggestive of primary lymphoma lesions. However, the characteristics have not been fully elucidated. We herein present an AL-HGBL-MBR case and conducted a literature review using PubMed to clarify the feature of this disease.

Case presentation

The condition of a 69-year-old Japanese woman was good until she developed remittent fever for one week. She had no previous history of lymphoma and presented to our institution with fever and increasing systemic bone pain. A physical examination showed no lymphadenopathy or hepatosplenomegaly. Laboratory tests showed a white blood cell count of 4.7×10^9/L, hemoglobin level of 119 g/L, platelet count of 104×10^9/L, and lactate dehydrogenase (LDH) level of 12,623 IU/L. A peripheral blood smear revealed leukoerythroblastosis with 7.5% blastoid cells. F-18-fluorodeoxyglucose (FDG) positron emission tomography (PET) detected the relatively strong accumulation of FDG in the liver, spleen, vertebrae, and bilateral clavicles, humeri, ilia, and femora (maximum standardized uptake value (SUVmax) 4.8~13.0) (Fig. 1a). A BM examination revealed that more than 90% of nuclear cells were medium-sized blastoid cells with fine chromatin (Fig. 1b). A flow cytometric analysis showed that the cells were positive for CD10, CD19, CD20, HLA-DR, and surface IgMκ, but were negative for CD3, CD5, CD13, CD33, CD34, and TdT. The patient was tentatively diagnosed with mature B-cell leukemia and admitted to our hospital. She received R-hyper CVAD/MA (rituximab plus cyclophosphamide, vincristine, doxorubicin, dexamethasone/methotrexate, and cytarabine). Although her serum LDH levels decreased to approximately 1000 IU/L after two courses of the intensive regimen, blastoid cells remained in the BM. Therefore, we changed the regimen to dose-adjusted EPOCH-R (rituximab plus etoposide, prednisolone, vincristine, cyclophosphamide, and doxorubicin). After two courses of dose-adjusted EPOCH-R, leukemic cells remained and lost the expression of CD20. She died seven months after the diagnosis because of disease progression.

Histological and immunohistochemical analyses on BM specimens

We morphologically reviewed BM specimens using hematoxylin and eosin (HE) staining. Immunohistochemistry (IHC) was also performed on formalin-fixed, paraffin-embedded sections. The monoclonal antibodies used for IHC were CD10 (56C6) (Nichirei, Tokyo, Japan), CD20 (L26) (Dako, Glostrup, Denmark), BCL2 (124) (Dako), BCL6 (P1F6) (Nichirei), MIB-1 (Dako), and MYC (Y60) (Abcam, Cambridge, UK). The MIB-1 index was calculated as the percentage of MIB-1-stained nuclei, which were counted among total 500 nuclei in three different visual fields.

The BM was massively infiltrated by medium-sized blastoid cells with fine chromatin and inconspicuous nucleoli (Fig. 1b). There were no paratrabecular lymphocyte aggregates, which are typically observed in FL [9, 11]. The blasts were strongly positive for CD20, CD10, BCL2, and the MYC protein and weakly positive for BCL6, indicating a GC B-cell phenotype (Fig. 1b). The MIB-1 index was unexpectedly low, at approximately 60% (Fig. 1b). This case was not diagnosed with DLBCL and suspected to have AL-HGBL-MBR.

Cytogenetic and fluorescence in situ hybridization studies

Standard G-banding and fluorescence in situ hybridization (FISH) analyses were performed. The probes used for the FISH analysis were a Vysis® LSI® *IGH/BCL2* dual-color, dual-fusion translocation probe, Vysis® LSI® *IGH/MYC/* CEP8 tri-color dual fusion probe, and Vysis® LSI® *MYC*

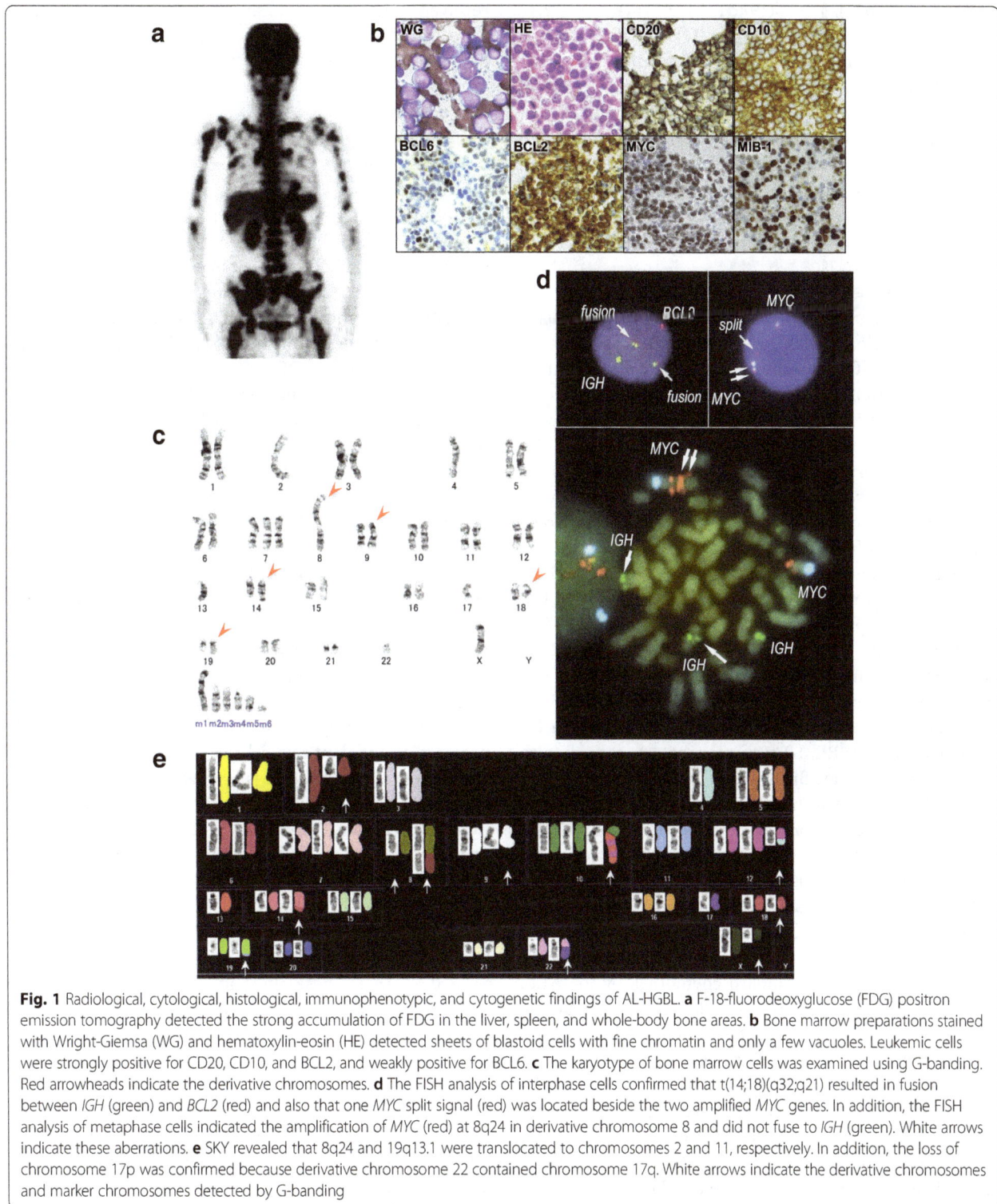

Fig. 1 Radiological, cytological, histological, immunophenotypic, and cytogenetic findings of AL-HGBL. **a** F-18-fluorodeoxyglucose (FDG) positron emission tomography detected the strong accumulation of FDG in the liver, spleen, and whole-body bone areas. **b** Bone marrow preparations stained with Wright-Giemsa (WG) and hematoxylin-eosin (HE) detected sheets of blastoid cells with fine chromatin and only a few vacuoles. Leukemic cells were strongly positive for CD20, CD10, and BCL2, and weakly positive for BCL6. **c** The karyotype of bone marrow cells was examined using G-banding. Red arrowheads indicate the derivative chromosomes. **d** The FISH analysis of interphase cells confirmed that t(14;18)(q32;q21) resulted in fusion between *IGH* (green) and *BCL2* (red) and also that one *MYC* split signal (red) was located beside the two amplified *MYC* genes. In addition, the FISH analysis of metaphase cells indicated the amplification of *MYC* (red) at 8q24 in derivative chromosome 8 and did not fuse to *IGH* (green). White arrows indicate these aberrations. **e** SKY revealed that 8q24 and 19q13.1 were translocated to chromosomes 2 and 11, respectively. In addition, the loss of chromosome 17p was confirmed because derivative chromosome 22 contained chromosome 17q. White arrows indicate the derivative chromosomes and marker chromosomes detected by G-banding

dual-color breakapart rearrangement probe (Abbott Molecular, Des Plaines, IL). The FISH analysis was applied to interphase and metaphase cells. Spectral karyotyping (SKY) was also performed for the aid of the interpretation of G-banded metaphase cells.

A G-banding analysis of BM specimens detected a complex karyotype including t(14;18)(q32;q21) and add(8)(q24) (Fig. 1c). A chromosomal segment of an unknown origin was translocated to the telomeric side of 8q24. The karyotype was 46,X,-X,-2,-4,+7,-8,add(8)(q24),inv(9)(p12q13),-

13,t(14;18)(q32;q21),-17,add(19)(q13.1),-22,+mar1,+mar2,+mar3,+mar4,+mar5,+mar6 [18] (Fig. 1c). The FISH analysis of interphase and metaphase cells confirmed the fusion between *IGH* and *BCL2* and the split and extra copies of *MYC* at 8q24 (Fig. 1d). Furthermore, SKY identified that 8q24 and 19q13.1 were translocated to chromosomes 2 and 11, respectively. G-banding and SKY confirmed the loss of chromosome 17p (Fig. 1c, e). Taken together, this case was diagnosed with AL-HGBL-MBR with the extra copies of *MYC* and loss of chromosome 17p.

Literature review

We selected the cases with BM involvement (at least ≥20% of nuclear cells) of non-centroblastic, non-immunoblastic TdT-negative blastoid B cells harboring both t(14;18)(q32;q21) and 8q24/*MYC* translocations, which was confirmed by G-banding and/or FISH analyses. The cases with either of them were excluded. Although secondary AL-HGBL-MBR arising from FL was also found, we selected only de novo cases to evaluate the survival from diagnosis because the onset and outcome were clearly recorded in each report.

We have identified further 47 de novo AL-HGBL-MBR cases from the published data (Table 1).[8–33] The median age at presentation is 61 years (range, 27–86); the male/female ratio was 2.0. Although 10 cases (21%) had a modest mass lesion at extranodal sites, the rest showed the clinical picture of ALL. In addition, 14 (36%) of 39 available cases showed central nervous system involvement. Unlike BL, L2-type morphology according to the French-American-British classification was observed in 14 (33%) of 42 available cases (Table 1). The immunophenotype of leukemic cells was positive for CD10, CD19, and CD20 in most cases (Table 1). Cytogenetic studies showed that loss of 17p and translocations at 2p12–13, 3q27, 9p13 are frequently observed as additional chromosomal aberrations, and at least nine (20%) cases had loss of 17p (Table 1). Most patients reported prior to 2003 received standard chemotherapy for ALL, whereas patients reported since 2003 were frequently treated with rituximab-combined chemotherapy for lymphomas (Table 1). Nevertheless, 42 patients (88%) died because of disease progression at the time of publication. Median survival of 46 cases, the observation period of which is well documented, was only five months (range 0.1–18 months) from the diagnosis. Their survival distribution was illustrated in Fig. 2a. The survival curves were determined using the Kaplan-Meier method. All analyses were performed using EZR (Saitama Medical Center, Jichi Medical University, ver.1.33) [34]. There was no significant difference in survival between older (≥60 years, n = 25) and younger (<60 years, n = 21) patients (log-rank test, P = 0.198) (Fig. 2b). Among the examined 46 cases, 44 cases

received chemotherapy, and their survival durations were significantly improved by rituximab use (log-rank test, P = 0.0294) (Fig. 2c).

Discussion

Based on the previous history and histopathology, our case was diagnosed with de novo AL-HGBL-MBR. Bone pain at the initial presentation was likely caused by rapid cell proliferation and the sudden onset of the disease in the BM. The literature review revealed that around 80% of de novo AL-HGBL-MBL cases had a typical clinical picture of ALL, and the features of present case were consistent with those of ALL. The noticeable behavior of this case is the unresponsiveness to R-hyper CVAD/MA and dose-adjusted EPOCH-R, which are expected to be effective regimens for not only BL but also HGBL-MBR [7, 35]. Indeed, DLBCL-type HGBL-MBR is reported to have a better prognosis than that of BL-like HGBL-MBR, which seems to have common clinical features with AL-HGBL-MBR [36]. The differences of cell morphology in HGBL-MBR may influence the therapeutic efficacy of the conventional regimens. The median survival of the collected cases suggests that AL-HGBL-MBR may show the most unfavorable prognosis in any type of B-cell lymphomas. Despite the disastrous consequence, the present review showed that rituximab use had a positive impact on survival in HGBL-MBR cases.

t(14;18)-harboring FL arising from GC B cells usually presents an indolent clinical behavior, while this type of lymphoma often undergoes clonal evolution.[37] AL-HGBL-MBR also develops from FL, and the clinical features of secondary AL-HGBL-MBR are nearly the same as those of de novo cases [9, 11, 15, 32] The prognosis of secondary AL-HGBL-MBR is likewise very poor [9, 11, 15, 32]. Besides alterations in *MYC*, disruptions in p53 and p14^{ARF}, and an additional 3q27/*BCL6* translocation are considered to be the dominant changes in transformed FL [37]. These alterations overlap with those of de novo AL-HGBL-MBR cases [9, 11, 15, 32] Although these abnormalities may incrementally accumulate during disease progression in FL, our case suggest that t(14;18)-carrying B cells suddenly develop into AL-HGBL-MBR when they have simultaneously acquired gene rearrangements and the amplification of *MYC* as well as the loss of 17p at the BM. If not, t(14;18)-carrying B cells may develop into a common FL. Even though this acquisition is a temporally distinct event, the accumulation of additional genetic abnormalities in t(14;18)-carrying B cells may eventually develop AL-HGBL. This situation is similar to that of ALL with *BCR/ABL1*. ALL with *BCR/ABL1* develops primarily and also arises from the blast crisis of chronic myelogenous leukemia. In AL-HGBL-MBR, the first hit is t(14;18), while the aggressive

Table 1 Clinicopathologic features of published cases with de novo acute lymphoblastic leukemia-like disease of high grade B-cell lymphoma with MYC and BCL2 and/or BCL6 rearrangements

Case (ref. n)	Age/sex	Extramedullary lesion at presentation	CNS	FAB criteria	CD10	CD19	CD20	sIg	Main cytogenetic abnormalities	IGH-BCL2	MYC	Curative therapy	Survival
					Immunophenotype					FISH or gene analysis			
1 (8)	57/F	bone	+	L3	+	+	–	ND	t(8;22)(q24;q12ª),t(14;18)(q32;q21)	NA	NA	ALL regimen	7 mo
2 (9)	74/M	palate, L (cervical, pretracheal)	–	L3	NA	+	NA	μ	t(8;22)(q24;q11),t(14;18)(q32;q21)	NA	NA	ALL regimen	3 mo
3 (9)	37/M	none	–	L2	–	+	+	IgMλ	t(8;22)(q24;q11),t(14;18)(q32;q21)	NA	NA	ALL regimen	12 mo
4 (9)	73/M	none	+	L3	+	+	+	IgMκ	t(8;22)(q24;q11),t(14;18)(q32;q21)	NA	NA	ALL regimen	8 mo
5 (10)	62/M	H, S	–	L3	+	+	+	ND	t(8;14)(q24;q32),t(14;18)(q32;q21)	NA	NA	ALL regimen	3 mo
6 (11)	35/M	none	–	L3	+	+	NA	ND	t(14;18)(q32;q21)	GR (+)	GR (+)	ALL regimen	0.3 mo
7 (12)	27/M	L (IP, RP)	+	L3	+	+	–	ND	t(8;22)(q24;q11),der(14)t(14;18)(q32;q21)	NA	NA	ALL regimen	5 mo
8 (13)	67/M	none	–	L3	NA	+	+	IgGκ	t(8;22)(q24;q11),t(14;18)(q32;q21)	NA	NA	none	0.1 mo
9 (14)	71/M	none	–	L3	–/+	+	+	IgMλ	t(1;3;11)(q42.3;q27.1;q23.1),der(8)t(8;9)(q24.2;p13.3),t(14;18)(q32.3;q21.3),der(17)t(17;?)(p13;?)	GR (+)	GR (+)	none	0.1 mo
10 (15)	36/F	IP mass	–	NA	+	+	NA	ND	t(8;22)(q24;q11),t(14;18)(q32;q21)	NA	GR (–)	ALL regimen	3 mo
11 (15)	60 M	none	+	L2	NA	NA	NA	NA	t(8;22)(q24;q11),t(14;18)(q32;q21),+der(14)t(14;18)(q32;q21)	NA	GR (–)	ALL regimen	6 mo
12 (16)	40/M	GL, paravertebral mass	–	L2	+	+	+	NA	der(6)t(6;8)(q17;q24),add(8)(q24),der(9)t(8;9)(q24;p17),t(14;18)(q32;q21),del(17)(p11)	NA	NA	ALL regimen	1 mo
13 (17)	69/M	H	–	L3	–	+	+	IgMκ	der(7;17)(q10;q10),+der(8)t(8;14;18)(q24;q32;q22),add(14)(q32),del(18)(q21)	GR (+)	NA	ALL regimen	5 mo
14 (18)	41/F	none	–	L3	+	+	+	NA	t(2;3)(p12;q27),del(8)(q24),t(14;18)(q32;q21)	GR (+)	GR (+)	ALL regimen	10 mo
15 (19)	50/F	GL	–	L2	+	+	+	IgMκ	t(3;4)(q27;p13),t(8;14;18)(q24;q32;q21),+ider(8)(q10)t(8;14;18)(q24;q32;q21)	GR (+)	GR (+)	ALL regimen	0.1 mo
16 (19)	44/M	GL, S	+	NA	+	+	+	IgMκ	t(3;13)(q27;q14),t(8;22)(q24;q11),t(14;18)(q32;q21),+der(18)t(14;18)(q32;q21)	GR (+)	GR (–)	NCVBP, IVAM, ASCT	7 mo
17 (19)	46/F	GL, S, Asc, PE	+	L2	+	+	+	IgMκ	t(2;3)(p12;q27),add(8)(q24),der(14)t(8;14)(q24;q32),der(18)t(14;18)(q32;q21)	GR (+)	GR (+)	ACVBP, allo-SCT	3 mo
18 (20)	62/F	none	NA	L3	NA	NA	NA	NA	t(2;8)(p12;q24),t(14;18)(q32;q21)	NA	NA	none	0.1 mo
19 (21)	48/M	GL	–	L2	NA	NA	NA	NA	t(8;9)(q24;p13),t(14;18)(q32;q21)	NA	NA	R-CHOP	3.5 mo
20 (22)	72/M	H, S	–	L2	+	NA	+	IgGκ	t(8;9)(q24;p13),t(14;18)(q32;q21)	NA	NA	R-EPOCH	4 mo
21 (23)	71/M	S (mild)	–	L2	–	+	+	γ	t(1;2)(q22-23;p13),t(8;14)(q24;q32),t(14;18)(q32;q22)	GR (+)	GR (+)	ALL regimen	2 mo
22 (24)	50/F	L (axillary), SC mass	–	L3	+	+	NA	ND	t(2;3)(p12;q27),t(8;22)(q24;q11),t(14;18)(q32;q21),-17	fusion (+)	split (+)	ALL regimen	7 mo

Table 1 Clinicopathologic features of published cases with de novo acute lymphoblastic leukemia-like disease of high grade B-cell lymphoma with MYC and BCL2 and/or BCL6 rearrangements (Continued)

Case (ref. n)	Age/ sex	Extramedullary lesion at presentation	CNS	FAB criteria	Immunophenotype				Main cytogenetic abnormalities	FISH or gene analysis		Curative therapy	Survival
					CD10	CD19	CD20	sIg		IGH-BCL2	MYC		
23 (25)	29/M	none	−	L3	+	+	+	NA	+8,t(8;22)(q24;q11),t(14;18)(q32;q21)	NA	split (+)	R-CHOP, R-ICE, R-hyper-CVAD/MA	5 mo
24 (25)	72/M	none	−	L3	+	+	+	NA	t(8;22)(q24;q11.2),t(14;18)(q32;q21)	NA	NA	R-hyper-CVAD/MA	11 mo[b]
25 (25)	50/F	none	+	L3	+	+	+	NA	t(8;22)(q24;q11),t(14;18)(q32;q21)	fusion (+)	split (+)	R-hyper-CVAD/MA	3 mo
26 (25)	32/M	L (mesenteric)	+	L3	+	+	+	NA	t(1;3)(p32;q26.2),t(8;22)(q24;q11),add(14)(q32),t(14;18)(q32;q21)	fusion (+)	split (+)	hyper-CVAD/MA	8 mo
27 (25)	67/M	L (P), small intestine	+	L3	+	+	+	NA	t(8;14)(q24;q32),der(8)t(8;14)t(14;18)(q32;q21),der(14)t(8;14),+add(14)(q32),i(17)(q10)	fusion (+)	split (+)	R-hyper-CVAD/MA, velcade	9 mo
28 (25)	61/M	L (RP), colon, prostate	+	L3	NA	NA	NA	NA	t(8;22)(q24;q11),t(14;18)(q32;q21),+der(14)t(14;18)	fusion (+)	NA	hyper-CVAD/MA, MOAP	9 mo
29 (25)	42/F	small intestine, omentum, breast	−	L3	+	+	+	NA	t(8;14)(q24;q32),t(14;18)(q32;q21),der(17)t(10;17)(q22;q10)	fusion (+)	NA	proMACECytaBOM, CHOP, ESHAP, hyper-CVAD/MA, SCT, RT	12 mo
30 (25)	63/M	testis, lip	−	L3	+	+	+	NA	NA	fusion (+)	split (+)	hyper-CVAD	18 mo
31 (26)	57/F	none	NA	NA	+	+	−	NA	der(3)t(3;14;?)(q27;q32;?),t(8;14)(q24;q32),der(18)t(14;18)(q32;q21)	fusion (+)	split (+)	CODOX-M/IVAC	2.5 mo
32 (26)	60/M	none	NA	L3	+	+	+	D	t(2;8)(p12;q24),der(8)t(2;8)(p12;q24),t(14;18)(q32;q21),?i(17)(q10)	fusion (+)	split (+)	hyper-CVAD, CODOX-M	3 mo
33 (26)	63/M	GL, S (mild)	NA	L3	−	+	+	D	der(3)t(1;3)(q23;q27),t(8;22)(q24;q11),t(14;18)(q32;q21)	fusion (+)	split (+)	CODOX-M/IVAC	6 mo
34 (26)	76/F	none	NA	L3	+	+	NA	D	t(8;22)(q24;q11),t(14;18)(q32;q21)	fusion (+)	split (+)	VAD	6 mo
35 (26)	59/F	none	NA	L2	+	NA	NA	NA	t(8;9)(q24;p13),t(14;18)(q32;q21)	fusion (+)	split (+)	ALL regimen	1.5 mo
36 (26)	69/M	L (IP), H	NA	L3	+	+	+	D	t(14;18)(q32;q21)	fusion (+)	split (+)	ALL regimen	1.5 mo
37 (26)	86/F	none	NA	L2	+	+	+	ND	add(9)(p13),t(14;18)(q32;q21)	fusion (+)	split (+)	none	0.5 mo
38 (27)	43/F	pancreas	+	L3	+	+	+	IgMλ	t(8;14)(q24;q32),t(14;18)(q32;q21)	fusion (+)	split (+)	R-CODOX-M/IVAC	5 mo
39 (28)	61/M	GL, S, PE	−	L3	+	+	+	γ	t(3;5)(q27;q15),t(8;14;18)(q24;q32;q21),+der(8)t(8;14;18),+der(18)t(8;14;18)	fusion (+)	split (+)	R-hyper-CVAD,	NA[c]
40 (29)	42/M	L (IP), S	+	L2	+	+	+	κ	der(8)del(8)(q12.1q12.3)del(8)(q24.21q24.21)t(8;12)(q24.21;p12.1),	fusion (+)	split (+)	R-CHOP, ALL regimen	7 mo

Table 1 Clinicopathologic features of published cases with de novo acute lymphoblastic leukemia-like disease of high grade B-cell lymphoma with *MYC* and *BCL2* and/or *BCL6* rearrangements *(Continued)*

Case (ref. n)	Age/sex	Extramedullary lesion at presentation	CNS	FAB criteria	CD10	CD19	CD20	sIg	Main cytogenetic abnormalities	IGH-BCL2	MYC	Curative therapy	Survival
41 (30)	72/M	bone, liver	+	NA	+	NA	+	NA	der(12)del(12)(p12.1p12.1)t(8;12)(q24.21;p12.1),t(14;18)(q32;q21)	fusion (+)	split (+)	ALL regimen	NA[c]
42 (31)	64/M	L (NA)	−	NA	+	+	+	NA	t(3;8)(q27;q24),t(14;18)(q32;q21)	fusion (+)	split (+)	R-EPOCH	1.7 mo[c]
43 (31)	72/M	L (NA)	−	NA	+	NA	+	NA	NA	fusion (+)	split (+)	R-EPOCH	1.6 mo[c]
44 (32)	74/F	none	+	L2	+	+	+	κ	t(3;22)(q27;q11.2),t(8;14)(q24;q32),t(14;18)(q32;q21), −8,del(11)(q23q25),del(13)(q12q14),t(14;18)(q32;q21),+18	fusion (+)	split (+)	R-CHOP	3 mo
45 (32)	67/M	colon	−	L3	+	+	−/+	κ	NA	fusion (+)	split (+)	R-CHOP	11 mo[d]
46 (32)	71/M	L (mediastinal)	−	L3	+	+	+	κ	der(8)t(8;14)(q24;q32q21),der(14)t(8;14)(q24.1;q32),der(18)t(14;18)(q32;q21)	fusion (+)	split (+)	R-EPOCH, R-ICE, ASCT	14 mo
47 (33)	60/M	GL	NA	L2	+	+	+	λ	+8,inv(8)(p11.2q24)×2,t(14;18)(q32;q21),−17	fusion (+)	split (+)	R-hyperCVAD, ofatumumab + EPOCH	18 mo
48 (present case)	69/F	none	−	L2	+	+	+	IgMκ	add(8)(q24),t(14;18)(q32;q21),−17	fusion (+)	split (+), EC (+)	R-hyper-CVAD/MA, R-EPOCH	7 mo

Abbreviations: Ref n reference number, FAB criteria blastoid cell morphology according to the French-American-British classification, CNS development of central nervous system involvement, sIg surface immunoglobulin, M male, F female, L lymphadenopathy, H hepatomegaly, S splenomegaly, SC subcutaneous, IP intraperitoneal, RP retroperitoneal, GL generalized lymphadenopathy, Asc ascites, PE pleural effusion, P pelvic, ND not detected, D detected, NA not available, GR gene rearrangement, EC extra copies, ALL regimen multidrug chemotherapy for acute lymphoblastic leukemia, NCVBP mitoxantrone, cyclophosphamide, vinblastine, bleomycin, and prednisone, IVAM ifosfamide, etoposide, cytarabine, and methotrexate, ASCT autologous stem cell transplantation, ACVBP doxorubicin, cyclophosphamide, vinblastine, bleomycin, and prednisone, allo-SCT allogeneic stem cell transplantation, R rituximab, CHOP cyclophosphamide, doxorubicin, vincristine, and prednisone, EPOCH etoposide, prednisone, vincristine, cyclophosphamide, and doxorubicin, ICE ifosfamide, carboplatin, and etoposide, hyper-CVAD/MA cyclophosphamide, vincristine, doxorubicin, dexamethasone alternating with methotrexate and cytarabine, MOAP methotrexate, vincristine, asparaginase, and prednisone, proMACEcytaBOM prednisone, methotrexate, doxorubicin, cyclophosphamide, etoposide, cytarabine, and bleomycin, ESHAP etoposide, methylprednisolone, cytarabine, and cisplatin, RT radiation therapy, CODOX-M/IVAC cyclophosphamide, vincristine, doxorubicin, methotrexate alternating with ifosfamide, etoposide, and cytarabine, VAD vincristine, doxorubicin, and dexamethasone, POMP prednisone, vincristine, methotrexate, and mercaptopurine

[a] This description is according to original work [8]

[b] Alive (disease status was not described)

[c] Alive with disease at the time of publication

[d] Alive with no evidence of disease at the time of publication

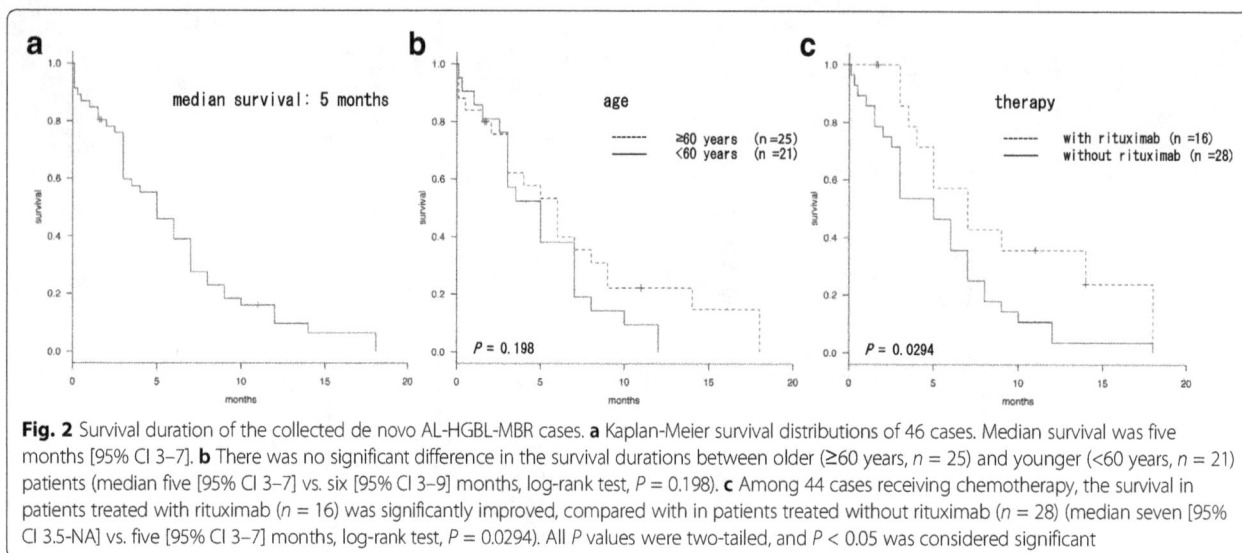

Fig. 2 Survival duration of the collected de novo AL-HGBL-MBR cases. **a** Kaplan-Meier survival distributions of 46 cases. Median survival was five months [95% CI 3–7]. **b** There was no significant difference in the survival durations between older (≥60 years, n = 25) and younger (<60 years, n = 21) patients (median five [95% CI 3–7] vs. six [95% CI 3–9] months, log-rank test, P = 0.198). **c** Among 44 cases receiving chemotherapy, the survival in patients treated with rituximab (n = 16) was significantly improved, compared with in patients treated without rituximab (n = 28) (median seven [95% CI 3.5-NA] vs. five [95% CI 3–7] months, log-rank test, P = 0.0294). All P values were two-tailed, and P < 0.05 was considered significant

nature may be provided by further aberrations including the deregulation of *MYC* and disruption of p53. Therefore, FISH analyses regarding *MYC* and *TP53* should be evaluated, when HGBL-MBR is suspected, in t(14;18)-harboring neoplasms.

The leukemic cells in the present case strongly expressed the MYC protein, which precludes entry into the G0 phase. However, many of them remained in the G0 phase, in which the MIB-1 antibody failed to stain the nucleus [38, 39]. This condition indicates that the G0/G1 switch regulation was also impaired in the present case. In spite of the overexpression of MYC, MIB-1 index in HGBL-MBR cases was reported to vary from 25% to 100% [40, 41]. The suboptimal response to the R-hyper CVAD/MA and EPOCH-R regimens may be explained by the existence of MIB-1-negative and BCL2-positive cells. Recent in vitro studies suggested that concurrent inhibition of BCL2 and MYC may have therapeutic potential for the treatment of AL-HGBL-MBR patients [42, 43]. This strategy may overcome the resistance to conventional chemoimmunotherapy.

Conclusions

Our case and a review of the literature indicate that de novo AL-HGBL-MBR is a rare but may be a distinct clinical condition in HGBL-MBR. AL-HGBL-MBR may be the most aggressive disease among all t(14;18)-harboring neoplasms. Because conventional chemotherapeutic regimens are ineffective, other therapeutic strategies, such as using inhibitors against BCL2 and MYC, may elicit the potential to overcome the chemoresistance. The further accumulation of molecular evidences to illustrate AL-HGBL-MBR is needed.

Abbreviations
AL-HGBL-MBR: ALL-like disease of HGBL-MBR; ALL: Acute lymphoblastic leukemia; BL: Burkitt lymphoma; BM: Bone marrow; DLBCL: Diffuse large

B-cell lymphoma; EPOCH-R: Etoposide, prednisolone, vincristine, cyclophosphamide, doxorubicin, and rituximab; FDG: F-18-fluorodeoxyglucose; FISH: Fluorescence in situ hybridization; FL: Follicular lymphoma; GC: Germinal center; HE: Hematoxylin and eosin; HGBL-MBR: High grade B-cell lymphoma with *MYC* and *BCL2* and/or *BCL6* rearrangements; IHC: Immunohistochemistry; LDH: Lactate dehydrogenase; PET: Positron emission tomography; R-CHOP: Rituximab, cyclophosphamide, doxorubicin, vincristine, and prednisone; R-hyper CVAD/MA: rituximab, cyclophosphamide, vincristine, doxorubicin, and dexamethasone/methotrexate and cytarabine; SKY: Spectral karyotyping; SUVmax: Maximum standardized uptake value; TdT: Terminal deoxynucleotidyl transferase; WHO: World Health Organization classification

Acknowledgments
The authors thank the following physicians for collecting clinical data: Dr. Yasuyuki Inoue, Dr. Yoshinori Suzuki, Dr. Manabu Matsunawa, Dr. Yuka Tsuruoka, Dr. Satoshi Yokoi, and Dr. Kazuyuki Satoh.

Funding
This work was not supported by any grant.

Authors' contributions
AU and YI equally contributed to this work. AU, YI, YU, and MI designed the study and collected and analyzed data. YI, YN, HS, and MK examined and treated the patient. KO performed and analyzed the data of cytogenetic studies. MH and MT performed and reviewed the histopathological study. The manuscript was written by AU, YI, and MI and approved by all authors prior to its submission.

Competing interests
The authors declare that they have no competing interests.

Author details
[1]Division of Hematology & Oncology, Department of Internal Medicine, St. Marianna University School of Medicine, 2-16-1 Sugao, Miyamae-ku, Kawasaki, Kanagawa 216-8511, Japan. [2]Department of cytogenetics, SRL Diagnostics, Hachioji Laboratory, Tokyo, Japan. [3]Department of Pathology, St. Marianna University School of Medicine, Kawasaki, Japan.

References

1. Küppers R. Mechanisms of B-cell lymphoma pathogenesis. Nat Rev Cancer. 2005;5:251–63.
2. Swerdlow SH, Campo E, Harris NL, et al. WHO classification of tumours of haematopoietic and lymphoid tissues. In: Bosman FT, Jaffe ES, Lakhani SR, Ohgaki H, editors. World Health Organization Classification of Tumours. IARC: Lyon, France; 2008.
3. Greisman HA, Lu Z, Tsai AG, et al. IgH partner breakpoint sequences provide evidence that AID initiates t(11;14) and t(8;14) chromosomal breaks in mantle cell and Burkitt lymphomas. Blood. 2012;120:2864–7.
4. Swerdlow SH, Campo E, Pileri SA, et al. The 2016 revision of the World Health Organization classification of lymphoid neoplasms. Blood. 2016;127:2375–90.
5. Aukema SM, Siebert R, Schuuring E, et al. Double-hit B-cell lymphomas. Blood. 2011;117:2319–31.
6. Aukema SM, Kreuz M, Kohler C, et al. Biological characterization of adult MYC-translocation-positive mature B-cell lymphomas other than molecular Burkitt lymphoma. Haematologica. 2014;99:726–35.
7. Howlett C, Snedecor SJ, Landsburg DJ, et al. Front-line, dose-escalated immunochemotherapy is associated with a significant progression-free survival advantage in patients with double-hit lymphomas: a systematic review and meta-analysis. Br J Haematol. 2015;170:504–14.
8. Gluck WL, Bigner SH, Borowitz MJ, Brenckman Jr WD. Acute lymphoblastic leukemia of Burkitt's type (L3 ALL) with 8;22 and 14;18 translocations and absent surface immunoglobulins. Am J Clin Pathol. 1986;85:636–40.
9. Thangavelu M, Olopade O, Beckman E, et al. Clinical, morphologic, and cytogenetic characteristics of patients with lymphoid malignancies characterized by both t(14;18)(q32;q21) and t(8;14)(q24;q32) or t(8;22)(q24;q11). Genes Chromosomes Cancer. 1990;2:147–58.
10. Matsuzaki H, Hata H, Asou N, et al. Establishment and characterization of acute B-cell lymphocytic leukemia cell line showing (8;14) and (14;18) chromosome translocation. Acta Haematol. 1990;84:156–61.
11. Kramer MH, Raghoebier S, Beverstock GC, de Jong D, Kluin PM, Kluin-Nelemans JC. De novo acute B-cell leukemia with translocation t(14;18): an entity with a poor prognosis. Leukemia. 1991;6:473–8.
12. Marosi C, Bettelheim P, Chott A, et al. Simultaneous occurrence of t(14;18) and t(8;22) common acute lymphoblastic leukemia. Ann Hematol. 1992;64:101–4.
13. Smith SR, Bown N, Wallis JP. Acute lymphoblastic leukemia of Burkitt type (L3) with a (14;18) and an atypical (8;22) translocation. Cancer Genet Cytogenet. 1992;62:197–9.
14. Nacheva E, Dyer MJS, Fischer P, et al. C-MYC translocations in de novo B-cell lineage acute leukemias with t(14;18) (cell lines Karpas 231 and 353). Blood. 1993;82:231–40.
15. Karsan A, Gascoyne RD, Coupland RW, et al. Combination of t(14;18) and a Burkitt's type translocation in B-cell malignancies. Leuk Lymphoma. 1993;10:433–41.
16. Lillington DM, Monard S, Johnson PW, et al. The t(14;18) in a patient with de novo acute lymphoblastic leukemia is associated with t(8;9). Leukemia. 1994;8:560–3.
17. van Ooteghem RBC, Smit EME, Beishuizen A, et al. A new B-cell line showing a complex translocation (8;14;18) and BCL2 rearrangement. Cancer Genet Cytogenet. 1994;74:87–94.
18. Berger R, Flexor M, Le Coniat M, Larsen C-J. Presence of three recurrent chromosomal rearrangements, t(2;3)(p12;q27), del(8)(q24), and t(14;18), in an acute lymphoblastic leukemia. Cancer Genet Cytogenet. 1996;86:76–9.
19. Stamatoullas A, Buchonnet G, Lepretre S, et al. De novo acute B cell leukemia/lymphoma with t(14;18). Leukemia. 2000;14:1960–6.
20. Velangi MR, Reid MM, Bown M, et al. Acute lymphoblastic leukaemia of the L3 subtype in adults in the northern healthe region of England 1983-99. J Clin Pathol. 2002;55:591–5.
21. Dunphy CH, van Deventer HW, Carder KJ, Rao KW, Dent GA. Mature B-Cell acute lymphoblastic leukemia with associated translocations (14;18)(q32; q21) and (8;9)(q24;p13). A Burkitt variant? Arch Pathol Lab Med. 2003;127:610–3.
22. Yoshida I, Takeuchi M. De novo acute lymphocytic leukemia with t(14;18) complicated by tumor lysis syndrome. J Jpn Soc Int Med 2003; 92: 865–867 (in Japanese).
23. Greer WL, Lee CLY, Callanan MB, Zayed E, Sadek I. Case of acute lymphoblastic leukemia presenting with t(14;18)/BCL2, t(8;14)/cMYC, and t(1; 2)/FCGR2B. Am J Hematol. 2003;74:112–8.
24. Fujii S, Miyata A, Tkeuchi M, Yoshino T. Acute lymphoblastic leukemia (L3) with t(2;3)(p12;q27), t(14;18)(q32;q21), and t(8;22)(q24;q11). Jpn J Clin Hematol. 2005; 46: 134–140 (in Japanese).
25. Kanungo A, Medeiros LJ, Abruzzo LV, Lin P. Lymphoid neoplasms associated with concurrent t(14;18) and 8q24/c-MYC translocateon generaly have a poor prognosis. Mod Pathol. 2006;19:25–33.
26. D'Achille P, Seymour JF, Campbell LJ. Translocation (14;18)(q32;q21) in acute lymphoblastic leukemia: a study of 12 cases and review of the literature. Cancer Genet Cytogenet. 2006;171:52–6.
27. Fujishima N, Fujishima M, Inomata M, et al. Early relapse of Burkitt's lymphoma with t(8;14) and t(14;18) after rituximab-combined CODOX-M and IVAC therapy. Jpn J Clin Hematol 2007; 48: 326–331 (in Japanese).
28. Liu D, Shimonov J, Primanneni S, Lai Y, Ahmed T, Seiter K. T(8;14;18): a 3-way chromosome translocateon in two patients with Burkit's lymphoma/leukemia. Mol Cancer. 2007;6:35.
29. Boström H, Leuchowius K-J, Hallböök H, et al. U-2973, a novel B-cell line established from a patient with a mature B-cell leukemia displaying concurrent t(14;18) and MYC translocation to a non-IG gene partner. Eur J Haematol. 2008;81:218–25.
30. Motlló C, Grau J, Junca J, et al. Translocation (3;8)(q27;q24) in two cases of triple hit lymphoma. Cancer Genet Cyrogenet. 2010;203:328–32.
31. Wang W, Hu S, Lu X, Young KH, Medeiros J. Triple-hit B-Cell lymphoma with MYC, BCL2, and BCL6 translocations/rearrangements. Clinicopathologic features of 11 cases. Am J Surg Pathol. 2015;39:1132–9.
32. Moench L, Sachs Z, Aasen G, Dolan M, Dayton V, Courville EL. Double- and triple-hit lymphomas can present with features suggestive of immaturity, including TdT expression, and create diagnostic challenges. Leuk Lymphoma. 2016;57:2626–35.
33. Chen Z, MYC HS. BCL2 double-hit lymphoma/leukemia mimicking acute leukemia at initial presentation. Blood. 2016;127:1072.
34. Kanda Y. Investigation of the freely available easy-to-use software 'EZR' for medical statistics. Bone Marrow Transplant. 2013;48:452–8.
35. Friedberg JW. How I treat double-hit lymphoma. Blood. 2017;130:590–6.
36. Johnson NA, Savage KJ, Ludkovski O, et al. Lymphomas with concurrent BCL2 and MYC translocations: the critical factors associated with survival. Blood. 2009;114:2273–9.
37. Kridel R, Sehn LH, Gascoyne RD. Pathogenesis of follicular lymphoma. J Clin Invest. 2012;122:3424–31.
38. Bretones G, Delgado MD, Léon J. Myc and cell cycle control. Biochim Biophys Acta. 1849;2015:506–16.
39. Gerdes J, Lemke H, Baisch H, Wacker HH, Schwab U, Stein H. Cell cycle analysis of a cell proliferation-associated human nuclear antigen defined by the monoclonal antibody Ki-67. J Immunol. 1984;133:1710–5.
40. Tomita N, Tokunaga M, Nakamura N, et al. Clinicopathological features of lymphoma/leukemia patients carrying both BCL2 and MYC translocations. Haematologica. 2009;97:935–43.
41. Snuderl M, Kolman OK, Chen YB, et al. B-cell lymphomas with concurrent IGH-BCL2 and MYC rearrangements are aggressive neoplasms with clinical and pathologic features distinct from Burkitt lymphoma and diffuse large B-cell lymphoma. Am J Surg Pathol. 2010;34:327–40.
42. Johnson-Fareley N, Veliz J, Bhagavathi S, et al. ABT-199, a BH3 mimetic that specifically targets Bcl-2, enhances the antitumor activity of chemotherapy, bortezomib and JQ1 in "double hit" lymphoma cells. Leuk Lymphoma. 2015;56:2146–52.
43. Cinar M, Rosenfelt F, Rokhsar S, et al. Concurrent inhibition of MYC and BCL2 is a potentially effectivetreatment strategy for double hit and triple hit B-cell lymphomas. Leuk Res. 2015;39:730–8.

22

The study of calcified atherosclerotic arteries: an alternative to evaluate the composition of a problematic tissue reveals new insight including metakaryotic cells

Silvia Fittipaldi[1,2]*, Francesco Vasuri[1], Alessio Degiovanni[1], Rodolfo Pini[1], Mauro Gargiulo[1], Andrea Stella[1], Gianandrea Pasquinelli[1], William G. Thilly[2] and Elena V. Gostjeva[2]

Abstract

Background: Calcifications of atherosclerotic plaques represent a controversial issue as they either lead to the stabilization or rupture of the lesion. However, the cellular key players involved in the progression of the calcified plaques have not yet been described. The primary reason for this lacuna is that decalcification procedures impair protein and nucleic acids contained in the calcified tissue. The aim of our study was to preserve the cellular content of heavily calcified plaques with a new rapid fixation in order to simplify the study of calcifications.

Methods: Here we applied a fixation method for fresh calcified tissue using the Carnoy's solution followed by an enzymatic tissue digestion with type II collagenase. Immunohistochemistry was performed to verify the preservation of nuclear and cytoplasmic antigens. DNA content and RNA preservation was evaluated respectively with Feulgen staining and RT-PCR. A checklist of steps for successful image analysis was provided. To present the basic features of the F-DNA analysis we used descriptive statistics, skewness and kurtosis. Differences in DNA content were analysed with Kruskal-Wallis and Dunn's post tests. The value of $P < 0.05$ was considered significant.

Results: Twenty-four vascular adult tissues, sorted as calcified (14) or uncalcified (10), were processed and 17 fetal tissues were used as controls (9 soft and 8 hard). Cells composing the calcified carotid plaques were positive to Desmin, Vimentin, Osteocalcin or Ki-67; the cellular population included smooth muscle cells, osteoblasts and osteoclasts-like cells and metakaryotic cells. The DNA content of each cell type found in the calcified carotid artery was successfully quantified in 7 selected samples. Notably the protocol revealed that DNA content in osteoblasts in fetal control tissues exhibits about half (3.0 ng) of the normal nuclear DNA content (6.0 ng).

Conclusion: Together with standard histology, this technique could give additional information on the cellular content of calcified plaques and help clarify the calcification process during atherosclerosis.

Keywords: DNA quantification, Atherosclerosis, Calcification, Osteogenesis, Immunohistochemistry, Metakaryotic cells

* Correspondence: sv.fittipaldi@gmail.com
[1]Department of Experimental, Diagnostic and Specialty Medicine (DIMES); S. Orsola-Malpighi Hospital, Bologna University, Via Massarenti 9, I 40139 Bologna, Italy
[2]Laboratory in Metakaryotic Biology (LIMB), Department of Biological Engineering, Massachusetts Institute of Technology, Cambridge, MA, USA

Background

Considered for decades a passive process, calcification is now seen as an active mechanism sharing many similarities with embryonic bone formation [1, 2]. The most recent mechanism proposed to elucidate arterial calcification is the possible role of resident or circulating stem cells that differentiate into chondro-osteogenic cells [3]. Nowadays, the clinical impact of arterial calcification is still unclear [4]; indeed the extent of calcification is associated with either a good or bad prognosis. For example, in the coronary arteries small calcifications increase the risk of plaque rupture whereas bigger deposits seem to stabilize the plaque [5]. On the other hand, calcified carotid plaques are considered a low athero-embolic risk [6]. In our recent study, we observed that plaques with massive calcifications showed the same incidence of histological complications but without influencing clinical symptomatology [7].

A big issue in analysing calcified plaques is the deterioration of the carotid tissues due to the strong pre-treatment used to dissolve minerals (ethylenediaminetetraacetic acid (EDTA) or chloride acid (HCl) prior to histopathological processing [8].

Previous studies attempted to process calcified tissue with alternative decalcification solutions or treatments as ultrasound, however the major issue was maintaining the whole cellular morphology together with an intact DNA content [9, 10]; indeed the use of strong acids hydrolyses the DNA molecule. We hereby apply a parallel approach to standard histology methods to preserve and study the cellular content of heavily calcified plaques. Our aim was to validate and optimized the techniques for the study of calcified arterial tissues. Additionally to calcified plaques, the technique was also tested on a wide series of tissues from soft to hard (bone).

Methods

Tissue sampling

All samples were obtained under a protocol approved in advance by the Massachusetts Institute of Technology, Committee on the Use of Humans as Experimental Subjects. No persons, including minors/children, were enrolled in MIT studies. Only surgical discards from patients anonymous to MIT researchers were received from collaborating hospitals. These comprised fixed tissues from a variety of organs. The Massachusetts Institute of Technology IRB reviewed and approved the several collaborative relationships specifically indicating that the arrangements were in the US NIH "exempt" category for the requirement for informed consent (COUHES approval number 0804002679). Anonymous surgical discards were fixed immediately upon surgical removal in Carnoy's solution as described and stored under refrigeration in 70 % ethanol [11]. A total of 41 tissue samples were finally collected from 26 cases, 16 fetuses and 10 adults.

Experimental parameters were optimized for two different types of samples, soft and hard. Hard adult samples were defined as "undissectable" with standard procedures without previous decalcification, commonly in Osteodec, Bio-optical (EDTA, calcium's chelates, 40 to 60 min dependent on the tissue dimension). Of the 41 tissue samples retrieved, 22 were hard and 19 were soft, sorted in:

- 8 hard fetal samples; 3 femoral, 1 nasal bone, 1 elbow, 1 hip bone and 1 knee bone, and 1 chondroid tissue.
- 9 fetal soft samples; 3 guts, 3 brains, 2 muscles, and 1 eye retinae.
- 14 hard adult samples; 13 calcified carotid plaques and 1 calcified abdominal aortic aneurism.
- 10 soft adult samples; 9 uncalcified carotid plaques and 1 uncalcified abdominal aortic aneurism.

Spreading method

All 41 tissue samples were fixed in cold Carnoy at 4 °C (3 ml Ethanol 100 % and 1 ml glacial acetic acid per <0.25 cm^2 within 30 min from surgical removal. Carnoy solution was changed after 60 and 120 min for a total of 3 hours fixation. Sample were then stored at -20 °C in 70 % ethanol [12]. Subsequent enzymatic tissue treatments with collagenase, type II (Clostridium histolyticum, ≥200 collagenase units/mg, Calbiochem, Merck Chemicals Ltd, UK) were tested with different incubation times and concentrations at 37 °C to define satisfactory conditions for various tissue types (Table 1). The most notable requirement is the need for up to 24 h of collagenase treatment to achieve unfolding of the hard tissues.

Collagenase-treated tissue samples were subsequently macerated in 500 ul of 45 % acetic acid (Table 1). Macerated tissue samples were minced with surgical scissors creating pieces no greater than 0.3 mm in length. Each piece was transferred to a slide

Table 1 Specifications for satisfactory spreading of soft versus calcified tissue samples in adult vascular tissues and fetal samples

Type of tissue	Collagenase II digestion time	Collagenase II working concentration (U^a/ml)	Acetic acid 45 % maceration time	Spread sections size (max)
Adult hard	24 h	10U/1 ml	30 min	0.1 mm
Adult soft	18 h	10U/1.5 ml	10 min	0.3 mm
Fetal hard	12 h	10U/1.5 ml	20 min	0.2 mm
Fetal soft	1–4 h	10U/1.5 ml	10 min	0.3 mm

^{a}One CDU unit is defined as the amount of enzyme that will release 1.0 nmol Leu equivalent from collagenase per min at 37 °C, pH 7.2

in a drop of 45 % acetic acid. To spread the macerated tissue into a monolayer, several thicknesses of filter paper were placed on the coverslip and a tweezer handle was moved steadily in one direction with a delicate pressure. Intermittent microscopic examination during the spreading process was used to determine when satisfactory spreading had been achieved. Increased pressure on the stacked filter paper was required for the harder bone-containing samples. Cover slips were removed after direct immersion in liquid nitrogen, and slides were air dried for 1 h. Spread slides were stored at 4 °C, in the dark, and subsequently used for different forms of analyses: Von Kossa, Feulgen-Giemsa staining, immunohistochemistry, Feulgen reaction for DNA quantification and RNA extraction.

Histochemistry
Histochemistry included Von Kossa staining for the identification of calcified matrix: sections were hydrated, treated with 1.5 % silver nitrate (AgNO3) solution and placed in front of a 100 W lamp for 1 h. Sections were therefore rinsed in distilled H_2O (dH_2O), counterstained with nuclear-fast Red, dehydrated and mounted.

The Feulgen-Giemsa staining was used to test the preservation of the nuclei after the collagenase digestion and the subsequent DNA quantification. Briefly, the slides were placed in a Coplin jar filled with HCl 1 N at 60 °C for 8 min, for partial hydrolysis of the macromolecules and DNA depurination. Hydrolysis was stopped by washing the slides in cold dH_2O. After carefully drying, sections were placed in Schiff's reagent (#3952016, Sigma-Aldrich, St. Louis MO, US) for 1 h at room temperature, washed twice with 2x standard saline citrate (trisodium citrate 8.8 g/L, sodium chloride 17.5 g/L), washed again with dH_2O and thereafter counterstained

with 1 % Giemsa solution (#GS500, Sigma-Aldrich, St. Louis MO, US) for 5 min. Slides were dehydrated in graded step of alcohol and mounted with Canada Balsam (Sigma- Aldrich C1795).

Feulgen DNA quantification
Feulgen densitometry relies on the premise that the amount of stain bound to DNA is proportional to the amount of DNA present in the nucleus with a 1:1 ratio. Feulgen reaction is specific for DNA and does not stain RNA [11, 13].

DNA quantification using Feulgen reaction (without Giemsa) was carried out in 3 fetal and 4 adult samples, each equally distributed as hard and soft areas (Table 2, raw data are included in the Additional file 1). Nuclei of chicken red blood cells (cRBC, #IC05-0810, Innovative Research, Novi, MI, US) were used as an internal standard for DNA quantification (one nucleus of RBC contains a diploid quantity of DNA equivalent to 2C = 2.5 pg). Slides are Feulgen stained in groups (25 to 100 slides) with the same reagents, lots, conditions and standards. Image acquisition and segmentation were performed with the Carl Zeiss Vision AxioVision software: these are the critical steps for a precise DNA quantification. All steps are presented in details in the Additional file 2. The measure features for each nucleus are the densitometric sum, the densitometric area and the densitometric standard deviation. The quantity of stain is determined based on the absorbance (Optical Density OD) evaluated by the transmitted light (T).

$$OD = log_{10}(1/T) \qquad (1)$$

As nuclear DNA stain is heterogeneous, a single point (OD) would not be representative. Thus it is necessary

Table 2 Descriptive statistics for Feulgen-DNA content and mean nuclear area

	Origin	Cell type	Nuclei Nr	Skewness	Kurtosis	DNA pg	SD	Mean µm²	SD	CV	SE	CI
1	Adult	Hard	137	0.4	-0.6	6.0	3.1	72.7	36.9	50.8 %	3.2	66.5–79.0
2	Adult	Soft	306	1.1	1.8	4.3	2.1	57.5	25.9	45.2 %	1.5	54.6–60.4
3	Adult	Soft	48	1.4	2.8	5.6	2.2	66.1	24.7	36.8 %	3.5	59.0–73.1
4	Adult	Soft	92	0.6	0.5	7.0	2.8	68.4	27.	40.4 %	2.9	62.7–74.1
5	Fetus	Hard	145	1.6	2.7	3.1	1.6	46.9	25.3	53.9 %	2.1	42.7–51.0
6	Fetus	Hard	46	1.5	1.7	1.7	0.9	31.4	16.8	53.5 %	2.5	26.4–36.3
7	Fetus	Soft	120	1.1	0.5	4.8	2.4	63.8	32.7	51.2 %	2.9	57.9–69.7
Total			894					59.2	30.2	51.1 %	1.0	57.2–61.2
cRBC	Control		339	-0.1	1.2	2.5[a]		25.9	5.9	22.6 %	0.3	25.3–26.5

SD standard deviation, CV coefficient of variation, SE standard error, CI confidence interval. Characteristics' of samples: 1, calcified atherosclerotic carotid; 2, soft atherosclerotic carotid; 3, healthy carotid; 4, abdominal aortic aneurism: 5, Femoral bone 11 weeks; 6, chondroid tissue 14 weeks; 7, fetal aorta 15 weeks
[a]Constant known quantity of DNA for the standard cRBC (the chicken red blood cells used as internal standards in each sample). Raw data are presented in the Additional file 1

to evaluate the whole nucleus as the integrated optical density (IOD):

$$IOD = \sum_{i=1}^{n} log_{10}(1/Ti) \qquad (2)$$

The scale of each image was 95.04 pixel/ μm^2. Additionally to nuclear IOD, the measured features were the nuclear area (μm^2) and the total number of nuclei evaluated.

Calculation of genome size DNA

To convert IOD in genome size in pg we used the primary standard of RBC (1 C = 1.25 pg). Smears were processed with the same way as samples and were included in each experiment. To calculate DNA content a standard curve (IOD *vs* known C-value) was generated and used to verify that the stain was accurate:

DNA pg per nuclei in sample = 2.5 pg / mean IOD standard
x IOD sample

Immunohistochemistry technique on Carnoy-fixed spread tissue

Table 3 summarizes the antibody characteristics and the blocking/antigen unmasking procedures used. Indeed, due to the Carnoy fixation, some modifications in the antigen retrieval procedures were optimized.

In addition to Von Kossa staining, immunostaining for Osteocalcin (OCN) was used to spot the main components of the bone matrix as well as the osteoblasts.

Samples were immunostained for Ki-67 antigen in order to assess the chromatin preservation after the procedure and the cell proliferation. Finally, in order to verify the preservation of specific cytoplasmic antigens, Desmin and Vimentin immunostaining was performed. Carnoy-fixed spread tissue was rehydrated through graded steps of ethanol absolute (100 %, Methanol 3 %

H_2O_2, 95 %, 70 %, H_2O). Endogenous peroxidase activity was neutralized with 3 % H_2O_2 in absolute methanol at room temperature (rt), in the dark. Antigen-antibody reaction was developed with the NovoLink® Polymer Detection Kit (Novocastra, Newcastle, UK). To reduce nonspecific antibody bindings, hydrophobic binding sites were blocked with Casein 0.4 % (Novolink Protein Block). Sections were incubated 1 h in a wet chamber at rt with the primary antibodies.

To detect primary antibody bound to tissue, sections were incubated with NovoLink® Polymer (8 mg/L) for 30 min at rt. Spreadings were further incubated with chromogen/substrate, 3,3 - diaminobenzidine NovoLink® (DAB pre-diluted 1:20), 30 s for fetal tissue and 2 min for adult tissue, at rt, Cell nuclei were counterstained with Mayer's haematoxylin (Sigma Chemicals). Fetal tissue was used as positive controls [12]. As negative controls primary antibodies were omitted. Washing steps were all performed with PBS. After dehydration in graded steps of ethanol, samples were mounted onto glass slides using Canada Balsam (Sigma-Aldrich C1795). The sections were observed under a light microscope (Axio Imager Z1 Zeiss, Germany) connected with a charge-coupled device (CCD) camera.

RNA content: RT-PCR
RNA extraction
The RNA was extracted from Carnoy fixed spread sections (monolayer). A commercial kit was used for RNA extraction (RNeasy® FFPE, Cat No. 73504, QIAGEN GmbH, Hilden, Germany); the protocol was slightly modified to increase RNA yield and purity. Spread tissue was recovered from the slides with a scalpel by adding 5 µl of Proteinase K buffer (PKD), under RNase free conditions. Retrieved tissues were combined into a single nuclease-free screw cap tube, dissolved in 245 µl of PKD and followed by centrifugation for 1 min at 10 000 rpm. For cell lysis, we added

Table 3 Technical characteristics of the antibodies used for imunohistochemistry

Antibodies	Type	Antigen specifications	Company	Locus-Clone	Dilution	Endogenous peroxidase blocking	Antigen unmasking treatment
Ki-67	Mouse Monoclonal	Perichromosomal layer protein. Identifies cells in G1-S-G2-M phases.	Dako A/S, Copenhagen, Denmark	10q26.2 MIB-1	1:100	20 min	Citrate Buffer, heat mediated (4 cycles 750 W, 5 min each)
Osteocalcin	Rabbit Polyclonal	Bone specific protein. Synthesized by osteoblasts, accumulates in the bone matrix.	Millipore USA	1p22	1:100	30 min	Tryton 0.5 % 4 min
Desmin	Mouse Monoclonal	Muscle specific intermediate filament type III protein.	Millipore USA	2q35 D33	1:100	20 min	Citrate Buffer, heat mediated (4 cycles 750 W, 5 min each)
Vimentin	Mouse Monoclonal	Intermediate filament type III protein expressed in mesenchymal cells.	Millipore USA	10p13 V9	1:80	20 min	Not required

20 μL of protease K; the mixture was incubated for 30 min at 56 °C, mixed at 850 rpm, and then incubated again at 80 °C for 15 min. The protocol was followed as stated by manufacturer's instruction. Finally the RNA was eluted in 22 μl of RNAse free-water, heated at 65 °C for 5 min in order to be denatured and to inactivate RNases, and stored at -80 °C until used. RNA integrity and concentration were measured by using an ND-1000 spectrophotometer (NanoDrop, Fisher Thermo, Wilmington, DE, USA). The ratio of the readings at 260 nm and 280 nm (A260/A280) provides an estimate of the purity of RNA with respect to the contaminants that absorb in the UV spectrum, such as protein. Pure RNA has an A260/A280 ratio of 1.9–2.1.

RT-PCR assay

To assess the possibility of extracting RNA from Carnoy-fixed spread tissue as template for retrotranscription and gene expression, we amplified by RT-PCR the housekeeping gene beta-glucuronidase (GUSB) for both femur bone and intestine. GUSB is considered an housekeeping gene required for the maintenance of basic cellular function and expressed in all cells [14].

We also amplified the transcription factor Osterix (OSX) essential for osteoblast differentiation and bone formation [15] and the carcinoembryonic antigen-related cell adhesion molecule 5 (CEACAM 5) normally produced in gastrointestinal tissue during fetal development [16].

The reverse transcription assay was performed using 2 μg of total RNA per 20 μl of mix, following the manufacturer's protocol (High capacity cDNA Archive kit, Applied Biosystem). The cDNA was stored at -20 °C until RT-PCR was performed. RT-PCR was carried out following MasterMix TaqMan® Protocol (TaqMan Univ PCR MasterMix, Applied Biosystems). Two μl of neat cDNA were amplified using specific probes for GUSB (NM_000181.3), CEACAM5 (NM_004363.2) and Osterix (NM_001173467.1) in the RT-PCR mix (TaqMan® Gene Expression Assay, Applied Biosystems, respective ID assay: Hs00939627_m1, Hs00237075_m1, Hs00541729_m1). Reactions were run on ABI PRISM 7900HT Sequence Detection System (Applied Biosystems). The cycling conditions were performed as follows: 10 min at 95 °C, 45 cycles at 95 °C for 15 s and 60 °C for 60 s. Each assay was carried out in triplicate and the transcription level was normalized using GUSB as a reference gene. The threshold was set at 0.2 in order to be in the exponential phase. The values were expressed as DCT (= > CT Target – CT GUSB).

Statistics

To present the basic features of the F-DNA analysis we used descriptive statistics: mean, standard deviation, coefficient of variation, standard error, confidence interval stated at 95 %, skewness and kurtosis. Differences in DNA content in pg and fluctuations of DNA (expressed as DNA content variation, DCV) [17] between samples were analysed with Kruskal-Wallis (non parametric-unmatched) and Dunn's post tests. The value of $P < 0.05$ was considered significant.

Results

Immunohistochemistry

Samples of all 41 tissues specifically including the 22 "hard" tissues containing calcified sections were satisfactorily spread for further analyses. Methods of decalcification, i.e. EDTA treatment, was required in tissue processed with the standard procedure but was not required in the spread method using collagenase.

The Fig. 1 compared the results obtained with EDTA treatment (Fig. 1a and b) *versus* collagenase digestion of a calcified carotid artery (Fig. 1d and e). Fig. 1a showed a Haematoxylin-Eosin section of calcified artery fixed in carnoy, embedded in paraffin and decalcified with EDTA. Precipitates of calcium were very basophilic so calcification areas were easily visible in violet (asterisk in Fig. 1). In the insert of figure A, we also noticed an empty area (white asterisk), where the calcified material was lost. Figure 1b showed the same tissue of Fig. 1a immunostained for osteocalcin. The Fig. 1c showed the standard section fixed in formalin, EDTA treated and stained for Osteocalcin, while Fig. 1d and e displays the same tissue treated with collagenase and stained for Osteocalcin. The immunohistochemistry (IHC) for Osteocalcin evidenced osteoblasts and synthesized matrix in the adult calcified artery (Fig. 1d and e). All fetal cases and two calcified adult cases showed multinucleated osteoclasts-like cells positive to Osteocalcin. Von Kossa histochemical stain evidenced the same calcified tissues in adult samples, but was negative in fetal samples, where no osteogenic calcification was present yet.

Antigen for cytoplasmic intermediates Desmin (Fig. 2) and Vimentin (not shown) were found in all preparations. Desmin and Vimentin showed a reliable positivity indicating that the collagenase digestion of samples and the other treatments did not damage the cytoplasmic intermediate filaments. Figure 2a and B show the good preservation of the smooth muscle cells expressing Desmin in the spread tissue. IHC for Ki-67 confirmed also the good preservation of the chromatin in the spread tissue (Fig. 3c-f). Surprisingly, Ki-67 was also detected in some cells in heavily calcified tissues: for example, case #1 (calcified atherosclerotic carotid, Fig. 3a) was described as acellular during routine IHC analysis by means of standard 2.5 μM sections. However, the monolayer IHC analysis revealed the presence of a heterogeneous population of cells (Fig. 3b), including Ki-67 positive cells (Fig. 3c and d). Mitotic figures were easily spotted with ki-67 staining (Fig. 3d). To verify the specificity of ki-67 staining in the spread artery, a tissue with

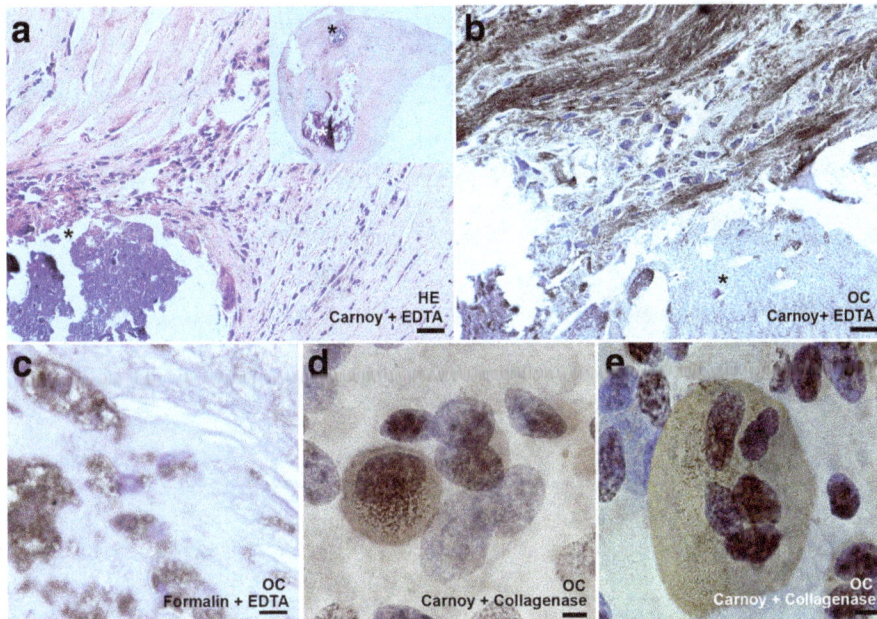

Fig. 1 Adult calcified carotid artery sections EDTA treated (**a-b-c**) and collagenase treated (**c-d**). **a** Haematoxylin-Eosin (HE) staining of a standard section fixed in carnoy and EDTA treated (scale bar 40 μm). The insert in figure **a** shows the whole arterial section with a diameter of 4 mm, * asterisks highlights the calcified areas. **b** osteocalcin immunostain of the same tissue fixed in carnoy (scale bar 20 μm) or (**c**) fixed in formalin (scale bar 10 μm). **d-e** Osteocalcin immunostaining of the collagenase treated tissue fixed in carnoy. **d** positive osteoblast and (**e**) positive osteoclast-like cells, scale bar 5 μm. Nucleus and cytoplasmatic structure are clearly visible in collagenase spread tissue compared to standard section (**a** and **b**)

a high rate of proliferative cells (fetal tissues) was selected and stained with ki-67 (Fig. 3e-f).

Nuclear DNA content of spread tissues

The Feulgen DNA quantification was performed in the 7 cases listed in Table 2: a total of 894 nuclei were evaluated for IOD and nuclear areas. Overall sample mean IOD was $2.3 \pm 1.3 \times 10^7$, overall mean nuclear area was 59.2 ± 30.2 μm^2. In the standard cRBC a total of 339 nuclei were examined: mean IOD was $1.2 \pm 0.3 \times 10^7$, mean nuclear area was 25.9 ± 5.9 μm^2. Feulgen absolute

DNA content was successfully calculated in all 7 cases, both soft and hard tissues. In particular, the heavily calcified carotid artery lesion (case #1), had a mean DNA quantity of 6.0 pg, concomitant with the known DNA diploid content of human cells (2C = 6 pg) (Fig. 4a, Table 2). Kurtosis and skewness analysis showed that samples had a unimodal, near-Gaussian distribution of the diploid F-DNA (2C) (Table 2, Fig. 4a). The nuclear size was directly proportional to the DNA content of the cells in the 7 cases. Indeed, Fig. 4b shows that the quantity of DNA within each cell of the calcified carotid

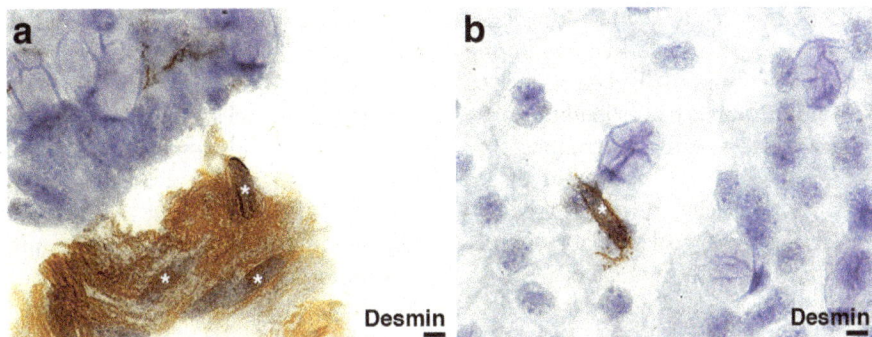

Fig. 2 Desmin IHC staining in spread fetal tissue. **a** group of desmin positive smooth muscle cells (SMC) and (**b**) a single SMC in the fetal bowel crypts. *SMC are indicated by a white asterisk and showed the typical elongated "cigar-shaped" nuclei. The SMC along the crypts show a moderate to strong cytoplasmatic staining reaction, scale bar 10 μm

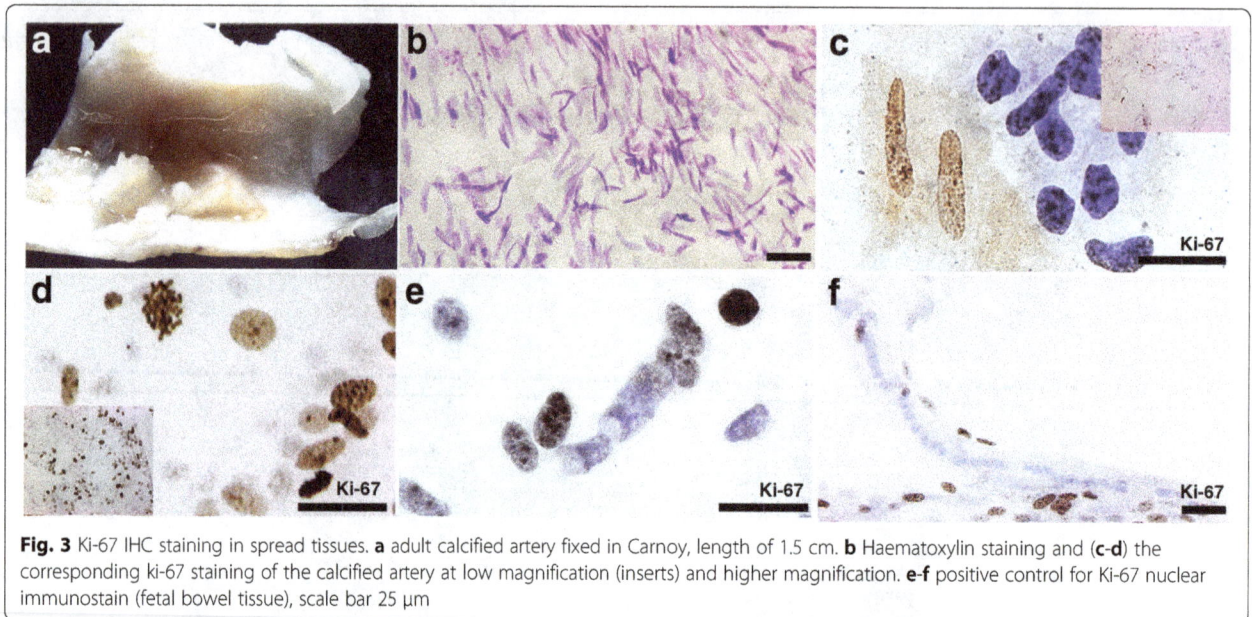

Fig. 3 Ki-67 IHC staining in spread tissues. **a** adult calcified artery fixed in Carnoy, length of 1.5 cm. **b** Haematoxylin staining and (**c-d**) the corresponding ki-67 staining of the calcified artery at low magnification (inserts) and higher magnification. **e-f** positive control for Ki-67 nuclear immunostain (fetal bowel tissue), scale bar 25 μm

artery (#1) was significantly proportional to the area of the nucleus ($R^2 = 0.97$, Pearson correlation $p < 0.0001$). This means that there is a good preservation of the nuclear structures also in the heavily calcified tissues after the procedure.

Adult and fetal tissues showed a significant DNA content variation (DCV, Table 2) within cells, except for DNA content in soft healthy adult arteries (#3, 5.6 pg, CV 36.8 %) compared to DNA content in fetal aortic cells (#7, 4.8 pg, CV 51.2 %). Both samples contained a homogenous population of smooth muscle cells. Of note, soft tissue from healthy carotid arteries #3 had the lowest adult CV (5.6 pg, 36.8 %). DCV significantly differs between pathological atherosclerotic soft arteries (45.2 %) and calcified arteries (50.8 %). Highest DCV were found in all fetal tissues (range 51.2 to 53.9 %).

In particular, two cases showed significant unexpected lower mean DNA content per nucleus compared to adult samples; case #5 (fetal femoral bone) with 3.1 ± 1.6 pg and case #6 (chondroid tissue) with 1.7 ± 0.9 pg ($p < 0.0001$, Table 2, Fig. 4c). In those cases we decided to perform detailed analyses of the DNA in each single cell composing the tissues (the AxioVision software marked each nucleus with a single identification number corresponding to its IOD). We noticed that case #5 was mainly composed of osteoclasts and case #6 of syncytia (Fig. 4d and e). By measuring the DNA content per nucleus we observed unexpected results. Nuclei outside osteoclasts and syncytial formations showed a constant DNA content of 6 pg. In osteoclasts, DNA content per nucleus ranged from 2 to 3 pg. In the syncytia formations, nucleus showed a DNA content ranging from 1 to 2 pg per nucleus. Surprisingly the mean DNA content per syncytium (sum of nuclear DNA nucleus in the whole syncytia) was 6.6 ± 1.4 pg.

RNA preservation (RT-PCR)

Additionally to the housekeeping gene GUSB, we evaluated the expression of CEA for intestinal fetal tissue and Osterix for calcified/osteogenic tissues. The total mean extracted mRNA from fetal intestine tissue (FI) and femur bone (FB) was 7374 ng and 1430 ng respectively. A260/A280 ratio was 1.94 for both fetal intestine and fetal bone showing the absence of contamination of the RNA extracted (standard ratio range from 1.9 to 2.1). The mean threshold cycle (CT) values of endogenous control GUSB were 30.34 ± 0.18 in FI and 37.34 ± 0.24 in FB. Mean CT for tested gene OSX and CEA were 38.52 ± 0.10 and 35.34 ± 0.31 respectively. ΔCT CEA and ΔCT OSX were 5.02 and 1.18 respectively (Table 4).

Additional cellular component observed in arteries

Figure 5a shows a standard histological staining of the carotid plaques section (#1); of note the rupture of the endothelium (marked with an asterisk) and the presence of extensive calcification. However, the spread of the same sample (#1) allowed the identifications of a disclosed and complex cellular content. Besides the majority of the cells that have a spindle shaped nucleus (Fig. 3b), cells with a particular balloon shaped nucleus were identified in the calcified carotid plaque (in 2 cases, Fig. 5b and c). Also, we noticed that Ki-67 antigen stained some of the metakaryotic nuclei in the mononuclear forms (data not shown). The same cells were also arranged in a tubular form that reminds syncytial structure (Fig. 5d). In syncytium, Ki-67 highlighted only the cells located in the extremities (Fig. 3e and f) and nuclei inside syncytia were negative to Ki-67. This type of cells, named metakaryotic cells [12], with a typical

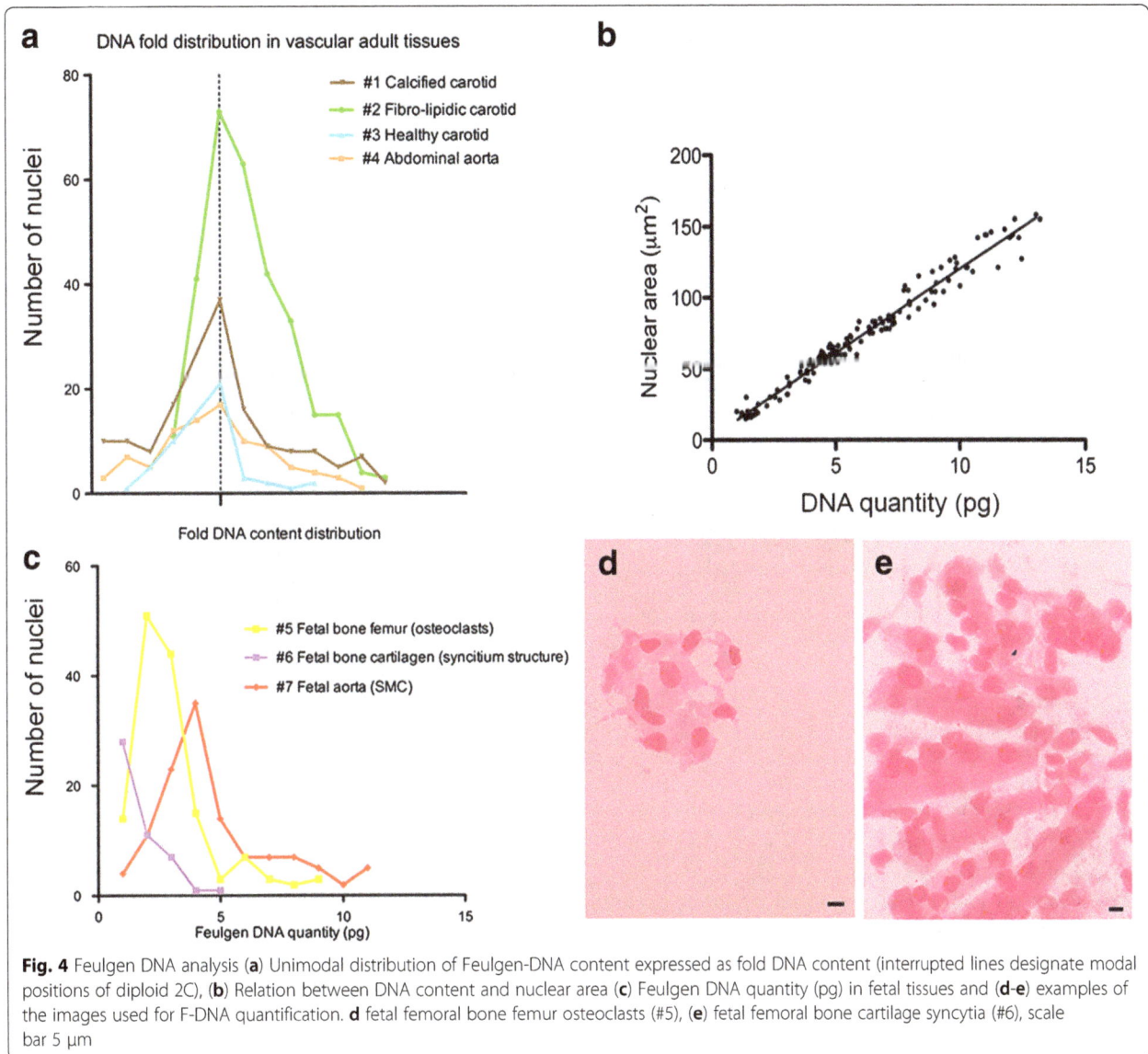

Fig. 4 Feulgen DNA analysis (**a**) Unimodal distribution of Feulgen-DNA content expressed as fold DNA content (interrupted lines designate modal positions of diploid 2C), (**b**) Relation between DNA content and nuclear area (**c**) Feulgen DNA quantity (pg) in fetal tissues and (**d-e**) examples of the images used for F-DNA quantification. **d** fetal femoral bone femur osteoclasts (#5), (**e**) fetal femoral bone cartilage syncytia (#6), scale bar 5 μm

Table 4 Threshold cycle (Ct) values for GUSB, OSX and CEA in fetal tissues

Micro-dissected sample	Threshold cycle values		
	β-glucuronidase GUSB	Osterix OSX	Carcino-embryonic antigen CEA
Fetal femur bone 12w	37.06	38.42	-
	37.50	38.63	
	37.45	38.51	
Fetal intestine 9w	30.03	-	35.70
	30.32		35.15
	30.37		35.17

hollow bell-shaped nucleus, was found in our study in all fetal tissues both in the syncytial form (Fig. 5d) and in the mononuclear form (Fig. 5e) while in the adult arteries, these cells were spotted in 6 cases.

Discussion

The spreading technique showed a good reproducibility and accuracy in the evaluation of cell protein expression and single-cell DNA content in calcified carotid arteries. The IHC markers were selected in order to check the integrity of the different cellular compartments: nucleus (Ki-67) and cytoplasm (Desmin, Vimentin, Osteocalcin). To verify the reliability of the techniques we used fetal tissues sample as positive control since this tissue was already validated [12]. As standard for the Feulgen DNA quantification we chose cRBC, since they are convenient, easy to isolate and they have a constant known DNA

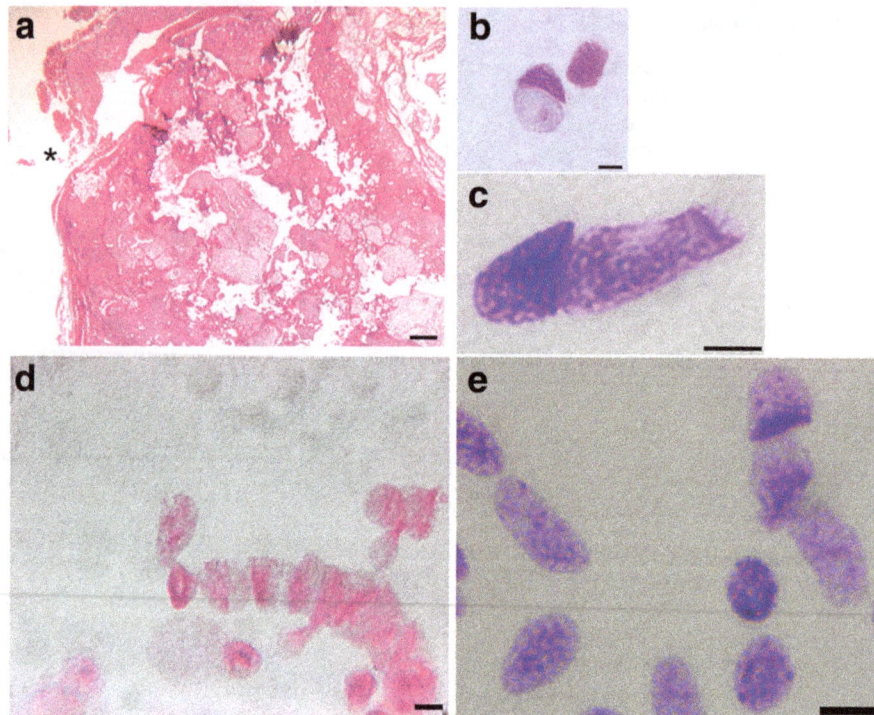

Fig. 5 Standard 2.5 μm sections and collagenase spread of calcified tissues. **a** Haematoxylin-Eosin staining of adult calcified carotid arteries, scale bar 400 μm. **b-c** Feulgen staining of spread tissue of adult calcified carotid arteries showing examples of metakaryotic nuclei. **d-e** Feulgen staining of spread tissues showing nuclei in syncytium (fetal femoral tissue), scale bar 5 μm

content [18, 19]. Our results confirmed the reliability of the standard as cRBC genome size was proportional to the area of the cells and CV% was low (23 %). The digestion times with collagenase requested by the spreading technique varied considerably according to the different tissues (see Table 1). Nevertheless, the adult and fetal DNA content distribution curves were all Gaussian with the same trend, showing that collagenase did not influence the DNA content, regardless the digestion times. The Carnoy-fixed spread tissue also allows to extract preserved RNA, without any contaminations by proteins or phenols, and the sigmoid-shaped curves obtained at RT-PCR showed a typical PCR gene amplification.

The technique could also give new information regarding the study of calcification and osteogenesis. Usually DNA quantity is evaluated in the whole tissue; unfortunately one disadvantage is the loss of information on the single cell profile. Moreover standard decalcification procedures degrade the DNA content in calcified arteries. First this protocol avoids the use of formalin to fix the arteries and also avoids the use of strong acid to decalcify the arteries. This allows extracting directly from the slides of spread tissue the RNA and DNA and evaluates the gene expression in calcified tissues from a very small quantity of sample. Moreover the protocol preserved the morphology of the nucleus and allowed the visualization of the nuclear organization. As already

reported, some cases of atherosclerotic carotid tissues contain bone lacunae-like mature structure in development with lamellar bone. In these cases, the protocol is of great help to open the "core" of the bone structure and visualize the cellular content. It is very difficult with the standard histological techniques to obtain a monolayer of cells. Surprisingly our data revealed and confirmed that the calcified part of arteries contains a heterogeneous population of cells composed by smooth muscle cells, osteoclasts-like cells and osteoblasts. Moreover the IHC revealed that some of the cells, composing the core of the calcification, were actively dividing. The observation is in line with other studies suggesting that arterial calcification is an active process [5].

Feulgen on calcified arteries spread allows spotting the peculiarity of the single cell. For example, we observed that two cases of fetal bone (#5 and #6) showed the lowest DNA absolute quantities. By reviewing the literature only a few groups spotted this paradox in DNA content. Solari et al. reported that osteoclasts undergo amitotic division by a budding mechanism in vitro [20]. Then Sundaram in 2004 demonstrated the existence of a set of cells dividing through neosis [21] and in 2014, Thilly et al. showed that the cells in syncytia divide by an amitotic mechanism with a dsRNA/DNA intermediate [22]. As Feulgen only stains DNA and not RNA [11, 13] we can hypothesize that the nuclei in the syncytia of fetal bone tissue undergo dsRNA/DNA intermediate during replication, thus explaining the lower mean quantity of DNA (1 pg to 3 pg) and the negativity to Ki-67.

Of fluctuations of DNA, defined as an increased range of DNA content, were observed both in the cell populations and within the single cells. The lowest CV variation was found in the healthy soft sample (#3) characterized by a homogenous population of SMC. Conversely the major CV in adult tissue was counted in the calcified tissue. This is likely to reflect a heterogeneous cell population in the fetal and adult pathologic tissues, compared to the cytological homogeneity of the smooth muscle cells in healthy arteries.

In conclusion, thanks to the preservation of the nuclear morphology the technique allowed to disclose osteoclasts-like cells and others cells type with a bell-shaped nucleus, recognised as metakaryotic cells [23]. These particular cells are very difficult to identify due to the loss of nuclear morphology when using strong acid for decalcification. Mainly studied in the progression of tumours [12], we can hypothesis that these cells are also a key player in atherosclerosis [24].

Conclusion

The spread gently preserves the original morphology of each single cell in the calcified vascular tissues. The presented protocol will be used to study the calcification or osteogenic process occurring during atherosclerosis and to evaluate the single cell DNA content on a large series of calcified plaques. The opportunity to extract and amplify intact nucleic acid from the cells of heavily calcified arteries opens the possibility to study calcification on a larger scale. This is not doable when arteries are treated with decalcification reagents.

Abbreviations
CEACAM 5, carcinoembryonic antigen-related cell adhesion molecule 5; cRBC, chicken red blood cells; CT, threshold cycle; CV, content variation; DCV, DNA content variation; EDTA, ethylenediaminetetraacetic acid; F-DNA, Feulgen DNA; GUSB, beta-glucuronidase; HCl, chloride acid; IOD, the integrated optical density; OCN, osteoclacin; OD, optical density; OSX, osterix; PKD, proteinase K buffer; RT, room temperature

Acknowledgements
Research at MIT (SF, EVG, WGT) was supported by a grant from United Therapeutics Corporation (UTC) (www.unither.com), Silver Springs Md, USA, to study metakaryotic biology under MIT No. 6915390.

Funding
United Therapeutics Corporation.

Authors' contributions
SF, AD, EVG, GP designed the experiments, performed the experiments, analysed the data and wrote the paper. RP, MG, AS, EVG, WGT designed the experiments, selected and provided the samples. SF and FV analysed the data and wrote the paper. SF, FV, WGT interpreted the data and revised paper. EVG, AS and FA provided the samples, analyzed the data and revised the paper. EVG and GP revised the paper. critically. All authors read and approved the final manuscript.

Competing interest
The authors declare they have no competing interests.

References
1. Karwowski W, Naumnik B, Szczepański M, Myśliwiec M. The mechanism of vascular calcification – a systematic review. Med Sci Monit. 2012;18(1):RA1–11.
2. Demer LL, Tintut Y. Vascular calcification: pathobiology of a multifaceted disease. Circulation. 2008;117:2938–48.
3. Pal SN, Golledge J. Osteo-progenitors in vascular calcification: a circulating cell theory. J Atheroscler Thromb. 2001;18:551–9.
4. Vasuri F, Fittipaldi S, Pasquinelli G. Arterial calcification: Finger-pointing at resident and circulating stem cells. World J Stem Cells. 2014;6(5):540–51.
5. Vengrenyuk Y, Carlier S, Xanthos S, Cardoso L, Ganatos P, Virmani R, Einav S, Gilchrist L, Weinbaum S. A hypothesis for vulnerable plaque rupture due to stress-induced debonding around cellular microcalcifications in thin fibrous caps. Proc Natl Acad Sci USA. 2006;103:14678–83.
6. Nandalur KR, Baskurt E, Hagspiel KD, Phillips CD, Kramer CM. Calcified carotid atherosclerotic plaque is associated less with ischemic symptoms than is noncalcified plaque on MDCT. AJR Am J Roentgenol. 2005;184(1):295–8.
7. Vasuri F, Fittipaldi S, Pini R, Degiovanni A, Mauro R, D'Errico-Grigioni A, Faggioli G, Stella A, Pasquinelli G. Diffuse calcifications protect carotid plaques regardless of the amount of neoangiogenesis and related histological complications. J Biomed Biotechnol January. 2015;8.
8. Sarsfield P, Wickham CL, Joyner MV, Ellard S, Jones DB, Wilkins BS. Formic acid decalcification of bone marrow trephines degrades DNA: alternative use of EDTA allows the amplification and sequencing of relatively long PCR products. Mol Pathol. 2000;53(6):336.
9. Prasad P, Donoghue M. A comparative study of various decalcification techniques. Indian J Dent Res. 2013;24(3):302–8.
10. Hatta H, Tsuneyama K, Nomoto K, Hayashi S, Miwa S, Nakajima T, Nishida T, Nakanishi Y, Imura J. A simple and rapid decalcification procedure of skeletal tissues for pathology using an ultrasonic cleaner with D-mannitol and formic acid. Acta Histochem. 2014;116(5):753–7.
11. Mello MLS. Cytochemistry of DNA, RNA and nuclear proteins. Braz J Genet. 1997;20(2):257–64.
12. Gostjeva EV, Zukerberg L, Chung D, Thilly WG. Bell-shaped nuclei dividing by symmetrical and asymmetrical nuclear fission have qualities of stem cells in human colonic embryogenesis and carcinogenesis. Cancer Genet Cytogenet. 2006;164:16–24.
13. Kasten FH. The chemistry of Schiff's reagent. Int Rev Cytol. 1960;10:1–100.
14. Naz H, Islam A, Waheed A, Sly WS, Ahmad F, Hassan I. Human β-glucuronidase: structure, function, and application in enzyme replacement therapy. Rejuvenation Res. 2013;16(5):352–63.
15. Baek WY, Lee MA, Jung JW, Kim SY, Akiyama H, de Crombrugghe B, Kim JE. Positive regulation of adult bone formation by osteoblast-specific transcription factor osterix. J Bone Miner Res. 2009;24(6):1055–65.
16. Han SU, Kwak TH, Her KH, Cho YH, Choi C, Lee HJ, Hong S, Park YS, Kim YS, Kim TA, Kim SJ. CEACAM5 and CEACAM6 are major target genes for Smad3-mediated TGF-beta signaling. Oncogene. 2008;27(5):675–83.
17. Westra JW, Rivera RR, Bushman DM, Yung YC, Peterson SE, Barral S, Chun J. Neuronal DNA content variation (DCV) with regional and individual differences in the human brain. J Comp Neurol. 2010;518(19):3981–4000.
18. Bloch D, Beaty N, Fu CT, Chin E, Smith J, Pipkin Jr JL. Flow-cytometric analysis of chicken red blood cells. J Histochem Cytochem. 1978;26(3):170–86.
19. Hardie DC, Gregory TR, Hebert PD. From pixels to picograms: a beginners' guide to genome quantification by Feulgen image analysis densitometry. J Histochem Cytochem. 2002;50(6):735–49.
20. Solari F, Domenget C, Gire V, Woods C, Lazarides E, Rousset B, Jurdic P. Multinucleated cells can continuously generate mononucleated cells in the absence of mitosis: a study of cells of the avian osteoclast lineage. J Cell Sci. 1995;108(Pt 10):3233–41.
21. Sundaram M, Guernsey DL, Rajaraman MM, Rajaraman R. Neosis: a novel type of cell division in cancer. Cancer Biol Ther. 2004;3(2):207–18.
22. Thilly WG, Gostjeva EV, Koledova VV, Zukerberg LR, Chung D, Fomina JN, Darroudi F, Stollar BD. Metakaryotic stem cell nuclei use pangenomic dsRNA/DNA intermediates in genome replication and segregation. Organogenesis. 2014;10(1):44–52.

23

Comparison of a microsphere-based platform with a multiplex flow cytometric assay for determination of circulating cytokines in the mouse

Alain Stricker-Krongrad*, Catherine Shoemake, Miao Zhong, Jason Liu and Guy Bouchard

Abstract

Background: Measuring expression profiles of inflammatory biomarkers is important in monitoring the polarization of immune responses; therefore, results should be independent of quantitation methods if they are to be accepted as validated clinical pathology biomarkers. To evaluate effects of differing quantitation methods, the seven major circulating Th1/Th2/Th17 cytokines interleukin 2 (IL-2), interferon γ (IFN-γ), tumor necrosis factor α (TNF-α), IL-4, IL-6, IL-10 and IL-17A were quantified in plasma of lipopolysaccharide (LPS)-treated mice with two different multiplex platforms.

Methods: Female C57BL6 mice were treated orally with vehicle or dexamethasone, followed by LPS intravenously. Plasma samples were analyzed 0.5, 1, 2, 4, and 6 h post-LPS challenge with assays at Myriad-RBM and compared to assays performed on a BD Accuri C6 flow cytometer.

Results: IL-17A response to LPS was limited but sustained, and the response for the remaining cytokines were early and transient; dexamethasone reduced expression of all 7 cytokines. TNF-α and IL-6 levels were similar across both assays, and IL-4 levels were generally very low. Plasma levels of remaining cytokines were variably lower with BD assays than Myriad-RBM assays.

Conclusions: The present findings demonstrate that quantitation of circulating biomarkers of inflammation can be achieved using multiplexed flow cytometry, but careful consideration must be taken for assay validation when cross-referencing with another multiplexed assay.

Background

A number of cytokines, such as interleukin 2 (IL-2), interferon γ (IFN-γ), tumor necrosis factor α (TNFα), IL-4, IL-6, IL-17A and IL-10, become elevated in tissues in response to inflammation. These cytokines are also key regulators of immune responses and elevations of these different cytokines are individually associated with responses of specific T helper cell (Th) lineages. IFN-γ, IL-2, and TNFα are associated with the Th1 response. IL-4, IL-6 and IL-10 are associated with the Th2 response. IL-6 and IL-17A are associated with the Th17 response. Since these variabilities exist, measuring expression profiles of these cytokines is important to monitor the polarization of the immune response.

Lipopolysaccharide (LPS) administration reliably induces an acute inflammation that is associated with increases of a number of inflammatory cytokines in the peripheral blood of LPS-treated animals [1]. Additionally, dexamethasone (DEX) administration inhibits the effects of LPS on cytokine synthesis in animal models [2]. These properties of LPS and DEX can then be used for evaluation of anti-inflammatory drug effects or, as in the present case, comparison and validation of cytokine identification and quantitation methods. The objective of the present study was to implement and validate bench top flow cytometry for the ex vivo quantitation of circulating cytokine levels in multiplex assay formats.

* Correspondence: astricker@sinclairresearch.com
Sinclair Research Center, LLC, 562 State Rd. DD, Auxvasse, MO 65231, USA

Cytokine quantitation was performed on a Becton Dickson (BD) Accuri C6 flow cytometer, and results were compared to those produced by a commercial biomarker testing laboratory performing rodent multi-analyte profile (MAP) assays.

Methods

Test system

Female C57BL/6 mice, approximately 6–9 weeks of age and weighing 17–20 g, were purchased from Charles River Laboratories. The mice were housed 2–3 per cage in shoebox cages in a room with temperature maintained between 64 and 80 °F (18–29 °C) and with a 12-h light/12-h dark photoperiod. The animals had ad libitum access to Harlan Teklad Global Rodent Diet 2018 and deep well water. All study procedures were reviewed and approved by Sinclair Research Center's Institutional Animal Care and Use Committee. Housing and animal care conformed to the guidelines of the Guide for the Care and Use of Laboratory Animals, 8th edition published by the U.S. National Institutes of Health and to applicable institutional standard operating procedures. Euthanasias were performed in accordance with the American Veterinary Medical Association's published guidelines [3].

After being acclimated for 3 days, mice were randomized into groups with 6 mice in the untreated group, 32 mice in a group treated with LPS, and 32 mice in a group treated with LPS plus DEX. Identification of each animal was maintained using ear notches and cage cards.

Methyl cellulose, DEX, and LPS were obtained from Sigma-Aldrich (St Louis, Missouri). Methyl cellulose was dissolved in sterile water (Hospira, Lake Forest, Illinois) overnight to form a 0.5% solution for use as the vehicle. DEX was suspended overnight in 0.5% methyl cellulose at a concentration of 0.5 mg/mL and then sonicated briefly before dosing. LPS was prepared the day before dosing in 0.9% saline for injection (Hospira) at a concentration of 0.04 mg/mL.

Mice in the untreated group were bled for plasma without any treatment. Mice in the LPS treatment group were administered 0.5% methyl cellulose at 10 mL/kg via oral gavage, and then were treated 1.5 h later with 0.2 mg/kg LPS intravenously (IV) at a volume of 5 mL/kg. The LPS plus DEX groups were administered 5 mg/kg dexamethasone via oral gavage, and then underwent the same IV LPS treatment as above 1.5 h later. Six to eight mice from each treatment group were bled for plasma at 0.5, 1, 2, 4, and 6 h following LPS challenge.

Plasma preparation and analysis

All blood samples were collected into K_2EDTA tubes (0.5 mL, Greiner Bio-One North America, Inc. Monroe, North Carolina). Filled tubes were placed on wet ice and were processed within 30 min after blood collections.

The samples were centrifuged at 3000 rpm for 15 min at 4 °C; plasma was then drawn off and placed into separate vials. Plasma samples were separated into two sets and placed on dry ice and stored at –70 °C before being analyzed for cytokine profiles.

One set of plasma samples were shipped on dry ice to Myriad RBM, Inc. (Austin, TX) for cytokine profiling with Mouse Cytokine Panels A & B (4-h time point) and Rodent MAP V3.0 Antigen (0.5-, 1, 2, and 6-h time points) assays (based on a Multiplexed Luminex Platform).

Seven cytokines (IL-2, IFN-γ, TNFα, IL-4, IL-6, IL-17A, and IL-10) were analyzed at the 2- and 4- h time points in the second set of collected plasma samples with a cytometric bead array (CBA) mouse Th1/Th2/Th17 cytokine kit (BD Biosciences) on a BD Accuri C6 flow cytometer. The CBA Mouse Th1/Th2/Th17 Cytokine Kit Manual (BD Biosciences) was followed for the assay procedure. Plasma samples were thawed at room temperature and then placed on wet ice for duration of analysis. One vial of mixed standards was freshly reconstituted in 2.0 mL of assay diluent, and then was serial diluted. The concentrations of standards for each cytokine were 0, 20, 40, 80, 156, 312.5, 625, 1250, 2500, and 5000 pg/mL. Seven types of cytokine capture beads were freshly mixed in equal amounts (10 µL bead per assay tube) in a master tube. To perform the assay, 50 µL of the mixed beads were incubated with 50 µL of standards or samples along with 50 µL of Phycoerythrin (PE) Detection Reagent in a MultiScreen filter plate (1.2 µm pore size, EMD Millipore, Darmstadt, Germany) at room temperature for 2 h. At the end of incubation, the plate was drained on a vacuum manifold. The beads in each of the individual wells of the plate were resuspended in 120 µL of wash buffer, and were then analyzed on the BD Accuri C6 flow cytometer. The seven distinct fluorescence beads were sorted with fluorescence signals captured in FL4 channel. PE intensity of individual beads was captured in FL2 channel. Approximately 200 events for each bead group were acquired (based on experience in generating data in previous experiments). The acquired data were subsequently analyzed for individual cytokine concentrations in each sample using the FCAP Array software (BD Biosciences).

Results for the 7 cytokines IL-2, IFN-γ, TNFα, IL-4, IL-6, IL-17A, and IL-10 were compared between BD Biosciences and Myriad RBM assays. Concentrations for individual cytokines were expressed as mean ± standard deviation. Effects of DEX on LPS-induced plasma cytokine changes were evaluated with a two-way student t-test.

Results

Levels of the selected cytokines in plasma of normal mice

For flow cytometry using BD CBA, a set of mixed standards for the 7 cytokines (IL-2, IFN-γ, TNF-α, IL-4, IL-6,

IL-17A and IL-10) were freshly prepared with serial dilution. When recombinant standards were diluted in normal mouse plasma, the data showed that each of the 7 cytokines was quantitated in the linear range between the expected concentrations of 20–5000 pg/mL. Circulating concentrations of the same cytokines were measured in 6 untreated normal mouse plasma samples. None of the 7 cytokines could be detected or quantified with the CBA or the Myriad RBM assays in the normal plasma, indicating that the background of cytokine levels were below the lower limit of detection.

Time-course of cytokines stimulation after LPS administration

The pharmacodynamics effects of LPS on Th1/Th2/Th17 circulating cytokines as quantitated with the Myriad RBM Assay are indicated in Table 1. After acute IV administration of 0.2 mg/kg LPS in mice, classical stimulatory responses were observed with a TNF-α peak at 1–2 h, followed by peaks of IFN-γ, IL-10 and IL-6 at 2 h, and gradual decline over the following 4 h. [4]. These time course data were used to select two critical time points, 2- and 4-h post LPS stimulation, to conduct further comparative analyses of the two analytical methods.

Comparative levels of the selected cytokines in plasma of LPS treated mice

For flow cytometry using BD CBA, the 7 cytokines were detected in diluted plasma for the 2-h samples and in undiluted plasma for the 4-h samples. IL-2 and IL-4 were below the lower limit of detection (LLOD) in both 2- and 4- h samples (data not shown). IL-17A was detectable only in the 4-h samples, but was below the lower limit of quantification (LLOQ). The other 4 cytokines (IFN-γ, TNF, IL-6, and IL-10) were detected within the defined concentration ranges. IL-6 was the only cytokine that needed to be quantitated in the diluted plasma. It was shown that 10× dilution was appropriate for the 2-h samples and 5× dilution potentially for the 4-h samples. Variations in concentrations of cytokines were consistent and acceptable when

determined in diluted plasma samples with BD CBA assay. Minimum required dilution was evaluated at the 2-h time point since the linear range of the BD CBA assay was limited to 20–5000 pg/mL. Coefficient of variations for dilutions of IL-10, TNF-α, and IL-6 were 12.5%, 11.2%, and 11.1% respectively in the LPS treated samples, and were 2.5%, 5.5%, and 6.2% respectively in the LPS plus DEX treated samples (Table 2).

In the Myriad RBM platform, while LPS was shown to increase plasma TNF-α to similar levels in both 2- and 4- h samples (Table 3), DEX had much weaker inhibition in 4-h samples than in 2-h samples (Table 4). Plasma IFN-γ was increased as previously reported [1] following LPS challenge in the Myriad RBM assays, while an increase did not occur in the BD CBA assay (Tables 3 and 4). IL-10 was quantified at lower plasma levels with a less potent inhibition of DEX in BD CBA assay than in Myriad-RBM assay.

In a comparison of both the Myriad RBM and BD Biosciences multiplex platforms, DEX was shown to inhibit plasma concentrations of IFN-γ, TNF-α, IL-6, and IL-10 in both 2- and 4- h samples. A similar inhibitory effect of DEX was also observed for IL-17A in the 4-h samples. However, variations were observed between the two assay platforms in terms of cytokine concentrations, time course effects of LPS, and magnitudes of DEX inhibition. IL-6 was the only cytokine that was detected comparably with Myriad-RBM assays and BD CBA assay, as demonstrated by the direct relationship between the two assays (Fig. 1).

Discussion

Plasma TNF-α has previously been shown to peak at 1 h post-LPS challenge and then to gradually decrease over time in treated mice [5]. In the BD CBA assay, a similar LPS effect on TNF-α was observed in the 2- and 4- h plasma samples, and the DEX inhibitions were comparable between the 2- and 4- h plasma samples. In the Myriad-RBM platform, while LPS was shown to increase plasma TNF-α to similar levels in both the 2- and 4- h samples, DEX had much weaker inhibition in the 4-h

Table 1 Time Course Effects of LPS on Th1/Th2/Th17 Cytokine Plasma Levels in LPS-Treated Mice Quantitated with Myriad Assay

Cytokines	Time post-LPS exposure				
	0.5[a] Hours	1.0[a] Hours	2.0[a] Hours	4.0[b] Hours	6.0[a] Hours
IL-2 (pg/mL)	–	–	245	68	–
IL-4 (pg/mL)	–	–	–	80	–
IL-6 (pg/mL)	176	4597	24,667	2936	1066
IL-10 (pg/mL)	697	5013	7717	3878	1646
IL-17A (ng/mL)	–	0.025	0.083	0.080	0.031
INF-γ (pg/mL)	–	447	1347	287	341
TNF-α (ng/mL)	0.22	1.82	0.42	0.40	0.15

[a] n = 6, [b] n = 8

Table 2 Quantitation of Circulating IL-6, IL-10, & TNF-α in Diluted 2-Hour Plasma Samples with the BD CBA Assay

Cytokines	Treatments							
	LPS				LPS + Dexamethasone			
	10× dilution	5× dilution	2× dilution	%CV[a]	10× dilution	5× dilution	2× dilution	%CV[a]
IL-6 (pg/mL)	33,926	39,860	32,419	11.1	10,537	11,032	11,906	6.2
IL-10 (pg/mL)	344	426	435	12.5	351	342	334	2.5
TNF-α (ng/mL)	1.8	2.2	2.3	11.2	0.2	0.2	0.3	5.5

[a]%CV = coefficient of variation

samples than in the 2-h samples. Therefore, this would suggest that the BD CBA assay was more accurate in measuring biologically-relevant TNF levels than Myriad RBM assays. In addition, this is supported by the lack of direct relationship between the two assays as illustrated in Fig. 2.

Plasma IFN-γ was shown to increase through 4 h post-LPS challenge in treated mice [1]. A similar LPS effect on IFN-γ was observed in the 2- and 4- h plasma samples with the BD CBA assay, whereas an opposite trend for the IFN-γ secretion was observed in the same samples with the Myriad RBM assays.

Plasma IL-10 was quantified at lower levels in the BD CBA assay than in Myriad RBM assays. DEX was shown to be less potent to inhibit IL-10 with BD CBA assay than with Myriad RBM assays. No other differences were found for IL-10 quantification between the two assay platforms, although the relationship between the two assays was weak (Fig. 3). LPS and DEX are frequently used in rodent studies evaluating various inflammatory diseases, responses, and chemical or medical agents. Their respective effects and responses in various scenarios have been described in publications such as those by NO Al-Harbi, F Imam, MM Al-Harbi, MA Ansari, KM Zoheir, HM Korashy, MM Sayed-Ahmed, SM Attia, OA Shabanah and SF Ahmad [6].

In the BD CBA assay, the time course effect of LPS on plasma TNF-α was consistent with what was previously

reported [5], and the DEX inhibitions were comparable between the 2- and 4- h plasma samples. Reproducible circulating IL-6 was obtained for plasma samples of the LPS treated mice with the assays from both Myriad-RBM and BD Biosciences. IL-6 was the only cytokine that was quantified comparably between the BD CBA and the Myriad-RBM assays, and also the only cytokine that needed be quantitated in diluted plasma when using the BD CBA assay, an indication of a high level of stimulation. IL-4 was the signature Th2 cytokine [7] which was supposed to not be induced by LPS treatment. The lack of signal in IL-4 quantification with BD CBA assay reflected the specificity of this kit in IL-4 measurement.

The BD CBA cytokine assay was not as sensitive as the Myriad RBM assays in detecting and quantitating circulating IL-2, IL-10, and IL-17A levels in the LPS treated mice, but was more biologically-accurate in measuring circulating IL-4, TNF-α, and IFN-γ levels. Differences and similarities between these two assays may relate to the format of these multiplexed assays but also to the nature of the immunological reagents used to capture and detect these cytokines. Although unknown at this time, it is quite possible that the antibodies used for the two assay platforms are identical when IL-6 is considered and different when TNF-α and IL-10 are measured.

There are well-accepted methods for the validation of biomarkers [8, 9], although some form of consensus

Table 3 Concentrations of the Circulating Th1/Th2/Th17 Cytokines in LPS-Treated Mice Quantitated with Myriad and BD CBA Assays

Cytokines	Time post-LPS exposure			
	2 h		4 h	
	Myriad	BD CBA	Myriad	BD CBA
IL-2 (pg/mL)	245	–	68	–
IL-4 (pg/mL)	–	–	80	–
IL-6 (pg/mL)	24,667	35,402	2935	5925
IL-10 (pg/mL)	7717	402	3878	238
IL-17A (ng/mL)	0.083	–	0.080	–
INF-γ (pg/mL)	1347	0.8	287	41
TNF-α (ng/mL)	0.42	2.09	0.40	0.35

Table 4 Concentrations of the Circulating Th1/Th2/Th17 Cytokines in LPS plus Dexamethasone-Treated Mice Quantitated with Myriad and BD CBA Assays

Cytokines	Time post-LPS exposure			
	2 h		4 h	
	Myriad	BD CBA	Myriad	BD CBA
IL-2 (pg/mL)	120	–	68	–
IL-4 (pg/mL)	–	–	53	–
IL-6 (pg/mL)	6482	11,158	314	629
IL-10 (pg/mL)	4060	343	1438	164
IL-17A (ng/mL)	0.037	–	0.020	–
INF-γ (pg/mL)	690	–	82	–
TNF-α (ng/mL)	0.11	0.20	0.18	0.05

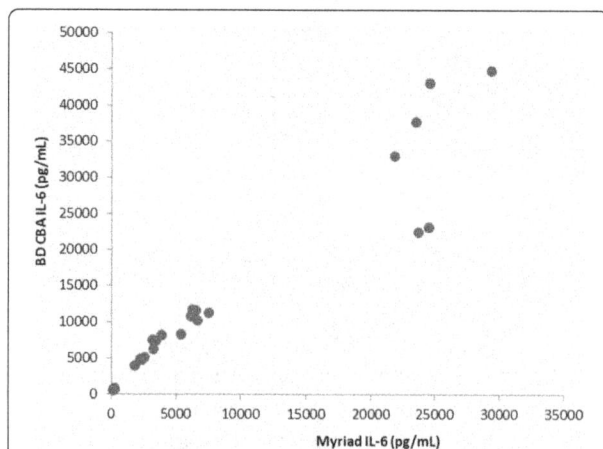

Fig. 1 Comparison between Myriad and BD CBA assays in measuring individual circulating IL-6 levels in mice exposed to acute LPS administration with/without dexamethasone suppression

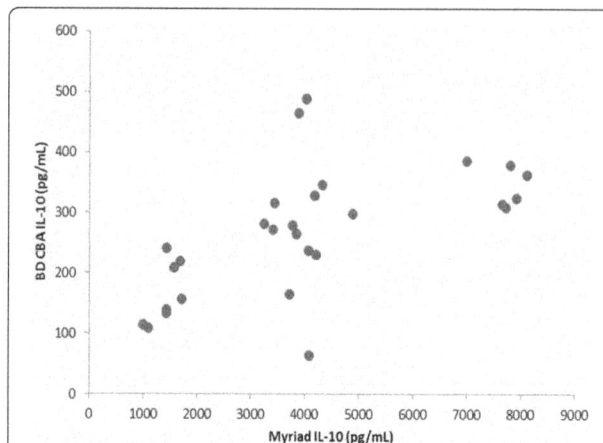

Fig. 3 Comparison between Myriad and BD CBA assays in measuring individual circulating IL-10 levels in mice exposed to acute LPS administration with/without dexamethasone suppression

still needs to be reached on standardization and validation of multi-parametric flow cytometry assays [10] and there are challenges surrounding both clinical specimen analysis and technical variations between instruments [11]. As a general rule, multiplex cytokine assays are cross-validated with or referenced to single analyte immunoassays [12] and more studies comparing different multiplex platform are needed to enable users to determine which are best for a particular study [13]. Previous studies have highlighted the intrinsic differences in reproducibility and accuracy between these technologies [14, 15] and our present report supports the current notion that careful consideration must be taken before generalization of biomarker clinical data when generated on a specific multiplex platform.

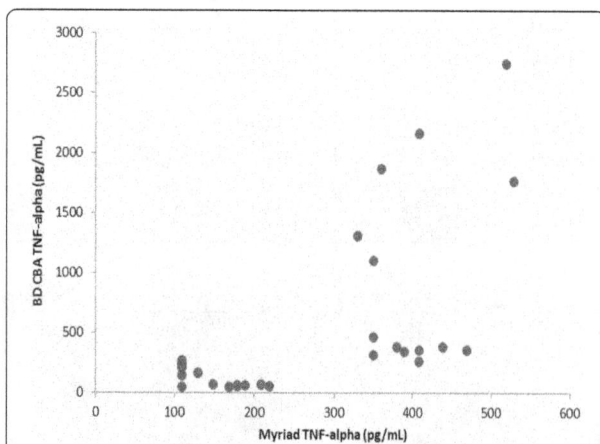

Fig. 2 Comparison between Myriad and BD CBA assays in measuring individual circulating TNF-α levels in mice exposed to acute LPS administration with/without dexamethasone suppression

Conclusion

In conclusion, reproducible quantitation of circulating TNF-α and IL-6 levels were obtained from plasma samples of LPS treated mice with assays from both Myriad RBM and BD Biosciences. The BD CBA cytokine assay was not as sensitive as the Myriad RBM assays in detecting and quantitating circulating IL-2 and IL-4 and IL-17A levels in the LPS treated mice, but was more sensitive in measuring circulating IFN-γ levels. Reliable circulating IL-4 measurements were not achieved by either assay. The present data demonstrate that the quantitation of circulating biomarkers of inflammation can be achieved using multiplexed flow cytometry, but that careful considerations have to be made to the biological validation of the assays. This data also suggest that a multiplex assay cannot be used as a validation reference when implementing another multiplex assay on a different platform.

Abbreviations

BD: Becton Dickson; CBA: Cytometric bead array; DEX: Dexamethasone; IFN-γ: Interferon-γ; IL: Interleukin; IV: Intravenously; LLOD: Lower limit of detection; LLOQ: Lower limit of quantification; LPS: Lipopolysaccharide; MAP: Multi-analyte profile; PE: Phycoerythrin; Th: T helper cell; TNF-α: Tumor necrosis factor-α

Acknowledgements
The Authors would like to thank Amanda Teel for generating the artwork for the figures.

Funding
The present studies were funded by the Sinclair Research Center with no other sources of funding.

Authors' contributions

ASK conceived the study, designed the experiment, carried out the flow cytometric data analyses, participated in the cytokines data analyses and drafted the manuscript. CS participated in the design of the experiment, participated in the cytokines data analyses and drafted the manuscript. MZ carried out the animal experiment, carried the flow cytometry experiment, conducted the cytokines data analyses and participated in the drafting of the manuscript. JL participated in the design and coordination of the study and helped to draft the manuscript. GB participated in the design and coordination of the study and helped to draft the manuscript. All authors read and approved the final manuscript.

Competing interests

The authors are employees of Sinclair Research Center, a private research organization. The Sinclair Research Center did not have any influence on the outcome the study or the interpretation of the data.

References

1. Pini M, Castellanos KJ, Rhodes DH, Fantuzzi G. Obesity and IL-6 interact in modulating the response to endotoxemia in mice. Cytokine. 2013;61(1):71–7.
2. Goodwin JE, Feng Y, Velazquez H, Zhou H, Sessa WC. Loss of the endothelial glucocorticoid receptor prevents the therapeutic protection afforded by dexamethasone after LPS. PLoS One. 2014;9(10):e108126.
3. Leary S, Underwood W, Anthony R, Cartner S, Corey D, Grandin T, Greenacre CB, Gwaltney-Bran S, McCrackin MA, Meyer R. AVMA Guidelines for the Euthanasia of Animals, 2013 Edition. Schaumburg: American Veterinary Medical Association; 2013.
4. Biesmans S, Meert TF, Bouwknecht JA, Acton PD, Davoodi N, De Haes P, Kuijlaars J, Langlois X, Matthews LJ, Ver Donck L, et al. Systemic immune activation leads to neuroinflammation and sickness behavior in mice. Mediat Inflamm. 2013;2013:271359.
5. Dinges MM, Schlievert PM. Role of T cells and gamma interferon during induction of hypersensitivity to lipopolysaccharide by toxic shock syndrome toxin 1 in mice. Infect Immun. 2001;69(3):1256–64.
6. Al-Harbi NO, Imam F, Al-Harbi MM, Ansari MA, Zoheir KM, Korashy HM, Sayed-Ahmed MM, Attia SM, Shabanah OA, Ahmad SF. Dexamethasone attenuates LPS-induced acute lung injury through inhibition of NF-kappaB, COX-2, and pro-inflammatory mediators. Immunol Investig. 2016;45(4):349–69.
7. Raphael I, Nalawade S, Eagar TN, Forsthuber TG. T cell subsets and their signature cytokines in autoimmune and inflammatory diseases. Cytokine. 2015;74(1):5–17.
8. Chau CH, Rixe O, McLeod H, Figg WD. Validation of analytic methods for biomarkers used in drug development. Clin Cancer Res. 2008;14(19):5967–76.
9. Lee JW, Devanarayan V, Barrett YC, Weiner R, Allinson J, Fountain S, Keller S, Weinryb I, Green M, Duan L, et al. Fit-for-purpose method development and validation for successful biomarker measurement. Pharm Res. 2006;23(2):312–28.
10. Barnard RM. Flow cytometry: a flexible tool for biomarker research. Bioanalysis. 2012;4(20):2471–83.
11. Wu DY, Patti-Diaz L, Hill CG. Development and validation of flow cytometry methods for pharmacodynamic clinical biomarkers. Bioanalysis. 2010;2(9):1617–26.
12. NC dP, Wang K, Wadhwa PD, Culhane JF, Nelson EL. Validation and comparison of luminex multiplex cytokine analysis kits with ELISA: determinations of a panel of nine cytokines in clinical sample culture supernatants. J Reprod Immunol. 2005;66(2):175–91.
13. Richens JL, Urbanowicz RA, Metcalf R, Corne J, O'Shea P, Fairclough L. Quantitative validation and comparison of multiplex cytokine kits. J Biomol Screen. 2010;15(5):562–8.
14. Moncunill G, Campo JJ, Dobano C. Quantification of multiple cytokines and chemokines using cytometric bead arrays. Methods Mol Biol. 2014;1172:65–86.
15. Djoba Siawaya JF, Roberts T, Babb C, Black G, Golakai HJ, Stanley K, Bapela NB, Hoal E, Parida S, van Helden P, et al. An evaluation of commercial fluorescent bead-based luminex cytokine assays. PLoS One. 2008;3(7):e2535.

24

Accuracy of cervical cytology: comparison of diagnoses of 100 Pap smears read by four pathologists at three hospitals in Norway

Sveinung Wergeland Sørbye[1*], Pål Suhrke[2], Berit Wallem Revå[2], Jannicke Berland[3], Ramona Johansen Maurseth[4] and Khalid Al-Shibli[4]

Abstract

Background: Cervical cancer can be prevented by early detection and treatment for precancerous lesions. Since 1995, there has been a national cervical cancer screening program in Norway, where women aged 25–69 years are recommended to take Pap smears every three years. There are 17 cytology laboratories covering a population of 5 million people. The detection rate of cervical abnormalities varies from laboratory to laboratory. We wanted to investigate the accuracy of cytology diagnoses by four different pathologists at three different hospitals in Norway.

Methods: One hundred Pap smears (20 Normal, 20 ASC-US, 20 LSIL, 20 ASC-H and 20 HSIL) screened at UNN in 2015 were evaluated by four pathologists at three hospitals in Norway. All patients were followed up through December 2016. Histologically confirmed high-grade dysplasia (CIN2+) was considered as study endpoint.

Results: The number of Pap smears evaluated as abnormal (ASC-US+) by the four pathologists varied from 61 to 85. The number of high-grade cytology (ASC-H+) varied from 26 to 50. There was moderate agreement (weighted kappa 0.45–0.58) between the observers. There were 32 women with high-grade histology (CIN2+) in the follow-up, including 19 CIN2, 12 CIN3 and one squamous cell carcinoma (SCC). Using high-grade cytology (ASC-H+) as cut-off, the sensitivity for CIN2+ varied from 68.8% to 93.8% (mean 77.4%) and specificity from 70.6% to 95.6% (mean 81.3%). The pathologist with the highest sensitivity for CIN2+ had the highest false positive rate and the lowest specificity ($p<0.05$). The accuracy for CIN2+ varied from 74.1% to 83.8% (mean 79.4%). The Pap smear from the woman with cervical cancer was diagnosed as high-grade (ASC-H+) by one of the four pathologists.

Conclusions: Cervical cancer screening based on cytology has limited accuracy. The study revealed a moderate agreement between the observers, along with a trade-off between sensitivity and specificity. This might indicate that hospitals with high detection rates of cervical cytology have higher sensitivity for CIN2+ but lower specificity.

Background

Cervical cancer is caused by human papillomavirus (HPV) and develops over many years through a series of precancerous steps [1, 2]. The disease can be prevented by using the HPV vaccine or by screening with HPV test or Pap smears [3, 4]. Since 2009, there has been a HPV vaccination program for 12-year-old girls in Norway.

The program's coverage is around 80% [5]. Since November 2016, there has been an ongoing two-year catch-up vaccination program for 20–25 years old women where the expected coverage rate is 40–45% (www.fhi.no). Since 2015, there has been a pilot for HPV testing in primary screening in four counties [6]. In this pilot, women 34 years and older are randomized to Pap smear every three years or HPV test every five years [6]. However, in most parts of Norway, the cervical screening program is still based on cervical cytology [5].

* Correspondence: sveinung.sorbye@unn.no
[1]Department of Clinical Pathology, University Hospital of North Norway, 9038 Tromsø, Norway
Full list of author information is available at the end of the article

Since 1995, there has been a national cervical cancer screening program in Norway, where women aged 25–69 years are recommended to take Pap smears every three years [5]. Women with high-grade cytology (ASC-H / HSIL) are referred to a gynecologist for colposcopy and biopsy. HPV test is used in triage of women with low-grade cytology (ASC-US / LSIL). The cervical screening program has a coverage of 60% after 3.5 years. The Norwegian Cancer Registry sends a reminder to women without a Pap smear after three years and a new reminder after four years. The coverage is 80% after 5 years [5]. Most Pap smears are taken by GPs, while some samples are taken by gynecologists. There are 17 different laboratories involved in the screening program, and most of these use liquid-based cytology (ThinPrep or SurePath).

It is well known that cervical cytology has limited sensitivity and reproducibility [7–12]. Diagnoses may vary from cytotechnician to cytotechnician, from pathologist to pathologist and from lab to lab [9, 11, 12]. All cervical cytology diagnoses, results of HPV tests and biopsies from all laboratories in Norway are reported to the Norwegian Cancer Registry, which drafts annual reports with feedback to each laboratory, including the distribution of their diagnoses compared with the national average [5] (Table 1).

There is a high variability in detection rates across hospitals. This may be due to higher sensitivity, lower specificity, differences in HPV prevalence, cervical dysplasia and cancer in some parts of the country compared to other parts of the country, or a combination of these causes. We wanted to investigate the accuracy of cytology diagnoses by four different pathologists at three different hospitals in Norway.

Methods

One hundred cervical cytological samples screened at UNN in 2015 with the diagnoses normal, ASC-US, LSIL, ASC-H and HSIL were sent to the Departments of Pathology in Bergen (HUS), Bodø (Nordland), Fredrikstad (Østfold), Stavanger (SUS) and Tønsberg (Vestfold). The pathologist at the Department of Pathology in Bergen did not have time to participate in the study, and he forwarded the slides to Stavanger without looking at them. Two cytotechnologist at the Department of Pathology in Fredrikstad diagnosed the slides, but they were trained to screen SurePath samples. Their results were therefore excluded from this study based on ThinPrep samples.

All slides were first screened by a cytotechnologist at UNN and then evaluated by a pathologist at UNN (P1, reference). The abnormal cells were marked on the slides before being dispatched for the study. The slides were not screened at the other hospitals. The four other pathologists (P2–P5) at other hospitals were to only evaluate the abnormal cells marked on the slides. The other pathologists were blinded for age, previous findings, clinical information and HPV result. Diagnoses from each of the four pathologists were compared with diagnoses from the three other pathologists. Women with abnormal findings at UNN were followed up according to national guidelines. In Norway, the Bethesda System for Reporting Cervical Cytology is used by all laboratories. All patients were followed up through December 2016. Histologically confirmed high-grade dysplasia (CIN2+) was considered as study endpoint (gold standard). When calculating the sensitivity and specificity, women with normal Pap smears, and women with low-grade cytology (ASC-US / LSIL) and negative HPV test without histology, were considered free of high-grade dysplasia (CIN1-).

All analyses were done in IBM SPSS Statistics, version 23, with Chi-square test for categorical variables and t-test for continuous variables. For accuracy of cytological diagnoses between different observers, we used weighted kappa with linear weights.

Table 1 Distribution (%) of selected cytological diagnoses in different labs in Norway in 2015

Lab	Normal	ASC-US	LSIL	ASC-H	HSIL
OUS	86.9	5.0	0.9	1.0	1.1
Lab for pat/Furst	92.6[2]	3.0[3]	0.7	0.5	0.6[3]
HUS[1]	83.6	5.0	2.4	0.8	1.4[2]
St.Olav[1]	84.0	8.0[2]	1.1	1.8[2]	1.1
Molde	86.6	2.9	1.0	0.4	1.1
Gyn lab/unilabs	89.9	4.9	0.8	0.7	0.6[3]
Østfold	87.0	4.6	0.9	0.9	0.8
UNN	79.2[3]	4.8	4.6[2]	1.4[2]	1.1
Telemark	88.7	3.2	2.3	0.3	1.0
Innlandet,Lillehammer	93.0[2]	3.4	0.9	0.6	0.6
Vestre Viken	91.1	3.6	1.8	0.6	0.9
Ålesund	91.4[2]	5.1	1.4	0.5	0.6[3]
Nordland	86.4	3.6	1.9	1.1	0.8
SUS[1]	84.6	4.9	2.5	0.6	1.3[2]
Sørlandet	89.1	3.0	1.1	0.7	0.8
AHUS	93.4[2]	2.5	1.5	0.8	1.0
Vestfold	83.0	8.5[2]	2.1	2.0[2]	0.9
Total	88.1	4.3	1.6	0.9	0.9

Adapted from the Norwegian Cancer Screening Programme – annual report 2015 [5]
[1]Laboratories included in HPV primary screening pilot where women 34 years and older are randomized to Pap smear every three years or HPV test every five years
[2]Significantly higher than the average for Norway ($p<0.05$)
[3]Significantly lower than the average for Norway ($p<0.05$)

Results

Of the 100 cervical cytology samples, 20 were diagnosed Normal, 20 ASC-US, 20 LSIL, 20 ASC-H and 20 HSIL at UNN. There were 32 women with high-grade histology

Table 2 Cytology diagnoses at UNN with HPV tests and biopsies

Diagnoses	Samples	HPV test	HPV pos	HPV pos (%)	Biopsy	CIN2+	PPV (%)
Normal	20	1	0	0.0	0	0	0.0
ASC-US	20	19	8	42.1	6	1	5.0
LSIL	20	19	15	78.9	17	3	15.0
ASC-H	20	17	16	94.1	20	10	50.0
HSIL	20	14	13	92.9	20	18	90.0
Total	100	70	52	74.3	63	32	32.0

ASC-US atypical squamous cells of undetermined significance, *LSIL* low-grade squamous intraepithelial lesion, *ASC-H* atypical squamous cells cannot exclude HSIL, *HSIL* high-grade squamous intraepithelial lesion, CIN2+ = CIN2, CIN3 and cancer, *PPV* positive predictive value

(CIN2+) in the follow-up, including 19 CIN2, 12 CIN3 and one squamous cell carcinoma (SCC). There were no CIN2+ in women with Normal diagnosis, one CIN2+ in women with ASC-US diagnoses, three women with CIN2+ in the LSIL group, 10 CIN2+ in the ASC-H group and 18 CIN2+ in the HSIL group (Table 2). Using high-grade cytology (ASC-H+) as cut-off, the sensitivity for CIN2+ at UNN was 87.5% (28/32).

The number of samples diagnosed as "Normal" varied from 15 to 39 by the four pathologists, with a mean of 28.8. One pathologist (P2) had significantly fewer "Normal" cases than the average of the four pathologists ($p<0.05$) (Table 3). The corresponding variation of ASC-US, LSIL, ASC-H and HSIL were 17 to 24 (mean 19.8), 9 to 20 (mean 14.0), 10 to 18 (mean 13.3) and 16 to 32 (mean 24.0), respectively (Table 3), none of which were significant. There was moderate agreement between the observers (weighted kappa 0.45–0.58) (Table 4). The kappa statistics were not statistically different.

The agreement of the different diagnoses was higher for "Normal" and "HSIL" samples than the other diagnoses (ASC-US, LSIL and ASC-H) (Additional file 1: Tables S1–S5). The number for high-grade cytology (ASC-H+) varied from 26 (P4) to 50 (P2). Of 61 women with at least one high-grade cytology, 17 samples (27.9%) were considered high-grade by all four observers (Additional file 1: Figure S1). The number of true positive (CIN2+) using ASC-H+ as a cut-off varied from 22 to 30 (mean 24.8) (Additional file 1: Figure S2 and Table 5).

The corresponding sensitivity for CIN2+ varied from 68.8% to 93.8% (mean 77.4%). One pathologist (P2) had significantly higher sensitivity than the average of the four pathologists ($p<0.05$) (Table 5). Of 32 women with CIN2+, 15 samples (46.9%) were considered high-grade by all four observers (Additional file 1: Figure S2). One woman with CIN2 was not considered to have high-grade cytology by any of the four observers (patient 57, Additional file 1: Table S3). The number of true negative (CIN1-) using LSIL- as a cut-off varied from 48 to 65 (mean 55.3). The corresponding specificity ranged from 70.6% to 95.6% (mean 81.3%) (Table 5). One pathologist (P2) had significantly lower specificity and one pathologist (P4) had significantly higher specificity than the average of the four pathologists ($p<0.05$) (see Table 5). The pathologist (P2) with the highest sensitivity for CIN2+ had the highest false positive rate and the lowest specificity (Table 5). The accuracy for CIN2+ varied from 74.1% to 83.8% (mean 79.4%). There were no statistically significant differences in accuracy (Table 5). The Pap smear from the woman with cervical cancer (SCC) was diagnosed as high-grade (ASC-H+) by one of the four pathologists (P2), while three pathologists diagnosed her as ASC-US (Additional file 1: Table S5). The woman had a positive HPV test for HPV type 16 (data not shown).

Discussion

The study's purpose was to investigate the accuracy of cytology diagnoses by four different pathologists at three

Table 3 Distribution of diagnoses per pathologist

Observer	Normal	ASC-US	LSIL	ASC-H	HSIL	Total
P1 (ref)	20	20	20	20	20	100
P2	15[1]	19	16	18	32	100
P3	23	19	20	14	24	100
P4	39	24	11	10	16	100
P5	38	17	9	11	25	100
Mean (P2–P5)	28.8	19.8	14.0	13.3	24.0	100.0

ASC-US atypical squamous cells of undetermined significance, *LSIL* low-grade squamous intraepithelial lesion, *ASC-H* atypical squamous cells cannot exclude HSIL, *HSIL* high-grade squamous intraepithelial lesion
[1]Significantly lower than the average for P2–P5 ($p<0.05$)

Table 4 Agreement between observers (weighted kappa)

Observer	P2	P3	P4	P5
P2	-	0.53	0.48	0.45
P3	0.53	-	0.50	0.49
P4	0.48	0.50	-	0.58
P5	0.45	0.49	0.58	-

< 0.00 = No agreement
0.00–0.20 = Slight agreement
0.21–0.40 = Fair agreement
0.41–0.60 = Moderate agreement
0.61–0.80 = Substantial agreement
0.81–1.00 = Almost perfect agreement

Table 5 True positive, true negative, sensitivity and specificity for CIN2+ per pathologists using ASC-H+ as cut-off

Observer	TP	TN	FP	FN	SE (%)	SP (%)	AU (%)	PPV (%)	NPV (%)
P1 (ref)	28	56	12	4	87.5	82.4	85.0	70.0	93.3
P2	30	48	20	2	93.8[1]	70.6[2]	82.2	60.0	96.0[1]
P3	24	54	14	8	75.0	79.4	77.2	63.2	87.1
P4	23	65	3	9	71.9	95.6[1]	83.8	88.5[1]	87.8
P5	22	54	14	10	68.8	79.4	74.1	61.1	84.4
Mean (P2–P5)	24.8	55.3	12.8	7.3	77.4	81.3	79.4	68.2	88.8

TP true positive, *TN* true negative, *FP* false positive, *FN* false negative, *SE* sensitivity, *SP* specificity, AU = AUROC = accuracy = (SE+SP)/2, *PPV* positive predictive value, *NPV* negative predictive value, ASC-H+ = ASC-H and HSIL, CIN2+ = CIN2, CIN3 and cancer
[1]Significantly higher than the average for P2–P5 ($p<0.05$)
[2]Significantly lower than the average for P2–P5 ($p<0.05$)

hospitals using 100 Pap smears with different cytological diagnoses screened at UNN. The agreement of the cytological diagnoses between the four pathologists in this study was "moderate." A moderate agreement is better than "fair," but worse than "substantial." The kappa statistics were not statistically different.

In Norway there are 17 cytology laboratories covering a population of 5 million people [5]. All the laboratories receive most of their samples from general practitioners in primary screening. The population in Norway is quite homogenous, where Norwegian women in the different parts of Norway are mostly the same. The differences between the various laboratories are probably caused by different interpretation of the Bethesda criteria. Two pathologists (P4 and P5) were from the same laboratory but still used very different diagnoses for the same patients.

In the ATHENA study, the sensitivity of cytology varied from 42.0% to 73.0% [12]. In our study, the sensitivity for CIN2+ varied from 68.8% to 93.8%, but all the smears were first screened at the same hospital, and abnormal cells were marked on the slide. It is easy to find abnormal cells on a slide full of marks. In a population with a given prevalence of CIN2+, the sensitivity of cytology is dependent on the detection rate. In the ATHENA study, the positivity rate of cytology in primary screening varied from 3.8% to 9.9% while the detection rate of HPV DNA test (Cobas 4800) varied from

10.9% to 13.4% [12]. In our study, the detection rate of high-grade cytology (ASC-H / HSIL) varied from 26.0% to 50.0%, while the detection rate of HPV DNA test (Cobas 4800) was 74.3% (52/70).

In our study, the accuracy varied from 74.1% to 83.8% (mean 79.4%). In five published studies the accuracy varied from 64.2% to 78.4% (mean 76.1%) (Table 6). There was less variation between the four pathologists in our study than between the five published studies. The mean accuracy of the four pathologists in our study was significantly higher than the mean of the five published studies (79.4% vs 76.1%, $p<0.05$).

There is a trade-off between sensitivity and specificity in cervical cancer screening. In our study the pathologist with the significantly highest sensitivity for CIN2+ had the significantly lowest specificity. In general, laboratories with a high detection rate of cytology also have higher sensitivity for CIN2+. If the sensitivity is higher, the hospital detects more women with CIN2/3 that can be treated, and fewer women develop cervical cancer before the next screening round. When women with low-grade cytology (ASC-US / LSIL) are triaged with HPV test, a high detection rate of low-grade cytology should not be considered as a major problem. A false positive ASC-US will have a negative HPV test and does not need follow-up. A false negative "Normal" cytology has no indication for HPV testing, according to Norwegian guidelines (www.kreftregisteret.no).

Table 6 True positive, true negative, sensitivity and specificity for CIN2+ in different studies using ASC-US+ as cut-off

Study	TP	TN	FP	FN	SE (%)	SP (%)	AU (%)	PPV (%)	NPV (%)
Katki 2011 [10]	1 226	318 093	11 415	1 084	53.1[2]	96.5[1]	78.4[1]	9.7[2]	99.7[1]
Dillner 2008 [15]	242	22 883	1 031	139	63.5[1]	95.7[2]	79.6[1]	19.0[1]	99.4[2]
Castle 2012 [16]	136	18 190	926	260	34.3[2]	95.2[2]	64.7[2]	12.8[1]	98.6[1]
Szarewski 2008 [17]	256	236	444	17	93.8[1]	34.7[2]	64.2[2]	36.6[1]	93.3[2]
Sørbye 2011 [18]	48	92	77	8	85.7[1]	54.4[2]	70.1[2]	38.4[1]	92.0[2]
Total	1 908	359 494	13 893	1 508	55.9	96.3	76.1	12.1	99.6

TP true positive, *TN* true negative, *FP* false positive, *FN* false negative, *SE* sensitivity, *SP* specificity, AU = AUROC = accuracy = (SE+SP)/2, *PPV* positive predictive value, *NPV* negative predictive value, ASC-US+ = ASC-US, LSIL, ASC-H and HSIL, CIN2+ = CIN2, CIN3 and cancer
[1]Significantly higher than the average ($p<0.05$)
[2]Significantly lower than the average ($p<0.05$)

Cytology is subjective with poorly reproducible criteria. HPV testing is more objective with strictly defined criteria. Co-testing with both cytology and HPV test may reduce the risk of false negative cytology when the pathologists take the HPV result in consideration when evaluating the cytological slide. In our study, only the observer at UNN (P1, reference) knew the HPV result. All other observers were blinded for clinical information and HPV result, which might explain the lower sensitivity for CIN2+ for some of the other pathologist. Originally, in the ATHENA study, cytology was reviewed blinded to HPV status. When the same slides were re-reviewed unblinded to HPV status, the sensitivity for CIN3+ of co-testing increased from 54.1% to 62.4% (P = 0.0015) [13]. In our study, the mean sensitivity for CIN2+ for the four external pathologists was 77.4% based on slides screened at the same hospital.

The present study also has other weaknesses. For P1 the diagnoses were set in normal routine work, while the cases for the other four pathologists had to be diagnosed in addition to normal workload. This might affect the interpretation. In addition, only P1 at UNN had access to the initial diagnoses suggested by the cytotechnician. In daily practice the pathologist usually compares his or her initial impression with the diagnosis suggested by the cytotechnician. If there is discrepancy, the slide is reviewed. This might explain the lower sensitivity of some of the other pathologist. In normal routine work, difficult cases will be discussed with other pathologists. In this study, the pathologists reviewed all the slides alone.

Out of the 100 women in this study, there was one woman with cervical cancer. Three of the four pathologists diagnosed her cytology as ASC-US. According to Norwegian guidelines, women with ASC-US and a positive HPV result should be followed up with a new cytology and HPV test after 6–12 months. Only women with persistent HPV infection should be referred to a gynecologist for colposcopy and biopsy (www.kreftregisteret.no). This may delay diagnosis, treatment and worsen her prognosis.

There were statistically significant differences in sensitivity and specificity ($p<0.05$) for CIN2+ between the observations, but not in accuracy. In a low resource setting, specificity is important to reduce colposcopy workload. In a high resource setting like Norway, sensitivity is more important to reduce the number of cervical cancer. Specificity of cytology can be improved by HPV test in a triage of ASC-US / LSIL. The costs of a high number of HPV tests are of minor importance in a high resource setting. In the USA, co-testing (cytology and HPV test) every five years is recommended for women 30–60 years of age [10, 14].

Conclusions
Cervical cancer screening based on cytology has limited accuracy. The study revealed a moderate agreement between the observers, along with a trade-off between sensitivity and specificity. This might indicate that hospitals with high detection rate of cervical cytology have higher sensitivity for CIN2+, but lower specificity.

Additional file

Additional file 1: Table S1. Diagnoses per pathologist (P2–P5) in samples with Normal cytology at UNN. **Table S2.** Diagnoses per pathologist (P2–P5) in samples with ASC-US cytology at UNN. **Table S3.** Diagnoses per pathologist (P2–P5) in samples with LSIL cytology at UNN. **Table S4.** Diagnoses per pathologist (P2–P5) in samples with ASC-H cytology at UNN. **Table S5.** Diagnoses per pathologist in samples with HSIL cytology at UNN. **Figure S1.** Distribution of high-grade cytology (ASC-H+) diagnoses by observer (P2–P5) in women with at least one high-grade cytology (N=61). **Figure S2.** Distribution of high-grade cytology (ASC-H+) diagnoses by observer (P2–P5) in women with histological CIN2+ in follow-up (N=32).

Abbreviations
ASC-H: Atypical squamous cells – cannot exclude HSIL; ASC-US: Atypical squamous cells of undetermined significance; CIN: Cervical intraepithelial neoplasia, also known as cervical dysplasia; CIN1, CIN2, CIN3: Cervical intraepithelial neoplasia grade 1, 2 or 3, also known as low-grade, moderate or severe cervical dysplasia; CIN2+, CIN2, CIN3: Adenocarcinoma in situ (ACIS) or cervical cancer; DNA: Deoxyribonucleic acid; HPV DNA test: Cobas 4800 detects DNA from 14 high-risk HPV types (16, 18, 31, 33, 35, 39, 45, 51, 52, 56, 58, 59, 66 and 68) at clinically relevant infection levels; HPV: Human papillomavirus; HSIL: High-grade squamous intraepithelial lesion; LBC: Liquid-based cytology; LSIL: Low-grade squamous intraepithelial lesion; NPV: Negative predictive value; Pap smear: the Papanicolaou test, also known as Pap test, cervical smear or cervical cytology; PPV: Positive predictive value; RNA: Ribonucleic acid; WHO: The World Health Organization.

Acknowledgements
This study was initiated by Gry Andersen, Director, Division of Diagnostic Services, University Hospital of North Norway. We want to thank Lars Uhlin-Hansen and Liv Hansen, at the Department of Clinical Pathology at University Hospital of North Norway, who were involved with the study's design. We are grateful Teresa Grid, Renate Veronica Hansen and the other pathologists, cytotechnicians and staff members at the departments of pathology in Bodø, Fredrikstad, Stavanger, Tromsø and Tønsberg who made this study possible. We also want to thank Frode Skjold for his assistance with the statistics.

Funding
Not applicable.

Authors' contributions
SWS participated in the study's design. TS, RJM and JB screened all PAP smears. SWS performed the statistical analysis. SWS, PS and KAS drafted the manuscript. All authors read and approved the final manuscript.

Authors' information
Not applicable.

Competing interests
The authors declare that they have no competing interests.

Author details
[1]Department of Clinical Pathology, University Hospital of North Norway, 9038 Tromsø, Norway. [2]Department of Pathology, Vestfold Hospital, Tønsberg, Norway. [3]Jannicke Berland, Stavanger University Hospital, Stavanger, Norway. [4]Nordlandssykehuset HF, Department of Pathology, Bodø, Norway.

References
1. Munoz N, Bosch FX, de SS, Herrero R, Castellsague X, Shah KV, et al. Epidemiologic classification of human papillomavirus types associated with cervical cancer. N Engl J Med. 2003;348:518–27.
2. Walboomers JM, Jacobs MV, Manos MM, Bosch FX, Kummer JA, Shah KV, et al. Human papillomavirus is a necessary cause of invasive cervical cancer worldwide. J Pathol. 1999;189:12–9.
3. de Blasio BF, Neilson AR, Klemp M, Skjeldestad FE. Modeling the impact of screening policy and screening compliance on incidence and mortality of cervical cancer in the post-HPV vaccination era. J Public Health (Oxf). 2012; 34:539–47.
4. Saslow D, Solomon D, Lawson HW, Killackey M, Kulasingam SL, Cain J, et al. American Cancer Society, American Society for Colposcopy and Cervical Pathology, and American Society for Clinical Pathology screening guidelines for the prevention and early detection of cervical cancer. Am J Clin Pathol. 2012;137:516–42.
5. Skare GB, Lonnberg S, Bjorge T, Trope A: The Norwegian cervical cancer screening programme. Annual report 2015. The Cancer Registry of Norway 2016.
6. Andreassen T, Vogt C. Screening for cervical cancer–future perspectives. Tidsskr Nor Laegeforen. 2014;134:1122–3.
7. Arbyn M, Buntinx F, Van Ranst M, Paraskevaidis E, Martin-Hirsch P, Dillner J. Virologic versus cytologic triage of women with equivocal Pap smears: a meta-analysis of the accuracy to detect high-grade intraepithelial neoplasia. J Natl Cancer Inst. 2004;96:280–93.
8. Arbyn M, Roelens J, Simoens C, Buntinx F, Paraskevaidis E, Martin-Hirsch PP et al.: Human papillomavirus testing versus repeat cytology for triage of minor cytological cervical lesions. Cochrane Database Syst Rev 2013, 3: CD008054.
9. Bigras G, Wilson J, Russell L, Johnson G, Morel D, Saddik M. Interobserver concordance in the assessment of features used for the diagnosis of cervical atypical squamous cells and squamous intraepithelial lesions (ASC-US, ASC-H, LSIL and HSIL). Cytopathology. 2013;24:44–51.
10. Katki HA, Kinney WK, Fetterman B, Lorey T, Poitras NE, Cheung L, et al. Cervical cancer risk for women undergoing concurrent testing for human papillomavirus and cervical cytology: a population-based study in routine clinical practice. Lancet Oncol. 2011;12:663–72.
11. Stoler MH, Schiffman M. Interobserver reproducibility of cervical cytologic and histologic interpretations: realistic estimates from the ASCUS-LSIL Triage Study. JAMA. 2001;285:1500–5.
12. Wright TC Jr, Stoler MH, Behrens CM, Sharma A, Sharma K, Apple R. Interlaboratory variation in the performance of liquid-based cytology: insights from the ATHENA trial. Int J Cancer. 2014;134:1835–43.
13. Wright TC Jr, Stoler MH, Aslam S, Behrens CM. Knowledge of Patients' Human Papillomavirus Status at the Time of Cytologic Review Significantly Affects the Performance of Cervical Cytology in the ATHENA Study. Am J Clin Pathol. 2016;146:391–8.
14. Massad LS, Einstein MH, Huh WK, Katki HA, Kinney WK, Schiffman M, et al. updated consensus guidelines for the management of abnormal cervical cancer screening tests and cancer precursors. Obstet Gynecol. 2012; 2013(121):829–46.
15. Dillner J, Rebolj M, Birembaut P, Petry KU, Szarewski A, Munk C, et al. Long term predictive values of cytology and human papillomavirus testing in cervical cancer screening: joint European cohort study. BMJ. 2008;337:a1754.
16. Castle PE, Glass AG, Rush BB, Scott DR, Wentzensen N, Gage JC, et al. Clinical human papillomavirus detection forecasts cervical cancer risk in women over 18 years of follow-up. J Clin Oncol. 2012;30:3044–50.
17. Szarewski A, Ambroisine L, Cadman L, Austin J, Ho L, Terry G, et al. Comparison of predictors for high-grade cervical intraepithelial neoplasia in women with abnormal smears. Cancer Epidemiol Biomarkers Prev. 2008;17:3033–42.
18. Sorbye SW, Arbyn M, Fismen S, Gutteberg TJ, Mortensen ES. Triage of women with low-grade cervical lesions–HPV mRNA testing versus repeat cytology. PLoS One. 2011;6:e24083.

25

The expression of MDM2 in gastrointestinal stromal tumors: immunohistochemical analysis of 35 cases

Boubacar Efared[1]*(iD), Gabrielle Atsame-Ebang[1], Layla Tahiri[1], Ibrahim Sory Sidibé[1], Fatimazahra Erregad[1], Nawal Hammas[1,2], Samia Arifi[3,4], Ihsane Mellouki[4,5], Abdelmalek Ousadden[4,6], Khalid Mazaz[4,6], Hinde El Fatemi[1,2] and Laila Chbani[1,2]

Abstract

Background: Gastrointestinal stromal tumors (GIST) are the most common primary mesenchymal tumors of the digestive system. The assessment of their biological behavior still remains a scientific challenge. To date, there are no well-established biological prognostic markers of GIST. Our aim is to study the expression of the MDM2 oncoprotein in GIST through an immunohistochemical analysis.

Methods: It was a retrospective study of 35 cases of GIST diagnosed from 2009 to 2012 in the department of pathology of Hassan II university hospital, Fès, Morocco. MDM2 immunohistochemical staining was performed on archival paraffin-embedded and formalin-fixed specimens (with a threshold of nuclear positivity > 10%). Analysis of correlations between MDM2 immunoexpression and clinicopathological features of GIST has been performed.

Results: The mean age was 55.23 years (range 25–84 years) with a male predominance (sex ratio = 1.5). The stomach was the main site of GIST, with 17 cases (48.57%) followed by the small bowel (9 cases, 25.71%). The spindle cell type GIST was the most frequent morphological variant (29 cases, 82.85%). Tumor necrosis was present in 8 cases (22.85%). Two patients (5.71%) had very low risk GIST, 5 (14.28%) had low risk GIST, 7 patients (20%) had intermediate risk tumors. The remaining 21 cases (60%) had high risk GIST. At the time of diagnosis, 9 patients (25.71%) had metastatic tumors. At immunohistochemical analysis, 40% of cases (14 patients) stained positive for MDM2. Of these MDMD2-positive tumors, 11/14 (78.57%) had high risk tumors and 8/14 cases (57.14%) presented with metastatic GIST. MDM2 positivity was significantly associated with the metastatic status ($p = 0.001$).

Conclusion: The current study suggests that MDM2 immunohistochemical expression is a negative histoprognostic factor in GIST with a statistically significant correlation with metastasis.

Keywords: Gastrointestinal stromal tumors (GIST), MDM2, Immunohistochemistry, Histoprognosis

Background

Gastrointestinal stromal tumors (GIST) are the most common primary mesenchymal tumors of the digestive system [1, 2]. They constitute a wide spectrum of neoplasms with characteristic histological, immunohisto-chemical and molecular features. The most common genetic alterations found in GIST include mutations of growth factors genes such as *KIT* (70–80%) and *PDGFRA* (platelet-derived growth factor A) (5–15%) [2–

6]. To date, much is known about the histological, immunohistochemical and molecular aspects of GIST especially in diagnostic purposes, it is however obvious that little is known about the clinicopathological features that can predict the biological behavior of these tumors. In fact, several features of GIST have been postulated in the past to predict their clinical behavior [1, 7–10]. The widely accepted risk stratification of GIST is known as AFIP (Armed Forces Institute of Pathology) criteria, reported by Miettinen et al. This system of risk stratification is in fact a modification of a NIH (National Institutes of Health) consensus criteria [1, 9, 10]. To

---

* Correspondence: befared2013@gmail.com
[1]Department of pathology, Hassan II university hospital, Fès, Morocco
Full list of author information is available at the end of the article

determine the risk of recurrence, the AFIP criteria takes into account tumor size and mitotic count/50 HPF (high power field), according to the anatomic location of the tumor. Thus, GIST are subdivided into very low, low, intermediate and high risk tumors [1]. Beside these systems of risk stratification, several attempts have been made to identify molecules or genetic alterations that can have a prognostic value in determining GIST behavior [11–13]. As a mesenchymal tumor, alterations of oncogenes (or their products) like *MDM2* (Murine Double Minute 2) or *TP53*, have been widely investigated through various techniques in GIST [11, 12]. In a similar perspective, herein we have tried to study the immunohistochemical overexpression of MDM2 in GIST, and its correlations with other clinicopathological parameters.

Methods

A part of this study has been presented as an E-poster (E-PS-06-036: MDM2 as a prognostic marker for GIST: A retrospective study of 43 cases) at the 28th European Congress of Pathology and published as an abstract (Virchows Arch (2016) 469 (Suppl 1):S1–S346).

Patients selection

The histological sections have been retrospectively retrieved from 35 patients diagnosed with gastrointestinal stromal tumors (GIST) from 2009 to 2012 in the department of pathology of Hassan II University hospital, Fès, Morocco. Clinical and histopathological data have been recorded from pathology requests forms and the patients' medical records. The initial diagnosis of GIST has been made on paraffin-embedded and formalin-fixed specimens after staining with hematoxylin-eosine-safran (HES) (Figs. 1a, b and 2). In all cases, the diagnosis of GIST has been retained after immunohistochemical analysis that showed unequivocal diffuse and intense membranous or cytoplasmic expression of CD117 (Fig. 3a), and after excluding potential differential diagnosis by using commonly utilized panel of antibodies such as

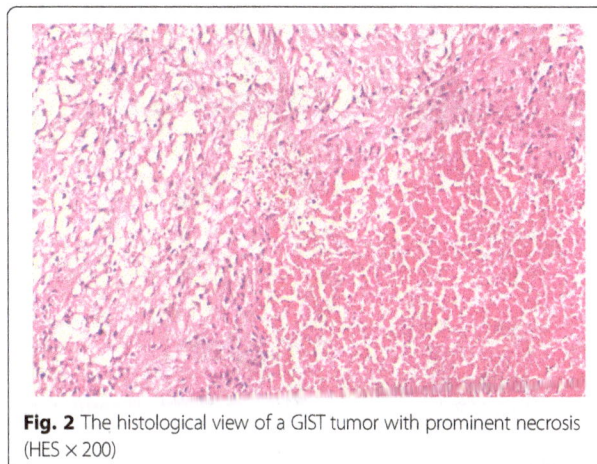

Fig. 2 The histological view of a GIST tumor with prominent necrosis (HES × 200)

anti-CD34, anti-S-100 protein and anti-SMA (smooth muscle actin) [1–4, 6]. The risk assessment of GIST has been based on the AFIP criteria [1].

Immunohistochemistry

MDM2 immunohistochemical staining was performed on archival paraffin-embedded and formalin-fixed specimens from all the 35 patients previously diagnosed with GIST. We have used the anti-MDM2 antibody according to the manufacturer's guidelines, with an automated immunohistochemical stainer (Ventana BenchMark ULTRA®). A threshold of nuclear positivity > 10% has been fixed as a positive MDM2 staining (Fig. 3b).

Statistics

The statistical analysis was performed by using SPSS® 20.0. The chi-square test or the Fisher exact test when appropriate, have been used to assess correlations between MDM2 immunoexpression with different features of GIST (risk assessment, metastatic status, tumor site, size, tumor necrosis and mitotic count). Results were statistically significant when $p < 0.05$.

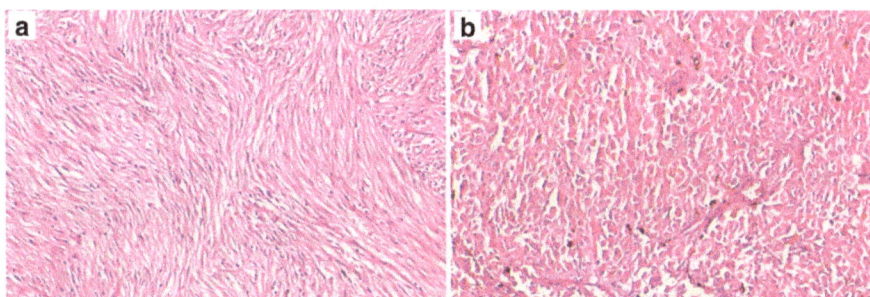

Fig. 1 The histomorphological types of gastrointestinal stromal tumors (GIST) in our study. **a** A spindle cells type with fusocellular cells disposed in intersected fascicles. **b** The epithelioid GIST variant shows a solid architecture with cohesive polygonal cells and oval nucleis. (HES × 200)

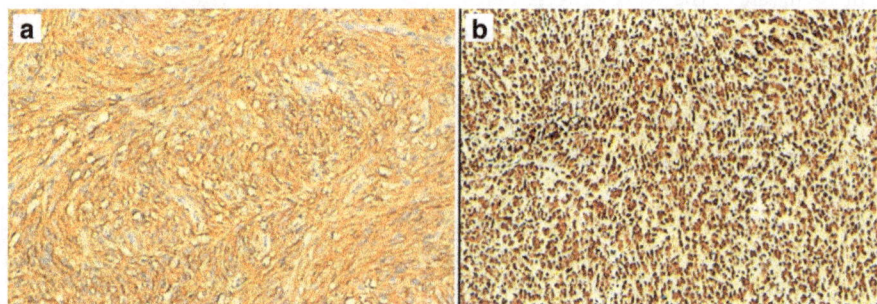

Fig. 3 a Example of a diffuse cytoplasmic immunoexpression of CD117 by a case of GIST in our study. **b** A case of GIST showing intense nuclear staining with anti-MDM2 antibody. (× 200)

Results

Table 1 summarizes the clinicopathological features of our 35 patients. The diagnosis of GIST has been made on 13 biopsies and on 22 surgical resected specimens (Fig. 4). The mean age was 55.23 years (range of 25-84 years); there was a slight male predominance, with 21 male patients and 14 women (sex ratio = 1.5). The stomach was the main site of GIST, with 17 cases (48.57%), followed by the small bowel with 9 cases (25.71%) (Fig. 4) and the peritoneum (5 cases, 14.28%). The duodenum and the colon were rarely affected, respectively in 8.57% (3 patients) and 2.85% (1 patient). The spindle cell type (Fig. 1a) was the most frequent histological variant of GIST in our study, with 29 cases (82.85%) while the epithelioid variant was found in only one patient (Fig. 1b). The mixed variant, spindle and epithelioid cell type was seen in 5 cases (14.28%). Tumor necrosis was present in 8 cases (22.85%).

According to the AFIP criteria of the risk assessment, 2 patients (5.71%) had very low risk GIST, 5 (14.28%) had low risk GIST, 7 patients (20%) had intermediate risk tumors. The remaining 21 cases (60%) had high risk GIST. At the time of diagnosis, 9 patients presented with synchronous metastasis. The peritoneal metastasis were the most frequent (4 cases, 11.42%). Other organs like the liver, the lung and the adrenal gland, have been involved by metastatic tumors (Table 1).

The immunohistochemical analysis showed 14 cases positive for MDM2 (40%) (Fig. 3b).

Among the 9 metastatic GIST, 8 had MDM2-positive tumors, showing a statistical significant correlation of MDM2 positivity with metastatic status ($p = 0.001$). Also, our current study showed that MDM2-positive GIST had a tendency to have a higher size (> 10 cm) as well as a higher mitotic count (> 5 mitosis/50 HPF) ($p = 0.08$ and 0.06 respectively) (Table 2).

Discussion

The epidemiological and histological characteristics of our current study are approximately similar to what has

been previously reported [1–4]. The mean age was 55.23 years with a slight male predominance (21 men for 14 women). All of our patients were adults, with age ranging from 25 to 84 years. Gastrointestinal stromal tumors (GIST) are usually encountered in middle-aged or elderly adults, affecting very rarely the pediatric population [3]. Unlike in adults where GIST usually affect equally both sex, in young patients the female predominance is common and tumors present as a component of cancer predisposing syndroms (Carney triad and Carney-Stratakis syndrom) [1, 3, 14]. The stomach is the most site of GIST followed by the small intestine, other parts of the gastrointestinal tract such as the colon or the esophagus are rarely affected [2, 4]. However, a small subset of GIST has been found to occur in extraintestinal wall, generally in the vicinity of the gastrointestinal tract (GI tract), especially in the omentum, the mesentery, or the retroperitoneum. These tumors are termed as extragastrointestinal stromal tumors (EGIST) and have histological and genetic features similar to those of the common GIST [3, 15, 16]. We have found 5 cases of peritoneal EGIST among our 35 patients. The vast majority of GIST were located in the stomach (17 cases, 48.57%) and in the small bowel (9 cases, 25.71%).

The histological features of our patients were consistent with those previously reported in the literature [1, 3]. The spindle cells variant is the most frequent histological subtype of GIST, followed by the epithelioid variant. We have recorded 29 cases (82.85%) of spindle cells GIST, 1 case of epithelioid variant and 5 mixed-subtypes (14.28%) showing admixture of epithelioid and spindle tumoral cells. We have not recorded rare morphologic variants like the sclerosing epithelioid or spindle cells subtype, the sarcomatoid variants or the palisading vacuolated spindle cell subtype. In our study, tumor necrosis was found in 22.45% (8 cases), and approximately 22–37% of GIST are associated with necrosis as reported in the literature [1]. On immunohistochemistry, GIST stain positive for CD117 (95%), with a small subset (5%) that can be negative for this marker. DOG1 is almost

Table 1 Clinicopathological features of our 35 patients diagnosed with GIST

Cases	Age (year)	Sex	Site	Histol type	Necrosis	Risk	Metastatic site	MDM2
1	40	F	Stomach	Sp cel	–	High	Peritoneum	+
2	53	M	Stomach	Sp cel	–	High	Peritoneum, Liver	+
3	65	F	Peritoneum	Sp + Ep cel	+	High	Liver, lung	+
4	42	M	Small bowel	Sp cel	–	Low	–	–
5	40	F	Duodenum	Sp cel	+	Intermediate	Peritoneum	+
6	50	F	Small bowel	Sp cel	–	Low	–	+
7	35	M	Small bowel	Sp cel	–	Intermediate	–	–
8	84	M	Small bowel	Sp cel	+	High	Liver	+
9	60	M	Peritoneum	Sp cel	–	High	–	+
10	50	M	Duodenum	Sp cel	–	Intermediate	–	+
11	43	F	Stomach	Sp cel	+	High	–	–
12	56	M	Small bowel	Sp + Ep cel	+	High	Peritoneum	+
13	64	F	Colon	Sp cel	–	Low	–	–
14	54	F	Stomach	Ep cel	+	High	–	–
15	72	M	Stomach	Sp cel	–	High	Peritoneum, liver, lung, adrenal gland	+
16	60	F	Stomach	Sp cel	–	High	–	+
17	52	M	Small bowel	Sp cel	–	High	–	+
18	70	M	Stomach	Sp cel	–	Intermediate	–	+
19	55	M	Small bowel	Sp cel	–	High	–	–
20	50	M	Stomach	Sp + Ep cel	–	High	Peritoneum	+
21	50	M	Stomach	Sp cel	–	Very low	–	–
22	48	M	Duodenum	Sp cel	–	Low	–	–
23	45	M	Stomach	Sp + Ep cel	+	High	–	+
24	83	M	Stomach	Sp cel	–	High	–	–
25	70	M	Small bowel	Sp cel	–	High	Lung, liver	–
26	25	F	Small bowel	Sp cel	–	Low	–	–
27	70	F	Stomach	Sp + Ep cel	–	Intermediate	–	–
28	49	M	Stomach	Sp cel	–	Intermediate	–	–
29	58	F	Peritoneum	Sp cel	–	High	–	–
30	52	M	Stomach	Sp cel	–	Intermediate	–	–
31	64	M	Stomach	Sp cel	–	High	–	–
32	56	M	Peritoneum	Sp cel	–	High	–	–
33	30	F	Peritoneum	Sp cel	+	High	–	–
34	57	F	Stomach	Sp cel	–	Very low	–	–
35	37	F	Stomach	Sp cel	–	High	–	–

F female, *M* male, *Sp cel* spindle cells type, *Sp + Ep cel* spindle and epithelioid type, *Ep* epithelioid type, – absent, negative, + present, positive

constantly expressed by GIST regardless of the mutational status [2–4]. Muscle markers and the S-100 protein can be weakly expressed by GIST, the CD34 immunoexpression is frequent in GIST, varying around 50–100% [1, 6]. In fact, these markers are not a "gold standard" for the positive diagnosis of GIST but can prove useful in order to rule out potential differential diagnosis. The most valuable markers are CD117 and DOG1 for the positive diagnosis [17]. In our study, for

the diagnostic purpose, we have used an immunohistochemical panel comprising antibodies against CD117, CD34, SMA and S-100 protein. All of our cases (100%) showed a diffuse and strong membranous or cytoplasmic staining for CD117, 27 cases (77.14%) were positive for CD34, 6 cases (17.14%) had a weak staining for SMA, whereas 1 case was weakly positive for S-100. The fact that we have not used DOG1 at the time of our study has certainly limited the chance of recording CD117-

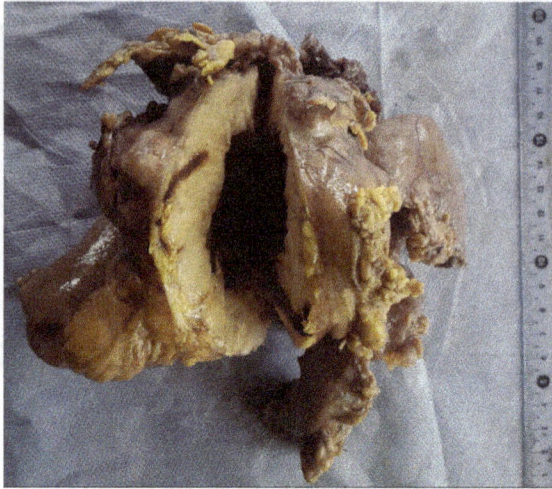

Fig. 4 A resected specimen of a small bowel GIST. The tumor arises typically in the intestinal wall and presents a cystic cavitation

Table 2 Correlation of MDM2 immunostaining with tumor site, size, mitotic count, necrosis, tumor risk, and metastastatic status

Variables	MDM2 negative (%)	MDM2 positive (%)	P value
Tumor site:			
Stomach	11/17 (64.70%)	6/17 (35.29%)	0.87
S. bowel	5/9 (55.55%)	4/9 (44.44%)	
Peritoneum	3/5 (60%)	2/5 (40%)	
Duodenum	1/3 (33.33%)	2/3 (66.66%)	
Colon	1/1 (100%)	0/1 (0%)	
Size (cm):			
≤ 5	7/8 (87.5%)	1/8 (12.5%)	0.08
5' S ≤ 10	7/17 (41.17%)	10/17 (58.82%)	
> 10	7/10 (70%)	3/10 (30%)	
Mitotic count/50 HPF:			
≤ 5	11/14 (78.57%)	3/14 (21.42%)	0.06
> 5	10/21 (47.61%)	11/21 (52.38%)	
Necrosis:			
Absent	18/27 (66.66%)	9/27 (33.33%)	0.14
Present	3/8 (37.5%)	5/8 (62.5%)	
Risk:			
Very low	2/2 (100%)	0/2 (0%)	0.34
Low	4/5 (80%)	1/5 (20%)	
Intermediate	5/7 (71.42%)	2/7 (28.57%)	
High	10/21 (47.61%)	11/21 (52.38%)	
Metastasis:			
Absent	20/26 (76.92%)	6/26 (23.07%)	0.001
Present	1/9 (11.11%)	8/9 (88.88%)	

negative GIST, especially the epithelioid subtype that can be CD117-negative in certain cases with *PDGRA* mutations or in other genetic alterations [2].

Like many cancers, the prognosis of GIST is based upon the occurrence of metastasis. In the past, a number of systems have been designed to assess the risk of recurrence or metastasis occurence in GIST [1, 7–10]. The AFIP criteria, reported by Miettienen et al. is widely used to assess the prognosis of GIST [1]. According to this system, 60% of patients (21 cases) in our study had high risk tumors, 7 patients (20%) had intermediate risk GIST, while the remaining cases had low risk and very low risk tumors (14.28% and 5.71% respectively). As synchronous metastasis have been diagnosed in 25.71% of our patients (9 cases), we have tried to correlate this clinical aggressive behavior with MDM2 immunoexpression. Although the AFIP criteria remains the most widely accepted model of predicting GIST behavior, other systems of risk stratification have been proposed, especially by Joensuu et al. These authors have suggested to consider the tumor rupture as a prognostic criteria along with the tumor site and the mitotic count [7, 9].

Concurrently, many attempts have been made to find prognostic biological markers to predict the behavior of GIST [11–13]. As a stromal tumor with a potential risk of malignancy (high risk tumors), GIST have been expected to harbor molecular or genetic disorders commonly found in various sarcomas. One of the most investigated molecular aspect in GIST is the MDM2-p53 pathway [11, 12, 18, 19]. *MDM2* is amplified in many human sarcomas, and at least 50% of human cancers harbor *TP53* mutations [19, 20]. In fact, *MDM2* is an oncogene that mainly exerts its activity by downregulating the *TP53* tumor suppressor gene activity and its product, p53. MDM2 negatively regulates p53 through its E3 ubiquitin ligase property. In fact, MDM2 binds to p53 and leads to its proteasomal degradation [18, 19, 21]. In 2005, Tornillo et al. found that around 10% of high risk/malignant GIST showed amplification of *MDM2* oncogene, and concluded that this fact may have a prognostic relevance in GIST [11]. However, more recently Wallander et al. found that amplification of *MDM2* is uncommon in GIST and it did not correlate with the tumoral behavior [12]. These studies have focused on *MDM2* amplification by using fluorescent in situ hybridization (FISH) analysis. In fact, MDM2 oncoprotein overexpression can be a result of either its gene mutation or a consequence of other post-transcriptional regulatory mechanisms [18, 19]. The proteomic approach is a best indicator of overexpression of oncoproteins like MDM2, regardless of biological mechanisms underlying their overproduction. Unfortunately this approach has been rarely applied to GIST [22]. We thought that immunohistochemistry, by showing overexpression of a given antigen, reflects partially the proteomic approach. In our current study, we have tried to assess overexpression of the MDM2 oncoprotein and its correlations with clinicopathological features of GIST. We found that 40% (14 cases) of GIST has shown immunohistochemical overexpression of MDM2, with 11/14 cases harboring high risk tumors and 8/14 cases presented with metastatic tumors. MDM2 immunohistochemical overexpression has been significantly associated with the metastatic status ($p = 0.001$). Despite the small size of our sample, we suggest that MDM2 immunohistochemical expression may have a prognostic significance in GIST, and this fact emphasizes the need for large studies to show the exact prognostic value of MDM2 oncoprotein. Recent studies have shown a great therapeutic promise of pharmacologic agents that modulate the MDM2-p53 pathway in GIST and in other types of cancers [23–25]. Interestingly, a new favorable prognostic biomarker of GIST, named pfetin has been discovered and its immunohistochemical assessment has proven useful in predicting recurrences or metastasis in GIST [22, 26]. The next years will probably provide significant insights about the identification of relevant prognostic biomarkers of GIST through robust scientific evidences.

Conclusion

Gastrointestinal stromal tumors (GIST) are common mesenchymal tumors of the gastrointestinal tract, with characteristic histopathological features. However the assessment of their biological behavior still remains a significant challenge. The current study suggests that MDM2 immunohistochemical expression is a negative histoprognostic factor in GIST and is significantly associated with the metastatic risk. These findings emphasize the urgent need for large studies in this way as the therapeutic modulation of MDM2-p53 pathway shows a consistent promise.

Abbreviations
AFIP: Armed Forces Institute of Pathology; GIST: Gastrointestinal stromal tumors; HES: Hematoxylin-eosin-safran; MDM2: Murine double minute 2; PDGFRA: Platelet-derived growth factor receptor A

Acknowledgements
Not applicable.

Funding
The authors received no specific funding for this study.

Authors' contributions
BE wrote the article and made substantial contributions to conception and design of the article; GAE, LT, ISS, FE, NH, AS, IM, AO, KM and HEF made critical assessment of the article; LC has been involved in drafting the manuscript and revising it critically for important intellectual content. All authors read and approved the final version of the manuscript.

Competing interest
All authors declare that they have no competing interest.

Author details
[1]Department of pathology, Hassan II university hospital, Fès, Morocco. [2]Laboratory of biological and translational research, Faculty of pharmacology and medicine, Sidi Mohamed Ben Abdellah University, Fès, Morocco. [3]Department of medical oncology, Hassan II university hospital, Fès, Morocco. [4]Faculty of pharmacology and medicine, Sidi Mohamed Ben Abdellah University, Fès, Morocco. [5]Department of hepatogastroenterology, Hassan II university hospital, Fès, Morocco. [6]Department of general and visceral surgery, Hassan II university hospital, Fès, Morocco.

References
1. Miettinen M, Lasota J. Gastrointestinal stromal tumors: pathology and prognosis at different sites. Semin Diagn Pathol. 2006;23(2):70–83.
2. Rubin BP, Heinrich MC. Genotyping and immunohistochemistry of gastrointestinal stromal tumors: an update. Semin Diagn Pathol. 2015;32(5):392–9.
3. Yamamoto H, Oda Y. Gastrointestinal stromal tumor: recent advances in pathology and genetics. Pathol Int. 2015;65(1):9–18.
4. Lamba G, Gupta R, Lee B, Ambrale S, Liu D. Current management and prognostic features for gastrointestinal stromal tumor (GIST). Exp Hematol Oncol. 2012;1(1):14.
5. Nannini M, Astolfi A, Urbini M, Indio V, Santini D, Heinrich MC, et al. Integrated genomic study of quadruple-WT GIST (KIT/PDGFRA/SDH/RAS pathway wild-type GIST). BMC Cancer. 2014;14:685.
6. Shidham VB, Chivukula M, Gupta D, Rao RN, Komorowski R. Immunohistochemical comparison of gastrointestinal stromal tumor and solitary fibrous tumor. Arch Pathol Lab Med. 2002;126(10):1189–92.
7. Joensuu H. Risk stratification of patients diagnosed with gastrointestinal stromal tumor. Hum Pathol. 2008;39(10):1411–9.
8. Gronchi A. Risk stratification models and mutational analysis: keys to optimising adjuvant therapy in patients with gastrointestinal stromal tumour. Eur J Cancer. 2013;49(4):884–92.
9. Joensuu H, Vehtari A, Riihimäki J, Nishida T, Steigen SE, Brabec P, et al. Risk of recurrence of gastrointestinal stromal tumour after surgery: an analysis of pooled population-based cohorts. Lancet Oncol. 2012;13(3):265–74.
10. Racz JM, Brar SS, Cleghorn MC, Jimenez MC, Azin A, Atenafu EG, et al. The accuracy of three predictive models in the evaluation of recurrence rates for gastrointestinal stromal tumors. J Surg Oncol. 2015;111(4):371–6.
11. Tornillo L, Duchini G, Carafa V, Lugli A, Dirnhofer S, Di Vizio D, et al. Patterns of gene amplification in gastrointestinal stromal tumors (GIST). Lab Investig. 2005;85(7):921–31.
12. Wallander ML, Layfield LJ, Tripp SR, Schmidt RL. Gastrointestinal stromal tumors: clinical significance of p53 expression, MDM2 amplification, and KIT mutation status. Appl Immunohistochem Mol Morphol. 2013;21(4):308–12.
13. Dorn J, Spatz H, Schmieder M, Barth TF, Blatz A, Henne-Bruns D, et al. Cyclin H expression is increased in GIST with very-high risk of malignancy. BMC Cancer. 2010;10:350.
14. Janeway KA, Weldon CB. Pediatric gastrointestinal stromal tumor. Semin Pediatr Surg. 2012;21(1):31–43.
15. Arabi NA, Musaad AM, Ahmed EE, Abdo AA, Elhassan AM, Hassan H, et al. Primary extragastrointestinal stromal tumour of the whole abdominal cavity, omentum, peritoneum and mesentery: a case report and review of the literature. J Med Case Rep. 2014;8:337.
16. Saeed Z, Taleb S, Evans-Molina C. A case of extragastrointestinal stromal tumor complicated by severe hypoglycemia: a unique presentation of a rare tumor. BMC Cancer. 2016;16(1):930.
17. Novelli M, Rossi S, Rodriguez-Justo M, Taniere P, Seddon B, Toffolatti L, et al. DOG1 and CD117 are the antibodies of choice in the diagnosis of gastrointestinal stromaltumours. Histopathology. 2010;57(2):259–70.
18. Zhao Y, Yu H, Hu W. The regulation of MDM2 oncogene and its impact on human cancers. Acta Biochim Biophys Sin Shanghai. 2014;46(3):180–9.
19. Wade M, Li YC, Wahl GM. MDM2, MDMX and p53 in oncogenesis and cancer therapy. Nat Rev Cancer. 2013;13(2):83–96.
20. Flørenes VA, Maelandsmo GM, Forus A, Andreassen A, Myklebost O, Fodstad O. MDM2 gene amplification and transcript levels in human sarcomas: relationship to TP53 gene status. J Natl Cancer Inst. 1994;86(17):1297–302.

21. Inoue K, Fry EA, Frazier DP. Transcription factors that interact with p53 and Mdm2. Int J Cancer. 2016;138(7):1577–85.
22. Kondo T, Suehara Y, Kikuta K, Kubota D, Tajima T, Mukaihara K, et al. Proteomic approach toward personalized sarcoma treatment: lessons from prognostic biomarker discovery in gastrointestinal stromal tumor. Proteomics Clin Appl. 2013;7(1–2):70–8.
23. Henze J, Mühlenberg T, Simon S, Grabellus F, Rubin B, Taeger G, et al. p53 modulation as a therapeutic strategy in gastrointestinal stromal tumors. PLoS One. 2012;7(5):e37776.
24. Zanjirband M, Edmondson RJ, Lunec J. Pre-clinical efficacy and synergistic potential of the MDM2-p53 antagonists, Nutlin-3 and RG7388, as single agents and in combined treatment with cisplatin in ovarian cancer. Oncotarget. 2016;7(26):40115–34.
25. Pishas KI, Neuhaus SJ, Clayer MT, Schreiber AW, Lawrence DM, Perugini M, et al. Nutlin-3a efficacy in sarcoma predicted by transcriptomic and epigenetic profiling. Cancer Res. 2014;74(3):921–31.
26. Kubota D, Mukaihara K, Yoshida A, Suehara Y, Saito T, Okubo T, et al. The prognostic value of pfetin: a validation study in gastrointestinal stromal tumors using a commercially available antibody. Jpn J Clin Oncol. 2013; 43(6):669–75.

26

Differential expression of CK20, β-catenin, and MUC2/5AC/6 in Lynch syndrome and familial colorectal cancer type X

Stefan Haraldsson[1][*] (iD), Louise Klarskov[2], Mef Nilbert[3,4], Inge Bernstein[5,6], Jesper Bonde[7] and Susanne Holck[8]

Abstract

Background: Hereditary non-polyposis colorectal cancer comprises Lynch syndrome and familial colorectal cancer type X (FCCTX). Differences in genetics, demographics and histopathology have been extensively studied. The purpose of this study is to characterize their immunoprofile of markers other than MMR proteins.

Methods: We compared the expression patterns of cytokeratins (CK7 and CK20), mucins (MUC2/5 AC/6), CDX2 and β-catenin in Lynch syndrome and FCCTX.

Results: Differences were identified for CK20 and nuclear β-catenin, which were significantly more often expressed in FCCTX than in Lynch syndrome ($p < 0.001$), whereas MUC2, MUC5AC and MUC6 were overexpressed in Lynch syndrome tumors compared with FCCTX tumors ($p = 0.001$, < 0.01, and < 0.001, respectively). We observed no differences in the expression patterns of CK7 and CDX2.

Conclusions: In summary, we identified significant differences in the immunoprofiles of colorectal cancers linked to FCCTX and Lynch syndrome with a more sporadic-like profile in the former group and a more distinct profile with frequent MUC6 positivity in the latter group.

Keywords: Hereditary non-polyposis colorectal cancer, Fcctx, Lynch syndrome, Immunohistochemical profile

Background

Identification of hereditary colorectal cancer provides an unprecedented possibility for cancer prevention through inclusion of family members at increased risk into surveillance programs. Identification and diagnostics of hereditary colorectal cancer requires joint efforts from clinicians, pathologists and geneticists. Hereditary non-polyposis colorectal cancer (HNPCC) represents the most common subset of hereditary colorectal cancer and comprises the major subsets Lynch syndrome and familial colorectal cancer type X (FCCTX). Germline mutations in one of the mismatch repair (MMR) genes and resultant microsatellite instability (MSI) characterize Lynch syndrome, whereas retained MMR function and unknown genetic causes characterize FCCTX [1–3]. Lynch syndrome shows a lower mean age at onset, an abundance of right-sided colon tumors and more frequent extracolonic tumors, whereas FCCTX is predominantly characterized by tumors in the distal colon and the rectum and shows a somewhat higher mean age at onset. Histologic differences include a "pushing" growth pattern, lymphocytic reactions, poor differentiation with mucinous and medullary growth patterns in Lynch syndrome and an infiltrative growth pattern, tumor budding, "dirty" necrosis, glandular differentiation and frequent node positivity in FCCTX [4–6].

The purpose of this study is to record the immunoprofile of markers well-described in colorectal carcinoma in general but, hitherto, incompletely studied in hereditary colorectal carcinomas. These include cytokeratins, mucin glycoproteins, and CDX2. Specifically, its discriminatory utility in FCCTX- vs Lynch syndrome cases is addressed, as is the feasibility of identifying FCCTX among colorectal carcinomas in general. Additionally, β-catenin is included, to compare the extent of the wnt pathway activation in the two hereditary cohorts, as Wnt-signaling genes are shown to be upregulated in FCCTX tumors.

* Correspondence: stebbihar@gmail.com
[1]Department of Gastroenterology, Copenhagen University Hospital, Kettegaard Alle 29, DK-2650 Hvidovre, Denmark
Full list of author information is available at the end of the article

Methods

Patient identification and accrual of samples

Patients were identified through the national Danish HNPCC register (http://www.hnpcc.dk). In Denmark, patients with suspected or verified hereditary colorectal cancer are reported to this register by laboratories and responsible clinicians. In Denmark, colorectal cancer diagnostics includes reflex testing for MMR protein expression using antibodies against MLH1, PSM2, MSH2 and MSH6. Cases with loss of expression are, if applicable, and implying the patient provides consent, referred to genetic counselling. Genetic counselling is performed by clinical genetic counsellors and clinical geneticists at 4 departments countrywide. Following genetic diagnostics, Lynch syndrome was defined as presence of disease-predisposing MMR gene variants (classes 4 and 5) and FCCTX was defined as families that fulfilled the Amsterdam criteria, but had tumors with retained MMR function and for the majority of families also genetic MMR gene testing without mutations. The histopathological profiles of the 2 cohorts have been presented in Klarskov et al. [4]. In total, 65 colorectal cancers from 60 individuals in 41 FCCTX families and 68 Lynch syndrome tumors from 62 individuals in 41 families were studied including 2 synchronous and 3 metachronous tumor pairs. Hematoxylin & eosin stained slides from the formalin fixed-paraffin embedded (FFPE) tissue samples selected were reviewed to ensure representation of the deep tumor margin [7]. Clinical data were collected from the pathology reports and tumor location was classified as proximal or distal in relation to the splenic flexure. Tumor differentiation was classified as poorly differentiated/undifferentiated or highly/moderately differentiated.

The study was granted ethical permission by the Region Hovedstaden ethical review board (H-D-2007-032).

Immunohistochemical staining

Immunohistochemical stainings were performed on fresh 4-μm sections from FFPE tissue that was deparaffinized in Tissue clear. Antigen retrieval was achieved by PT-Link and 3-in-1 buffer, pH 9 (Dako). The sections were processed in a Dako autostainer (Dako, Denmark), applying the antibodies targeting CK7/20, MUC2/5 AC/6, CDX2, and β-catenin (Table 1). The Envision Detection Kit (DakoCytomation) was used according to the manufacturer's instructions and tissue sections were counterstained with Meyer's hematoxylin, dehydrated, mounted on coated slides, and dried 1 h at 60°. The immunostainings were scored semiquantitatively by two independent pathologists (LK, SH), blinded to mutational status. A 5-tier scale was applied, using the following categories; no staining, < 5%, 5–50%, 51–95% and > 95% stained tumor cells. In the analyses, the stainings were dichotomized into negative (< 5% staining) and positive (≥ 5% staining). For

Table 1 Antibodies

Antibody	Clone	Dilution	Manufacturer
CK7	OV-TL 12/30	RTU	Dako, DK
CK20	KS20.8	RTU	Dako, DK
MUC2	Ccp58	1:25	Novocastra/Leica, UK
MUC5Ac	CLH2	1:200	Novocastra/Leica, UK
MUC6	CLH5	1:50	Novocastra/Leica, UK
β-catenin	β-catenin 1	RTU	Dako, DK
Cdx2	Dak-CDX2	RTU	Dako, DK

RTU ready to use

CDX2 only strong expression, equivalent to the intensity of the normal mucosa was considered, for the other immunostainings, labelling intensity was not considered. Where interpretative doubts arose and in case of diverse readings, which rarely exceeded one category, consensus was reached by conference.

Statistics

All data were entered in duplicate in Epidata and exported to SPSS 17.0 for statistical analysis. Statistical differences between the groups were determined using Pearson's χ^2-test for categorical and independent samples, t-test for continuous parametric data. P-values less than 0.05 were considered statistically significant.

Results

Clinical data

Clinical data are summarized in Table 2. Significant differences applied as regards age (younger mean age in Lynch syndrome, $p < 0.001$), tumor location (78% of FCCTX tumors were left-sided versus 26% of Lynch syndrome, $p < 0.001$) and extent of differentiation (54% of Lynch syndrome poorly differentiated/undifferentiated versus 17% of FCCTX tumors ($p < 0.001$)).

Table 2 Demographics and tumor differentiation

Variables	FCCTX ($n = 65$)	Lynch ($n = 68$)	P value
Median age, (range), years	60 (28–83)	52 (25–82)	< 0.001
Gender, male	34 (52%)	28 (41%)	NS
Tumor site[a]			< 0.001
Right	13 (20%)	48 (71%)	
Left	51 (78%)	18 (26%)	
Not indicated	1 (2%)	2 (3%)	
Histological differentiation			< 0.001
High/moderate	54 (83%)	31 (56%)	
Poor/undifferentiated	11 (17%)	37 (54%)	

NS not significant

[a] Cut-off: splenic flexure

Immunohistochemistry

The immunohistochemical profiles for five of the seven markers studied significantly differed between colorectal cancers linked to FCCTX and Lynch syndrome (Tables 3 and 4). Aberrant, nuclear staining for β-catenin (Fig. 1a) was more common in FCCTX tumors, whereas the β-catenin staining more often was normal, i.e. confined to the cell membranes (Fig. 1b), in Lynch syndrome ($p < 0.001$). Compared to FCCTX tumors, Lynch syndrome tumors displayed significantly more often expression of the tested MUC glycoproteins. The difference in MUC expression was particularly prominent for MUC6 (Fig. 2) ($p < 0.001$), less so for MUC2 (Fig. 3) ($p = 0.001$), and MUC5AC ($p < 0.01$). FCCTX tumors showed more frequent CK20 expression than did Lynch syndrome tumors ($p < 0.001$) with an equal distribution in right and left side of the large bowel. In Lynch syndrome tumors, CK20 expression patterns correlated to tumor location with more frequent expression of CK20 in right-sided tumors (77%) than in the left-sided tumors (50%) ($p = 0.03$).

The CK7 expression rate was 12 and 15% in FCCTX and Lynch syndrome, respectively.

The combined CK7/20 patterns showed significant differences between Lynch syndrome tumors and FCCTX tumors (Table 4). The prevailing CK7−/CK20+ profile was identified in 83% of the FCCTX cases and in 63% of the Lynch syndrome tumors. CK7+/CK20+ profile was the second most common combination (12%) in FCCTXs, but was rare (4%) in Lynch syndrome tumors, which more often (22%) showed a CK7−/CK20− profile.

Expression of CDX2 was abundant without statistical significant differences between Lynch syndrome and FCCTX (93 and 99%, respectively).

Discussion

Immunohistochemical staining is commonly applied as adjunct diagnostics in colorectal cancer. To this end profiles for the expression of cytokeratins, CDX2 and mucin glycoproteins are well-established markers [8–11] that are available in colorectal cancer diagnostics in most pathology laboratories. Since application of such

Table 3 Immunoprofiles of FCCTX and Lynch syndrome-associated CRC

Marker	FCCTX (n = 65)	Lynch (n = 68)	P value
CK20, n (%)	62 (95)	46 (68)	< 0.001
CK7, n (%)	8 (12)	10 (15)	NS
MUC2, n (%)	42 (65)	60 (88)	0.001
MUC5AC, n (%)	7 (11)	20 (29)	< 0.01
MUC6, n (%)	2 (3)	17 (25)	< 0.001
CDX2, n (%)	·64 (99)	63 (93)	NS
β-catenin, nuclear, n (%)	34 (52)	11 (16)	< 0.001

NS not significant

Table 4 Combined CK7/CK20-profiles of FCCTX and Lynch syndrome-associated CRC

Combination	FCCTX (n = 65)	Lynch (n = 68)	P value
CK7−/CK20+, n (%)	54 (83)	43 (63)	0.01
CK7+/CK20+, n (%)	8 (12)	3 (4)	NS
CK7−/CK20-, n (%)	3 (5)	15 (22)	0.003
CK7+/CK20-, n (%)	0 (0)	7 (10)	0.008

NS not significant

profiles may be relevant also in hereditary cancer diagnostics, our aim was to define these profiles in the two major HNPCC subsets of colorectal cancer. Moreover, immunohistochemical profiling may contribute to the molecular understanding of these subsets. Herein, a large fraction of FCCTX tumors has been shown to harbour *APC* (adenomatous polyposis coli) mutations [12], which motivated evaluation of β-catenin staining as a candidate marker.

Tumors linked to Lynch syndrome and FCCTX showed significant differences, primarily related to frequent expression of CK20 and nuclear β-catenin in FCCTX and relative over-expression of MUC2, MUC5AC and MUC6 in Lynch syndrome. Sánchez-Tomé et al. likewise reported differences in the immunoprofile of FCCTX carcinomas (27 cases) – and Lynch syndrome carcinomas (18 cases) based on markers selected to analyze colorectal carcinogenesis, including SMAD4, COX2, MUC1, and P53 [13]. Despite differences in the selected immunopanels in these two studies the differences between the two hereditary cohorts in both studies are remarkable, and suggest that these profiles may be of clinical diagnostic relevance. We further found that FCCTX tumors generally mimicked the profile of the non-neoplastic colorectal mucosa, with CK20+, MUC5AC- and MUC6-, which contrasted to the expression pattern in the Lynch syndrome tumors.

Frequent (70–100%) expression of CK20 has been reported in unselected colorectal cancers [8, 14–20]. The reduced expression of CK20 observed in Lynch syndrome is in line with reduced CK20 levels in MSI tumors [9] and in poorly differentiated tumors (54% of Lynch syndrome carcinomas vs 17% in the FCCTX cases in the present material were poorly differentiated). In this context, it is noteworthy that cytokeratin filaments are relatively stable during transformation to carcinoma [21], a quality that is lost in a proportion of the Lynch syndrome carcinomas. CK20 expression has also been reported to correlate with the anatomical location with more abundant expression in the distal colon [17, 22]. This distribution pattern was, however, not observed in the current cohorts, which showed no side differences in FCCTX and higher expression in proximal than in distal Lynch syndrome tumors.

218

New Frontiers in Clinical Pathology

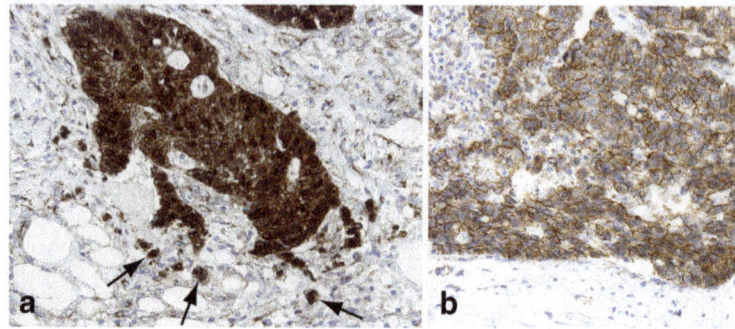

Fig. 1 β-catenin expression In a FCCTX carcinoma (**a**) and in a Lynch syndrome carcinoma (**b**): The invasive front of FCCTX carcinoma (**a**) with prominent nuclear labelling of the single, budding tumor cells (some are arrowed) and in most tumor cells sited in the more coherent group. This aberrant profile characterized 52% of the FCCTX cohort, but only 16% of the Lynch syndrome tumors. Note additionally the infiltrative quality of the invasive front of the tumor, another feature of FCCTX tumors [4]. The invasive front of a Lynch syndrome carcinoma (**b**) with normal staining pattern, i.e. labelling confined to the tumor cell membranes, specifically absence of nuclear labelling. Note the pushing quality of the invasive border (below) and absence of budding cells, additional features of Lynch syndrome carcinomas [4]

CK7 expression did not differ between Lynch syndrome tumors and FCCTX tumors and paralleled the expression levels (10–22%) in unselected and sporadic colorectal cancers reported in the literature [8, 15, 17].

The prevailing CK7−/CK20+ cytokeratin profile is reported in 55–77% of colorectal cancer in general [9] and was also the predominant profile in the hereditary subsets, though more frequent in FCCTX compared to Lynch syndrome. The second most common cytokeratin profile in unselected tumors is the CK7+/CK20+ combination identified in 15% of tumors [8, 9, 23]. This pattern was also the second leading profile in the FCCTX cases. In Lynch syndrome tumors the CK7−/CK20− profile was the second most common pattern, conceivably reflecting a higher frequency of poorly differentiated tumors [4, 24], speculatively a result of the hypermutated state of MSI tumors. Of further note is the CK7+/20− combination in 10% of our Lynch syndrome tumors. Bayrak et al. [8] reported this rare pattern in only 2% of unselected cases, whereas this profile specifically was noted in high grade, right-sided colorectal cancers, properties suggestive of Lynch syndrome. According to our results, this unusual profile seems to exclude FCCTX and might suggest Lynch syndrome. Additionally, the CK7−/20− combination makes FCCTX unlikely. The other combinations of CK7 and CK20 lack, however, discriminatory value.

Loss of expression of CDX2 in colorectal cancer has been reported as a negative prognostic marker [25]. CDX2 expression in the HNPCC-associated colorectal cancers in the present study was high, which is in accordance with the relatively good prognosis characterizing these cancers, and did not differ from some series on colorectal carcinoma in general [23, 26–28]. Diversities in study design, specifically use of tissue micro array, can readily contribute to the lower values noted in other reports of colorectal cancers [15, 29, 30].

Our study on the secreted gel-forming mucins (MUC2, MUC5AC, and MUC6) demonstrated significantly higher values in the Lynch syndrome than in the FCCTX tumors. In this context, the idea that the MSI status may influence mucus production, by altering the genes involved [31] is noteworthy. Mucinous differentiation, though it may not reach the 50% required for

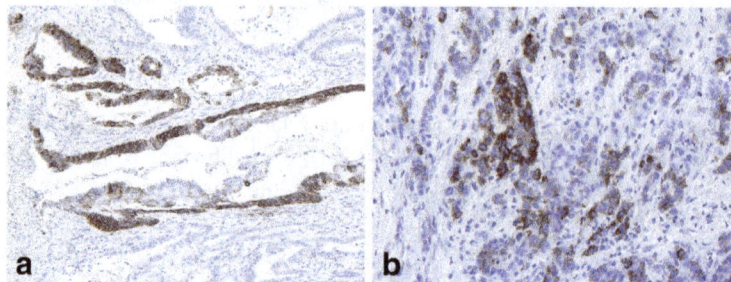

Fig. 2 Focal MUC6 expression in two LS carcinomas (**a** and **b**): 25% of the Lynch syndrome carcinomas were focally positive. This profile was noted in highly/moderately differentiated examples (prominent glandular component) (**a**), as well as in poorly differentiated/undifferentiated cases (absence of glandular elements) (**b**). Merely 3% of the FCCTX cohort displayed MUC6 expression

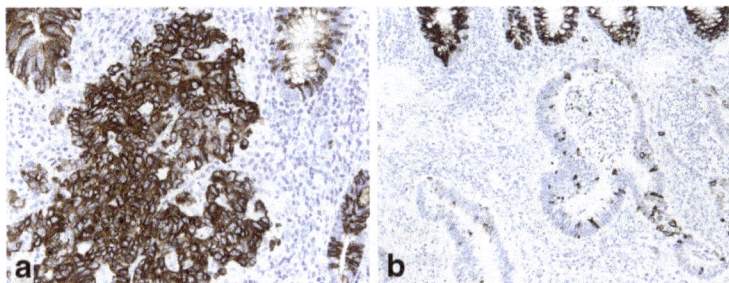

Fig. 3 MUC2 expression in a Lynch syndrome carcinoma (**a**) and in a FCCTX carcinoma (**b**): 88% of the Lynch syndrome carcinomas were MUC2 positive, compared to 65% of the FCCTX cases. The Lynch syndrome carcinoma illustrated in A, is extensively decorated (portions of non-neoplastic crypts appear to the right). The FCCTX carcinoma, illustrated in B, comprises only few scattered immunopositive cells. Top of the field displays basis of several non-neoplastic crypts

classification of a mucinous tumor, is frequent in Lynch syndrome tumors. Of note is the observation that MUC expression levels identified in Lynch syndrome tumors were higher than described in reported series of mucinous tumors [32–34]. MUC6 expression has been suggested to inhibit tumor invasion in pancreatic cancer [35], which may apply to colorectal cancer as well and could play a role in the favourable prognosis known to characterize Lynch syndrome tumors. Indeed, a recent report on the clinical significance of secreted gel-forming MUCs in colorectal carcinomas demonstrated a favorable influence on the outcome in case of gain in aberrant MUC expression, particularly of MUC6 expression [36]. The MUC profile in the FCCTX subset was more akin to that of unselected colorectal cancers with MUC2 expression reported in 40–54%, MUC5AC in 6–10% and MUC6 in 4% [17, 37].

Nuclear translocation of β-catenin is a marker of dysregulated Wnt signalling. Diverse mechanisms may induce this event in colorectal carcinoma, the major cause being dysfunction of the *APC* gene [38]. In total, 52% of the present FCCTX tumors showed aberrant nuclear β-catenin, which is in line with unselected and MMR-proficient series [26, 39]. The findings also roughly correlate with those of Franscisco et al. [12] who reported *APC* mutation in 62% of their FCCTX cases. Other MMR-mutation negative, familial series (including 20, 24, and 44 cases) have reported lower frequencies of nuclear β-catenin [40–42]. Given the presumed heterogeneity of FCCTX tumors, partial inclusion of MSI tumors, differences in study design and limited-size series disparities can be anticipated [12]. *β-catenin* mutation, another cause of aberrant β-catenin, probably contributes to the occasional aberrant β-catenin expression in Lynch syndrome tumors. Based on the current immunohistochemical study, nuclear β-catenin expression in Lynch syndrome tumors is uncommon compared to its prevalence in FCCTX (16% vs. 52%). In concert, nuclear β-catenin expression was previously recorded in merely

19% of colorectal cancer from 118 Lynch syndrome patients in a study conducted by some of us [43]. Further markers of the wnt-signalling pathway may be of interest in future studies of FCCTX tumors.

Distinct gene expression patterns have been demonstrated in colorectal cancers linked to Lynch syndrome and FCCTX and overall support that FCCTX tumors mimic sporadic MMR-proficient tumors [44, 45]. These data and the immunohistochemical expression differences we describe herein suggest that evaluation of key markers should be exploited for future diagnostic application. FCCTX tumors are characterized by chromosomal instability and deregulation of genes and proteins involved in e.g. chromosomal segregation, genomic stability, apoptosis, proliferation, growth inhibition, angiogenesis and migration [44]. The limited data available point to involvement of pathways related to G protein-coupled signaling, proliferation and migration. In line with this, FCCTX tumors frequently show infiltrative growth patterns and presence of dirty necrosis [45]. Lynch syndrome tumors show frequent deregulation of genes involved in the cell cycle progression and in the oxidative phosphorylation pathway as well as immune response genes. Regarding the latter, studies are currently exploring the role of immunohistochemical evaluation of specific immune checkpoint proteins in the context of immunotherapy in colorectal cancer. The role for DNA methylation changes remains to be defined, though the gene-specific methylation of MLH1 is a hallmark of the hypermutable phenotype in sporadic MSI tumors and global hypomethylation has been demonstrated in FCCTX and has been shown to interfere with chromosomal instability.

The strengths of the present study include clinically well-defined and relatively large study populations, immunohistochemical evaluations on whole sections in contraposition to the limited areas available by tissue micro arrays (the latter a potential source of error, as previously pinpointed [23]), and evaluation by two pathologists who were blinded to patient data. The study design allows for descriptive analyses only, which is a limitation and data on somatic mutations of KRAS, NRAS and BRAF are not included.

Conclusions

Significant differences in the immunohistochemical profiles of colorectal cancers linked to Lynch syndrome and FCCTX are not restricted to MMR-proteins. In particular, CK20, MUC2, MUC5AC, MUC6 and β-catenin showed disparate expression patterns that may in part be ascribed to clinicopathologic factors such as tumor location, mucinous components, differentiation, and MSI-status, conceivably reflecting diverse underlying genetic mechanism(s). The chosen antibody panel did not allow differentiation between FCCTX and colorectal carcinoma in general. As knowledge on FCCTX genetic(s) emerges, translation into novel biomarkers, useful in discriminating FCCTX from its sporadic counterpart can be anticipated.

Abbreviations
APC: Adenomatous polyposis coli; CDX: Caudal type homeobox; CK: Cytokeratin; FCCTX: Familial Colorectal Cancer Type X; FFPE: Formalin fixed paraffin embedded; HNPCC: Hereditary non-polyposis colorectal cancer; MMR: Mismatch repair; MSI: Microsatellite instability; MUC: Mucin

Acknowledgements
Not applicable

Funding
Financial support was granted by the Beckett Foundation.

Authors' contributions
SH supervised the study, participated in study design, was one of the blinded pathologists who examined the slides and participated in the writing of the manuscript. LLK participated in study design, was one of the blinded pathologists who examined the slides, participated in data analysis and in the writing of the manuscript. StH analysed the data, performed statistical analysis and participated in the writing of the article. MN, IB and JB provided key technical and scientific input and contributed in writing the manuscript. All authors read and approved the final manuscript.

Competing interests
The authors declare that they have no competing interests.

Author details
[1]Department of Gastroenterology, Copenhagen University Hospital, Kettegaard Alle 29, DK-2650 Hvidovre, Denmark. [2]Department of Pathology, Herlev-Gentofte Hospital, Herlev, Denmark. [3]Clinical Research Centre, HNPCC register, Copenhagen University Hospital, Hvidovre, Denmark. [4]Institute of Clinical Sciences, Division of Oncology, Lund University, Lund, Sweden. [5]HNPCC register, Copenhagen University Hospital, Hvidovre, Denmark. [6]Department of Surgical Gastroenterology, Aalborg University Hospital, Aalborg, Denmark. [7]Department of Pathology and Clinical Research Center, Copenhagen University Hospital, Hvidovre, Denmark. [8]Department of Pathology, Copenhagen University Hospital, Hvidovre, Denmark.

References
1. Lindor NM, Rabe K, Petersen GM, Haile R, Casey G, Baron J, Gallinger S, Bapat B, Aronson M, Hopper J, et al. Lower cancer incidence in Amsterdam-I criteria families without mismatch repair deficiency: familial colorectal cancer type X. JAMA. 2005;293(16):1979–85.
2. Vasen HF, Mecklin JP, Khan PM, Lynch HT. The international collaborative group on hereditary non-polyposis colorectal cancer (ICG-HNPCC). Dis Colon Rectum. 1991;34(5):424–5.
3. Vasen HF, Watson P, Mecklin JP, Lynch HT. New clinical criteria for hereditary nonpolyposis colorectal cancer (HNPCC, lynch syndrome) proposed by the international collaborative group on HNPCC. Gastroenterology. 1999;116(6):1453–6.
4. Klarskov L, Holck S, Bernstein I, Nilbert M. Hereditary colorectal cancer diagnostics: morphological features of familial colorectal cancer type X versus lynch syndrome. J Clin Pathol. 2012;65(4):352–6.
5. Halvarsson B, Muller W, Planck M, Benoni AC, Mangell P, Ottosson J, Hallen M, Isinger A, Nilbert M. Phenotypic heterogeneity in hereditary non-polyposis colorectal cancer: identical germline mutations associated with variable tumour morphology and immunohistochemical expression. J Clin Pathol. 2007;60(7):781–6.
6. Jenkins MA, Hayashi S, O'Shea AM, Burgart LJ, Smyrk TC, Shimizu D, Waring PM, Ruszkiewicz AR, Pollett AF, Redston M, et al. Pathology features in Bethesda guidelines predict colorectal cancer microsatellite instability: a population-based study. Gastroenterology. 2007;133(1):48–56.
7. Laurent C, Svrcek M, Flejou JF, Chenard MP, Duclos B, Freund JN, Reimund JM. Immunohistochemical expression of CDX2, beta-catenin, and TP53 in inflammatory bowel disease-associated colorectal cancer. Inflamm Bowel Dis. 2011;17(1):232–40.
8. Bayrak R, Yenidunya S, Haltas H. Cytokeratin 7 and cytokeratin 20 expression in colorectal adenocarcinomas. Pathol Res Pract. 2011;207(3):156–60.
9. McGregor DK, Wu TT, Rashid A, Luthra R, Hamilton SR. Reduced expression of cytokeratin 20 in colorectal carcinomas with high levels of microsatellite instability. Am J Surg Pathol. 2004;28(6):712–8.
10. Olsen AK, Coskun M, Bzorek M, Kristensen MH, Danielsen ET, Jorgensen S, Olsen J, Engel U, Holck S, Troelsen JT. Regulation of APC and AXIN2 expression by intestinal tumor suppressor CDX2 in colon cancer cells. Carcinogenesis. 2013;34(6):1361–9.
11. Yao T, Tsutsumi S, Akaiwa Y, Takata M, Nishiyama K, Kabashima A, Tsuneyoshi M. Phenotypic expression of colorectal adenocarcinomas with reference to tumor development and biological behavior. Gann. 2001;92(7):755–61.
12. Francisco I, Albuquerque C, Lage P, Belo H, Vitoriano I, Filipe B, Claro I, Ferreira S, Rodrigues P, Chaves P, et al. Familial colorectal cancer type X syndrome: two distinct molecular entities? Familial Cancer. 2011;10(4):623–31.
13. Sanchez-Tome E, Rivera B, Perea J, Pita G, Rueda D, Mercadillo F, Canal A, Gonzalez-Neira A, Benitez J, Urioste M. Genome-wide linkage analysis and tumoral characterization reveal heterogeneity in familial colorectal cancer type X. J Gastroenterol. 2015;50(6):657–66.
14. Chu PG, Weiss LM. Keratin expression in human tissues and neoplasms. Histopathology. 2002;40(5):403–39.
15. Kim MJ, Hong SM, Jang SJ, Yu E, Kim JS, Kim KR, Gong G, Ro JY. Invasive colorectal micropapillary carcinoma: an aggressive variant of adenocarcinoma. Hum Pathol. 2006;37(7):809–15.
16. Lagendijk JH, Mullink H, van Diest PJ, Meijer GA, Meijer CJ. Immunohistochemical differentiation between primary adenocarcinomas of the ovary and ovarian metastases of colonic and breast origin. Comparison between a statistical and an intuitive approach. J Clin Pathol. 1999;52(4):283–90.
17. Lee MJ, Lee HS, Kim WH, Choi Y, Yang M. Expression of mucins and cytokeratins in primary carcinomas of the digestive system. Mod Pathol. 2003;16(5):403–10.
18. Moll R, Lowe A, Laufer J, Franke WW. Cytokeratin 20 in human carcinomas. A new histodiagnostic marker detected by monoclonal antibodies. Am J Pathol. 1992;140(2):427–47.
19. Park SY, Kim HS, Hong EK, Kim WH. Expression of cytokeratins 7 and 20 in primary carcinomas of the stomach and colorectum and their value in the differential diagnosis of metastatic carcinomas to the ovary. Hum Pathol. 2002;33(11):1078–85.
20. Tot T. The role of cytokeratins 20 and 7 and estrogen receptor analysis in separation of metastatic lobular carcinoma of the breast and metastatic signet ring cell carcinoma of the gastrointestinal tract. APMIS. 2000;108(6):467–72.
21. Omary MB, Ku NO, Strnad P, Hanada S. Toward unraveling the complexity of simple epithelial keratins in human disease. J Clin Invest. 2009;119(7):1794–805.

22. Saad RS, Silverman JF, Khalifa MA, Rowsell C. CDX2, cytokeratins 7 and 20 immunoreactivity in rectal adenocarcinoma. Appl Immunohistochem Mol Morphol. 2009;17(3):196–201.

23. Barbareschi M, Murer B, Colby TV, Chilosi M, Macri E, Loda M, Doglioni C. CDX-2 homeobox gene expression is a reliable marker of colorectal adenocarcinoma metastases to the lungs. Am J Surg Pathol. 2003;27(2):141–9.

24. Pancione M, Di Blasi A, Sabatino L, Fucci A, Dalena AM, Palombi N, Carotenuto P, Aquino G, Daniele B, Normanno N, et al. A novel case of rhabdoid colon carcinoma associated with a positive CpG island methylator phenotype and BRAF mutation. Hum Pathol. 2011;42(7):1047–52.

25. Dalerba P, Sahoo D, Paik S, Guo X, Yothers G, Song N, Wilcox-Fogel N, Forgo E, Rajendran PS, Miranda SP, et al. CDX2 as a prognostic biomarker in stage II and stage III colon cancer. N Engl J Med. 2016;374(3):211–22.

26. Logani S, Oliva E, Arnell PM, Amin MB, Young RH. Use of novel immunohistochemical markers expressed in colonic adenocarcinoma to distinguish primary ovarian tumors from metastatic colorectal carcinoma. Mod Pathol. 2005;10(1):19–23.

27. Moskaluk CA, Zhang H, Powell SM, Cerilli LA, Hampton GM, Frierson HF Jr. Cdx2 protein expression in normal and malignant human tissues: an immunohistochemical survey using tissue microarrays. Mod Pathol. 2003;16(9):913–9.

28. Werling RW, Yaziji H, Bacchi CE, Gown AM. CDX2, a highly sensitive and specific marker of adenocarcinomas of intestinal origin: an immunohistochemical survey of 476 primary and metastatic carcinomas. Am J Surg Pathol. 2003;27(3):303–10.

29. Baba Y, Nosho K, Shima K, Freed E, Irahara N, Philips J, Meyerhardt JA, Hornick JL, Shivdasani RA, Fuchs CS, et al. Relationship of CDX2 loss with molecular features and prognosis in colorectal cancer. Clin Cancer Res. 2009;15(14):4665–73.

30. Lugli A, Tzankov A, Zlobec I, Terracciano LM. Differential diagnostic and functional role of the multi-marker phenotype CDX2/CK20/CK7 in colorectal cancer stratified by mismatch repair status. Mod Pathol. 2008;21(11):1403–12.

31. Messerini L, Vitelli F, De Vitis LR, Mori S, Calzolari A, Palmirotta R, Calabro A, Papi L. Microsatellite instability in sporadic mucinous colorectal carcinomas: relationship to clinico-pathological variables. J Pathol. 1997;182(4):380–4.

32. Shin JH, Bae JH, Lee A, Jung CK, Yim HW, Park JS, Lee KY. CK7, CK20, CDX2 and MUC2 Immunohistochemical staining used to distinguish metastatic colorectal carcinoma involving ovary from primary ovarian mucinous adenocarcinoma. Jpn J Clin Oncol. 2010;40(3):208–13.

33. Ishizu H, Kumagai J, Eishi Y, Takizawa T, Koike M. Mucin core protein expression by colorectal mucinous carcinomas with or without mucus hyperplasia. J Gastroenterol. 2004;39(2):125–32.

34. Chu PG, Chung L, Weiss LM, Lau SK. Determining the site of origin of mucinous adenocarcinoma: an immunohistochemical study of 175 cases. Am J Surg Pathol. 2011;35(12):1830–6.

35. Leir SH, Harris A. MUC6 mucin expression inhibits tumor cell invasion. Exp Cell Res. 2011;317(17):2408–19.

36. Betge J, Schneider NI, Harbaum L, Pollheimer MJ, Lindtner RA, Kornprat P, Ebert MP, Langner C. MUC1, MUC2, MUC5AC, and MUC6 in colorectal cancer: expression profiles and clinical significance. Virchows Arch. 2016; 469(3):255–65.

37. Fujimoto Y, Nakanishi Y, Sekine S, Yoshimura K, Akasu T, Moriya Y, Shimoda T. CD10 expression in colorectal carcinoma correlates with liver metastasis. Dis Colon Rectum. 2005;48(10):1883–9.

38. Hao X, Frayling IM, Willcocks TC, Han W, Tomlinson IP, Pignatelli MN, Pretlow TP, Talbot IC. Beta-catenin expression and allelic loss at APC in sporadic colorectal carcinogenesis. Virchows Arch. 2002;440(4):362–6.

39. Lugli A, Zlobec I, Minoo P, Baker K, Tornillo L, Terracciano L, Jass JR. Prognostic significance of the wnt signalling pathway molecules APC, beta-catenin and E-cadherin in colorectal cancer: a tissue microarray-based analysis. Histopathology. 2007;50(4):453–64.

40. Abdel-Rahman WM, Ollikainen M, Kariola R, Jarvinen HJ, Mecklin JP, Nystrom-Lahti M, Knuutila S, Peltomaki P. Comprehensive characterization of HNPCC-related colorectal cancers reveals striking molecular features in families with no germline mismatch repair gene mutations. Oncogene. 2005;24(9):1542–51.

41. Sanchez-de-Abajo A, de la Hoya M, van Puijenbroek M, Tosar A, Lopez-Asenjo JA, Diaz-Rubio E, Morreau H, Caldes T. Molecular analysis of colorectal cancer tumors from patients with mismatch repair proficient hereditary nonpolyposis colorectal cancer suggests novel carcinogenic pathways. Clin Cancer Res. 2007;13(19):5729–35.

42. Balaz P, Plaschke J, Kruger S, Gorgens H, Schackert HK. TCF-3, 4 protein expression correlates with beta-catenin expression in MSS and MSI-H colorectal cancer from HNPCC patients but not in sporadic colorectal cancers. Int J Color Dis. 2010;25(8):931–9.

43. Isinger-Ekstrand A, Therkildsen C, Bernstein I, Nilbert M. Deranged Wnt signaling is frequent in hereditary nonpolyposis colorectal cancer. Familial Cancer. 2011;10(2):239–43.

44. Dominguez-Valentin M, Therkildsen C, Veerla S, Jonsson M, Bernstein I, Borg A, Nilbert M. Distinct gene expression signatures in lynch syndrome and familial colorectal cancer type x. PLoS One. 2013;8(8):e71755.

45. Dominguez-Valentin M, Therkildsen C, Da Silva S, Nilbert M. Familial colorectal cancer type X: genetic profiles and phenotypic features. Mod Pathol. 2015;28(1):30–6.

27

Histopathological techniques for the diagnosis of combat-related invasive fungal wound infections

Sarah M. Heaton[1], Amy C. Weintrob[1,2,3], Kevin Downing[1], Bryan Keenan[1], Deepak Aggarwal[2,3], Faraz Shaikh[2,3], David R. Tribble[2], Justin Wells[1*] and the Infectious Disease Clinical Research Program Trauma Infectious Disease Outcomes Study Group

Abstract

Background: Effective management of trauma-related invasive fungal wound infections (IFIs) depends on early diagnosis and timely initiation of treatment. We evaluated the utility of routine staining, histochemical stains and frozen section for fungal element identification.

Methods: A total of 383 histopathological specimens collected from 66 combat-injured United States military personnel with IFIs were independently reviewed by two pathologists. Both periodic acid-Schiff (PAS) and Gomori methenamine silver (GMS) stains were used on 74 specimens. The performance of the two special stains was compared against the finding of fungal elements via any histopathological method (ie, special stains or hematoxylin and eosin). In addition, the findings from frozen sections were compared against permanent sections.

Results: The GMS and PAS results were 84 % concordant (95 % confidence interval: 70 to 97 %). The false negative rate of fungal detection was 15 % for GMS and 44 % for PAS, suggesting that GMS was more sensitive; however, neither stain was statistically significantly superior for identifying fungal elements ($p = 0.38$). Moreover, 147 specimens had frozen sections performed, of which there was 87 % correlation with permanent sections (60 % sensitivity and 98 % specificity). In 27 permanent sections, corresponding cultures were available for comparison and 85 % concordance in general species identification was reported.

Conclusions: The use of both stains does not have an added benefit for identifying fungal elements. Furthermore, while the high specificity of frozen section may aid in timely IFI diagnoses, it should not be used as a stand-alone method to guide therapy due to its low sensitivity.

Keywords: Invasive fungal infections, Invasive mold infections, Combat-related infections, Histopathology, Histochemical stains for fungus

Background

Trauma-related invasive fungal wound infections (IFIs) are characterized by high mortality (up to 38 %) and substantial morbidity (eg, surgical amputations). Consequently, early diagnosis and timely initiation of treatment are critical for the successful management of the disease [1–7]. While use of cultures to identify specific pathogens remains an effective diagnostic method, fungal organisms may take weeks to grow, if they grow at all. Therefore, IFIs are often diagnosed through routine histopathological examination of tissue specimens, which is a process that can be completed and interpreted within 24-48 h when expedited [8–11]. Although histopathology is useful for differentiating between fungal colonization and infection through the identification of tissue invasion or inflammation [8], ascertainment of the organism's genus and species is limited [9, 12, 13].

The most common type of histopathological examination involves using permanent (paraffin-embedded)

* Correspondence: Justin.m.wells8.mil@mail.mil
[1]Department of Pathology, Walter Reed National Military Medical Center, 8901 Wisconsin Avenue, Bethesda, MD 20814, USA
Full list of author information is available at the end of the article

sections of biopsy tissue stained with hematoxylin and eosin (H&E). Although H&E is capable of staining the fungal cell wall, it is easy to overlook fungal organisms due to limited staining differential from background tissue. Moreover, when fungal organisms are observed with H&E, it can be difficult to identify characteristics useful for classification (eg, septate versus aseptate) [9, 14]. Therefore, if an IFI is suspected, but organisms are either not identified or are poorly visualized with H&E, the use of additional stains, particularly Gomori methenamine silver (GMS) and/or periodic acid-Schiff (PAS), can be used to either rule out a fungal infection or identify morphologic characteristics. Both GMS and PAS stains provide greater contrast by highlighting the fungal cell wall; however, misidentification, false-positives and false-negatives, do occur with these techniques. Specifically, GMS may result in poor staining when there is fragmentation or necrosis of fungal elements [9]. A further limitation is that GMS masks the natural color of mold, making it difficult to identify hyaline organisms from dematiaceous [15]. When PAS is used, background tissue components may also be stained along with the fungal cell wall [9, 16].

Another form of histopathological examination is an intraoperative consultation or frozen section, which provides a more rapid result than permanent sections. This technique involves freezing a portion or the entire debridement specimen, which allows for expedient cutting, slide mounting, and staining. Typically, these results can be obtained within twenty minutes of tissue submission from the operating room. Nonetheless, this expedited turn-around time comes at a cost as the histological quality is significantly compromised [17].

During the recent war in Afghanistan, clinicians observed a higher than expected proportion of combat-related IFIs among wounded United States (U.S.) military personnel [7]. In general, diagnosis of the combat-related IFIs was not dependent upon mold growth from wound cultures, but more commonly the result of identification of fungal elements on histologic examination. Overall, 70 % of IFI patients were diagnosed in this manner [18].

There is limited literature regarding the use of frozen and permanent sections for the diagnosis of IFIs in this setting. The use of GMS and PAS as supplemental staining also needs further elucidation. Our objective was to survey pathologic information collected from U.S. military personnel with combat-related IFIs to determine the utility of GMS and PAS stains for IFI diagnosis. We also examined the role of frozen sections in aiding the diagnosis of IFIs. Lastly, we evaluated the correlation between fungal morphology, as observed with light microscopy, and culture-based identification.

Methods

Study population

Data were collected from U.S. military personnel with combat-related injuries sustained between June 1, 2009 and August 31, 2011 and medically evacuated to Landstuhl Regional Medical Center (LRMC) in Germany. Following initial treatment, patients were subsequently transferred to a participating military hospital in the U.S.: Walter Reed Army Medical Center in Washington, DC, National Naval Medical Center in Bethesda, MD, and Brooke Army Medical Center in San Antonio, TX. The overarching project is the U.S. Department of Defense (DoD) – Department of Veterans Affairs, Trauma Infectious Disease Outcomes Study (TIDOS), which collects longitudinal, prospective data in order to analyze infectious complications among service members with deployment-related trauma [19]. The study was approved by the Infectious Disease Institutional Review Board of the Uniformed Services University of the Health Sciences.

Invasive fungal infection case identification

The IFI patients were identified from the population of military personnel with combat-related trauma based upon evidence of recurrent wound necrosis after a minimum of two successive surgical debridements and fungal infection of viable tissue on either histopathology or culture [7, 18]. Histopathologic evidence included either fungal angioinvasion and/or fungal elements seen on routine histochemical staining (H&E and/or special stains). Inclusion in the study population also required a review of surgical pathology slides at the time of diagnosis.

Demographics and injury characteristics of patients who met the IFI case criteria were collected from the DoD Trauma Registry [20], while fungal culture and histopathological data were obtained through the supplemental TIDOS infectious disease module. Histopathology specimens associated with IFI patients were independently reviewed by two surgical pathologists. Furthermore, infectious disease and trauma surgery services case records were also examined.

Invasive fungal wound infection pathology

Tissue samples collected from U.S. military personnel with combat-related trauma IFIs were retrospectively examined to compare sensitivity and specificity of staining and preparatory methods. For each specimen with frozen sections, results were obtained from the final pathology report. All specimens required slides prepared with H&E as per routine surgical pathology handling. The GMS and/or PAS stains were performed on the specimen per primary pathologist discretion at time of diagnosis. Artisan GMS and PAS-green stain kits (Dako,

Carpinteria, CA) were used with Dako Artisan Link Special Staining System. After case completion, all slides were blindly and individually re-read by two pathologists, who upon disagreement on any data element would reach consensus during a multi-headed microscope review. Presence of invasive fungus, identification characteristics (described below), tissue type involved, presence of necrosis and special staining result were recorded for each case. A threshold for special stain positivity was set as easily discernible fungal wall staining as compared to background at 100x magnification. This threshold simplified interpretation and provided more clinically relevant staining data. Limited fungal identification was utilized as previously defined, including categories of aseptate, septate, yeast, or polymicrobial [9]. When available, histopathology was compared against results from cultures collected from the same wound site.

Statistical analysis

Due to the primary mechanism of injury (ie, dismounted blast), polytrauma was common among combat casualties and; therefore, multiple wounds with IFI may develop in an individual patient. Independency was assumed among all specimens, including those collected from the same patient (ie, specimens that were not collected from the same wound site on the same day). Stain performance was demonstrated by sensitivity for fungal detection of the GMS and PAS staining methods. The presence of fungal elements identified via any histopathological method (ie, GMS, PAS, and/or H&E) was used as the reference for the evaluation. Similarly, frozen identification was compared to permanent sections. Lastly, descriptions of fungal morphology reported by pathologists following examination of histologic specimens were compared to results of concurrent fungal cultures (± 3 days) taken from the same anatomic site. All comparisons were conducted using McNemar's test and Kappa's coefficient. Statistical analysis was conducted using SAS® version 9.3 (SAS, Cary, NC) and significance was defined as $p < 0.05$.

Results

Patient demographics and injury characteristics
From the population of wounded U.S. military personnel admitted to LRMC (June 2009 - August 2011), 66 IFI patients met the criteria for inclusion in the study population (ie, availability of surgical pathology slides reviewed at the time of diagnosis). The characteristics of these IFI cases have been previously described [7, 18]. All of the patients were young men (median age of 23 years) and the majority sustained moderate to severe injuries as indicated by the injury severity score (83 % $\geq$16), which is a summary score estimated from

injury values determined for the six main body regions [21]. Tissue specimens were examined in separate study population subset analyses based on the following criteria (Fig. 1): stained with both PAS and GMS (Analysis 1); having aseptate or septate organisms identified on permanent sections (Analysis 2); and having frozen sections available (Analysis 3).

Invasive fungal infection surgical pathology findings
A total of 383 specimens were collected from the 66 IFI patients (141 wound sites), of which 149 specimens (49 patients) displayed fungal organisms on permanent sections (ie, paraffin-embedded tissues stained for examination). Specimens sent for pathological examination were largely comprised of more than one type of tissue with the predominance containing fibroconnective tissue (91 %) followed by adipose (75 %), muscle (55 %), skin (17 %), and bone (7 %). Moreover, specimen sites were largely extremity wounds with 54 % of tissue samples collected from the lower extremities and 15 % from the upper. The remaining specimens were collected from the pelvis/hip (27 %), abdomen (4 %), and craniofacial area (0.3 %).

Staining methods (analysis 1)
All 383 tissue specimens were stained with routine H&E along with at least one of the special stains. An example of tissue with different stains with resulting visualized fungal organisms consistent with mold classified as septate and aseptate are presented in Figs. 2 and 3. For this subset analysis, 74 specimens (28 patients) that were stained with both PAS and GMS were examined (Table 1). Both stains decorated fungal elements in 20 (27 %) specimens, while fungal elements were not present with either stain (or H&E) in 49 (66 %) specimens. Of the five discordant results, one (1 %) specimen had fungal elements highlighted only with PAS stain and another four (5 %) only with GMS. Overall, there were no significant differences between the staining methods for visualizing fungal elements ($p = 0.38$) with concordance estimated to be approximately 84 % with a 95 % confidence interval range between 70 to 97 %. When GMS used alone was compared to GMS used in combination with PAS (Table 2), there was no significant difference in fungal detection ($p = \sim 1.0$).

Among 12 patients (14 wound sites), serial isolates were collected from the same wound site at multiple time points. An evaluation of these serial specimens (total of 14) found that two initially negative wound sites had fungal elements in subsequent biopsies with GMS; however, fungal elements were not visualized at any time using PAS stain for these specimens. In addition, one wound site that was initially negative with GMS had fungal elements in later tissue samples, while PAS

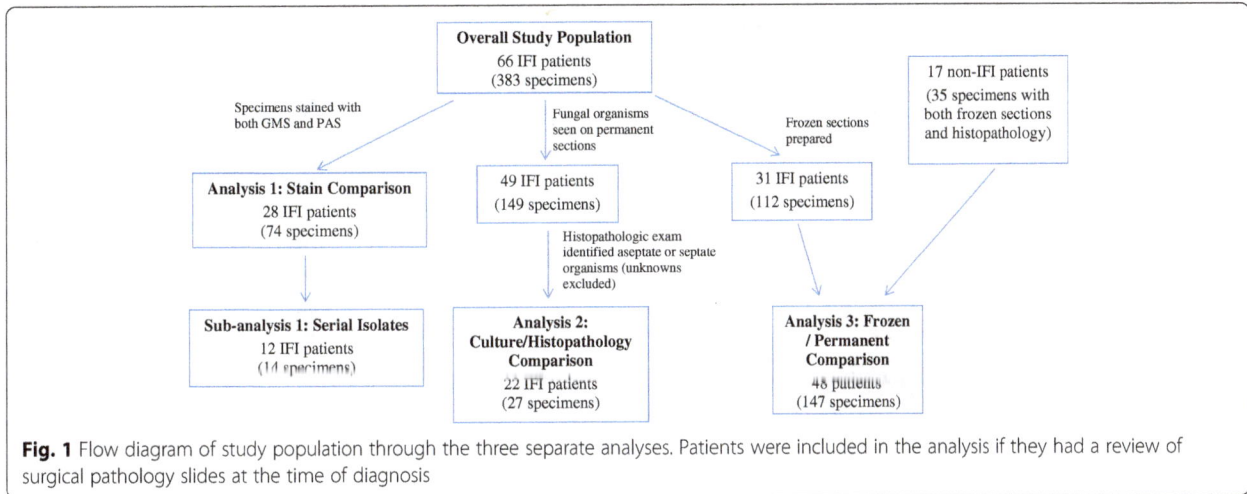

Fig. 1 Flow diagram of study population through the three separate analyses. Patients were included in the analysis if they had a review of surgical pathology slides at the time of diagnosis

stain identified fungal elements in both the initial and subsequent specimens. Using the total number of cases with fungal elements identified on histopathology (ie, H&E plus GMS and/or PAS) as the point of reference, the sensitivity for fungal detection was 56 % and 85 % for PAS and GMS, respectively, which translates to a false negative rate of 44 % and 15 %, respectively.

Mycology and histopathologic morphology comparison (analysis 2)

The histopathological findings of 27 specimens identified the mold as either aseptate, septate, or mixed (both septate and aseptate), which allowed for comparison of fungal morphology against tissue cultures collected from the same wound site (more than 55 % of wound cultures did not grow mold). Specimens with histopathological

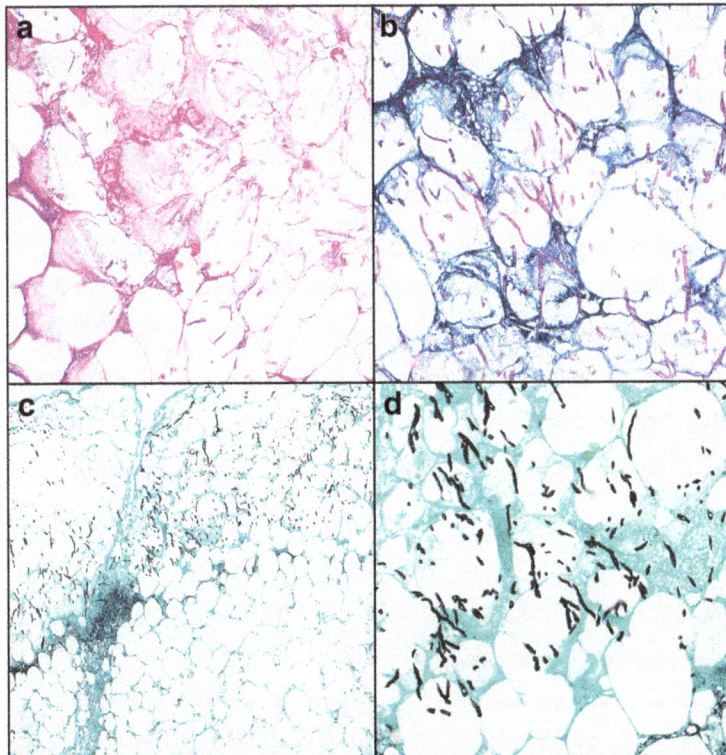

Fig. 2 Necrotic fibroadipose tissue with fungal organisms consistent with septate, acute angle branching morphology. (**a**) hematoxylin and eosin stain, 20X; (**b**) Periodic Acid-Schiff stain, 20X; (**c**) Gomori Methenamine Silver stain, 5X; (**d**) Gomori Methenamine Silver stain, 20X

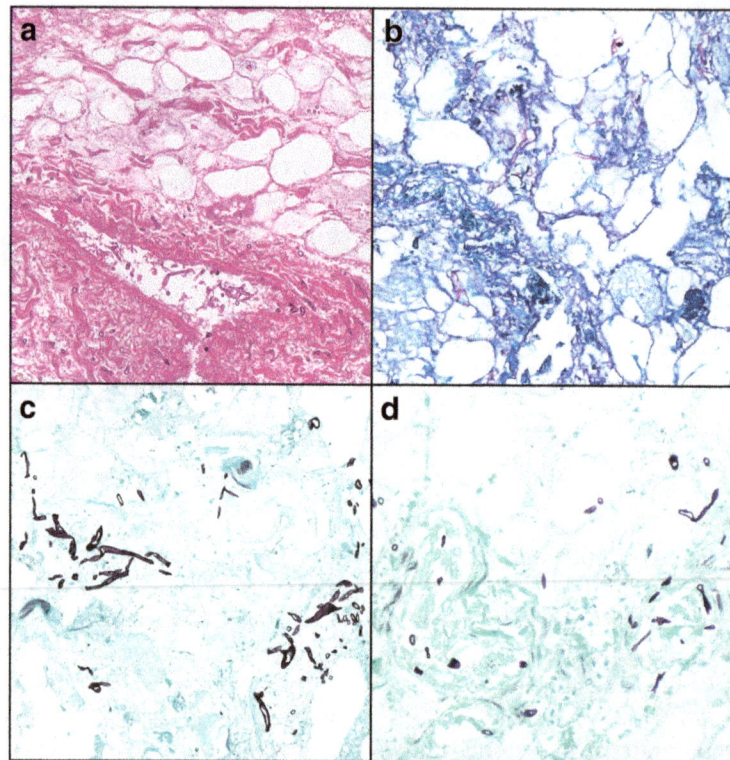

Fig. 3 Necrotic fibroadipose tissue with fungal organisms consistent with aseptate Zygomycete species (broad, ribbon-like hyphae). Angioinvasion can be seen in parts A and D. (**a**) hematoxylin and eosin stain, 20X; (**b**) Periodic Acid-Schiff stain, 20X; (**c** and **d**) Gomori Methenamine Silver stain, 20X

findings that could not clearly designate the mold as aseptate, septate, or mixed or did not have a corresponding tissue culture that grew mold were excluded from this analysis.

Among the wound cultures that grew mold, the following were identified: *Acrophialophora fusispora, Aspergillus* spp., *Fusarium* spp., *Graphium* spp., *Mucor* spp., and *Mycelia sterilia*. Between the permanent sections and cultures, there was correlation in 85 % (23 of 27) of the wounds (90 % in histopathologically classified septate organisms and 72 % in aseptate) (Table 3). Six histopathological specimens and three microbiological cultures had 'mixed' findings. Although the corresponding

culture and histopathology specimens always observed either septate or aseptate only, they were counted as concordant because at least one of the organisms from the mixed findings was identified.

Frozen sectioning (analysis 3)

Frozen sections were prepared on 147 specimens collected from 48 patients (Table 4). Fungal elements were identified in 24 (16 %) specimens on both frozen and permanent sections, while fungal elements were not visualized with either method in 105 (71 %) specimens. Using results of the permanent sections as the point of reference (40 with fungal elements and 107 with no

Table 1 Comparison of results with PAS and GMS staining for the identification of fungal elements[a]

Results with PAS stain	Results with GMS stain		
	Positive for fungal elements	Negative for fungal elements	Total
Positive for fungal elements	20	1	21
Negative for fungal elements	4	49	53
Total	24	50	74

[a] Kappa coefficient for comparison is 84 % (95 % confidence interval of 70-97 %); McNemar's test p-value =0.38

Table 2 Comparison of GMS staining alone versus PAS with GMS staining for identification of fungal elements[a]

GMS alone	GMS Plus PAS staining		
	Positive for fungal elements	Negative for fungal elements	Total
Positive for fungal elements	24	0	24
Negative for fungal elements	1	49	50
Total	25	49	74

[a] Kappa coefficient for comparison is 97 % (95 % confidence interval of 91-100 %); McNemar's test p-value ~1.0

Table 3 Comparison of results with permanent sections and fungal culture for the identification of fungal morphology

Morphology with permanent sections	Morphology with cultures			
	Non-*Mucorales* and septate fungi	*Mucorales*	Mixed (both septate and aseptate)	Total
Septate assumed non-*Mucorales*	9	1	0	10
Aseptate assumed *Mucorales*	3	5	3[a]	11
Mixed (both septate and aseptate)	3[a]	3[a]	0	6
Total	15	9	3	27

[a] 'Mixed' findings were counted as concordant with the 'septate/asepate only' results because at least one of the organisms observed in the specimens designated as mixed was identified in the corresponding histopathology specimens/cultures

visualized fungal elements), the positive and negative predictive values of frozen sections were 92 % and 87 %, respectively (Fig. 4). The sensitivity of frozen section was calculated to be 60 % and specificity was 98 %.

Of the 40 permanent sections with fungal elements, 20 specimens were identified to have aseptate growth, 11 with septate, and 9 with unspecified or multiple molds. Frozen sections identified 13 specimens with aseptate growth (35 % false negative rate), 4 with septate growth (64 % false negative rate), and 7 with unspecified/multiple molds.

Discussion

Between 2009 and 2011, 6.8 % of combat casualties admitted to LRMC and transferred to a TIDOS-participating hospital were diagnosed with IFIs [22]. A concentrated effort was made to promote earlier diagnosis, which involved collection of tissue samples for culture and histopathological examination from all patients considered to be at risk due to their mechanism and pattern of injury [23]. Although it is agreed that early diagnosis of IFIs is a crucial step in achieving a beneficial patient outcome, there is little experience with routine histopathology techniques in this setting. Therefore, our goal was to compare the utility of two special stains used

Table 4 Comparison of results with frozen and permanent sections for the identification of fungal elements[a]

Results with frozen sections	Results with permanent sections		
	Positive for fungal elements	Negative for fungal elements	Total
Positive for fungal elements	24	2	26
Negative for fungal elements	16	105	121
Total	40	107	147

[a] The specimens are collected from 48 patients, of which 31 were diagnosed with IFIs and 17 were non-IFI patients

for visualizing fungal elements, along with examining the results of frozen sections and cultures when compared with permanent section.

While our overall concordance is 85 %, disagreement between the results of morphology on slides and cultures is not uncommon. In general, accuracy of microscopic identification of fungal species using either histopathological or cytological specimens has been estimated to range from 20 % to 80 % [8, 9]. Morphology consistent with *Aspergillus* spp. is hyaline, thin (3-12 µm) septate hyphae with acute angle branching, while the order *Mucorales* is characterized by hyaline, wide (5-20 µm), thin-walled, aseptate, ribbon-like hyphae with right angle branching [9]. Nonetheless, *Aspergillus* spp. may occasionally display morphology consistent with the *Mucorales* order and vice versa resulting in misclassification [8, 9]. In particular, misclassification involving septate and aseptate hyphae may occur in situations with substantial necrosis as the hyphae may become swollen or distorted, making histopathological identification difficult. Moreover, fungal hyphae may be scant, folded, kinked, or fragmented so an accurate description of septation or branching is difficult [8]. Culture also has its limitations as results may be hindered by contamination and the inability to determine colonization from true infection without associated clinical indicators [13, 24]. The duration (ranging from days to weeks) required for mold growth and identification also severely limits use of cultures in acute situations where delay in treatment can result in poor outcomes. These results and the obvious limitations identified need to be considered by our clinical colleagues as they make treatment decisions.

We also evaluated the potential benefit of frozen section preparations in relation to IFI diagnostics [8, 9, 25]. Our data suggest that there is a finite role in identification of fungal organisms at the time of surgery. Specifically, when organisms are identified on frozen sections, this strongly supports an IFI diagnosis. In contrast, the usefulness of a negative result is questionable and should not be used to rule out an IFI if there is a strong clinical suspicion. Large false negative rates are not unexpected as this procedure suffers from inferior histology and is susceptible to sampling error [8, 25]. Unlike permanent sections where the entire tissue sample can be examined, frozen sections often only evaluate selected areas of a larger debridement specimen. Characterization as septate versus aseptate is also problematic as distorted histology and frozen artifacts makes this challenging diagnosis even more difficult. For example, freezing tends to balloon tissues, which may cause a thin hyphae to become broad, leading to inaccuracies [17]. Overall, the findings observed in this military setting are comparable with other publications, which found frozen

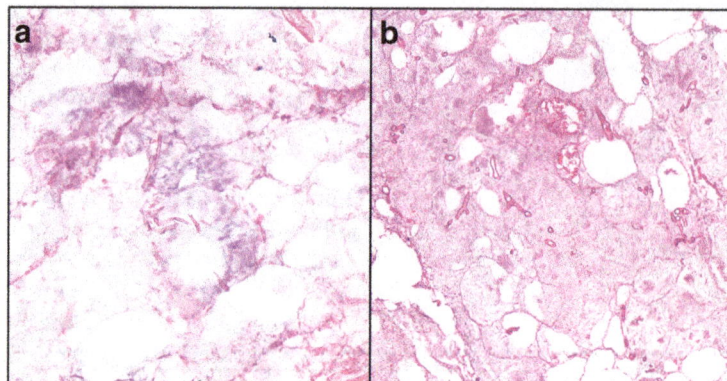

Fig. 4 Necrotic fibroadipose tissue with fungal organisms consistent with Zygomycete species (broad, ribbon-like hyphae). (**a**) Frozen section with hematoxylin and eosin stain, 20X; and (**b**) Corresponding permanent section with hematoxylin and eosin stain, 20X

sections to be largely predictive of IFIs in patients with rhinosinusitis [15, 25, 26]. Furthermore, an assessment of 33 specimens collected from a patient with fungal-infected bedsores found 68 % sensitivity and 100 % specificity of frozen sections in the soft-tissue margin evaluation in wound debridement [27], which is comparable to our findings.

During the combat-related IFI outbreak, pathologists involved with diagnosis often recommended that treatment decisions not be determined by special stains alone. Our findings support this belief. The ease of identification on GMS and PAS may cause pathologists to overlook or quickly review H&E slides. In actuality, rare cases early in the outbreak of IFIs were missed when special stains failed to highlight organisms. When the corresponding H&E was reviewed, organisms were readily found. In our analysis, PAS and GMS had false negative rates of 44 % and 15 %, respectively.

Methods of histologic evaluation to support diagnosis of the disease rapidly evolved following recognition of the unexpected outbreak of IFIs among wounded military personnel. Staining methods initially included both GMS and PAS to increase sensitivity; however, due to anecdotal evidence, pathologists began to reduce their reliance on PAS as they believed it was not as sensitive as GMS and added little additional benefit. Furthermore, the decision to focus on one stain was also based on factors related to cost and labor required to perform multiple stains on each tissue block. Our results demonstrated a high level of concordance between the special stains with GMS more sensitive in this series (GMS false negative rate of 15 % versus 44 % with PAS), indicating that GMS may be more suitable for identifying zygomycetes. Supporting this initial decision, the data also demonstrate that there is no significant benefit to using both stains in an effort to identify fungal elements. Therefore, we recommend use of GMS for fungal identification over PAS.

Routine histopathologic techniques and culture, as reported in our study, are still the most commonly used techniques for rapid fungal identification. Nonetheless, in our opinion, we believe that the future of early diagnosis with accurate speciation may ultimately be achieved through more complex testing in conjunction with histopathology, to include immunohistochemistry, in situ hybridization, PCR and Matrix-assisted laser desorption/ionization. These tests should be able to quickly and definitively identify fungal species in tissues and may better detect dual infections [9]. Investigations to determine the benefit of these modalities are underway.

While our clinical setting, specific to blast injuries sustained by soldiers serving in Afghanistan, seems narrow, we believe these data are applicable to other presentations. Recent examples of invasive fungal infections in the civilian setting include the occurrence of trauma-related IFIs following the Joplin tornado and the outbreak of mucormycosis associated with linens in a pediatric hospital [2, 28]. We hope that our report provides insight for pathologists and clinicians into a truly unfortunate problem.

Conclusions

Overall, the GMS and PAS staining for the identification of invasive fungal elements were 84 % concordant and neither stain was statistically significantly better with identifying fungal elements ($p = 0.38$). Despite their obvious advantages for supporting diagnosis of fungal infections, GMS and PAS had false negative rates for fungal detection of 15 % and 44 %, respectively, which stresses the importance of closely reviewing the H&E. Furthermore, the authors demonstrated that while frozen section had high specificity (98 %), it should not be used as a standalone method for the diagnosis of invasive fungal wound infections due to its low sensitivity.

Abbreviations
DoD, Department of Defense; GMS, Gomori methenamine silver; H&E, Hematoxylin and eosin; IFI, Invasive fungal wound infections; LRMC, Landstuhl Regional Medical Center; PAS, periodic acid-Schiff; TIDOS, Trauma Infectious Disease Outcomes Study; U.S., United States

Acknowledgments
We are indebted to the Infectious Disease Clinical Research Program Trauma Infectious Disease Outcomes Study team of clinical coordinators, microbiology technicians, data managers, clinical site managers, and administrative support personnel for their tireless hours to ensure the success of this project.

Funding
This work (IDCRP-024) was supported by the Infectious Disease Clinical Research Program (IDCRP), a Department of Defense program executed through the Uniformed Services University of the Health Sciences, Department of Preventive Medicine and Biostatistics. This project has been funded by the National Institute of Allergy and Infectious Diseases, National Institutes of Health, under Inter-Agency Agreement Y1-AI-5072, and the Department of the Navy under the Wounded, Ill, and Injured Program [HU001-10-1-0014].

Authors' contributions
SMH – study conception, pathological analysis, data interpretation, manuscript preparation. ACW – study conception, data interpretation, manuscript preparation. KD – data interpretation, manuscript preparation. BK – data interpretation, manuscript preparation. DA – assist with data interpretation, manuscript preparation. FS – data interpretation, manuscript preparation. DRT – study conception, data interpretation, manuscript preparation. JW – study conception, data collection, pathological analysis, data interpretation, manuscript preparation. All authors read and approved the final manuscript.

Competing interests
The authors declare that they have no competing interests.

Disclaimer
The view(s) expressed are those of the authors and does not necessarily reflect the official views of the Uniformed Services University of the Health Sciences, the Henry M. Jackson Foundation for the Advancement of Military Medicine, Inc., the National Institutes of Health or the Department of Health and Human Services, the Department of Defense (DoD) or the Departments of the Army, Navy, or Air Force. Mention of trade names, commercial products, or organizations does not imply endorsement by the U.S. Government. The identification of specific products or scientific instrumentation does not constitute endorsement or implied endorsement on the part of the author, DoD, or any component agency. While we generally excise references to products, companies, manufacturers, organizations, etc. in government produced works, the abstracts produced and other similarly situated research present a special circumstance when such product inclusions become an integral part of the scientific endeavor.

Author details
[1]Department of Pathology, Walter Reed National Military Medical Center, 8901 Wisconsin Avenue, Bethesda, MD 20814, USA. [2]Infectious Disease Clinical Research Program, Department of Preventive Medicine and Biostatistics, Uniformed Services University of the Health Sciences, Bethesda, MD, USA. [3]The Henry M. Jackson Foundation for the Advancement of Military Medicine, Inc., Bethesda, MD, USA.

References
1. Pfaller MA, Pappas PG, Wingard JR. Invasive fungal pathogens: Current epidemiological trends. Clin Infect Dis. 2006;43 Suppl 1:S3–S14.
2. Neblett Fanfair R, Benedict K, Bos J, Bennett SD, Lo YC, Adebanjo T, et al. Necrotizing cutaneous mucormycosis after a tornado in Joplin, Missouri, in 2011. N Engl J Med. 2012;367(23):2214–25.
3. Roden MM, Zaoutis TE, Buchanan WL, Knudsen TA, Sarkisova TA, Schaufele RL, et al. Epidemiology and outcome of zygomycosis: a review of 929 reported cases. Clin Infect Dis. 2005;41(5):634–53.
4. Vitrat-Hincky V, Lebeau B, Bozonnet E, Falcon D, Pradel P, Faure O, et al. Severe filamentous fungal infections after widespread tissue damage due to traumatic injury: six cases and review of the literature. Scand J Infect Dis. 2009;41(6-7):491–500.
5. Hajdu S, Obradovic A, Presterl E, Vecsei V. Invasive mycoses following trauma. Injury. 2009;40(5):548–54.
6. Lanternier F, Dannaoui E, Morizot G, Elie C, Garcia Hermoso D, Huerre M, et al. A global analysis of mucormycosis in France: the RetroZygo Study (2005-2007). Clin Infect Dis. 2012;54 Suppl 1:S35–43.
7. Warkentien T, Rodriguez C, Lloyd B, Wells J, Weintrob A, Dunne J, et al. Invasive mold infections following combat-related injuries. Clin Infect Dis. 2012;55(11):1441–9.
8. Sangoi AR, Rogers WM, Longacre TA, Montoya JG, Baron EJ, Banaei N. Challenges and pitfalls of morphologic identification of fungal infections in histologic and cytologic specimens: a ten-year retrospective review at a single institution. Am J Clin Pathol. 2009;131(3):364–75.
9. Guarner J, Brandt ME. Histopathologic diagnosis of fungal infections in the 21st century. Clin Microbiol Rev. 2011;24(2):247–80.
10. Schwarz J. The diagnosis of deep mycoses by morphologic methods. Hum Pathol. 1982;13(6):519–33.
11. Skiada A, Pagano L, Groll A, Zimmerli S, Dupont B, Lagrou K, et al. Zygomycosis in Europe: analysis of 230 cases accrued by the registry of the European Confederation of Medical Mycology (ECMM) Working Group on Zygomycosis between 2005 and 2007. Clin Microbiol Infect. 2011;17(12):1859–67.
12. Gomes MZ, Lewis RE, Kontoyiannis DP. Mucormycosis caused by unusual mucormycetes, non-Rhizopus, -Mucor, and -Lichtheimia species. Clin Microbiol Rev. 2011;24(2):411–45.
13. Schofield CM, Murray CK, Horvath EE, Cancio LC, Kim SH, Wolf SE, Hospenthal DR. Correlation of culture with histopathology in fungal burn wound colonization and infection. Burns. 2007;33(3):341–6.
14. Kaufman L. Immunohistologic diagnosis of systemic mycoses: an update. Eur J Epidemiol. 1992;8(9):377–82.
15. Hofman V, Castillo L, Betis F, Guevara N, Gari-Toussaint M, Hofman P. Usefulness of frozen section in rhinocerebral mucormycosis diagnosis and management. Pathology. 2003;35(3):212–6.
16. Anthony PP. A guide to the histological identification of fungi in tissues. J Clin Pathol. 1973;26(11):828–31.
17. Taxy JB. Frozen section and the surgical pathologist: a point of view. Arch Pathol Lab Med. 2009;133(7):1135–8.
18. Weintrob AC, Weisbrod AB, Dunne JR, Rodriguez CJ, Malone D, Lloyd BA, et al. Combat trauma-associated invasive fungal wound infections: epidemiology and clinical classification. Epidemiol Infect. 2015;143(1):214–24.
19. Tribble DR, Conger NG, Fraser S, Gleeson TD, Wilkins K, Antonille T, et al. Infection-associated clinical outcomes in hospitalized medical evacuees after traumatic injury: trauma infectious disease outcome study. J Trauma. 2011;71 Suppl 1:S33–42.
20. Eastridge BJ, Jenkins D, Flaherty S, Schiller H, Holcomb JB. Trauma system development in a theater of war: Experiences from Operation Iraqi Freedom and Operation Enduring Freedom. J Trauma. 2006;61(6):1366–72.
21. Linn S. The injury severity score–Importance and uses. Ann Epidemiol. 1995;5(6):440–6.
22. Rodriguez C, Weintrob AC, Shah J, Malone D, Dunne JR, Weisbrod AB, et al. Risk factors associated with invasive fungal infections in combat trauma. Surg Infect (Larchmt). 2014;15(5):521–6.
23. Lloyd B, Weintrob A, Rodriguez C, Dunne J, Weisbrod A, Hinkle M, et al. Effect of early screening for invasive fungal infections in U.S. service members with explosive blast injuries. Surg Infect (Larchmt). 2014;15(5):619–2.
24. Rodriguez CJ, Weintrob AC, Dunne JR, Weisbrod AB, Lloyd BA, Warkentien T, et al. Clinical relevance of mold culture positivity with and without recurrent wound necrosis following combat-related injuries. J Trauma Acute Care Surg. 2014;77(5):769–73.

28

Diagnostic guidelines for the histological particle algorithm in the periprosthetic neo-synovial tissue

G. Perino[1]*⦿, S. Sunitsch[2], M. Huber[3], D. Ramirez[1], J. Gallo[4], J. Vaculova[5], S. Natu[6], J. P. Kretzer[7], S. Müller[8], P. Thomas[9], M. Thomsen[10], M. G. Krukemeyer[11], H. Resch[12], T. Hügle[13], W. Waldstein[14], F. Böettner[15], T. Gehrke[16], S. Sesselmann[17], W. Rüther[18], Z. Xia[19], E. Purdue[20] and V. Krenn[8]

Abstract

Background: The identification of implant wear particles and non-implant related particles and the characterization of the inflammatory responses in the periprosthetic neo-synovial membrane, bone, and the synovial-like interface membrane (SLIM) play an important role for the evaluation of clinical outcome, correlation with radiological and implant retrieval studies, and understanding of the biological pathways contributing to implant failures in joint arthroplasty. The purpose of this study is to present a comprehensive histological particle algorithm (HPA) as a practical guide to particle identification at routine light microscopy examination.

Methods: The cases used for particle analysis were selected retrospectively from the archives of two institutions and were representative of the implant wear and non-implant related particle spectrum. All particle categories were described according to their size, shape, colour and properties observed at light microscopy, under polarized light, and after histochemical stains when necessary. A unified range of particle size, defined as a measure of length only, is proposed for the wear particles with five classes for polyethylene (PE) particles and four classes for conventional and corrosion metallic particles and ceramic particles.

Results: All implant wear and non-implant related particles were described and illustrated in detail by category. A particle scoring system for the periprosthetic tissue/SLIM is proposed as follows: 1) Wear particle identification at light microscopy with a two-step analysis at low ($\times 25$, $\times 40$, and $\times 100$) and high magnification ($\times 200$ and $\times 400$); 2) Identification of the predominant wear particle type with size determination; 3) The presence of non-implant related endogenous and/or foreign particles. A guide for a comprehensive pathology report is also provided with sections for macroscopic and microscopic description, and diagnosis.

Conclusions: The HPA should be considered a standard for the histological analysis of periprosthetic neo-synovial membrane, bone, and SLIM. It provides a basic, standardized tool for the identification of implant wear and non-implant related particles at routine light microscopy examination and aims at reducing intra-observer and inter-observer variability to provide a common platform for multicentric implant retrieval/radiological/histological studies and valuable data for the risk assessment of implant performance for regional and national implant registries and government agencies.

Keywords: Arthroplasty, Histological particle algorithm, Periprosthetic tissue, Synovial-like interface membrane, Orthopaedic implant wear particles, Non-implant related particles, Synovial crystals, Metallic wear particles, Ceramic wear particles, Polyethylene wear particles

* Correspondence: perinog@hss.edu
[1]Department of Pathology and Laboratory Medicine, Hospital for Special Surgery, 535 E 70th Street, New York, NY 10023, USA
Full list of author information is available at the end of the article

Background

The identification of particulate wear material of orthopaedic implants and its differential diagnosis with endogenous crystalline and non-crystalline materials in the periprosthetic capsular neo-synovial membrane, bone, and the synovial-like interface membrane (SLIM) is important for the evaluation of clinical outcome, correlation with radiological and implant retrieval studies, and understanding of the biological adverse reactions associated with implant failures. The role of wear particles was first recognized by Willert and Semlitsch in 1977 in the occurrence of bone resorption leading to aseptic loosening/osteolysis, one of the most frequent causes of orthopaedic implant failure up to the present time [1].

Wear in orthopaedic implants is considered a result of removal of material by mechanical action. Implant wear particles are derived from polyethylene, metallic alloys, ceramics, implant porous coatings, and polymethyl methacrylate orthopaedic cement (PMMA). The great majority of these particles are generated by two mechanisms: 1) The two-body adhesive/abrasion wear when material is removed or displaced from the softer surface by irregularities of the harder surface; 2) The three-body abrasion wear when some form of other particles generated by materials used to fasten the implant to the bone (e.g. PMMA) or particles generated by the wear of a primary implant components which remain after the implant failure and revision (e.g. ceramic particles after a fracture of a ceramic femoral head or liner) [2]. Particulate material can also be generated by tribochemical wear (tribocorrosion) mechanism and by other modality at the head-neck tapers such mechanically assisted crevice/fretting corrosion, pitting and intergranular corrosion, and etching which depend on the material, material couple, and alloy microstructure [3, 4].

In the histological examination of capsular neo-synovial membrane, bone and SLIM, wear particles can be of any size, shape, contour, colour, and chemical composition. The differential diagnosis with non-implant related exogenous particles can be difficult or sometimes even impossible by light microscopy (e.g. presence of minute particles of surgical suture or glove powder). Large wear particles can also represent aggregates of smaller particles, especially of nano-size and also admixed with or coated by adherent organic substance, such as blood-derived products or synovial fluid proteins forming a protein corona, which can define the immunogenic properties of the particles [5–7].

In the past forty years, histological classifications of implant wear particles at conventional light microscopy examination with and without polarized light have been published and used for clinical purposes and research studies, usually modifications of the classification reported by Mirra et al. in 1976 [8]. Although the proposed classification based on a semi-quantitative scale of particle number and size is to some extent still valid, the progressive evolution of implant and non-implant related material and technological developments in microscopy optics, microscope camera and imaging, and particle analysis techniques has made the original classification and its modifications not suitable to address all the current diagnostic challenges for surgical pathologists and in need of an up-to-date classification and a comprehensive, digital photographic documentation. Moreover, the identification of wear particles and the measurement of their total burden has become more difficult or impossible to be determined with accuracy by conventional light microscopy due to the size of most of the particulate material well below the resolution limit of the optic microscope, the morphological similarities of some of the material, and the mixture of particles from different material in the cytoplasm of the macrophages.

Histological examination of the periprosthetic tissue removed during implant revisions, although still not mandatory in many countries, has been considered instrumental in the classification, cell composition/subtyping, and grading of the adverse biological reactions to implant wear particles and the identification of new types [9–15]. These reactions can potentially carry vast medical and economic consequences for public health, as exemplified by the increasing number and type of joints replaced (hip, knee, shoulder, elbow, wrist, ankle), and the projected increased number of orthopaedic implant revisions in the future [16]. A recent example has come from the re-introduction of the metal-on metal (MoM) bearing surface either in hip resurfacing arthroplasty (HRA) or total hip arthroplasty (THA) with or without cobalt-chromium (CoCr) metallic adapter sleeve (MAS) and in Non-MoM THA implants with CoCr dual modular neck (DMN) followed by the unintended occurrence of adverse local tissue reactions resulting in a higher rate of revision operations and need of long-term follow-up [17].

The first analysis of the implant wear material and of the host reaction is almost always performed by conventional light microscopy on paraffin embedded tissue and usually by a general surgical pathologist. Therefore, a classification of the materials which is reproducible and accurate within the limits of the optic microscope resolution and also of limited methodological complexity is necessary for providing a standardized and comparable diagnostic tool which can be expanded further with the use of additional, sophisticated analytical techniques when necessary. A set of detailed criteria is presented with the intent of providing a useful and reproducible guide for the identification of wear particulate material (Fig. 1) and for the differential diagnosis with non-implant related endogenous materials such as crystal deposits and degradation

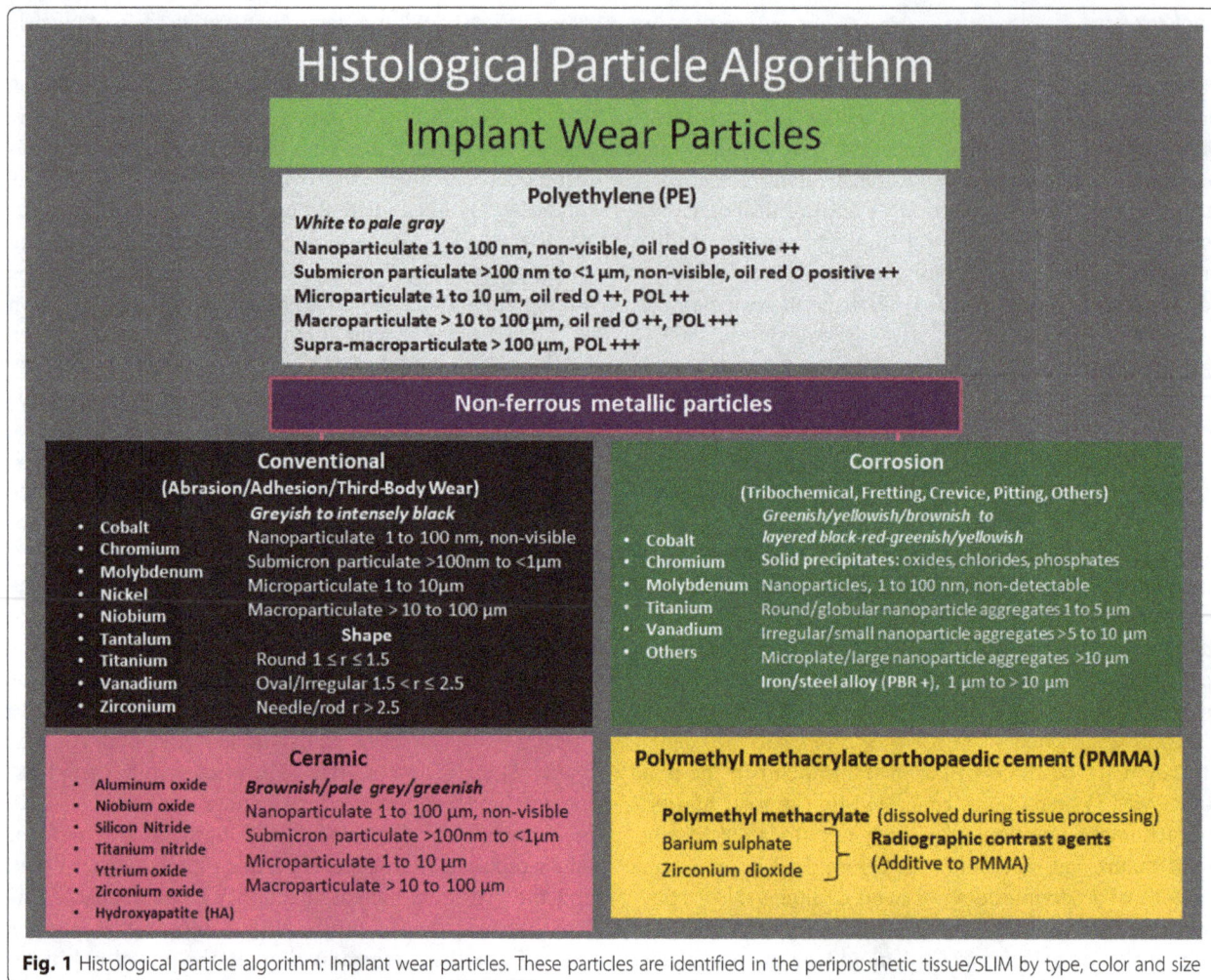

Fig. 1 Histological particle algorithm: Implant wear particles. These particles are identified in the periprosthetic tissue/SLIM by type, color and size

products of organic substances, especially blood-derived, as well as foreign particles/grafts from different sources (Fig. 2). These criteria can be applied to the decisional tree of the Histological Particle Algorithm (HPA) for the correct identification of the particles which has been reported before in a condensed version [18, 19] and more recently in a manual for the histological diagnosis of pathologies associated with orthopaedic implants [20].

Methods

The HPA is fully described and illustrated with examples of each category of implant wear particles and endogenous/foreign particles generated in different implanted joints. The cases were selected retrospectively from the pathology archives of the Hospital for Special Surgery, New York, NY, USA and the Centre with Focus on Orthopaedic Pathology, Trier, Germany. All cases were retrieved by histological diagnosis and presence of implant-wear or non-implant related material. The cases were selected on the basis of exhibiting ample evidence of presence of a specific type of particle and in some

cases of a certain size range for illustrative purposes. All cases were histologically examined by three orthopaedic pathologists (GP, SS, VK) with consensus agreement on the histological diagnosis. Approval for the use of the periprosthetic tissue was obtained by the Institutional Review Board, Hospital for Special Surgery (Protocol Number 26085) and the Ethics Commission of the Medical Board of Rheinland-Pfalz; Mainz, Germany [Case Number 837.230.15 (9998)]. All particle categories were described according to their size, shape, colour, and properties observed at conventional light microscopy with or without polarized light and after histochemical stains when necessary. The criteria used in the HPA for particle identification are based in large part on the ones previously described in the scientific literature and provided in the definitions of particle size and shape section below. The particle size ranges were determined using computer-aided interactive morphometric analysis, Leica DM 2005, microsystems framework 2007 by two of the three pathologists (VK and SS) and independently verified by the third pathologist (GP) using a similar

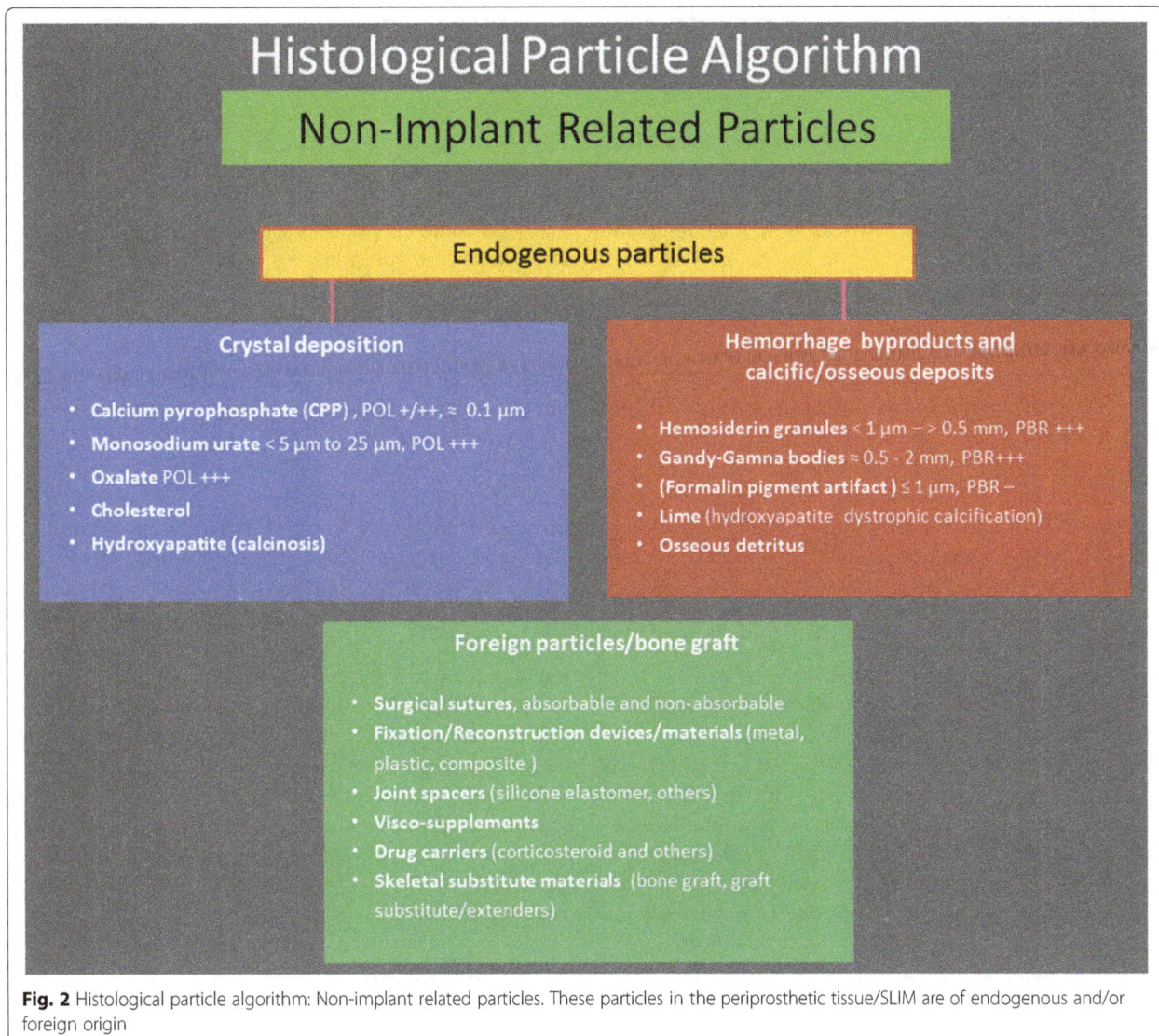

Fig. 2 Histological particle algorithm: Non-implant related particles. These particles in the periprosthetic tissue/SLIM are of endogenous and/or foreign origin

computer-aided system, Zeiss Axioskop 40, Jenoptik ProgRes microscope camera. The systems were calibrated using a standard micrometer glass slide with 1 mm horizontal scale, 100 divisions -10 μm intervals.

Implant data

The type of prosthesis and its time of implantation were known in each case and the removed implant components available for inspection at gross examination. The material composition of the joint prostheses covered the full range of the implant material spectrum (polyethylene, metals, ceramics, silicone, hydroxyapatite, polymethyl methacrylate orthopaedic cement).

Macroscopic examination and histological processing and staining of tissue samples

The fresh tissue collected at surgery was fixed in 10% buffered formalin. Macroscopic description of the

specimens was performed and depending on the wet tissue sample size/weight and/or tissue mapping locations, up to 10 tissue blocks (1–2 sections/block) were selected per case, processed and embedded according to a standard protocol, cut at 4 to 5 μm and stained with hematoxylin and eosin (H&E) and additional histochemical stains when necessary. The H&E staining and Prussian blue reaction (PBR) were carried out with a standard protocol using the Leica ST 4040 staining module; nuclear staining was undertaken with Harris hematoxylin (Harris hematoxylin, Surgipath, Richmond, IL, USA), the background staining was performed using eosin Y (Sigma-Aldrich, St. Louis, MO, USA). PBR reaction was performed manually according to the Mallory's method and Oil-red-O staining (Sigma-Aldrich, St. Louis, MO, USA) following a standard protocol [21]. In selected cases, 0.35 μm thick sections were stained with 0.1% toluidine blue in borax buffer after fixation in 2.5%

glutaraldehyde for 24 h and trimming with preservation of tissue orientation, transferred to sodium cacodylate buffer, processed through a standard cycle and embedded in epoxy resin.

We retain that sampling from multiple regions around large joints of periprosthetic tissue has value and can also provide more accurate information of the type of wear particles and their distribution as well as the quantitative and qualitative evaluation of the host cell response. This method has been previously described in detail [22] and has been used for the assessment of ALTR inflammatory infiltrate and the identification of large aggregates of corrosion particles/products [23, 24]. However, mapping for tissue sampling can be time consuming with a higher technical and professional cost to be applied routinely to all specimens and its benefits have also been recently investigated on non-MoM total hip and knee arthroplasty specimens showing comparable results with or without the use of a mapping chart [25].

Particle analysis
We found it challenging to match the wear particle lexicon used for retrieval analysis with the categories used in the histological classification and especially for the metal-on-metal and non-metal-on metal implants with wear particles generated at taper junctions between modular components. In particular, we faced the issue of separating metallic particles generated by adhesion/abrasion, tribocorrosion and mechanically assisted fretting/crevice and other types of corrosion. Therefore, we divided the metallic wear particles into two subcategories: 1) Conventional, as the most frequently occurring particles generated by adhesion/abrasion which can be predominantly composed of Co with variable amount of Cr, Mo, and Ti elements, varying in size and color from grey to jet black and responsible for the synovial fluid staining and macroscopic appearance clinically defined as "metallosis"; 2) Corrosion, as the particles of nanosize generated at the metal-on-metal bearing surface by tribocorrosion and composed of Cr with absent or minimal CoMo component distinctive of the MoM bearing surface and the particles generated by fretting, crevice, pitting, intergranular, etching, and possibly other types of corrosion at the taper junctions and composed of variable amounts of Cr, Co, Mo, Ti, and other metals used in the alloy and which usually appear at light microscopy of greenish/yellowish colour and less frequently brownish. This matter is further complicated by the fact that both sub-categories of particles can be observed simultaneously at histological examination of periprosthetic tissue and cannot be distinguished with certainty without tissue sampling for transmission electron microscopy (TEM)/scanning electron microscopy (SEM) and

subsequent particle nano-analysis. Corrosion particles have also been referred to as corrosion products or corrosion particulate material in the literature because of their composite nature of metallic particles admixed with organic substance [20, 23]. Although it would be difficult to separate them in the classification, we used the term "corrosion products" instead of "corrosion particles" in some illustrations when the particle aggregates were large and multi-layered with the addition or organic derivatives mainly from blood/synovial fluid proteins and cell debris.

Non-implant related particles present in the periprosthetic tissue are divided in two main categories: endogenous particles and foreign particles/bone grafts.

Endogenous particles are those microscopic particles in the periprosthetic tissue/SLIM which have been produced by the body, frequently secondary to metabolic diseases/disturbances or blood-derived products and degenerative processes. The majority of them are of crystalline nature and are detected either in the synovial fluid or in deposits into the articular soft tissues. For the analysis of endogenous particles, a light microscope fitted with polarized filters and a first order red compensator is sufficient [26]. Crystals are detected because of their birefringence which is evident with the use of compensated polarized light microscopy (CPLM).

Foreign particles are derived from absorbable and non-absorbable surgical sutures, fixation devices/scaffolding materials (metal, plastic, composite materials), joint spacers, skeletal substitute materials, visco-supplements, and drug carriers.

Definitions of particle size and shape
The most difficult issue of the classification of wear and prosthetic material particles generated by orthopedic implants is to translate the size range of the particles into equivalent words to provide a practical and easily reproducible classification. This issue is not trivial because different morphological features of the particles and in particular their size and irregular surface could lead to an increase in the activation of the macrophage inflammasome with subsequent cytokine release in vivo and therefore have an important clinical significance, at least for metallic particles, as shown in an in vitro study [27]. We propose a unified range of particle size, defined as a measure of length only, which includes five classes for PE particles, and four classes for metallic particles and ceramic particles (class 1 to 4): 1) Nanoparticles (1 to 100 nm), 2) Submicron particles (> 100 nm to < 1 μm), 3) Microparticles (1 μm to 10 μm), 4) Macroparticles (> 10 μm to 100 μm), and 5) Supra-macroparticles (> 100 μm). This particle range is supported by its use for characterization of GFV UHMWPE in vitro [28] and in the attempt to predict their functional biological activity [29, 30], of metallic

particles [31], and of ceramic particles [11]. It must also be taken into consideration that particles of large size, especially metallic wear debris, can be actually aggregates of particles of much smaller size with the possible addition of organic elements. For an approximate extimate of particle size at light microscopy examination, nanoparticle aggregates, submicron, and microparticles are usually present in macrophages, macro-particles in single or syncytial giant cells, and supra-macroparticles are surrounded by giant cells or free in the capsular neo-synovial stroma/SLIM. The use of a ruler reticle mounted on the eyepiece can be helpful for a more precise, still approximate measure of the particle sizes. It needs to be emphasized that light microscopy examination cannot provide a reliable estimate of particle size distribution for which other techniques such as laser diffraction, dynamic light scattering, and image analysis must be used after particle isolation or TEM/SEM for in vivo analysis of intracellular and extracellular particle content. Shape descriptors can also be used, although different terms are used for various materials [31–33]. The following sub-division is proposed for the most common wear material observed at light microscopy with the use of a polarizing filter when necessary and according to the size ranges detected for each material:

1) *Polyethylene*: nanoparticles, non-detectable (1 to 100 nm); submicron particles (> 100 nm to < 1 μm), non-detectable; microparticles (1 to 10 μm); macroparticles (> 10 μm to 100 μm); and supra-macroparticles (> 100 μm);

2) *Conventional metallic*: nanoparticles, non-detectable (1 to 100 nm); submicron particles (> 100 nm to < 1 μm), non-detectable; microparticles (1 to 10 μm); and macroparticles (> 10 μm). Their shape can be defined by the ratio (r) between the length and the width of the particles: round ($1 \leq r \leq 1.5$), oval/irregular ($1.5 < r \leq 2.5$), needle/rod shaped ($r > 2.5$) [33];

3) *Corrosion metallic*: nanoparticles (1 to 100 nm), non-detectable; round/globular nanoparticle aggregates (1 to 5 μm); irregular, small nanoparticle aggregates (1 to 10 μm), usually break-down fragments of larger aggregates; microplate, large nanoparticle aggregates (> 10 μm). Nanoparticles and small aggregates are usually associated with tribocorrosion and the larger aggregates to crevice/fretting corrosion;

4) *Ceramic*: nanoparticles, non-detectable (1 to 100 nm), submicron particles (> 100 nm to < 1 μm), non-detectable, microparticles (1 to 10 μm), macroparticles (> 10 μm);

5) *PMMA*: Large particles surrounded by giant cells dissolved during tissue processing cycle and appearing as empty lacunae with small aggregates of radiographic contrast agent present; medium and small size particles engulfed in giant cells and dissolved as well; particles of radiographic contrast agent in macrophages (barium sulphate, zirconium dioxide) especially numerous in cases of three-body wear failure.

Results

Implant wear particles

Wear particle characterization of orthopedic implant wear is the most challenging component of the histological examination of the periprosthetic tissue and it is often time consuming, especially when multiple specimens/case and several cases have to be examined in a single session. The most frequently used bearing surface couplings are: metal-on-polyethylene (MoP), ceramic on polyethylene (CoP), metal-on-metal (MoM), and ceramic-on-ceramic (CoC); a metallic adapter sleeve, made of CoCrMo or Ti has been added to large metallic heads (≥32 mm) and of Ti to large ceramic heads (≥32 mm). PMMA cement can be present around the femoral and/or the acetabular component. Each material can be a source of particulate debris.

Polyethylene (PE)

The term polyethylene usually refers today to its ultra-high molecular weight type (UHMWPE) with an exceptionally high molecular mass, defined by the American Society for testing and materials as a molecular weight higher than 3.1 million g/mol [34]. Today the most common subtypes analyzed at the time of revision according to the year of implantation and type of prosthetic device are the first and second generation of highly crossed-linked polyethylene (HXLPE) subject to different regimens of radiation for sterilization and remelting/thermal heating for oxidation stability and in the future also with the addition of an anti-oxidant stabilizer, such as vitamin E [35]. The use of highly crossed-linked polyethylene varies among the different joint implants and the detailed information of the dose of radiation and of the use of remelting or thermal heating is usually not available to the pathologist at the time of the histological examination. Although the occurrence of macro- or supra-macroparticles has been typically associated with first generation non-highly cross-linked polyethylene [36], particles of large size can still be observed in implants of more recent design [37]. PE particles of variable size are detected at light microscopy examination under polarized light:

Microparticles:

PE microparticles are usually located in the cytoplasm of the macrophages; they measure between 1 and 10 μm and are predominantly globular, elongated, and fibrillary/needle-shaped showing variable birefringent reactivity under polarized light (Fig. 3a). Scanning electron microscopy (SEM) analysis has shown that particles of

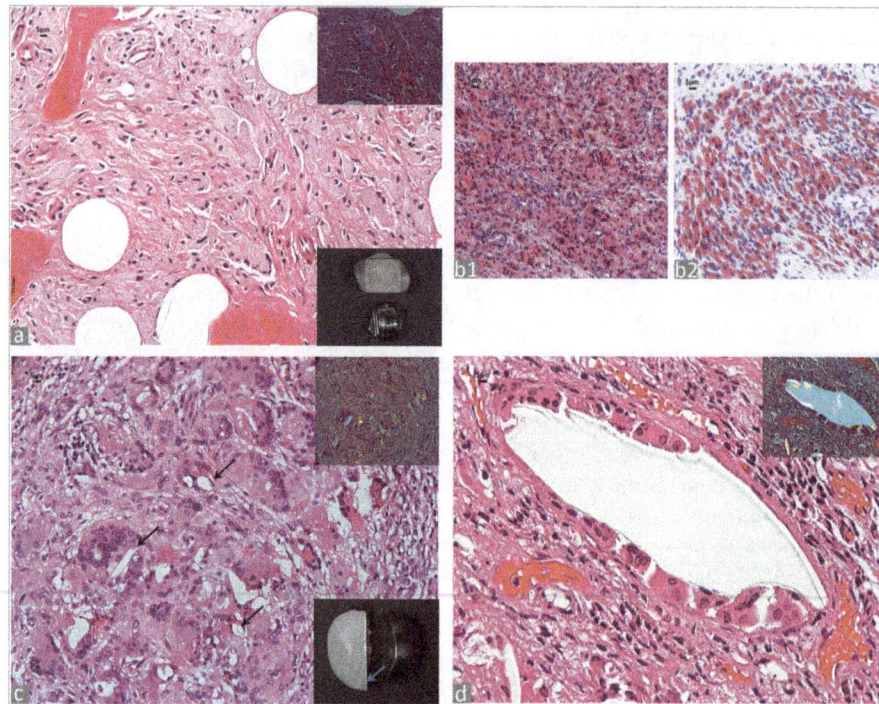

Fig. 3 Polyethylene (PE) particles. **a** Osteolysis with diffuse macrophage infiltrate containing PE micro-particles (H&E× 200), birefringent PE micro-particles under polarized light in the upper right inset (× 400), total ankle replacement implant in the lower right inset. **b1.** Oil red O positivity for macrophage cytoplasm containing PE micro- and submicron particles in a MoP TKA implant (× 200); **b2.** Oil red O positivity for macrophage cytoplasm containing tribocorrosion metallic particles in MoM HRA implant (× 200). **c** PE macroparticles (black arrows) in multinucleated giant cells (H&E × 200), birefringent particles under polarized light in the upper right inset (× 200), left unicompartmental knee implant with large area of PE abrasion/delamination (blue arrow) in the lower right inset. **d** PE supra-macroparticle lined by multinucleated giant cells in a case of failed total elbow prosthesis (H&E × 200), birefringent PE supra-macroparticle under polarized light in inset (× 200)

UHMWPE are round or elongated and that the former are in large majority submicron in size and therefore non-detectable at polarized light microscopy examination with predominance of the latter often around to 10 μm in length [38, 39]. They are visible at × 400 and × 200 under polarized light. The equivalent shape ratio (ESR) has been used in a recent study comparing UHMWPE to HXLPE particles in total ankle arthroplasty to characterize the particles which are classified as round (ESR < 1.5), elongated ($1.5 \leq ESR \leq 3$) and fibrillary ($3 < ESR$) [40]. The detectable number of particles is also dependent on the polarizer and analyzer components used for the analysis. Oil red O staining provides positive staining of cytoplasmic, micro-particulate PE (Fig. 3b1), although it is non-specific and stains also diffusely the cytoplasm of macrophages filled with metallic nanoparticles generated by tribocorrosion in MoM bearing surface implants (Fig. 3b2), most probably bound to lipids of phagosome membranes and/or lipoprotein component of the protein corona as recently described [41].

Macroparticles:

PE macro-particles measure between > 10 μm and < 100 μm; they are they exhibit variable shape from roundish

to oval or irregular with usually smooth contour (Fig. 3c). They are detected at × 100 and × 40 magnification.

Supra-macroparticles:

These particles are detectable at × 25 magnification, especially under polarized light. Their shape is variable and frequently curved and they are surrounded by multinucleated giant cells or free in the stromal tissue with size ranging from 100 μm up to > 2000 μm (Fig. 3d). Particles larger than 1000 μm may be also detected at macroscopic examination.

Non-ferrous metallic particles

Conventional metallic particles Non-ferrous metals and their alloys are used predominantly in joint endoprosthesis, where ferrous metals (i.e. steel) are used considerably less at the present time [42]. The most used non-ferrous metals in joint prosthesis are: aluminum (Al), cobalt (Co), chromium (Cr), molybdenum (Mo), nickel (Ni), niobium (Nb), tantalum (Ta), titanium (Ti), vanadium (Va), zirconium (Zr). These metals are used in various combinations and alloys. Conventional metallic wear particles are predominantly very small particles and have an average diameter ranging from 0.05 μm to < 5 μm and only occasionally are > 5 μm especially in cases of component displacement or massive abrasion by three-body wear. The shape is predominantly rod/needle-like, but can vary from round to polygonal, sharp-edged. Their colour varies from grey to jet black. Conventional metallic debris can be admixed with either polyethylene (Fig. 4a) or ceramic debris and appear in micro and macroparticulate form in cases of femoral neck impingement or marked edge loading of the acetabular rim (Fig. 4b). It is important to emphasize that CoCrMo metallic particles, either generated by tribocorrosion (corrosion particles in our classification and rich in Cr) or by abrasion/adhesion (conventional particles in our classification and rich in Cr and Co) at the MoM bearing surface of HRA and LHTHA hip implants can be also oxidized during H&E staining with Harris hematoxylin and appear pale green/yellowish or brownish at light microscopy examination, in contrast with the charcoal-grey/black appearance of the tissue at surgery and macroscopic examination (Fig. 4c). In this case, the whole blood level of Co was 91.6 µg/L and of Cr 96.5 µg/L at the time of revision. This difference in wear particles composition has been corroborated by the finding of a predominant group of amorphous particles smaller than 10 nm in the phagosomes and composed of Cr admixed with a small number of larger, high electron density needle-like particles of Cr with Co component (Cr particles density < CoCr particle density) in cases of MoM HRA when analysed by TEM and BSEM-analysis [43]. Similar findings have also been shown with particles generated by a MoM hip simulator in vitro [44]. Moreover, wear debris from implants classified under the ceramic category and composed of a wrought zirconium alloy oxidized by thermal diffusion to form a thin, surface layer of oxidized zirconium can also have a similar appearance.

Corrosion metallic particles Corrosion of orthopaedic implants was considered a serious clinical concern in the late nineties, although it was believed that the adverse clinical outcomes could be minimized with attention to variables related to the selection of the materials and implant configuration, and metallurgical processing [45]. A renewed attention has been recently devoted to implant corrosion particles/products because of the adverse local tissue reactions/adverse reaction to metallic debris (ALTR/ARMD) associated with MoM HRA and MoM THA [14, 46], MoM large head THA implants with or without CoCr MAS [47, 48], non-MoM THA implants with CoCr DMN [49–51] and other MoP THA configurations [52, 53]. They are predominantly produced by tribocorrosion at the MoM bearing surface (the intended wear mode) and by mechanically assisted fretting/crevice corrosion (the unintended wear mode) and other less frequent types of corrosion at the head/

neck junctions [54]. They have also been recently described in modular TKA implants [55, 56]. Direct inflammatory cell induced corrosion has also been reported [57]. This cellular mechanism, although of uncertain biological significance, could also contribute to the total wear particle load. Corrosion metallic particles can be associated with a variable amount of conventional metallic particles generated by adhesion/abrasion through edge loading or neck/ acetabular rim impingement. Their shape varies from round/globular to irregular or rod/needle-like and they usually appear characteristically greenish/yellowish. When observed in large aggregates of nanoparticles or macroparticles of variable size (1 µm to > 500 µm), they can appear as greenish microplates layered with black/reddish streaks (Fig. 4d). Their metal composition varies according to the type of implant and of the wear mechanism [44]. Semithin sections prepared for electron microscopy analysis show nanoparticle aggregates present in the cytoplasm of macrophages in MoM HRA (Fig. 4e), in MoM THA with CoCr MAS with a giant cell containing a large aggregate (Fig. 4f), and Non-MoM THA with CoCr DMN with a large aggregate in inset (Fig. 4g). Corrosion particles can be generated also at metallic interface of fixation device components, as shown in Fig. 4h.

Ceramic particles

Ceramics are generally employed in joint replacement arthroplasty as combinations of CoP bearing surface in hip, knee, shoulder, elbow, and ankle implants or CoC bearing surfaces in hip implants. They are classified as: 1) Oxidized ceramics, composed of aluminum oxide ceramic (Al_2O_3), zirconium dioxide ceramic (ZrO_2) or alumina matrix composite (mixed oxide ceramic) with components such as yttrium oxide (Y_2O_3), strontium oxide (SrO), and chromium oxide (Cr_2O_3); 2) Non-oxide ceramics such as silicon nitride (Si_3N_4); 3) Hard coating on metals, such as titanium nitride (TiN); 4) Surface modifications of metals such as a zirconium alloy with 2.5% of niobium through surface oxidation by thermal diffusion; 5) Calcium phosphate ceramics such as hydroxyapatite and tri-calcium phosphate [58, 59]. Wear-induced ceramic particles usually occur in the size range of 20–100 nm and only occasionally up to several micrometers. If only a few particles are present in the macrophages, they are difficult to be identified with certainty and they should be reported only as morphologically compatible with ceramic particulate debris. Abundant ceramic debris is shown in Fig. 5a and b. The larger microparticles observed in Fig. 5a are unusual and probably due to the fracture of the acetabular liner. The birefringence of the microparticles varies from absent to weak, and they exhibit variable shape from globular to irregular-polygonal with sharp edge and colour, from clear to translucent yellowish/greenish/brownish [12, 60,

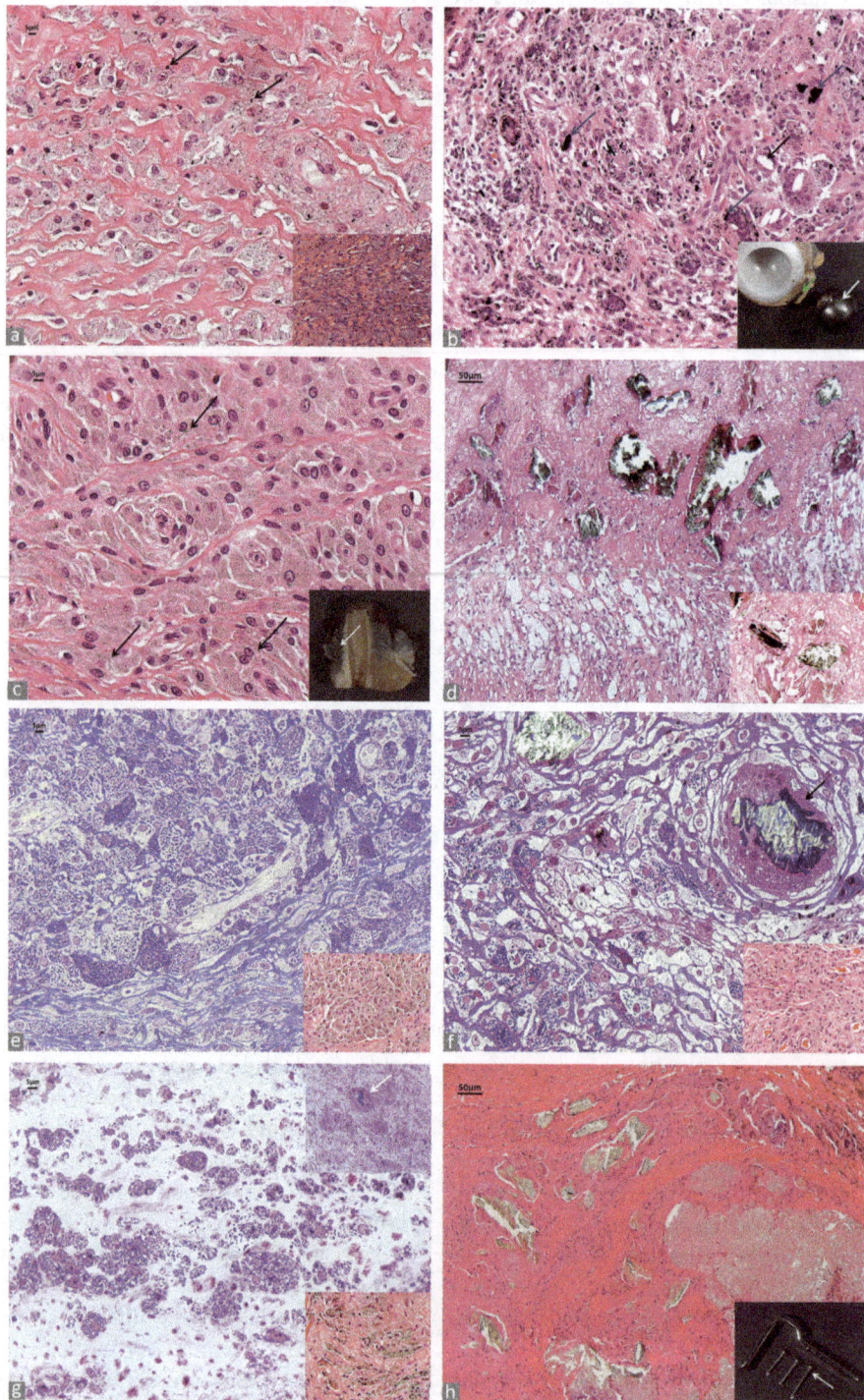

Fig. 4 (See legend on next page.)

(See figure on previous page.)

Fig. 4 Metallic non-ferrous particles. **a** Conventional black metallic particulate debris (black arrows) in MoP implant (H&E × 400), birefringent PE debris is evident as blue, granular and needle-shaped particles under polarized light in inset (× 400). **b** Macrophagic and giant cell reaction to conventional particulate metallic debris with irregular macroparticles in multinucleated giant cells (blue arrows) with empty lacunae of methyl methacrylate orthopedic cement (black arrow) (H&E × 200), CoCr femoral head with a large band of abrasion (white arrow) secondary to edge loading due to subluxation on the distorted and cemented Ti acetabular rim (green arrow) in inset. **c** Oxidized metallic particulate debris in MoM HRA implant macrophages filled with tribocorrosion nanoparticle aggregates and rod/needle-shaped larger abrasion microparticles (black arrows) (H&E × 400); femoral head with osteolytic cavity (white arrow) and neo-synovium with charcoal-gray color, indicative of conventional metallic debris from edge loading in inset. **d** Deposits of large aggregates of greenish corrosion products in enlarged trochanteric bursa of a MoM THA implant with MAS generated at head/neck junction by mechanically assisted fretting/crevice corrosion (H&E × 100), details of particles with green (CoCrMo), red (blood-derived) and black (Ti) layers in inset (H-E × 400). **e** Macrophagic infiltrate containing predominantly tribocorrosion metallic nanoparticles in MoM HRA implant, semithin section (toluidine blue × 400); macrophagic infiltrate in inset (H&E × 400). **f** Macrophage infiltrate containing predominantly tribocorrosion metallic nanoparticles (white arrow) and microplate of corrosion product from head-neck junction in a multinucleated giant cell (black arrow) of a MoM THA implant with MAS, semithin section (toluidine blue × 400); macrophage infiltrate in inset (H&E × 400). **g** Macrophage infiltrate containing irregular metallic nanoparticle aggregates in a non-MoM THA with CoCr DMN, semithin section (toluidine blue × 400) and giant cell with a large aggregate of nanoparticles/corrosion product (white arrow), semithin section, in the upper right inset (toluidine blue × 400), macrophage infiltrate in the lower right inset (H&E × 400). **h** Microplates of corrosion particle aggregates generated at fixation device screw-plate interface (H&E × 100). Metallic plate and metallic screws with corrosion observed at the screw head/threaded body junction (white arrow) in inset

61] or grey/black (oxidized metal, not shown) according to the type of ceramic of the implant component(s).

Hydroxyapatite (HA)

The HA surface coating often used in metal materials (mostly on metallic surfaces) facilitates the osteointegration process of the prosthesis. HA is usually completely replaced by the periprosthetic bone formation and can only be detected by hard grinding techniques in the early phase following implantation and very infrequently as a particulate material in the SLIM. Hydroxyapatite/beta tricalcium phosphates can also be used as bone augmentation agents and are synthesized in sizes ranging from hundreds nanometer to hundreds micrometers [62]. They can present as aggregates of nanoparticles to microparticles with morphological features similar to ceramic particles and can also be associated with calcium deposits and giant cell reaction, as shown in a case treated with hydroxyapatite agent for bone augmentation for massive osteolysis (Fig. 5c).

Polymethyl methacrylate orthopaedic cement particles (PMMA)

In the conventional histological tissue preparation, PMMA particles are chemically dissolved during tissue processing. They are identified at light microscopy as empty, multivacuolated cavities of variable size lined or engulfed by multinucleated giant cells (Fig. 5d).

Radiographic contrast agent (zirconium dioxide and barium sulfate) In the vacuoles of the PMMA, which has been dissolved during tissue processing, only the additive, radiological contrast agent zirconium dioxide or barium sulphate is identifiable (Fig. 5d). They are detectable as small, aciniform aggregates of round, slightly birefringent particles with a dark border and a clear center. They

can be numerous in the cytoplasm of macrophages, especially in cases of three body-wear and be an indicator of this mode of implant failure (Fig. 5e). Differentiation of zirconium dioxide from barium sulfate is not possible with certainty at light microscopy examination.

Non-implant related particles

The non-implant related particles present in the periprosthetic soft tissue and/or SLIM include endogenous particles, for the large majority crystals and material related to blood by-products and foreign particles, derived from surgical sutures, fixation/reconstruction devices, joint spacers, skeletal substitute materials, visco-supplements, and drug carriers.

Endogenous particles

Endogenous particles are identified by the use of polarized light for the identification of crystals and PBR for the identification of hemosiderin/blood products.

Calcium pyrophosphate Calcium pyrophosphate (CPP) exists in the form of characteristically rhomboid shaped crystals admixed to cuboid, parallelepiped, and also needle-shaped forms, approximately ≤1 μm to 1 μm in size [26]. CPP deposits exhibit a weak positive birefringence under compensated polarized light (pale yellow with the long axis perpendicular to the compensator and pale blue when parallel) and are characteristically embedded into a reddish, homogeneous matrix (Fig. 6a). In the periprosthetic soft tissue and/or the SLIM, deposits of calcium pyrophosphate crystals can also be detected in proximity to the macrophage/giant cell reaction to wear debris.

Urate Sodium urate crystals are present in the H&E section in the form of haphazardly arranged short fascicles of needle-shaped, empty spaces corresponding to dissolved

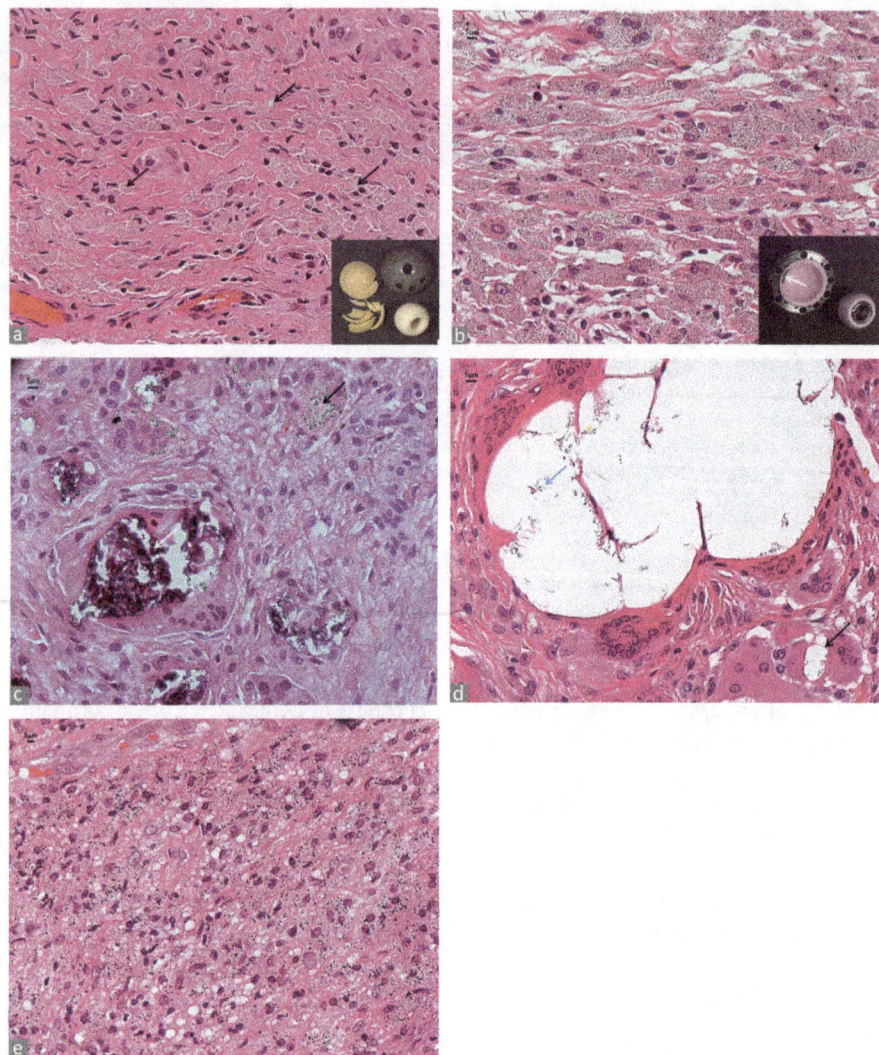

Fig. 5 Ceramic/ Polymethyl methacrylate orthopedic cement particles (PMMA). **a** Ceramic particulate debris, small and large microparticles (black arrows) (H&E × 400), fractured alumina ceramic liner in a ceramic-on-ceramic hip implant in inset. **b** Ceramic particulate debris and scattered black particles of conventional metallic debris (white arrows) (H&E × 400); the metallic debris is secondary to neck-to-rim impingement with metal transfer to the ceramic liner (white arrow) in a zirconia toughened alumina ceramic-on-ceramic hip implant with Ti metallic adapter sleeve in inset. **c** Hydroxyapatite. Macrophage/giant cell reaction to deposits of hydroxyapatite (black arrow) with calcification (white arrow) (H&E × 400). **d** PMMA. Large vacuoles of orthopaedic cement dissolved in tissue processing and containing residual particles of radiographic contrast agent (blue arrow) are lined by multinucleated giant cells (H&E × 200) and a smaller vacuole is engulfed by a multinucleated giant cell (black arrow) (H&E × 400). **e** Macrophage infiltrate containing numerous particles of radiographic contrast agent, indicative of third body wear implant failure (H&E × 400)

urate crystals, embedded into an amorphous, greyish matrix and surrounded by a macrophage/giant cell reaction (Fig. 6b). Since urate crystals are water-soluble, negatively birefringent urate crystals (bright blue with the long axis perpendicular to the compensator and bright yellow when parallel) may only be detected directly in the native preparation or in histological section before paraffin removal [26], although some residual crystal fascicles can be present after staining in large tophi. The particle size can range between 5 and 25 µm.

Oxalate Deposits of calcium oxalate in bone and other tissues is known as oxalosis and it is a secondary to the occurrence of primary hyperoxaluria (PH) due to an autosomal recessive hereditary disorder of the metabolism of glyoxylate, most frequently caused by a enzyme deficit of alanine-glyoxylate aminotransferase (PH type I) located in the hepatic peroxisomes which causes excessive oxalate production with involvement of the kidney, the excretory organ [63]. The crystals appear as pale green or pale yellow arranged in clusters of broken

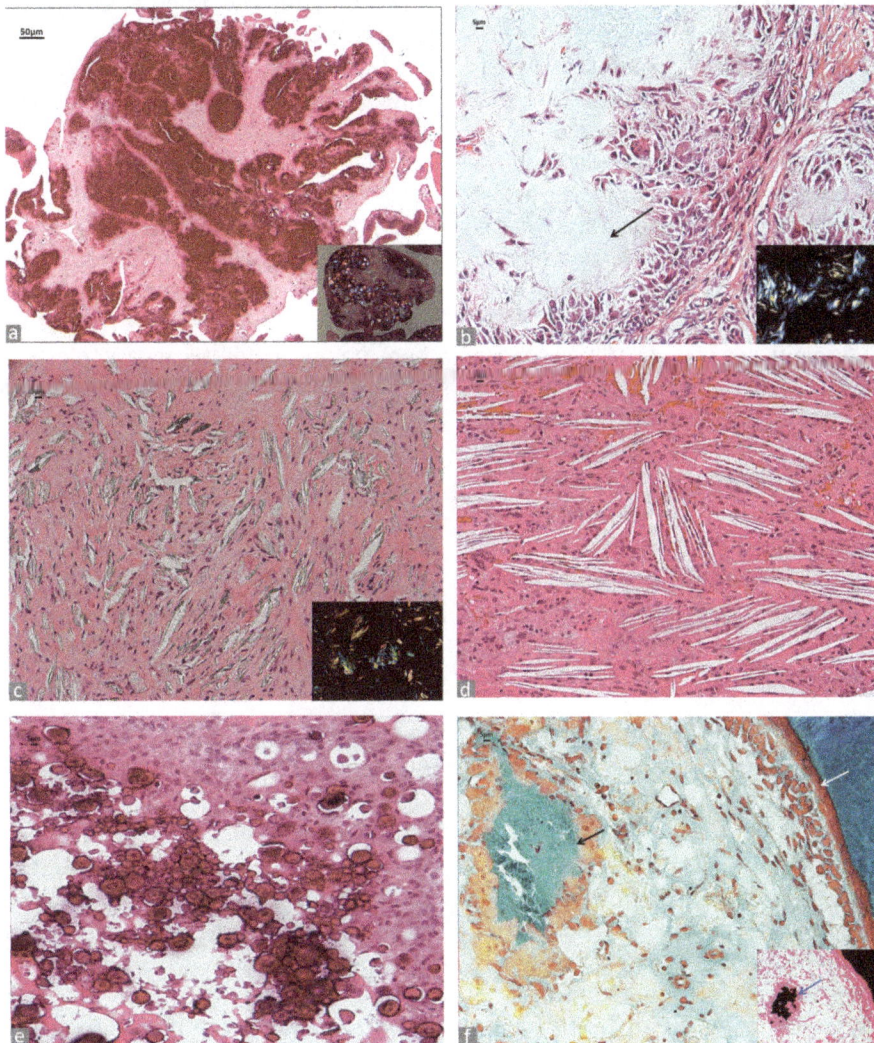

Fig. 6 Crystal Deposits. **a** Calcium pyrophosphate (CPP). Synovial sclerosis with large amount of CPP (× 100), CPP positive birefringent crystals with rhomboid shape under polarized light, inset (× 200). **b** Monosodium urate. Macrophage and giant cell reaction to fascicles of dissolved urate crystals (black arrow) (H&E × 200), residual negative birefringent crystals under polarized light in inset (× 400). **c** Oxalate. Deposition of oxalate crystals in bone marrow in a case of primary oxaluria (H&E × 200). Positive birefringent crystals under polarized light in inset (× 400). **d** Cholesterol. Clefts of cholesterol crystals in long-standing chronic bursitis with macrophage reaction with numerous foamy forms to particulate wear debris of MoM THA implant (H&E × 200). **e** Hydroxyapatite (calcinosis). Spherical and targetoid deposits of calcium hydroxyapatite in calcific bursitis of shoulder joint (H&E × 200). **f** Hydroxyapatite (calcinosis). Bone marrow stromal reaction to deposits of calcium hydroxyapatite (black arrow) with brisk osteoblatic activity and thick osteoid seam (white arrow) in a femoral head with periarticular tumoral calcinosis in a case of long-standing scleroderma. Undecalcified bone section (Goldner's Masson Trichrome × 200) with black calcium hydroxyapatite deposits evident in inset (blue arrow) (Von Kossa × 200)

plates or radial rosettes embedded in a fibrous stroma and are birefringent under polarized light (Fig. 6c).

Cholesterol Cholesterol crystals are dissolved during tissue processing and typically appear as haphazardly arranged small fascicles of empty clefts (Fig. 6d). The formation of the crystals in the periprosthetic neo-synovium occurs in arthroplasty after a relative long time of implantation and often in long-standing chronic

bursitis with a marked particle-laden macrophage infiltrate with abundant necrotic cell debris.

Hydroxyapatite (calcinosis) Soft tissue deposition of hydroxyapatite can occur in a single or multiple locations and can be related to a number of systemic disorders such as familial or idiopathic tumoral calcinosis, associated with autoimmune rheumatologic disorders and in particular scleroderma, and metabolic conditions such as renal failure with dialysis, hypervitaminosis D, and other disorders of the calcium/phosphorus homeo-stasis. Although almost any joint can be affected by cal-cinosis, the shoulder is the most commonly involved region where calcific tendinitis and/or bursitis can occur [64]. The crystals appear spherical and targetoid and are lined by a macrophage/giant cell reaction (Fig. 6e). De-posits with stromal reaction in the bone marrow associ-ated with brisk osteoblastic activity and thick osteoid seam can also be observed in cases of periarticular tu-moral calcinosis associated with scleroderma (Fig. 6f).

Hemosiderin Hemosiderin deposits, usually secondary to chronic bleeding in the periprosthetic soft tissue or traumatic events such as implant dislocation or peri-prosthetic fracture, appear as course, granular golden brown deposits in the macrophage cytoplasm (Fig. 7a). In the Prussian blue reaction, hemosiderin deposits stain intensely dark blue (Fig. 7a, inset). Hemosiderin deposits in macrophages of the SLIM may also be present in con-junction with prosthesis material wear particles and might be difficult to differentiate without the PBR stain from ceramic and/or metallic corrosion particles espe-cially if they have a granular size.

Gamna-Gandy bodies Gamna-Gandy (G-G) bodies are defined as small, spheroidal or irregular yellow-brown foci, consisting of dense fibrous tissue and collagenous fibers encrusted with iron pigments and calcium salts (Fig. 7b1 and b2). They were first described in the spleen early in the twentieth century and were erroneously con-sidered to be caused by fungal infection. Now G-G bod-ies are considered to result from organization of small hemorrhages and have been characterized by scanning electron microscopy and x-ray fluorescence spectroscopy with demonstration of their crystalline nature and chem-ical structure of $CaPO_4 \cdot FeOH$ [65]. G-G bodies are a well-recognized finding in atrial myxomas where they form linear arrays of mineral-encrusted fibers, often at the edge of resolving hemorrhages. Their definition has been expanded to include all the formations of connect-ive tissue fibers admixed to iron pigments and calcium salts, irrespective of size or form.

Formalin pigment This pigment is produced by acid acting upon hemoglobin and is also known as acid hematin. The appearance is black to brown with amorphous to microcrystalline granules (Fig. 7c). Forma-lin pigment granules can be present in the H&E stained histological sections of periprosthetic tissues fixed in for-malin having a low pH [66].

Lime (calcium carbonate) Calcium carbonate, as one of the most important forms of lime, appears in the form of basophilic, non-birefringent coagulative deposits (Fig. 7d).

Calcium carbonate is observed mostly embedded in a fiber-rich connective tissue with scant macrophage/multi-nucleated giant cell reaction and can be a consequence of an inflammatory process and/or tissue necrosis. The par-ticle size is usually larger than 1 mm.

Bone tissue detritus The bone tissue fragments are often surrounded by macrophages and osteoclast-like giant cells, particularly in detritus synovitis as a conse-quence of osteoarthritis, necrosis, and especially rapidly progressive osteoarthritis. In SLIM, the cause can be bone fragmentation secondary to osteolysis with or with-out fracture and also bone milling during surgery, the so-called cutting-grinding effect, as a by-product of the surgical operation. The particle size usually ranges from 5 to > 300 μm (Fig. 7e).

Foreign particles
Foreign particles are predominantly generated by fixation/reconstruction devices and by materials or substances used as fillers or carriers to alleviate the symptoms or complications of joint arthritis and arthrosis.

Surgical sutures (absorbable and non-absorbable) Surgical sutures are usually easy to identify because of their high birefringence and tubular structure in longitu-dinal, oblique, and cross section or even filamentous structure. Absorbable surgical sutures, however, can be more challenging especially when broken in small frag-ments because of their heterogeneous birefringence and appearance (Fig. 8a).

Fixation/reconstruction devices/materials Fixation de-vices which can break down and can represent a differ-ential diagnosis with supra-macroparticulate PE are fixation plastic screws and/or anchors and in our experi-ence birefringence is usually less intense and homoge-neous for fixation devices than for large PE particles (Fig. 8b).

Debris released by broken metallic devices, such as metallic plates or acetabular screws cannot be distin-guished from metallic wear debris and a clinical history and examination of the explanted hardware is essential for the correct histological diagnosis.

Among the reconstruction materials, an interesting ex-ample is represented by the Active Biosynthetic Com-posite Ligament (ABC), introduced as a scaffold class ligament in 1985 for primary reconstruction of the hu-man anterior cruciate ligament, composed of interwoven carbon and polyester unit material. The artificial liga-ment failure usually occurs because of stretching and breaking of the fibers secondary to mechanical or fatigue factors [67]. At histological examination carbon fibers appear jet black with a cylinder-like shape and do not

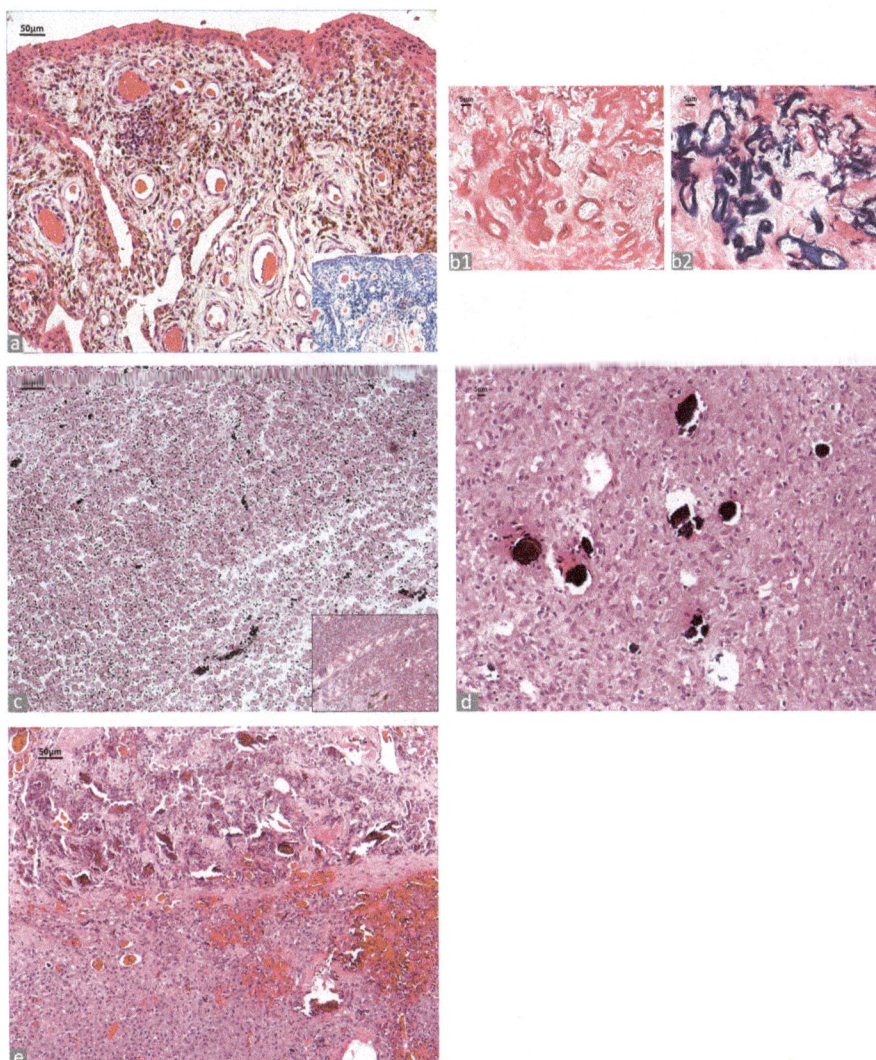

Fig. 7 Hemorrhage byproducts and calcific/osseous deposits. **a** Hemosiderin pigment in neo-synovium (H&E × 100), hemosiderin deposits positive for PBR in inset (PBR × 100). **b1** Gamna-Gandy bodies in failed MoP THA with hemorrhage secondary to multiple dislocations (× 400), **b2** positivity to PBR reaction, PBR stain in inset (× 400). **c** Formalin pigment artifact, negative for PBR reaction (PBR stain × 100) and with typical birefringence of the granules of formalin pigment under polarized light in inset (× 200). **d** Lime (dystrophic calcification) in periprosthetic neo-synovium of a case of hip implant failure (H&E × 200). **e** Neo-synovium of a failed MoP THA implant for aseptic loosening/osteolysis with abundant osseous detritus embedded in the superficial layer (H&E × 100)

polarize. The diameter is approximately 5–8 μm and the length of the fibers is variable; in the non-fragmented state, it can be up to several mm. They are embedded in a fibrous matrix, without presence of a macrophage response (Fig. 8c). A distinct granulomatous foreign body reaction has been described in a single case report [68]; however, examination of the histological picture provided shows only fibrous reaction around the carbon fibers without cellular response.

Joint spacers Silicone elastomer is the most common joint spacer and has been used for decades as an inert spacer for small and medium-size joints, such as fingers,

toes, metatarsal-phalangeal, thumb, wrist and elbow [69]. In the so-called silicone synovitis polycyclic, irregular and rectangular macroparticles up to several mm are present in synovial or capsular location, usually resulting from a fracture of the prosthesis with fragmentation and subsequent development of a foreign body giant cell reaction. These fragments are pale white and can be partially dissolved through tissue processing and histologic section staining. They exhibit a variable degree of birefringence under polarized light (Fig. 8d). Other materials have also been used as spacers causing a similar reaction, such as porous polyurethaneurea [70], shown in Fig. 8e.

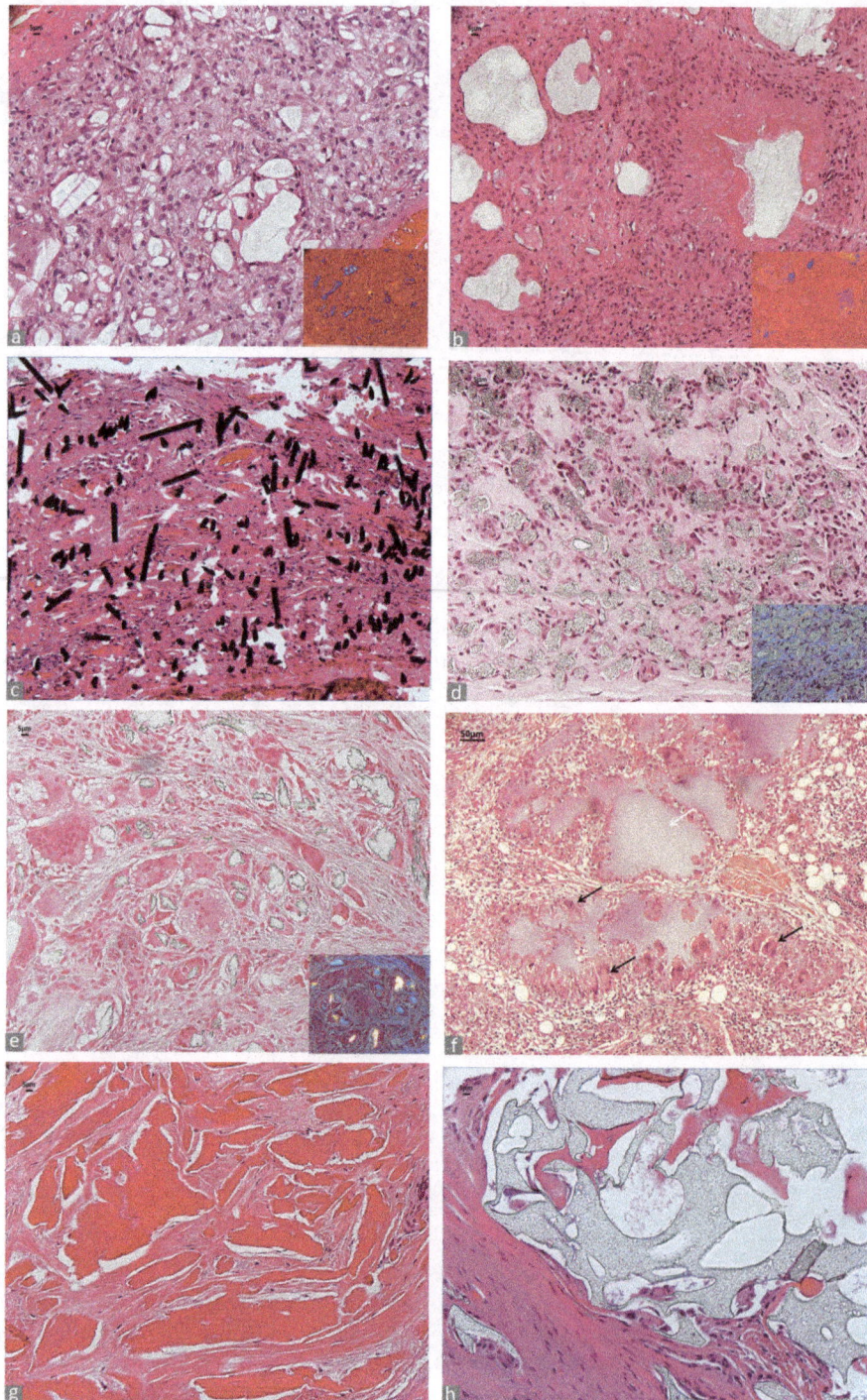

Fig. 8 Non-implant wear, foreign particles/bone graft. **a** Absorbable surgical suture. Macrophage/giant cell reaction to deposits of absorbable suture material (H&E × 200), birefringent suture under polarized light in inset (× 200). **b** Fixation device (interference plastic poly-DL-lactide screw). Macrophage/giant cell reaction with palisading macrophages to plastic screw material implanted for anterior cruciate ligament reconstruction (H&E × 200), focal birefringence under polarized light in inset (× 200). **c** Scaffold composite material (carbon and polyester). Reactive fibrous tissue with embedded fragments of carbon fibers from a scaffold class anterior cruciate ligament (H&E × 200). **d** Joint spacer material. Macrophage reaction to silicone elastomer particles from a finger prosthetic implant (H&E × 200); particles are non-reactive under polarized light in inset (× 400). **e** Joint spacer material. Florid giant cell reaction to particles of porous polyurethaneurea (H&E × 200); particles are birefringent under polarized light in inset (× 400). **f** Visco-supplement reaction. Palisading macrophages and giant cell (black arrows) reaction to hyaluronan deposits (white arrow) (H&E × 100). **g** Skeletal substitute material. Demineralized bone matrix of allograft implant with intervening fibrous tissue (H&E × 200). **h** Skeletal substitute material. Porous tricalcium phosphate bone substitute (H&E × 200)

Injected foreign materials (visco-supplements and drug carriers) Foreign body-induced cases of synovitis are typically observed following applications of intra-articular substances/drugs. Histologically, the specification of the material (in most cases the drug substrate) is not possible unless a detailed clinical history is available, although certain materials, such as visco-supplements, provide a distinctive foreign body reaction of palisading macrophages admixed to multinucleated giant cells [71] (Fig. 8f).

Skeletal substitute materials Although strictly not part of the particle algorithm, skeletal substitute materials are also used to fill voids around failed joint prostheses and/or increase osteointegration and their recognition at histological examination is important to interpret correctly the pathological findings of the specimen [72]. Among those frequently used are demineralized bone matrix (Fig. 8g) and soluble calcium-based granules (Fig. 8h).

Differential diagnosis of particle laden macrophages and other macrophage diseases in bone

A challenging differential diagnosis can occur in the presence of bone marrow macrophage infiltrates which are characteristic of other conditions, such as lysosomal storage diseases [73] and other macrophage disorders, such as Erdheim-Chester disease (polyostotic sclerosing histiocytosis) [74], especially when limited tissue is available or in consultation practice without a detailed clinical history. Although the diagnosis should be known clinically before the occurrence of a joint prosthetic revision, exceptions can occur because of mild forms of the storage diseases with adulthood onset or misdiagnosis because of their rare occurrence. However, careful examination of the macrophage infiltrate provides clues to differentiate these conditions at light microscopy. The particle laden macrophage infiltrate is usually composed of packed, polygonal macrophages with abundant cytoplasm infiltrating the bone marrow with an easily identifiable particle loading of PE, metal, orthopaedic cement, complex mixed wear; PE particles are seen in Fig. 9a with inset and conventional and tribocorrosion metallic particles are seen in Fig. 9b. The macrophages in the lysosomal storage diseases contain the substance which cannot be digested because of the enzymatic defect, such as in Gaucher's disease, in which they show characteristic crumpled tissue paper-like cytoplasm (Fig. 9c). In polyostotic sclerosing histiocytosis, the macrophages are

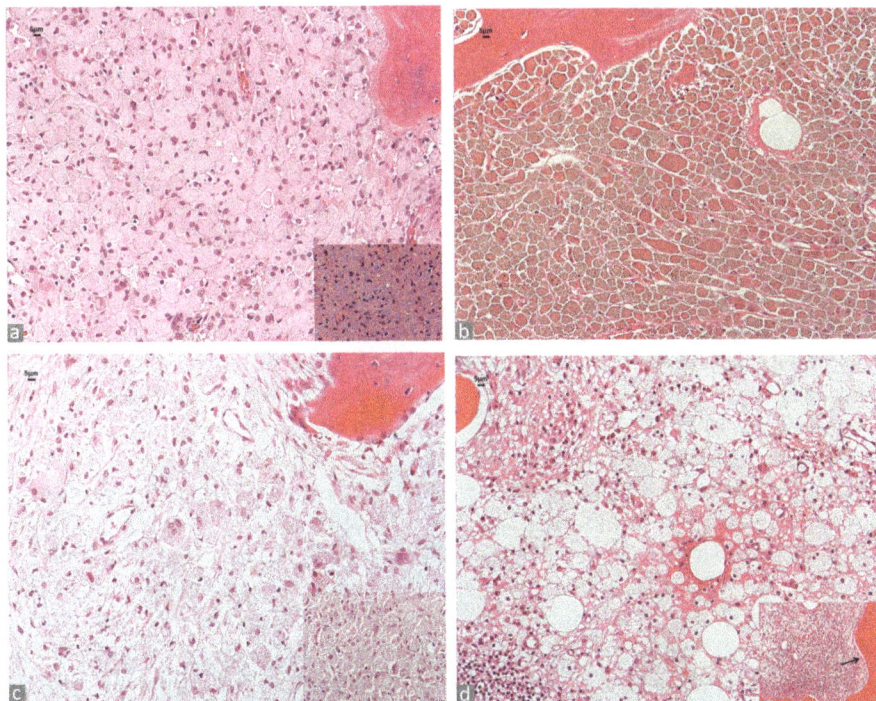

Fig. 9 Differential diagnosis between particle laden macrophagic infiltrate and other macrophagic diseases in bone. **a** Implant aseptic loosening (osteolysis). Dense macrophage infiltrate in the bone marrow in a MoP THA implant (H&E × 200) containing birefringent PE microparticles under polarized light in inset (× 400). **b** Implant aseptic loosening (osteolysis). Diffuse, brownish macrophage infiltrate containing tribocorrosion and conventional metallic particles in a femoral head of a MoM HRA implant (H&E × 200). **c** Gaucher's disease. Macrophage infiltrate in the bone marrow of a femoral head (H&E × 200) with details of the macrophage crumpled cytoplasm in inset (H&E × 400). **d** Erdheim-Chester disease. Bone marrow from proximal tibia with foamy macrophages and mixed chronic inflammatory infiltrate (H&E × 200) and mixed chronic inflammatory infiltrate and adjacent sclerotic cancellous bone with osteoblastic rimming in inset (H&E × 400)

lipid laden with abundant foamy cytoplasm and admixed to an inflammatory infiltrate predominantly composed of lymphocytes and plasma cells (Fig. 9d) and if present, the cancellous bone is sclerotic with evident osteoblastic rimming (Fig. 9d, inset).

Discussion

In general, an algorithm is a logical sequence of actions to be performed for solving a diagnostic or therapeutic problem and is widely used in guideline-oriented medical practice. We propose a histological particle algorithm based on particle-defining criteria which provide a guide to implant wear as well as non-implant related endogenous and foreign particle identification in the periprosthetic tissue and SLIM using conventional histology examined at light microscopy with the aid of polarized light and simple histochemical stains when necessary. This simple and comprehensive flow chart aims at providing complementary information to the diagnostic classification of the periprosthetic neo-synovial membrane, bone, and SLIM reaction to implant wear. The characterization of these particles is defined in accordance with a classification based on size and shape, staining characteristics, and properties under polarized light. The particle algorithm is also designed to assist general surgical pathologists, orthopaedic surgeons and the material scientists in the identification of particulate material in the periprosthetic neo-synovial membrane, bone, and SLIM with minimal methodical complexity.

It needs to be emphasized that the particle algorithm constitutes only a guide to identification of implant by-products on a descriptive level by conventional histological examination. Particularly for metallic and ceramic materials but also for the different types of UHMWPE, the definitive material identification, chemical composition and oxidative status is only possible through the use of physical, high-resolution procedures, for example energy dispersive X-ray spectroscopy (EDS) and Fourier transform infrared spectroscopy (FTIR) [53] or synchrotron micro X-ray absorption spectroscopy (XAS) and X-ray absorption near edge structure (XANES) [75]. For detection of low concentration elements in nano-size wear particles, even more sensitive analytical techniques need to be used, such as TEM and TEM-EDS element mapping, SEM, backscatter scanning electron microscopy (BSEM) and BSEM-EDS element mapping examination, X-Ray diffraction spectrometry (XRD) examination and single particle-inductively coupled plasma-mass spectrometry (SP-ICP-MS), as recently reported [43]. The use of analytical nano-technology is also advocated for complex cases in which several revisions have occurred with different bearing coupling and/or use of materials for implant adherence [76]. It needs also to be taken into account that wear particles are tridimensional objects and that for a

correct interpretation of their shape and volume, SEM stereoscopy has been shown to provide the most reliable results [77]. The use of these techniques is particularly important for research purposes and also for the determination of different toxicity/immunogenicity of the particles generated by in vitro wear simulation or in vivo for clinical purposes. It is also important to highlight that wear particles generated by new implant configurations can be missed or misdiagnosed at light microscopy examination. One recent, noteworthy example is represented by the metallic nanoparticles generated by MoM implants which were originally described in 2005 as "cytoplasmic pseudo-inclusions which did not resemble wear debris" [78] and therefore were not counted as metallic wear particles or considered as possible cause of the adverse reaction named aseptic lymphocyte-dominated vasculitis-associated lesion (ALVAL). The first study that correctly characterized the cytoplasmic pseudo-inclusions as metallic wear nanoparticles analysed by TEM and SEM was published six years later in 2011 [79] and later confirmed by a larger study including the same implant configuration [43].

The evaluation of the tissue response pattern(s) is also performed in addition to the identification of implant wear and non-implant related particles for a comprehensive pathological report. The correlation between type of particulate wear and inflammatory response can be important for the choice of the most host-compatible materials and tribological couplings [80]. Due to rapidly advancing developments in prosthesis materials and prosthesis design, new types of wear particles and associated inflammatory response patterns can be detected in the periprosthetic tissue and SLIM by histological examination. These response patterns are determined by biomechanical factors (prosthesis design, loading mode, positioning of implant components, and joint fluid waves), particle properties (composition, size, surface, total burden), and host factors (genetic, immunological, protein corona of particles). For the tissue response classification which goes beyond the scopes of this report, we refer to our previous publications which described it in detail [19, 20].

A particle scoring system is advisable to summarize the most important information for the material scientist and the orthopaedic surgeon: 1) Predominant prosthetic particle material; 2) Minor wear/non-wear components; 3) Non-implant related particle material type, if present. Wear particle assessment has been reported with the use of a semi-quantitative scale based on the number of particles/HPF (× 400 or × 500) or particles/macrophage [8, 81], even for small PE and metallic particles below the optic microscope resolution. Since the wear particles from PE components in MoP and CoP bearing surfaces, metallic in MoM and ceramic in CoC bearing surfaces occur mostly in the nano- and submicron size, it appears that only aggregates can be seen at light microscopy with H&E stain and polarized light without the possibility of a reliable count by number. Therefore the use of a practical semi-quantitative scale of five grades is suggested for the evaluation of the wear particle load within the macrophages with slight modifications from the one reported by Natu [13] and adapted from the assessment of iron overload in liver biopsies [82], following the simple principle of the optic microscope magnifications (eyepiece x objective lens): 0 - no identifiable particles at × 400; 1 - particles identifiable at × 400, 2 - particles identifiable at × 200; 3 - particles identifiable at × 100; 4 - particles identifiable at × 40 and × 25. Particle content is assessed in the areas of maximum macrophage density on 10 consecutive HPF starting at the lowest magnification. A web-based particle algorithm would be desirable for assuring the constant updating of particle identification associated to the inflammatory response patterns. This tool would be particularly useful to provide information on potential new alternative bearing materials in different stages of pre-clinical examination/use, such as polyethererether-ketone which has been recently described in animal/human retrieval studies [83]. The proposed particle algorithm will also need further studies for the assessment of its internal and external validity.

The differences in crystalline deposits in the SLIM, the wide variety of prosthesis materials and the diversity of material combinations and particle pathogenesis mechanisms explain the high level of morphological particle heterogeneity in the periprosthetic tissue/SLIM which makes the process of particle identification for diagnostic purposes challenging, especially when the particle burden is below the resolution power of the optic microscope.

A properly conducted and reported histopathological analysis of peri-implant tissue can provide indispensable information on in vivo performance and modalities of failure of orthopaedic implants [84]. The pathology report, issued primarily for the clinical practice and management of the patient and also in consultation practice for diagnostic and/or medico-legal purposes should include the sections below.

Macroscopic description
1) Neo-synovial and capsular tissue configuration, consistency, colour, three dimensional measurements, optional weight of the wet specimen, bone tissue sampling if present; 2) Description of the removed implant components if available with specification of manufacturer and type (basic prosthetic alloy, bearing pair, modularity, and component serial number optional

when available). Description of basic wear analysis at naked eye or with the use of a dissecting microscope and a digital camera may be added, according to the expertise of the examiner or with the assistance of a biomechanical engineer. However, it needs to be stressed that only basic surface characterization is possible and therefore no definitive conclusions should be drawn on the modality of implant failure with the use of this technique. The terminology used for the implant description should be as precise as possible, using the technical documentation provided by each manufacturer. Consultation of the operative report can also provide confirmatory or additional information on the implant components not removed at surgery. Photographic documentation of the revised components of each implant and of relevant soft tissue specimens can be useful at microscopic examination, for retrospective examination of the cases, and for educational purposes.

Microscopic description
1) Tissue morphology with presence/absence of tissue necrosis/infarction (thickness measurement) and apoptotic cell necrosis with semi-quantitative assessment (slight, moderate, marked); 2) The description of the wear particulate and non-wear particulate material, according to the criteria previously described and mention of the dominant and secondary implant wear material(s); 3) The description of all cell types present with semi-quantitative analysis and relation to the particle wear, including macrophages, fibroblasts, endothelial cells (flat, tall) and the inflammatory cells of the white series: neutrophils, lymphocytes, plasma cells, eosinophils, mast cells. Immunohistochemical and immunofluorescence studies can provide additional, more specific information when necessary.

Diagnosis
The diagnosis is centred on the type(s) of periprosthetic tissue/SLIM present according to the classification previously reported [20] with the optional addition of the particulate material(s) as described microscopically and the material of the revised implant component(s). A case comment can be added to highlight a discrepancy with the clinical diagnosis, special features, and indications for a specific clinical follow-up.

The concept of wear particle threshold has been proposed by several groups of investigators for polyethylene wear debris in relation to the occurrence of osteolysis and in particular for total hip replacements, suggested as a practical level of 0.05 mm/y for a 28 mm head size [85], although not universally accepted and with concerns related to its general applicability because of too short follow-up of many studies, inadequate definition of osteolysis, use of plain radiographs only for its determination, and consideration of other associated factors which might be more important than particle volume [86] such as the oxidative state of the particles [35].

Moreover, a systematic review of wear and osteolysis outcomes for first-generation HXLPE could not establish the risk for osteolysis for large diameter (≥ 32 mm) metallic femoral heads or ceramic femoral heads of any size and for TKA because of lack of a sufficient number of studies available [36]. For metallic wear nano-particles it has been reported that they can stimulate a higher inflammatory reaction which can be the result of complex biological factors depending on particle size, shape, composition, surface properties [87] and protein corona coating with lipoproteins [6, 41]. Adverse local tissue reactions recently reported in hip implants of different bearing surfaces could be more dependent on particle composition and aggregation than number and volume, as shown in a study comparing metallic particle generation and inflammatory response in three different configurations, MoM HRA, MoM THA, and Non-MoM THA with CoCr dual modular neck [43] and also development of osteolysis dependent on different cytokines according to particle composition and size and macrophage response [87]. Attempt to establish a threshold concentration of Co and Cr blood metal ion has been proposed and recently modified in an attempt to identify patients at risk for adverse tissue reaction progression [88]. To the best of our knowledge, no particle threshold value for osteolysis or other adverse tissue reactions has been reported for ceramic or polymethyl methacrylate orthopedic cement particulate debris. A final word of caution has to be spent for potential, long-term health effects of wear particles and in particular of metallic nano-particulate debris in distant tissues and in contact with bone marrow residing mesenchymal stromal cells [89] and hematopoietic stem cells.

Conclusions

Due to the continuous developments of new materials and combinations in orthopaedic prostheses, we believe that a web-based particle algorithm would be the ideal set up to assure the constant updating of the materials used for accurate particle identification in the periprosthetic tissue/SLIM.

The histological particle algorithm for detection and identification of implant wear and non-implant related particulate materials in joint arthroplasty should be considered a standard for the histological analysis. It provides a basic, useful tool for particle identification at routine light microscopy examination and it is time-saving and low-cost.

The algorithm can also be used to reduce intra-observer and inter-observer variability in order to provide a common platform for multicentric implant retrieval/radiological/histological studies and valuable data for the risk assessment of implant performance to regional and national implant registries and government agencies.

Abbreviations

ALTR: Adverse local tissue reaction; ALVAL: Aseptic lymphocytic vasculitis associated lesion; ARMD: Adverse reaction to metallic debris; BSEM: Backscatter scanning electron microscopy; CoC: Ceramic-on-ceramic; CoCr: Cobalt-chromium; CoP: Ceramic-on-plastic; CPLM: Compensated polarized light microscopy; CPP: Calcium pyrophosphate; DMN: Dual modular neck; EDS: Energy-dispersive X-ray spectroscopy; FITR: Fourier infrared transmission spectroscopy; H&E: Hematoxylin and eosin; HPA: Histological particle algorithm; HRA: Hip resurfacing arthroplasty; HXLPE: Highly crossed-linked polyethylene; LHTHA: Large head total hip arthroplasty; MAS: Metallic adapter sleeve; MoP: Metal-on-plastic; Non-MoM DMNTHA: Non-metal-on-metal hip dual modular neck total hip arthroplasty; PH: Primary oxalosis; PMMA: Polymethyl methacrylate orthopaedic cement; SDD: Silicon drift detector; SEM: Scanning electron microscopy; SLIM: Synovial-like interface membrane; SP-ICP-MS: Single particle-inductively coupled plasma–mass spectrometry; TEM: Transmission electron microscopy; THA: Total hip arthroplasty; TKA: Total knee arthroplasty; UHMWPE: Ultra-high molecular weight polyethylene; XANES: X-ray absorption near edge structure; XAS: Synchrotron micro X-ray absorption spectroscopy; XRD: X-ray diffraction spectrometry

Acknowledgements

We would like to acknowledge Lingxin Zhang, MD for critical proof reading of the manuscript; Simone Giak for her expert secretarial and editorial skills; Irina Shuleshko and Yana Bronfman for technical assistance in histology preparations; Philip Rusli for preparation of the illustrations.

Authors' contributions

GP– study conception, data collection, pathological analysis, data interpretation, manuscript preparation. SS – study conception, data collection, pathological analysis, data interpretation, manuscript preparation. MH – pathological analysis, data interpretation; DR – data collection, pathological analysis; JG, VJ, SN – critical review of the manuscript; KJP, MS, PT, MT, MGK, RH, TH – data interpretation for multidisciplinary assessment of HPA; WW, FB – data collection and interpretation; TG, SS, WR – clinical assessment of data interpretation; ZX – data preparation and particle nanoanalysis; EP- data collection, data interpretation; VK – study conception, pathological analysis, data interpretation, manuscript preparation. All authors read and approved the final manuscript.

Competing interests

The authors declare that they have no competing interests.

Author details

[1]Department of Pathology and Laboratory Medicine, Hospital for Special Surgery, 535 E 70th Street, New York, NY 10023, USA. [2]Medizinische Universität Graz, Institut für Pathologie, Graz, Austria. [3]Pathologisch-bakteriologisches Institut, Otto Wagner Spital, Wien, Austria. [4]Department of Orthopaedics, Faculty of Medicine and Dentistry, University Hospital, Palacky University Olomouc, Olomouc, Czech Republic. [5]Department of Pathology, Fakultni Nemocnice Ostrava, Ostrava, Czech Republic. [6]Department of Pathology, University hospital of North Tees and Hartlepool NHS Foundation Trust, Stockton-on-Tees, UK. [7]Labor für Biomechanik und Implantat-Forschung, Klinik für Orthopädie und Unfallchirurgie, Universitätsklinikum Heidelberg, Heidelberg, Germany. [8]MVZ-Zentrum für Histologie, Zytologie und Molekulare Diagnostik, Trier, Germany. [9]LMU Klinik, Klinik und Poliklinik für Dermatologie und Allergologie, Munich, Germany. [10]Baden-Baden Klinik, Baden-Baden, Germany. [11]Paracelsus-Kliniken Deutschland Gmbh, Osnabrück, Germany. [12]Universitätsklinik für Unfallchirurgie und Sporttraumatologie, Salzburg, Austria. [13]Hôpital Orthopédique, Lausanne, Switzerland. [14]Medizinische Universität Wien, AKH-Wien, Universitätsklinik für Orthopädie, Wien, Austria. [15]Adult Reconstruction and Joint Replacement Division, Hospital for Special Surgery, New York, NY, USA. [16]Helios Endo-Klinik, Hamburg, Germany.

[17]Orthopädische Universitätsklinik Erlangen, Erlangen, Germany. [18]Klinik und Poliklinik für Orthopädie, Universitätsklinikum Hamburg-Eppendorf, Hamburg, Germany. [19]Centre for Nanohealth, Swansea University Medical School, Singleton Park, Swansea, UK. [20]Hospital for Special Surgery, Research Institute, New York, NY, USA.

References

1. Willert HG, Semlitsch M. Reactions of the articular capsule to wear products of artificial joint prostheses. J Biomed Mater Res. 1977;11:157–64.
2. Williams JA. Wear and wear particles-some fundamentals. Tribology Int. 2005;38:863–70.
3. Mc Kellop HA, Hart A, Park SH, Hothi H, Campbell P, Skinner JA. A lexicon for wear of metal-on-metal hip prostheses. J Orthop Res. 2014;32:1221–33.
4. Hall DJ, Pourzal R, Lundberg HJ, Mathew MT, Jacobs JJ, Urban RM. Mechanical, chemical and biological damage modes within head-neck tapers of CoCrMo and Ti6Al4V contemporary hip replacements. J Biomed Mater Res Part B. 2018;106B:1672–85.
5. Monopoli MP, Åberg C, Salvati A, Dawson K. Biomolecular coronas provide the biological identity of nanosized materials. Nat Nanotechnol. 2012;7:779–86.
6. Tenzer S, Docter D, Kuharev J, Musyanovych A, Fetz V, Rouven H, Schlenk F, Fischer D, Klytaimnistra K, Reihardt C, Landfester K, Schild H, Maskos M, Knauer SK, Stauber RH. Rapid formation of plasma protein corona critically affects nanoparticle pathophysiology. Nat Nanotechnol. 2013;8:772–81.
7. Fleischer CC, Payne CK. Nanoparticle-cell interactions: molecular structure of the protein corona and cellular outcomes. Acc Chem Res. 2014;47:2651–9.
8. Mirra JM, Amstutz HC, Matos M, Gold R. The pathology of the joint tissues and its clinical relevance in prosthesis failure. Clin Orthop Rel Res. 1976;117: 221–40.
9. Ito S, Matsumoto T, Enomoto H, Shindo H. Histological analysis and biological effects of granulation tissue around loosened hip prostheses in the development of osteolysis. J Orthop Sci. 2004;9:478–81.
10. Scharf B, Clement C, Wu X, Morozova K, Zanolini D, Follenzi A, Larocca JN, Levon K, Sutterwala F, Rand J, Cobelli N, Purdue E, Hajjar KA, Santambrogio L. Annexin A2 binds to endosomes following organelle destabilization by particulate wear debris. Nat Commun. 2012;3:755. https://doi.org/10.1038/ncomms1754.
11. Pizzoferrato A, Stea S, Sudanese A, Toni A, Nigrisoli M, Gualtieri G, Squarzoni S. Morphometric and microanalytical analyses of alumina wear particles in hip prostheses. Biomaterials. 1992;14(8):583–7.
12. Savarino L, Baldini N, Ciapetti G, Pellacani A, Giunti A. Is wear debris responsible for failure in alumina-on-alumina implants? Acta Orthop. 2009; 80(2):162–7.
13. Natu S, Sidaginamale RP, Gandhi J, Langton DJ, Nargol AV. Adverse reactions to metal debris: histopathological features of periprosthetic soft tissue reactions seen in association with failed metal on metal hip arthroplasties. J Clin Pathol. 2012;65(5):409–18.
14. Campbell P, Ebramzadeh E, Nelson S, Takamura K, De Smet K, Amstutz HC. Histological features of pseudotumor-like tissues from metal-on-metal hips. Clin Orthop Relat Res. 2010;468(9):2321–7.
15. Mittal S, Revell M, Barone F, Hardie DL, Matharu GS, Davenport AJ, S M, Revell M, Barone F, Hardie DL, Matharu GS, Davenport AJ, Martin RA, Grant M, Mosselmans F, Pynsent P, Sumathi VP, Addison O, Revell PA, Buckley CD. Lymphoid aggregates that resemble tertiary lymphoid organs define a specific pathological subset in metal-on-metal hip replacements. PLoS One. 2013;8(5):e63470.
16. Kurtz SM, Ong KL, Lau E, Bozic KJ. Impact of the economic downturn on total joint replacement demand in the United States: updated projections to 2021. J Bone Joint Surg Am. 2016;96(8):624–30.
17. Matharu GS, Mellon SJ, Murray DW. Follow-up of metal-on-metal hip arthroplasty patients is currently not evidence based or cost effective. J ArthroplastJ Arthroplasty. 2015;30(8):1317–23.
18. Krenn V, Thomas P, Thomsen M, Kretzer JP, Usbeck S, Scheuber L, Perino G, Rüther W, vWelser R, Hopf F, Huber M. Histopathological particle algorithm. Particle identification in the synovium and the SLIM. Z Rheumatol. 2014; 73(7):639–49.
19. Krenn V, Morawietz L, Perino G, Kienapfel H, Ascherl R, Hassenpflug GJ, Thomsen M, Thomas P, Huber M, Kendoff D, Baumhoer D, Krukemeyer MG, Natu S, Boettner F, Zustin J, Kölbel B, Rüther W, Kretzer JP, Tiemann A, Trampuz A, Frommelt L, Tichilow R, Söder S, Müller S, Parvizi J, Illgner U, Gehrke T. Revised histopathological consensus classification of joint implant related pathology. Pathol Res Pract. 2014;210(12):779 86.
20. Krenn V, Perino G. Histological diagnosis of implant-associated pathologies. Germany: Springer-Verlag Berlin Heidelberg; 2017. ISBN 978-3
21. Hansen T, Otto M, Buchhorn GH, Schamweber D, Gaumann A, Delank KS, Eckardt A, Willert HG, Kriegsmann J, Kirkpatrick CJ. New aspects in the histological examination of polyethylene wear particles in failed total joint replacements. Acta Histochem. 2002;104:263–9. 662–54203-3
22. Fujishiro T, Moojen DJ, Kobayashi N, Dhert WJ, Bauer TW. Perivascular and diffuse lymphocytic inflammation are not specific for failed metal-on-metal hip implants. Clin Orthop Relat Res. 2011;469:1127–33.
23. Perino G, Ricciardi BF, Jerabek SA, Martignoni G, Wilner G, Maass D, Goldring SR, Purdue PE. Implant based differences in adverse local tissue reaction in failed total hip arthroplasties: a morphological and immunohistochemical study. BMC Clin Pathol. 2014;14(39) https://doi.org/10.1186/1472-6890-14-39.
24. Ricciardi BF, Nocon AA, Jerabek SA, Wilner G, Kaplowitz E, Goldring SR, Purdue PE, Perino G. Histopathological characterization of corrosion product associated adverse local tissue reaction in hip implants: a study of 285 cases. BMC Clin Pathol. 2016;16:3. https://doi.org/10.1186/s12907-016-0025-9.
25. Vaculova J, Gallo J, Hurnik P, Motyka O, Goodman S, Dvorackova J. Low intra-patient variability of histomorphological findings in periprosthetic tissues from revised joint arthroplasties. J Biomed Mater Res B Appl Biomater. 2017; https://doi.org/10.1002/jbm.b.33990.
26. Pascual E, Vega J. Synovial fluid analysis. Best Pract Res Cl Rh. 2005;19:371–86.
27. Caicedo MS, Samelko L, McAllister K, Jacobs JJ, Hallab NJ. Increasing both CoCrMo-alloy particle size and surface irregularity induces increased macrophage inflammasome activation in vitro potentially through lysosomal destabilization mechanisms. J Orthop Res. 2013;31:1633–42.
28. Tipper JL, Galvin A, Williams S, McEwen HMJ, Stone MH, Ingham E, Fisher J. Isolation and characterization of UHMWPE wear particles down to ten nanometers in size from in vitro hip and knee joint simulators. J Biomed Mater Res. 2006;3:473–80.
29. Fisher J, Bell J, Barbour PSM, Tipper JL, Matthews JB, Besong AA, Stone MH, Ingham E. A novel method for the prediction of functional biological activity of polyethylene wear debris. Proc Instn Mech Engrs. 2001;215:127–32.
30. Endo M, Tipper JL, Barton DC, Stone MH, Ingham E, Fisher J. Comparison of wear, wear debris, and functional biological activity of moderately crosslinked and non-crosslinked polyethylenes in hip prostheses. Proc Instn Mech Engrs. 2002;216:111–7.
31. Nine MJ, Choudhury D, Hee AC, Mootanah R, Osman NAA. Wear debris characterization and corresponding biological response: artificial hip and knee joints. Materials. 2014;7:980–1016.
32. Stratton-Powell AA, Tipper JL. Characterization of UHMWPE wear particles. In: UHMWPE Biomaterials Handbook. Ultra High Molecular Weight Polyethylene in Total Joint Replacement and Medical Devices. vol. 33. Amsterdam: Elsevier; 2015. p. 635–53.
33. Catelas I, Bobyn JD, Medley JB, Krygier JJ, Zukor DJ, Petit A, Huk OL. Effects of digestion protocols on the isolation of metal-metal wear particles. I. Analysis of particle size and shape. J Biomed Mater Res. 2001;55(3):320–9.
34. Sobieraj MC, Rimnac CM. Ultra-high molecular weight polyethylene: mechanics, morphology, and clinical behavior. J Mech Behav Biomed Mater. 2009;2:433–43.
35. Bracco P, Bellare A, Bistolfi A, Affatato S. Ultra-high molecular weight polyethylene: influence of the chemical, physical, and mechanical properties on the wear behavior. A review. Materials. 2017;10:1–22.
36. Kurtz SM, Gawel HA, Patel JD. History and systematic review of wear and Osteolysis outcomes for first-generation highly crosslinked polyethylene. Clin Orthop Relat Res. 2011;469:2262–77.
37. Schipper ON, Haddad SL, Pytel P, Zhou Y. Histological analysis of early osteolysis in total ankle arthroplasty. Foot Ankle Int. 2017;38:351–9.
38. Campbell P, Ma S, Yeom B, McKellop H, Schmalzried TP, Amstutz HC. Isolation of predominantly submicron-sized UHMWPE wear particles from periprosthetic tissues. J Biomed Mater Res. 1995;29:127–31.
39. Wolfarth DL, Han G, Bushar DW. Separation and characterization of polyethylene wear debris from synovial fluid and tissue samples of revised knee replacements. J Biomed Mater Res. 1997;34:57–61.
40. Schipper ON, Haddad SL, Fullam S, Pourzal R, Wimmer MA. Wear characteristics of conventional ultrahigh-molecular-weight polyethylene versus highly cross-linked polyethylene in total ankle arthroplasty. Foot Ankle Int. 2018;1:1071100718786501. https://doi.org/10.1177/1071100718786501
41. Muller J, Prozeller D, Ghazaryan A, Kokkinopoulou M, Volker M, Morsbach S,

Landfester K. Beyond the protein corona – lipids matter for biological response to nanocarriers. Acta Biomater. 2018;71:420–31.

42. Learmonth ID, Young C, Rorabeck C. The operation of the century: total hip replacement. Lancet. 2007;370:1508–19.

43. Xia Z, Ricciardi BF, Liu Z, von Ruhland C, Ward M, Lord A, Hughes L, Goldring SR, Purdue E, Murray D, Perino G. Nano-analyses of wear particles from metal-on-metal and non-metal-on-metal dual modular neck hip arthroplasty. Nanomedicine. 2017;13:1205–17.

44. Catelas I, Medley JB, Campbell PA, Huk OL, Boby DJ. Comparison of in vitro with in vivo characteristics of wear particles from metal-on-metal hip implants. J Biomed Mater Res Part B: Appl Biomater. 2004;70B:167–78.

45. Jacobs J, Gilbert JL, Urban RM. Corrosion of metal orthopaedic implants. J Bone Joint Surg Am. 1998;80:268–82.

46. Huber M, Reinisch G, Trettenhahn G, Zweymüller K, Lintner F. Presence of corrosion products and hypersensitivity-associated reactions in periprosthetic tissue after aseptic loosening of total hip replacements with metal bearing surfaces. Acta Biomater. 2009;5:172–80.

47. Langton DJ, Sidaginamale R, Lord JK, Nargol AV, Joyce TJ. Taper junction failure in large-diameter metal-on-metal bearings. Bone Joint Res. 2012;1: 56–63.

48. Meyer H, Mueller T, Goldau G, Chamaon K, Ruetschi M, Lohmann CH. Corrosion at the cone/taper Interface leads to failure of large-diameter metal-on-metal Total hip arthroplasties. Clin Orthop Relat Res. 2012;470: 3101–8.

49. Cooper HJ, Urban RM, Wixson RL, Meneghini RM, Jacobs JJ. Adverse local tissue reaction arising from corrosion at the femoral neck-body junction in a dual-taper stem with a cobalt-chromium modular neck. J Bone Joint Surg Am. 2013;95:865–72.

50. DeMartino I, Assini JB, Elpers ME, Wright TM, Westrich GH. Corrosion and fretting of a modular hip system: a retrieval analysis of 60 rejuvenate stems. J Arthroplast. 2015;30:1470–5. 36

51. Buente D, Huber G, Bishop N, Morlock M. Quantification of material loss from the neck piece taper junctions of a bimodular primary hip prosthesis. A retrieval study from 27 failed rejuvenate bimodular hip arthroplasties. Bone Joint J Br. 2015;97:1350–7.

52. Whitehouse MR, Endo M, Zachara S, Nielsen TO, Greidanus NV, Masri BA, Garbuz DS, Duncan CP. Adverse local tissue reactions in metal-on-polyethylene total hip arthroplasty due to trunnion corrosion. Bone Joint J Br. 2015;97:1024–30.

53. Pourzal R, Hall DJ, Ehrich J, McCarthy SM, Mathew MT, Jacobs JJ, Urban RM. Alloy microstructure dictates corrosion modes in THA modular junctions. Clin Orthop Relat Res. 2017;475(12):3026–43.

54. Catelas I, Wimmer MA. New insights into wear and biological effects of metal-on-metal bearings. J Bone Joint Surg Am. 2011;93(Suppl 2):76–83.

55. Arnholt C, Donald DW, Tohfafarosh M, Gilbert JL, Rimnac CL, Kurtz SM, the Implant Research Writing Committee, Klein G, Mont MA, Parvizi J, Cates HE, Lee GC, Malkani A, Kraay M. Mechanically assisted taper corrosion in modular TKA. J Arthroplast. 2014;29(9 Suppl):205–8.

56. Arnholt C, Donald DW, Malkani A, Klein G, Rimnac CL, Kurtz SM, the Implant Research Writing Committee, Kocagöz SB, Gilbert JL M. Corrosion damage and wear mechanisms in long-term retrieved CoCr femoral components for Total knee arthroplasty. J Arthroplast. 2016;31(12):2900–6.

57. Gilbert JL, Sivan S, Liu Y, Kocagöz SB, Arnholt CM, Kurtz SM. Direct in vivo inflammatory cell corrosion of CoCrMo alloy orthopedic implant surfaces. J Biomed Mater Res Part A. 2015;103A:211–23.

58. Bal SB, Garino J, Ries M, Rahaman MN. Ceramic materials in total joint arthroplasty. Semin Arthro. 2006;17:94–101.

59. Macdonald N, Bankes M. Ceramic on ceramic hip prostheses: a review of past and modern materials. Arch Orthop Trauma Surg. 2014;134:1325–35.

60. Hatton A, Nevelos JE, Nevelos AA, Banks RE, Fisher J, Ingham E. Alumina-alumina artificial hip joints. Part I: a histological analysis and characterisation of wear debris by laser capture microdissection of tissues retrieved at revision. Biomaterials. 2002;23:3429–40.

61. Esposito C, Maclean F, Campbell P, Walter WL, Walter WK, Bonar FS. Periprosthetic tissues from third generation alumina-on-alumina total hip arthroplasties. J Arthroplast. 2013;28:860–6.

62. Bohner M, Tadier S, van Garderen N, de Gasparo A, Döbelin N, Baroud G. Synthesis of spherical calcium phosphate particles for dental and orthopedic applications. Biomatter. 2013;3(2):e25103. https://doi.org/10.4161/biom.25103

63. Lorenzo V, Torres A, Salido E. Primary hyperoxaluria. Nefrologia. 2014;34(3): 398–412.

64. Pereira BPG, Chang EY, Resnick DL, Pathria MN. Intramuscular migration of calcium hydroxyapatite crystal deposits involving the rotator cuff tendons of the shoulder: report of 11 patients. Skelet Radiol. 2016;45:97–103.

65. Piccin A, Rizkalla H, Smith O, McMahon C, Furlan C, Murphy C, Negri G, Mc Dermott M. Composition and significance of splenic Gamna-Gandy bodies in sickle cell anemia. Human Pathol. 2012;43:1028–36.

66. Pizzolato P. Formalin pigment (acid hematin) and related pigments. Am J Med Technol. 1976;42(11):436–40.

67. Jadeja H, Yeoh D, Lal M, Mowbray M. Patterns of failure with time of an artificial scaffold class ligament used for reconstruction of the human anterior cruciate ligament. Knee. 2007;14:439–42.

68. Mortier J, Engelhardt M. Foreign body reaction in carbon fiber prosthesis implantation in the knee joint - case report and review of the literature. Z Orthop Ihre Grenzgeb. 2000;138(5):390–4.

69. Pugliese D, Bush D, Harrington T. Silicone synovitis. Longer term outcome data and review of the literature. J Clin Rheumatol. 2009;15:8–11.

70. Giuffrida AY, Gyuricza C, Perino G, Weiland AJ. Foreign body reaction to Artelon spacer: case report. J Hand Surg Am. 2009;34(8):1388–92.

71. Chen AL, Desai P, Adler EM, Di Cesare PE. Granulomatous inflammation after Hylan G-F 20 viscosupplementation of the knee: a report of six cases. J Bone Joint Surg Am. 2002;84-A:1142–7.

72. Bauer TW. An overview of the histology of skeletal substitute materials. Arch Pathol Lab Med. 2007;131:217–24.

73. James RA, Singh-Grewal D, Lee SJ, McGill J, Adib N. Lysosomal storage disorders: a review of the musculoskeletal features. J Paediatr Child Health. 2016;52:262–71.

74. Campochiaro C, Tomelleri A, Cavalli G, Berti A, Dagna L. Erdheim-Chester disease. Eur J Intern Med. 2015;26:223–9.

75. Di Laura A, Quinn PD, Panagiotopoulou VC, Hothi HS, Henckel J, Powell JJ, Berisha F, Amary F, Mosselmans JFW, Skinner JA, Hart AJ. The chemical form of metal species released from corroded taper junctions of hip implants: synchrotron analysis of patient tissue. Sci Rep. 2017;7:10952. https://doi.org/10.1038/s41598-017-11225-w.

76. Schoon J, Geißler S, Traeger J, Luch A, Tentschert J, Perino G, Schulze F, Duda GN, Perka C, Rakow A. Multi-elemental nanoparticle exposure after tantalum component failure in hip arthroplasty: in-depth analysis of a single case. Nanomedicine. 2017;13:2415–23.

77. Stachowiak GW, Pdsiadlo P. Characterization of wear particles and surfaces. Wear. 2001;249:194–200.

78. Willert HG, Buchhorn GH, Fayyazi A, Flury R, Windler M, Köster G, Lohmann CH. Metal-on-metal bearings and hypersensitivity in patients with artificial hip joints. J Bone Joint Surg Am. 2005;87(1):28–36.

79. Xia Z, Kwon YM, Mehmood S, Downing C, Jurkschat K, Murray DW. Characterization of metal-wear nanoparticles in pseudotumor following metal-on-metal hip resurfacing. Nanomedicine. 2011;7:674–81.

80. Hopf F, Thomas P, Sesselmann S, Thomsen MN, Hopf M, Hopf J, Krukemeyer MG, Resch H, Krenn V. CD3+ lymphocytosis in the peri-implant membrane of 222 loosened joint endoprostheses depends on the tribological pairing. Acta Orthop. 2017;88(6):642–8.

81. Doorn PF, Mirra JM, Campbell PA, Amstuz HC. Tissue reaction to metal on metal total hip prostheses. Clin Orthop Rel Res. 1996;329(Suppl):187–205.

82. Scheuer PJ, Lefkowich JH. Disturbances of copper and iron metabolism. In: Liver Biopsy Interpretation. Philadelphia: WB Saunders; 2000. p. 270e83.

83. Stratton-Powell AA, Pasko KM, Brockett CL, Tipper JL. The biologic response to Polyetheretherketone (PEEK) wear particles in total joint replacement: a systematic review. Clin Orthop Relat Res. 2016;474:2394–404.

84. Torosyan Y, Bowsher JG, Kurtz SM, Mihalko WM, Marinac-Dabic D. Opportunities and challenges in retrieval analysis: the role of standardized periprosthetic tissue and fluid analysis for assessing an aggravated host response. In: Mihalko WM, Lemons JE, Greenwald AS, Kurtz SM, editors. Beyond the implant: retrieval analysis methods for implant surveillance, ASTM STP1606. West Conshohocken: ASTM International; 2018. p. 215–28.

85. Dumbleton JH, Manley MT, Edidin AA. A literature review of the association between wear rate and osteolysis in total hip arthroplasty. J Arthroplast. 2002;17:649–61.

86. Harris WH. "The lysis threshold": an erroneous and perhaps misleading concept? J Arthroplast. 2003;18:506–10.

29

Cerebrospinal fluid pleocytosis level as a diagnostic predictor? A cross-sectional study

Anne Ahrens Østergaard[1], Thomas Vognbjerg Sydenham[2], Mads Nybo[3,4] and Åse Bengård Andersen[1,4,5]* (iD)

Abstract

Background: Lumbar puncture with quantification of leukocytes and differential count of cellular subsets in the cerebrospinal fluid is a standard procedure in cases of suspected neuroinfectious conditions. However, a number of non-infectious causes may result in a low leukocyte number (0–1000 cells/ml). We wanted to assess the diagnostic diversity of unselected adult patients with pleocytosis in the cerebrospinal fluid.

Methods: The study is based on data from cerebrospinal fluid (CSF) analyses of all adult patients (15 years or older) admitted to a large university hospital in Denmark during a two-year period (2008–2009). Data from the local patient administrative system supplied with data from patient charts were combined with laboratory data.

Results: A total of 5390 cerebrospinal fluid samples from 3290 patients were included. Pleocytosis >5 leucocytes/µl was found in samples from 262 patients of which 106 (40.5%) were caused by infection of the central nervous system (CNS), 20 (7.6%) by infection outside CNS, 79 (30.2%) due to non-infectious neurological diseases, 23 (8.8%) by malignancy, and 34 (13.0%) caused by other conditions. Significantly higher mean CSF leukocytes was found in patients suffering from CNS infection (mean 1135 cells/µl, *p*-value <0.0001).

Conclusions: CNS infection, non-infectious neurological disease, malignancy, and infection outside CNS can cause pleocytosis of the cerebrospinal fluid. Leukocyte counts above 100/µl is mainly caused by CNS infection, whereas the number of differential diagnoses is higher if the CSF leukocyte counts is below 50/µl. These conditions are most commonly caused by non-infectious neurological diseases including seizures.

Keywords: Cerebrospinal fluid, CSF, Pleocytosis, Lumbar puncture, Central nervous system infection, CNS infection, Seizures

Background

Migration of leukocytes to the cerebrospinal fluid (CSF) is a cardinal symptom of an infectious condition affecting the meninges or the cerebral parenchyma. Bacterial and viral meningitis cannot reliably be differentiated clinically and requires lumbar puncture to analyse the CSF [1, 2]. Patients suffering from viral meningitis present CSF leukocyte concentrations varying from 10 to 1000/µl, but typically below 500 [3]. In bacterial meningitis CSF leukocytes vary from below 100 to more than 10,000 leukocytes/µl, often between 1000 and 5000/µl [4]. However, pleocytosis in the CSF may also occur in other medical conditions, e.g. neurological, rheumatic or malignant disease [5, 6]. Some patients with pleocytosis in the CSF never obtain a final diagnosis and in many settings the proportion of patients with "suspected CNS infection" is larger than that of patients with proven aetiology [1].

Apart from the issue of a large overlap in leukocyte concentrations caused by viral and bacterial infections, the relative distributions of the non-infectious diagnoses are not well described. One reason for this is the fact that these patients are dealt with by different clinical specialities.

Methods

This study aimed at obtaining an overview of the relative contribution of the causes of cerebrospinal pleocytosis

* Correspondence: Aase.Bengaard.Andersen@regionh.dk
[1]Department of Infectious Diseases, Odense University Hospital, Odense, Denmark
[4]University of Southern Denmark, Odense, Denmark
Full list of author information is available at the end of the article

by a comprehensive method including all adult patients (regardless indication for lumbar puncture, requesting department, and symptomatology of the patient) admitted to a large university hospital in Denmark during a two-year period.

Pleocytosis is defined as increased cell count. In the following the term pleocytosis will be used to describe >5 leucocytes/µl in CSF. The study was performed at Odense University Hospital, a large regional hospital in Denmark with 1038 beds serving as referral hospital for 1.8 million inhabitants and holding all medical specialities including neurology, neurosurgery, rheumatology, oncology and haematology.

Data from CSF analyses performed at the Department of Clinical Biochemistry and Pharmacology from January 1st 2008 to December 31th 2009 (sample date, CSF leukocytes, CSF monocytes, CSF polymorphonuclear leukocytes, CSF protein, CSF glucose and plasma glucose) and data from the patient administration system of Funen County (FPAS; Fyns Patient Administrative System) (patient age, sex, hospital admission dates, discharge dates and discharge diagnoses) from 1994 to 2012 was retrieved. In addition, we obtained data from the electronic patient records on hospital admissions and CSF sample reports.

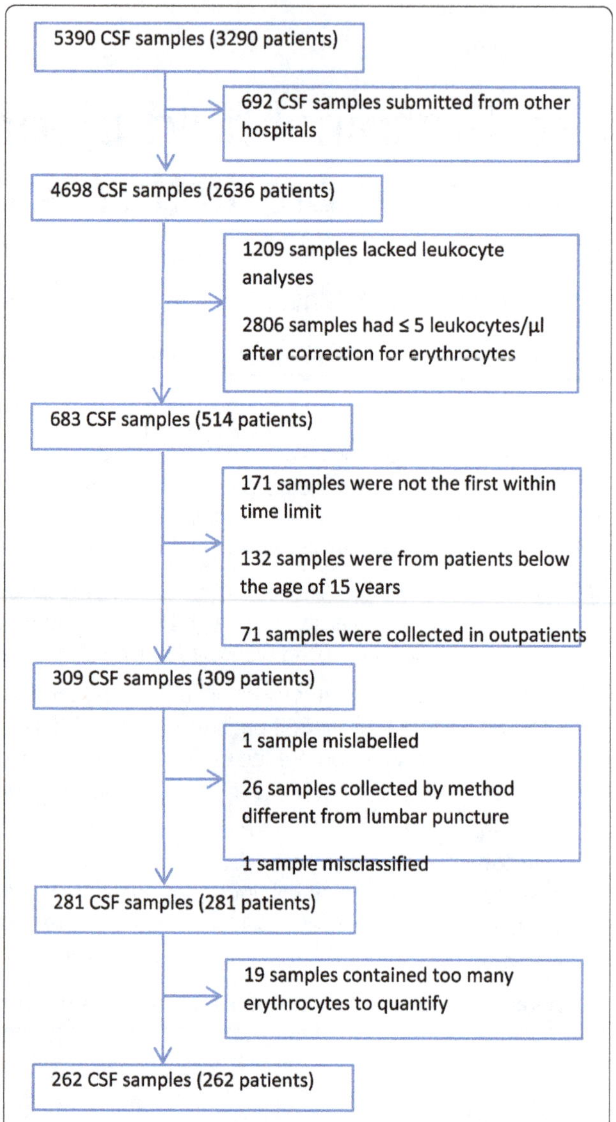

Only the initial CSF analysis requested with pleocytosis (>5 leukocytes/µl after correction for erythrocytes (1 leucocyte/1000 erythrocytes)) in hospitalized patients at age of 15 years or older were included. Exclusion criteria were: not the first CSF sample in the time period, wrong social security number, if the sample was not cerebrospinal fluid, if the erythrocytes were in layers or too numerous to quantify, if a sample was collected by a method different from lumbar puncture, or if the patient was transferred to another hospital with an uncertain diagnosis. If a sample was analysed more than once, the report given to the clinician was used (Fig. 1). Discharge diagnoses (ICD-10) were used to categorise the cause of pleocytosis. However, the cause of pleocytosis was adjusted in the following circumstances: 1) Discharge diagnosis was not verified para-clinically (magnetic resonance imaging (MRI)/computed tomography (CT), microbiological analyses, flow-cytometry, or autopsy) and the discharge summary mentioned a diagnosis in plain text not coded as a discharge diagnosis; the cause of pleocytosis was changed to this diagnosis. 2) a CNS infection was mentioned in the discharge summary but not included as a discharge diagnosis; Cause of pleocytosis was changed to *CNS infection*. 3) a discharge diagnosis was not verified nor was CNS infection but a secondary diagnosis was verified; the cause of pleocytosis was changed to this diagnosis. 4) Discharge diagnosis was "Observation for other suspected diseases and conditions" or "Observation for suspected nervous system

Fig. 1 Flowchart of study inclusion

disorder" and the suspected disorder was CNS infection; the cause of pleocytosis was changed to *CNS infection*, 5) the patient received full treatment for a CNS infection but this was not included in discharge summary; the cause of pleocytosis was changed to *CNS infection*. 6) the discharge diagnosis did not coincide with the patient chart or discharge summary; the cause of pleocytosis was changed to the cause mentioned in the chart. 7) a clear diagnosis was not made at time of discharge but was verified within 3 months after discharge date; this diagnosis was used as cause of pleocytosis.

The category *CNS infection* was further divided into 2 groups: *verified* and *probable*. A discharge diagnosis was considered *verified* if the diagnosis was verified by MRI, CT, microbiological analyses, or autopsy.

Charlson index score [7] was used to describe patients comorbidity. Charlson score estimating risk of death from comorbid disease in longitudinal studies by scoring each comorbid disease a score of 1, 2, 3, or 6.22 comorbidity conditions are included. Calculation was based on registered diagnoses in the patient administration system from years 1994 to 2009.

Statistical analysis

Data processing was performed in STATA version 13.1–14.0. Wilcoxon/Mann-Whitney (Mann-Whitney U/ Wilcoxon rank sum) test was performed for data not normally distributed (sex, Charlson score, CSF leukocytes, CSF protein, CSF monocyte proportion, and CSF polymorph nuclear leukocyte proportion). Student's t-test was used if data was normally distributed (age). All p-values were comparisons between the marked category and the other categories. Only significant p-values (≤ 0.05) were included.

Results

Out of 5390 unselected cerebrospinal fluid samples, 262 met the inclusion criteria (Fig. 1). The neurological department (56.5%), department of emergency admission

(14.9%), and the department of intensive care (7.3%) were the main contributors to CSF analyses.

Patients were divided into diagnosis categories of *CNS infection, Infection outside CNS, Non-infectious neurological diseases, Malignancy, Other*, and subgroups (Appendix A). *CNS infection* amounted to 40.5% of the causes of pleocytosis. *Infection outside CNS* to 7.6%, *Non-infectious neurological diseases* to 30.2%, *Malignancy* 8.8%, and *Other* 13.0%.

There was no significant difference in distribution of sex in any of the categories (Table 1). Significantly lower mean age was found in the *Non-infectious neurological diseases* category (mean age 46.1, p-value 0.0088). Mean Charlson score in the 262 patients was 0.9, range 0–11. Mean Charlson score was significantly lower in the *Non-infectious neurological diseases* category (mean 0.6, p-value 0.0125), while it was significantly higher in the *Malignancy* (mean 2.7, p-value <0.001) than in all other categories. In general, there was a tendency of high mean Charlson score in the categories with high mean age.

In 141 patients mean CSF/plasma glucose ratio was 0.6 (normal). Significantly lower CSF/plasma glucose ratio was found in the decreased interval (<0.46) for *CNS infection* (mean 0.2, p 0.0085). Significant higher

Table 1 Summery of baseline findings by diagnosis category

	Diagnosis category					
	CNS infection ($n = 106$)	Infection outside CNS ($n = 20$)	Non-infectious neurological diseases ($n = 79$)	Malignancy, all foci ($n = 23$)	Other ($n = 34$)	Total ($n = 262$)
Sex[a]	n (%)	n (%)	n (%)	n (%)	n (%)	n (%)
Male	49 (46.2)	11 (55.0)	43 (54.4)	14 (60.9)	16 (47.1)	133 (50.8)
Female	57 (53.8)	9 (45.0)	36 (45.6)	9 (39.1)	18 (52.9)	129 (49.2)
Age[b]	n (%)	n (%)	n (%)	n (%)	n (%)	n (%)
< 36 yrs	26 (24.5)	5 (25.0)	24 (30.6)	2 (8.7)	7 (20.6)	64 (24.4)
36-51 yrs	31 (29.3)		27 (34.2)	6 (26.1)*	7 (20.6)	71 (27.1)
52-64 yrs	20 (18.9)	4 (20.0)	14 (17.7)	9 (39.1)	13 (38.2)	60 (22.9)
≥ 65 yrs	29 (27.4)	11 (55.0)	14 (17.7)	6 (26.1)	7 (20.6)	67 (25.6)
Mean	50.4	58.5	46.1*	59.1	52.0	50.7
Range	15-88	17-91	20-89	28-81	17-95	15-95
Charlson score[a]	n (%)	n (%)	n (%)	n (%)	n (%)	n (%)
0	66 (62.3)	9 (45.0)	52 (65.8)	1 (4.4)	19 (55.9)	147 (56.1)
1	25 (23.6)	3 (15.0)	18 (22.8)	1 (4.4)	9 (26.5)	56 (21.4)
2	7 (6.6)	5 (25.0)	5 (6.3)	14 (60.9)	6 (17.7)	37 (14.1)
3	2 (1.9)	2 (10.0)	2 (2.5)	3 (13.0)		9 (3.4)
≥4	6 (5.7)	1 (5.0)	2 (2.5)	4 (17.4)		13 (5.0)
Mean	0.7	1.2	0.6	2.7**	0.6	0.9
Range	0-6	0-4	0-7	0-11	0-2	0-11

[a]Wilcoxon-Mann-Whitney test
[b]p-values calculated by Student's t-test
*p-value <0.01
**p-value <0.001

CSF/plasma glucose ratio was found in the decreased interval (<0.46) for *Non-infectious neurological diseases* (mean 0.4, *p* 0.0276).

The mean concentration of CSF leukocytes was 494/µl (Table 2). Significantly higher concentrations of mean CSF leukocytes were found in patients with *CNS infection* (mean 1135, *p*-value <0.001). In the category *CNS infection* no distinction between viral and bacterial neuroinfection was made. When only verified diagnoses were included, a higher concentration of CSF leukocytes were found in the category *Meningitis, acute bacterial* (*p*-value = 0.0002) (Table 5) compared to the others in *CNS infection*.

The proportion of patients in the *CNS infection* category increased with increasing CSF leukocyte concentration, and at leukocyte counts above 100/µl *CNS infection* was the most frequent cause of pleocytosis (Fig. 2). Eighty seven point three percent of the patients with more than 200 leukocytes were diagnosed with *CNS infection*.

In CSF samples with leukocytes below 50/µl especially non-infectious neurological diagnoses should be considered as differential diagnoses, since the proportion of *CNS infection* increased with increasing CSF leukocytes (Fig. 3). The category of *Other* seemed to occur mainly in patients with CSF leukocytes below 100/µl. *Infection outside CNS* occurred primarily when CSF leukocytes were below 50/µl. *CNS infection* was the only category present in all intervals.

The mean CSF protein concentration in all patients was 1.0 g/l (Table 2). CSF protein was normal (0.2–0.4 g/l) or decreased in 32.4% of all patients. All patients with *CNS infection* had a significantly higher level of protein in CSF (mean 1.4) (*p*-value <0.0001). CNS protein is known to be increased in meningitis, but also to be one of the least specific parameters in CSF [4].

Of the 106 patients with *CNS infection* 59 (55.7%) were paraclinically confirmed. For the categories of *malignancy* 20 (87.0%), *other* 15 (44.1%), *non-infectious neurologically disease* 37 (46.8%), and *other infection* 10 (50.0%) were paraclinically confirmed. Table 3 shows that more diagnoses in the CNS infection category were paraclinically verified as cell count increases. Mean protein level was higher in the verified CNS infections than in probable CNS infection. CSF/plasma glucose ratios shows a tendency of being lower in total in the verified category and are in both groups the lowest when cell count is high.

For six patients, seizures, epilepsy or status epilepticus was the cause of pleocytosis. Two patients had <10

Table 2 Summary of CSF findings by diagnosis category

| | Diagnosis category | | | | | | | | | | | |
| | CNS infection (n = 106) | | Infection outside CNS (n = 20) | | Non-infectious neurological diseases (n = 79) | | Malignancy, all foci (n = 23) | | Other (n = 34) | | Total (n = 262) | |
CSF leukocytes/µl[a]	n (%)	[mean]	n (%)	[mean]	n (%)	[mean]	n (%)	[mean]	n (%)	[mean]	n (%)	[mean]
6–10	11 (10.4)	8.1	10 (50.0)	7.3	32 (40.5)	7.3	8 (34.8)	7.4	14 (41.2)	7.2	75 (28.6)	7.4
>10–50	23 (21.7)	29.3	9 (45.0)	22.9	34 (43.0)	20.2	11 (47.8)	21.9	14 (41.2)	20.1	91 (34.7)	23.0
>50–100	8 (7.6)	84.0			3 (3.8)	66	2 (8.7)	62.5	5 (14.7)	69.8	18 (6.9)	74.7
>100–200	17 (16.0)	135.0			6 (7.6)	138			1 (2.9)	159	24 (9.2)	136.8
>200–400	13 (12.3)	266.4	1 (5.0)	221	2 (2.5)	247.5	1 (4.4)	347			17 (6.5)	266.2
>400–600	12 (11.3)	524.6			1 (1.3)	537					13 (5.0)	525.5
>600–800	2 (1.9)	744									2 (0.8)	744
>800–1000	3 (2.8)	896									3 (1.2)	896
>1000	17 (16.0)	6041.2			1 (1.3)	2015	1 (4.4)	1980			19 (7.3)	5615.5
Total	106 (100.0)	1135.5**	20 (100.0)	25.0*	79 (100.0)	63.2**	23 (100.0)	119.7	34 (100.0)	26.2*	262 (100.0)	494.3
CSF protein g/l[a]	n (%)	[mean]	n (%)	[mean]	n (%)	[mean]	n (%)	[mean]	n (%)	[mean]	n (%)	[mean]
<0.2					1 (1.3)	0.0			1 (2.9)	0.0	2 (0.8)	0.0
0.2–0.4	18 (17.0)	0.4	12 (60.0)	0.3	34 (43.0)	0.3	8 (34.8)	0.3	11 (32.4)	0.4	83 (31.7)	0.3
0.41–1.11	50 (47.2)	0.7	8 (40.0)	0.8	36 (45.6)	0.7	10 (43.5)	0.6	18 (52.9)	0.6	122 (46.6)	0.7
>1.11	38 (35.9)	2.8			8 (10.1)	2.5	5 (21.7)	2.9	4 (11.8)	2.6	55 (21.0)	2.8
Total	106 (100.0)	1.4**	20 (100.0)	0.5	79 (100.0)	0.7**	23 (100.0)	1.0	34 (100.0)	0.7	262 (100.0)	1.0

[a]Wilcoxon-Mann-Whitney test
[b]*p*-values by Student's t-test
p-value <0.01
**p*-value <0.001

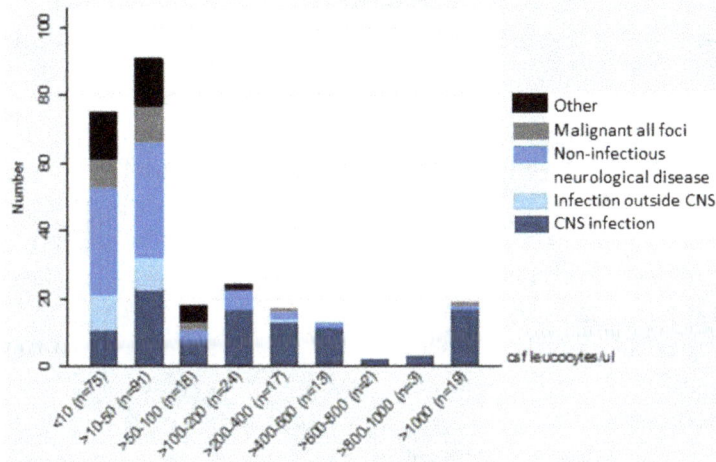

Fig. 2 Distribution of diagnose category per cell count. CNS infection is the only category present in all intervals. The category of Other occurs mainly in patients with CSF leukocytes below 100/µl. Infection outside CNS occurs primarily when CSF leukocytes were below 50/µl

leukocytes/µl and four patiens had 10–50 leukocytes/µl (Table 4). Pleocytosis has previosly been found in patientes after seizures [8]. Higher concentrations of CSF leukocytes were found in *Other neurological diseases*. One patient, who suffered from obstructive hydrocephalus, had >1000 leukocytes/µl in CSF (categorised as *Other neurological diseases*) but did not suffer from neuroinfection. No distinction between viral and bacterial meningitis was made. No patients had tuberculosis or fungal CNS infection as shown in the Appendix.

Discussion

The discharge diagnoses were retrospectively adjusted for 36 (13.7%) patients following discharge summary and patient chart review. We found it important to manually review the charts as also suggested by others in retrospective studies to secure that all relevant diagnoses were included [9, 10].

A wide span of diagnoses were included in the *Others* category including neurosarcoidosis and rheumatic diseases, which are known causes of pleocytosis [6, 11–13]. In the category *Other*, the mean CSF leukocyte concentration was 26/µl (SD 32.6). The patients in this category did not differ from the other patients in age, sex, or Charlson score. It could be speculated that some of these patients suffered from a benign viral infection either not detected by available diagnostic setups or not tested for.

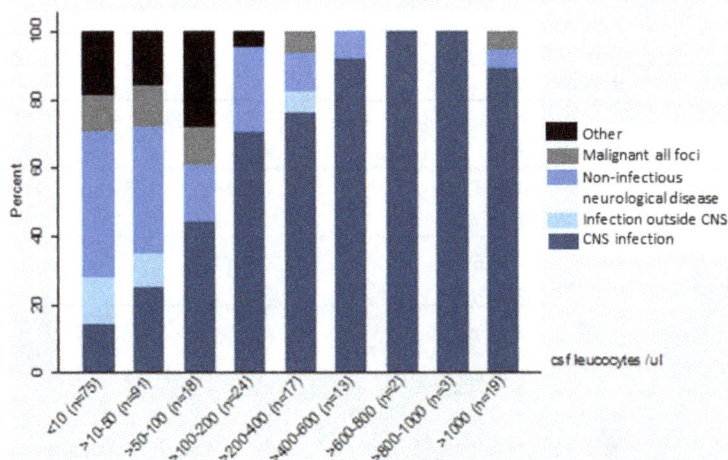

Fig. 3 Distribution of diagnose category as a percentage per cell count. The proportion of patients in the *CNS infection* category increased with increasing CSF leukocyte concentration, and at leukocyte counts above 100/µl *CNS infection* was the most frequent cause of pleocytosis

Table 3 CSF leukocyte count, mean protein and mean CSF/plasma glucose ratio in verified and probable CNS infection

CSF leukocytes /μl a	CNS infection, Verified			CNS infection, Probable			Total		
	n (% horizontal)	Protein g/l Mean (range)	Glucose ratio mean (range)	n (% horizontal)	Protein g/l mean (range)	Glucose ratio mean (range)	n (% vertical)	Protein g/l mean (range)	Glucose ratio mean (range)
6–10	4 (36.4)	0.6 (0.4–0.9)	-	7 (63.6)	0.7 (0.4–0.9)	0.7 (0.5–0.9)	11 (10.4)	0,6 (0.4–0.9)	0.7 (0.5–0.9)
>10–50	9 (39.1)	0.9 (0.3–2.2)	0,5 (0.4–0.7)	14 (60.9)	0.6 (0.3–2.2)	0.6 (0.3–1.0)	23 (21.7)	0.7 (0.2–2.2)	0.6 (0.3–1.0)
>50–100	5 (62.5)	1.0 (0.2–1.6)	0.6 (0.5–0.7)	3 (37.5)	0.6 (0.4–0.7)	0.4 (0.4–0.5)	8 (7.6)	0,8 (0.2–1.6)	0.5 (0.4–0.7)
>100–200	7 (41.2)	0.8 (0.3–1.3)	0.7 (0.5–0.7)	10 (58.8)	0.8 (0.4–1.7)	0.6 (0.6–0.8)	17 (16.0)	0.8 (0.3–1.7)	0.7 (0.6–1.0)
>200–400	8 (61.5)	1.3 (0.4–2.4)	0.5 (0.4–0.6)	5 (38.5)	0.9 (0.5–1.9)	0.6 (0.5–0.8)	13 (12.3)	1.1 (0.4–2.4)	0.6 (0.4–0.8)
>400–600	8 (66.7)	2.3 (0.7–6.8)	0.4 (0.0–0.6)	4 (33.3)	1.3 (0.6–2.8)	0.6 (0.4–0.9)	12 (11.3)	2.0 (0.6–6.8)	0.5 (0.0–0.9)
>600–800	2 (100.0)	1.4 (0.8–2)	0.5 (0.3–0.6)				2 (1.9)	1.4 (0.8–2.0)	0.5 (0.3–0.6)
>800–1000	2 (66.7)	1.2 (1.2–1.2)	0.7 (0.7–0.7)	1 (33.3)	1.4	0.4	3 (2.8)	1.3 (1.2–1.4)	0.5 (0.4–0.7)
>1000	14 (82.4)	4 (0.8–6.8)	0.1 (0.1–0.1)	3 (17.6)	4.4 (1.5–9.0)	0.2 (0.1–0.1)	17 (16.0)	3.6 (0.8–6.8)	0.2 (0.0–0.4)
Total	59 (55.7)	1.8 (0.2–6.8)	0.4 (0.0–1.0)	47 (44.3)	1.0 (0.2–9.0)	0.6 (0.1–1.0)	106 (100.0)	1.4 (0.2–9)	0.5 (0.0–1.0)

- missing data: CSV/plasma glucose ratio only available in 59 of 106 patients

In the *Non-infectious neurological diseases* category five patients suffered from *Migraine* or *Headache* and three patients from *Paralysis/paresis of facial nerve*. These eight patients could have suffered from a mild viral CNS infection or Lyme's disease, since viral CNS infection can present with similar symptoms [14, 15]. However, variation from the normal levels cannot be ruled out.

Three patients in the *Malignancy* category suffered from lung or oropharyngeal cancer. Previously, it has been found that patients can develop chemical meningitis (sterile and inflammatory) due to concurrent systemic and local chemotherapy [16]. This could explain pleocytosis in these patients. One patient in the *Malignancy* category was found with 1980 cells in CSF and suffered from agranulocytosis secondary to cancer chemotherapy but was not found to suffer from a CNS infection though the high cell count would suggest otherwise. Neither was the patient found to suffer from infection else where and was therefore categorized as *Malignancy*.

This explains the high mean cell count in the subgroup *Cancer, foci elsewhere* (Table 5).

Limitations
The study was performed retrospectively, which means that no actions of the treating staff or patients could influence the results. A limitation of the study is the fact that data only was available from registers and patient charts, which might have led to incorrect categorization of some of the patients. However, all patients charts have been reviewed and categorized as part of this study as described in the methods section. Not all diagnoses were paraclinically confirmed. This could be due to administration of antimicrobial therapy prior to lumbar puncture or due to insufficient sensitivity of the available methods.

Conclusions
This study correlates CSF findings to final diagnosis. CNS infection, non-infectious neurological disease,

Table 4 CSF leukocyte count in non-infectious neurological diseases subgroups

Non-infectious neurological diseases subgroup	CSF leukocytes/μl							
	≤10	>10–50	>50–100	>100–200	>200–400	>400–600	>600	Total
	n (%)	n (%)	n (%)	n (%)	n (%)	n (%)	n (%)	n (%)
Encephalitis/myelitis, non-infectious		8 (66.7)		2 (16.7)	1 (8.3)	1 (8.3)		12 (100.0)
Seizures/epilepsy/status epilepticus	2 (33.3)	4 (66.7)						6 (100.0)
Ischemia/infarction/stroke	4 (36.3)	4 (36.6)	1 (9.1)	2 (18.2)				11 (100.0)
Intracranial haemorrhage		1 (50.0)		1 (50.0)				2 (100.0)
Multiple sclerosis	8 (53.3)	7 (46.7)						15 (100.0)
Demyelinating disease/polyneuropathy	2 (40.0)	3 (60.0)						5 (100.0)
Paralysis/palsy of cranial nerve	2 (66.7)		1 (33.3)					3 (100.0)
Headache/migraine	3 (60.0)	2 (40.0)						5 (100.0)
Other neurological	11 (55.0)	5 (25.0)	1 (5.0)	1 (5.0)	1 (5.0)		1 (5.0)	20 (100.0)
Total	32 (40.5)	34 (43.0)	3 (3.8)	6 (7.6)	2 (2.5)	1 (1.3)	1 (1.3)	79 (100.0)

malignancy, and infection outside CNS can cause pleocytosis of the cerebrospinal fluid. Leukocyte counts above 100/µl are mainly caused by CNS infection, whereas the number of differential diagnoses is higher when CSF leukocytes levels are below 50/µl. These conditions are most commonly caused by non-infectious neurological diseases including seizures.

Appendix

Table 5 Summary of subgroups in the diagnosis categories

	Number	Percent	Mean CSF leukocytes/µl
CNS infection	106	40.5	1135.5
Meningitis. viral/unknown agent	38	35.9	617.0
Meningitis. acute bacterial	21	19.8	3591.3
Meningitis. borrelia/syphilis	25	23.6	150.6
Encephalitis. infectious	11	10.4	295.3
CNS abscess	3	2.8	4654.3
Other CNS infection (Including: Herpes zoster with other complication in CNS, Hydrocephalus caused by infectious or parasitic disease classified elsewhere, Meningoencephalitis due to toxoplasmosis, Polyneuropathy caused by infectious or parasitic disease classified elsewhere, Viral infection of CNS unspecified)	8	7.6	66.0
Infection outside CNS	20	7.6	25.0
Endocarditis	2	9.5	113.5
Sepsis	10	47.6	18.8
Other infection with foci outside CNS (including: Acute pharyngitis, Acute sinusitis, Analabsces, Other pneumonia due to other unspecified microorganism, Oral candidiasis, HIV with other infectious and parasitic disease, Erysiphelas, unspecified, Viralinfection, unspecified, Pilonidal cyst with abscess)	8	40.0	10.6
Non-infectious neurological diseases	79	30.2	63.2
Encephalitis/myelitis. Non-infectious	12	15.2	108.3
Seizures/epilepsy/status epilepticus	6	7.6	15.8
Ischemia/infarction/stroke	11	13.9	38.9
Intracranial haemorrhage	2	2.5	85.0
Multiple sclerosis	15	19.0	15.0
Demyelinating disease/ polyneuropathy	5	6.3	10.8
Paralysis/palsy of cranial nerve	3	3.8	29.7
Headache/migraine	5	6.3	10.2
Other neurological	20	25.3	129.1

Table 5 Summary of subgroups in the diagnosis categories *(Continued)*

(including: Acute transverse myelitis in demyelinating disease of central nervous system, Other extrapyramidal and movement disorders, Ventriculitis of the brain, unspecified, Sequelae of inflammatory diseases of central nervous system), Obstructive hydrocephalus, Spinal stenosis, Herniation of lumbar disc with radiculopathy, Disorder of central nervous system, unspecified, Symptom of central nervous system unspecified)			
Malignancy. all foci	23	8.8	119.7
Lymphoma	9	39.13	20.7
Leukaemia	3	13.04	16.3
CNS cancer	5	21.74	30.6
Cancer. foci elsewhere (Including: Malignant neoplasm of unspecified part of unspecified bronchus or lung, Malignant neoplasm of oropharynx, unspecified, Agranulocytosis secondary to cancer chemotherapy)	4	17.39	500.5
Carcinomatosis	2	8.7	181.0
Other	34	13.0	26.2
Sarcoidosis	4	11.4	54.5
Rheumatologic	2	5.7	89.0
Cardiologic. non-infectious	2	5.7	8.0
Observation for suspected/other or not specified findings	8	22.9	25.9
Others (Including: Acute respiratory failure, Fever, unspecified, Hypokalemia, Complications following infusion, transfusion and therapeutic injection, Care involving use of rehabilitation procedure, unspecified, Unspecified multiple injuries, Hypopituitarism, Benign paroxysmal vertigo)	18	52.9	15.1

Appendix

Abbreviations
CNS: Central nervous system; CSF: Cerebrospinal fluid; CT: Computed tomography; MRI: Magnetic resonance imaging; PCR: Polymerace chain reaction

Acknowledgements
We thank Michael Due Larsen, Center for Clinical Epidemiology, Odense University Hospital, for assisting the Charlson score calculations and Michala Kehrer, Department of Infectious Diseases, Odense University Hospital, for help with STATA calculations.

Funding
University of Southern Denmark Research Foundation (Syddansk Universitets Forskningsfond) sponsored the study.

Authors' contributions

ÅBA contributed with study design, interpretation, and supervised the study. TVS contributed with study design, acquisition, and analysis of the data. MN contributed with acquisition of data. AAØ contributed with conception, acquisition and analysis of data. All authors participated in preparing the manuscript. All authors read and approved the final manuscript.

Competing interests

The authors declare that they have no competing interests.

Author details

[1]Department of Infectious Diseases, Odense University Hospital, Odense, Denmark. [2]Department of Clinical Microbiology, Odense University Hospital, Odense, Denmark. [3]Department of Clinical Biochemistry and Pharmacology, Odense University Hospital, Odense, Denmark. [4]University of Southern Denmark, Odense, Denmark. [5]Department of Infectious Diseases 8632, Copenhagen University Hospital Rigshospitalet, Blegdamsvej 9, DK 2100 Copenhagen OE, Denmark.

References

1. Michael BD, Sidhu M, Stoeter D, Roberts M, Beeching NJ, Bonington A, Hart IJ, Kneen R, Miller A, Solomon T. Acute central nervous system infections in adults–a retrospective cohort study in the NHS north west region. QJM. 2010;103(10):749–58.
2. Logan SA, MacMahon E. Viral meningitis. BMJ (Clinical research ed). 2008; 336(7634):36–40.
3. Chadwick DR. Viral meningitis. Br Med Bull. 2005;75-76:1–14.
4. Mandell LG, Bennett EJ, Raphael D: Principles and practice of infectious diseases. , vol. 1, 7 Philidelphia: Elsevier; 2010.
5. Kumar R. Aseptic meningitis: diagnosis and management. Indian J Pediatr. 2005;72(1):57–63.
6. Zunt JR, Baldwin KJ. Chronic and subacute meningitis. Continuum (Minneapolis, Minn). 2012;18(6 Infectious Disease):1290–318.
7. Charlson ME, Pompei P, Ales KL, MacKenzie CR. A new method of classifying prognostic comorbidity in longitudinal studies: development and validation. J Chronic Dis. 1987;40(5):373–83.
8. Tumani H, Jobs C, Brettschneider J, Hoppner AC, Kerling F, Fauser S. Effect of epileptic seizures on the cerebrospinal fluid–a systematic retrospective analysis. Epilepsy Res. 2015;114:23–31.
9. Gradel KO, Nielsen SL, Pedersen C, Knudsen JD, Ostergaard C, Arpi M, Jensen TG, Kolmos HJ, Sogaard M, Lassen AT, et al. Low completeness of bacteraemia registration in the Danish National Patient Registry. PLoS One. 2015;10(6):e0131682.
10. Henriksen DP, Nielsen SL, Laursen CB, Hallas J, Pedersen C, Lassen AT. How well do discharge diagnoses identify hospitalised patients with community-acquired infections?–a validation study. PLoS One. 2014;9(3):e92891.
11. Segal BM. Neurosarcoidosis: diagnostic approaches and therapeutic strategies. Curr Opin Neurol. 2013;26(3):307–13.
12. Lo Monaco A, La Corte R, Caniatti L, Borrelli M, Trotta F. Neurological involvement in north Italian patients with Behcet disease. Rheumatol Int. 2006;26(12):1113–9.
13. Kawai M, Hirohata S. Cerebrospinal fluid beta(2)-microglobulin in neuro-Behcet's syndrome. J Neurol Sci. 2000;179(S 1–2):132–9.
14. Irani DN. Aseptic meningitis and viral myelitis. Neurol Clin. 2008;26(3): 635–55. vii-viii
15. Bremell D, Hagberg L. Clinical characteristics and cerebrospinal fluid parameters in patients with peripheral facial palsy caused by Lyme neuroborreliosis compared with facial palsy of unknown origin (Bell's palsy). BMC Infect Dis. 2011;11:215.
16. Chamberlain MC, Glantz MJ. Cerebrospinal fluid-disseminated meningioma. Cancer. 2005;103(7):1427–30.

Permissions

The contributors of this book come from diverse backgrounds, making this book a truly international effort. This book will bring forth new frontiers with its revolutionizing research information and detailed analysis of the nascent developments around the world.

We would like to thank all the contributing authors for lending their expertise to make the book truly unique. They have played a crucial role in the development of this book. Without their invaluable contributions this book wouldn't have been possible. They have made vital efforts to compile up to date information on the varied aspects of this subject to make this book a valuable addition to the collection of many professionals and students.

This book was conceptualized with the vision of imparting up-to-date information and advanced data in this field. To ensure the same, a matchless editorial board was set up. Every individual on the board went through rigorous rounds of assessment to prove their worth. After which they invested a large part of their time researching and compiling the most relevant data for our readers.

The editorial board has been involved in producing this book since its inception. They have spent rigorous hours researching and exploring the diverse topics which have resulted in the successful publishing of this book. They have passed on their knowledge of decades through this book. To expedite this challenging task, the publisher supported the team at every step. A small team of assistant editors was also appointed to further simplify the editing procedure and attain best results for the readers.

Apart from the editorial board, the designing team has also invested a significant amount of their time in understanding the subject and creating the most relevant covers. They scrutinized every image to scout for the most suitable representation of the subject and create an appropriate cover for the book.

The publishing team has been an ardent support to the editorial, designing and production team. Their endless efforts to recruit the best for this project, has resulted in the accomplishment of this book. They are a veteran in the field of academics and their pool of knowledge is as vast as their experience in printing. Their expertise and guidance has proved useful at every step. Their uncompromising quality standards have made this book an exceptional effort. Their encouragement from time to time has been an inspiration for everyone.

The publisher and the editorial board hope that this book will prove to be a valuable piece of knowledge for researchers, students, practitioners and scholars across the globe.

List of Contributors

Tom Were
Department of Clinical Medicine, University of Kabianga, Kericho, Kenya

Jesca O Wesongah
Department of Medical Laboratory Sciences, Jomo Kenyatta University of Agriculture and Technology, Juja, Kenya

Elly Munde and Collins Ouma
Department of Biomedical Sciences and Technology, Maseno University, Maseno, Kenya

Titus M Kahiga
Department of Pharmacy and Complementary Medicine, Kenyatta University, Nairobi, Kenya

Francisca Ongecha-Owuor
Department of Medicine, Therapeutics, Dermatology and Psychiatry, Kenyatta University, Nairobi, Kenya

James N Kiarie
Department of Obstetrics and Gynaecology, University of Nairobi, Nairobi, Kenya

Aabid A Ahmed
Bomu Hospital, Mombasa, Kenya

Ernest P Makokha
Centre for Virus Research, Kenya Medical Research Institute, Nairobi, Kenya

Valentine Budambula
Department of Environment and Health Sciences, Technical University of Mombasa, Mombasa, Kenya

Clarissa N. Amaya and Brad A. Bryan
Department of Biomedical Sciences, Paul L. Foster School of Medicine, Texas Tech University Health Sciences Center, El Paso, TX, USA

Janneke A Cox
Department of Clinical Sciences, Institute of Tropical Medicine, Nationalestraat 155, 2000 Antwerpen, Belgium
Infectious Diseases Institute, Makerere University College of Health Sciences, Kampala, Uganda

Robert Colebunders
Department of Clinical Sciences, Institute of Tropical Medicine, Nationalestraat 155, 2000 Antwerpen, Belgium
Faculty of Medicine, University of Antwerp, Antwerp, Belgium

Yukari C Manabe
Infectious Diseases Institute, Makerere University College of Health Sciences, Kampala, Uganda
Division of Infectious Diseases, Department of Medicine, Johns Hopkins University School of Medicine, Baltimore, Maryland

Robert L Lukande and Asafu Munema
Department of Pathology, College of Health Sciences, Makerere University, Kampala, Uganda

Sam Kalungi
Department of Pathology, College of Health Sciences, Makerere University, Kampala, Uganda
Department of Pathology, Mulago Hospital Complex, Kampala, Uganda

Koen Van de Vijver
Department of Diagnostic Oncology and Molecular Pathology, Netherlands Cancer Institute - Antoni van Leeuwenhoek Hospital, Amsterdam, The Netherlands

Eric Van Marck
Department of Pathology, University Hospital Antwerp, University of Antwerp, Antwerp, Belgium

Ann M Nelson
Joint Pathology Center, Silver Spring, USA

Margareta Heby, Jakob Elebro, Björn Nodin, Karin Jirström and Jakob Eberhard
Department of Clinical Sciences Lund, Division of Oncology and Pathology, Lund University, Skåne University Hospital, 221 85 Lund, Sweden

Claudio A. Mastronardi and Gilberto Paz-Filho
Department of Genome Sciences, The John Curtin School of Medical Research, The Australian National University, 131 Garran Rd, Canberra, Acton ACT 2601, Australia

Belinda Whittle and Robert Tunningley
Australian Phenomics Facility, The Australian National University, 117 Garran Rd, Canberra, Acton ACT 2601, Australia

Teresa Neeman
Statistical Consulting Unit, The Australian National University, 27 Union Lane, Canberra, Acton ACT 2601, Australia

Raju SR Adduri, Viswakalyan Kotapalli and Murali Dharan Bashyam
1Laboratory of Molecular Oncology, Centre for DNA Fingerprinting and Diagnostics, Nampally, Hyderabad 500001, India

Neha A Gupta
Laboratory of Molecular Oncology, Centre for DNA Fingerprinting and Diagnostics, Nampally, Hyderabad 500001, India
Currently at National Centre for Cell Science, Ganeshkhind, Pune, India

Swarnalata Gowrishankar and Umanath K Nayak
Apollo Hospitals, Jubilee Hills, Hyderabad, India

Mukta Srinivasulu and Mohammed Mujtaba Ali
MNJ Institute of Oncology and Regional Cancer Centre, Red Hills, Hyderabad, India

Subramanyeshwar Rao
MNJ Institute of Oncology and Regional Cancer Centre, Red Hills, Hyderabad, India
Currently at Basavatarakam Indo American Cancer Hospital and Research Institute, Hyderabad, India

Shantveer G Uppin
Nizam's Institute of Medical Sciences, Punjagutta, Hyderabad, India

Snehalatha Dhagam and Mohana Vamsy Chigurupati
Omega Hospitals, Jubilee Hills, Hyderabad, India

Michael Majores, Anne Schindler, Angela Fuchs, Johannes Stein and Glen Kristiansen
Institute of Pathology, University of Bonn, Sigmund-Freud-Str. 25, D-53127 Bonn, Germany

Lukas Heukamp
New Pathology, Cologne, Germany

Peter Altevogt
Skin Cancer Unit, German Cancer Research Center (DKFZ), Heidelberg, Germany
Department of Dermatology, Venereology and Allergology University Medical Center Mannheim, Ruprecht-Karl University of Heidelberg, Mannheim, Germany

Ru-Xin Melanie Foong, Osvaldo Borrelli, Eleni Volonaki, Robert Dziubak, Rosan Meyer and Mamoun Elawad
Paediatric Gastroenterology Department, Great Ormond Street Hospital, London WC1N 3JH, United Kingdom

Neil Shah
Paediatric Gastroenterology Department, Great Ormond Street Hospital, London WC1N 3JH, United Kingdom
Institute of Child Health/UCL, London WC1N 1EH, UK

Neil J. Sebire
Histopathology Department, Great Ormond Street Hospital, London, United Kingdom

Benjamin F. Ricciardi and Seth A. Jerabek
Department of Orthopedic Surgery, Hospital for Special Surgery, New York, NY, USA

Allina A. Nocon
Healthcare Research Institute, Hospital for Special Surgery, New York, NY, USA

Gabrielle Wilner, Elianna Kaplowitz, Steven R. Goldring and P. Edward Purdue
Division of Research, Hospital for Special Surgery, New York, NY, USA

Giorgio Perino
Department of Pathology and Laboratory Medicine, Hospital for Special Surgery, 535 East 70th Street, New York, NY 10021, USA

Sanna Huovinen, Marita Laurila, Sinikka Porre, Mika Tirkkonen and Paula Kujala
Department of Pathology, Fimlab Laboratories, Tampere University Hospital, Tampere, Finland

Teemu T Tolonen
Department of Pathology, Fimlab Laboratories, Tampere University Hospital, Tampere, Finland
Department of Cancer Biology, Institute of Biomedical Technology, University of Tampere, Tampere, Finland

Jorma Isola
Department of Cancer Biology, Institute of Biomedical Technology, University of Tampere, Tampere, Finland

Antti Kaipia
Department of Surgery, Satakunta Hospital district, Pori, Finland
Department of Urology, Tampere University Hospital, Tampere, Finland

Laura Koivusalo
Department of Surgery, Satakunta Hospital district, Pori, Finland
Department of Materials Science, Tampere University of Technology, Tampere, Finland

Jarno Riikonen
Department of Urology, Tampere University Hospital, Tampere, Finland

Will W Minuth and Lucia Denk
Department of Molecular and Cellular Anatomy, University of Regensburg, University Street 31, D-93053 Regensburg, Germany

Mohamed Allaoui, Adil Boudhas, Mustapha Azzakhmam, Mohammed Boukhechba, Abderrahmane Al Bouzidi and Mohamed Oukabli
Department of Pathology, Military General Hospital Mohammed V, Mohammed V Souissi University - Faculty of Medicine and Pharmacy of Rabat, Hay Riad, Rabat 10000, Morocco

Ilias Benchafai
Department of Clinical Haematology, Military General Hospital Mohammed V, Mohammed V Souissi University - Faculty of Medicine and Pharmacy of Rabat, Hay Riad, Rabat 10000, Morocco

El Mehdi Mahtat and Safae Regragui
Department of Otorhinolaryngology, Military General Hospital Mohammed V, Mohammed V Souissi University - Faculty of Medicine and Pharmacy of Rabat, Hay Riad, Rabat 10000, Morocco

Mukesh Verma, Tram Kim Lam, Elizabeth Hebert and Rao L Divi
Epidemiology and Genomics Research Program, Division of Cancer Control and Population Sciences, National Cancer Institute, National Institutes of Health, Rockville, MD 20850, USA

Giorgio Perino
Department of Pathology, Hospital for Special Surgery, 535 East 70th Street, New York, NY 10021, USA

Benjamin F Ricciardi and Seth A Jerabek
Department of Orthopedic Surgery, Hospital for Special Surgery, New York, NY, USA

Guido Martignoni
Department of Pathology and Diagnostics, University of Verona, Verona and Pederzoli Hospital, Peschiera, Italy

Gabrielle Wilner, Dan Maass, Steven R Goldring and P Edward Purdue
Division of Research, Hospital for Special Surgery, New York, NY, USA

Bernard Seshie
Department of Surgery, Tema General Hospital, Tema, Ghana

Nii Armah Adu-Aryee, Florence Dedey and Joe-Nat Clegg-Lamptey
Department of Surgery, School of Medicine and Dentistry, University of Ghana, Accra, Ghana

Benedict Calys-Tagoe
Department of Community Health, School of Public Health, University of Ghana, Accra, Ghana

Davis R Ingram and Dina Chelouche Lev
Departments of Surgical Oncology, M.D. Anderson Cancer Center, University of Texas, 1515 Holcombe Blvd, Houston, TX, USA

Lloye M Dillon and Todd W Miller
Departments of Pharmacology and Toxicology, Norris Cotton Cancer Center, Geisel School of Medicine at Dartmouth, Dartmouth-Hitchcock Medical Center, One Medical Center Drive, HB-7936, Lebanon, NH 03756, USA

Alexander Lazar
Departments of Surgical Pathology, M.D. Anderson Cancer Center, University of Texas, 1515 Holcombe Blvd, Houston, TX, USA

Burton L Eisenberg
Departments of Surgery, Norris Cotton Cancer Center, Geisel School of Medicine at Dartmouth, Dartmouth-Hitchcock Medical Center, One Medical Center Dr, Lebanon, NH, USA

Elizabeth G Demicco
Department of Pathology, Mount Sinai Medical Center, One Gustave L. Levy Pl, New York, NY, USA

Bjørn Westre, Anita Giske and Hilde Guttormsen
Department of Pathology, Ålesund Hospital, Møre and Romsdal Health Trust, Ålesund, Norway

Sveinung Wergeland Sørbye
Department of Clinical Pathology, University Hospital of North Norway, 9038 Tromsø, Norway

Finn Egil Skjeldestad
Research Group Epidemiology of Chronic Diseases, Department of Community Medicine, UiT The Arctic University of Norway, Tromsø, Norway

Kenneth O. Inaku
Department of Chemical Pathology, Faculty of Medicine, College of Medical Sciences, University of Calabar, Calabar, Cross River State, Nigeria

Obasola O. Ogunkeye and Christian O. Isichei
Department of Chemical Pathology, Faculty of Medical Sciences, University of Jos, Jos, Plateau State, Nigeria

Fayeofori M. Abbiyesuku
Department of Chemical Pathology, Faculty of Medicine, University of Ibadan, Ibadan, Oyo State, Nigeria

Evelyn K. Chuhwak
Department of Internal Medicine, Faculty of Medical Sciences, University of Jos, Jos, Plateau State, Nigeria

Lucius C. Imoh, Noel O. Amadu and Alexander O. Abu
Department of Chemical Pathology, University of Jos Teaching Hospital, Jos, Plateau State, Nigeria

Nur Fatiha Norhisham, Choi Yen Chong and Sabreena Safuan
School of Health Sciences, Universiti Sains Malaysia, 16150 Kubang Kerian, Kelantan, Malaysia

M. Abdulla Al-Mamun
Department of Biotechnology, The University of Tokyo, Bunkyo-ku, Tokyo, Japan
Protein Science Lab, Department of Genetic Engineering and Biotechnology, University of Rajshahi, Rajshahi 6205, Bangladesh

M. Ataur Rahman, M. Habibur Rahman, K.M.F. Hoque, Z. Ferdousi, Mohammad Nurul Matin and M. Abu Reza
Protein Science Lab, Department of Genetic Engineering and Biotechnology, University of Rajshahi, Rajshahi 6205, Bangladesh

Akiko Uchida, Yasushi Isobe, Yu Uemura, Yuji Nishio, Hirotaka Sakai, Masayuki Kato and Ikuo Miura
Division of Hematology and Oncology, Department of Internal Medicine, St. Marianna University School of Medicine, 2-16-1 Sugao, Miyamae-ku, Kawasaki, Kanagawa 216-8511, Japan

Kaori Otsubo
Department of cytogenetics, SRL Diagnostics, Hachioji Laboratory, Tokyo, Japan

Masahiro Hoshikawa and Masayuki Takagi
Department of Pathology, St. Marianna University School of Medicine, Kawasaki, Japan

Francesco Vasuri, Alessio Degiovanni, Rodolfo Pini, Mauro Gargiulo, Andrea Stella and Gianandrea Pasquinelli
Department of Experimental, Diagnostic and Specialty Medicine (DIMES); S. Orsola-Malpighi Hospital, Bologna University, Via Massarenti 9, I 40139 Bologna, Italy

Silvia Fittipaldi
Department of Experimental, Diagnostic and Specialty Medicine (DIMES); S. Orsola-Malpighi Hospital, Bologna University, Via Massarenti 9, I 40139 Bologna, Italy
Laboratory in Metakaryotic Biology (LIMB), Department of Biological Engineering, Massachusetts Institute of Technology, Cambridge, MA, USA

William G. Thilly and Elena V. Gostjeva
Laboratory in Metakaryotic Biology (LIMB), Department of Biological Engineering, Massachusetts Institute of Technology, Cambridge, MA, USA

Alain Stricker-Krongrad, Catherine Shoemake, Miao Zhong, Jason Liu and Guy Bouchard
Sinclair Research Center, LLC, 562 State Rd. DD, Auxvasse, MO 65231, USA

Sveinung Wergeland Sørbye
Department of Clinical Pathology, University Hospital of North Norway, 9038 Tromsø, Norway

Pål Suhrke and Berit Wallem Revå
Department of Pathology, Vestfold Hospital, Tønsberg, Norway

Jannicke Berland
Jannicke Berland, Stavanger University Hospital, Stavanger, Norway

Ramona Johansen Maurseth and Khalid Al-Shibli
Nordlandssykehuset HF, Department of Pathology, Bodø, Norway

Boubacar Efared, Gabrielle Atsame-Ebang, Layla Tahiri, Ibrahim Sory Sidibé and Fatimazahra Erregad
Department of pathology, Hassan II university hospital, Fès, Morocco

Nawal Hammas, Hinde El Fatemi and Laila Chbani
Department of pathology, Hassan II university hospital, Fès, Morocco
Laboratory of biological and translational research, Faculty of pharmacology and medicine, Sidi Mohamed Ben Abdellah University, Fès, Morocco

Samia Arifi
Department of medical oncology, Hassan II university hospital, Fès, Morocco
Faculty of pharmacology and medicine, Sidi Mohamed Ben Abdellah University, Fès, Morocco

Ihsane Mellouki
Faculty of pharmacology and medicine, Sidi Mohamed Ben Abdellah University, Fès, Morocco

Department of hepatogastroenterology, Hassan II
university hospital, Fès, Morocco

Abdelmalek Ousadden and Khalid Mazaz
Faculty of pharmacology and medicine, Sidi Mohamed
Ben Abdellah University, Fès, Morocco
Department of general and visceral surgery, Hassan II
university hospital, Fès, Morocco

Stefan Haraldsson
Department of Gastroenterology, Copenhagen
University Hospital, Kettegaard Alle 29, DK-2650
Hvidovre, Denmark

Louise Klarskov
Department of Pathology, Herlev-Gentofte Hospital,
Herlev, Denmark

Mef Nilbert
Clinical Research Centre, HNPCC register, Copenhagen
University Hospital, Hvidovre, Denmark
Institute of Clinical Sciences, Division of Oncology,
Lund University, Lund, Sweden

Inge Bernstein
HNPCC register, Copenhagen University Hospital,
Hvidovre, Denmark
Department of Surgical Gastroenterology, Aalborg
University Hospital, Aalborg, Denmark

Jesper Bonde
Department of Pathology and Clinical Research Center,
Copenhagen University Hospital, Hvidovre, Denmark

Susanne Holck
Department of Pathology, Copenhagen University
Hospital, Hvidovre, Denmark

**Sarah M. Heaton, Kevin Downing, Bryan Keenan
and Justin Wells**
Department of Pathology, Walter Reed National
Military Medical Center, 8901 Wisconsin Avenue,
Bethesda, MD 20814, USA

Amy C. Weintrob
Department of Pathology, Walter Reed National
Military Medical Center, 8901 Wisconsin Avenue,
Bethesda, MD 20814, USA
Infectious Disease Clinical Research Program,
Department of Preventive Medicine and Biostatistics,
Uniformed Services University of the Health Sciences,
Bethesda, MD, USA
The Henry M. Jackson Foundation for the Advancement
of Military Medicine, Inc., Bethesda, MD, USA

David R. Tribble
Infectious Disease Clinical Research Program,
Department of Preventive Medicine and Biostatistics,
Uniformed Services University of the Health Sciences,
Bethesda, MD, USA

Deepak Aggarwal and Faraz Shaikh
Infectious Disease Clinical Research Program,
Department of Preventive Medicine and Biostatistics,
Uniformed Services University of the Health Sciences,
Bethesda, MD, USA
The Henry M. Jackson Foundation for the Advancement
of Military Medicine, Inc., Bethesda, MD, USA

G. Perino and D. Ramirez
Department of Pathology and Laboratory Medicine,
Hospital for Special Surgery, 535 E 70th Street, New
York, NY 10023, USA

S. Sunitsch
Medizinische Universität Graz, Institut für Pathologie,
Graz, Austria

M. Huber
Pathologisch-bakteriologisches Institut, Otto Wagner
Spital, Wien, Austria

J. Gallo
Department of Orthopaedics, Faculty of Medicine and
Dentistry, University Hospital, Palacky University
Olomouc, Olomouc, Czech Republic

J. Vaculova
Department of Pathology, Fakultni Nemocnice Ostrava,
Ostrava, Czech Republic

S. Natu
Department of Pathology, University hospital of North
Tees and Hartlepool NHS Foundation Trust, Stockton-
on-Tees, UK

J. P. Kretzer
Labor für Biomechanik und Implantat-Forschung,
Klinik für Orthopädie und Unfallchirurgie,
Universitätsklinikum Heidelberg, Heidelberg,
Germany

S. Müller and V. Krenn
MVZ-Zentrum für Histologie, Zytologie und
Molekulare Diagnostik, Trier, Germany

P. Thomas
LMU Klinik, Klinik und Poliklinik für Dermatologie
und Allergologie, Munich, Germany

M. Thomsen
Baden-Baden Klinik, Baden-Baden, Germany

M. G. Krukemeyer
Paracelsus-Kliniken Deutschland Gmbh, Osnabrück, Germany

H. Resch
Universitätsklinik für Unfallchirurgie und Sporttraumatologie, Salzburg, Austria

T. Hügle
Hôpital Orthopédique, Lausanne, Switzerland

W. Waldstein
Medizinische Universität Wien, AKH-Wien, Universitätsklinik für Orthopädie, Wien, Austria

F. Böettner
Adult Reconstruction and Joint Replacement Division, Hospital for Special Surgery, New York, NY, USA

T. Gehrke
Helios Endo-Klinik, Hamburg, Germany

S. Sesselmann
Orthopädische Universitätsklinik Erlangen, Erlangen, Germany

W. Rüther
Klinik und Poliklinik für Orthopädie, Universitätsklinikum Hamburg-Eppendorf, Hamburg, Germany

Z. Xia
Centre for Nanohealth, Swansea University Medical School, Singleton Park, Swansea, UK

E. Purdue
Hospital for Special Surgery, Research Institute, New York, NY, USA

Anne Ahrens Østergaard
Department of Infectious Diseases, Odense University Hospital, Odense, Denmark

Åse Bengård Andersen
Department of Infectious Diseases, Odense University Hospital, Odense, Denmark
University of Southern Denmark, Odense, Denmark
Department of Infectious Diseases 8632, Copenhagen University Hospital Rigshospitalet, Blegdamsvej 9, DK 2100 Copenhagen OE, Denmark

Thomas Vognbjerg Sydenham
Department of Clinical Microbiology, Odense University Hospital, Odense, Denmark

Mads Nybo
Department of Clinical Biochemistry and Pharmacology, Odense University Hospital, Odense, Denmark
University of Southern Denmark, Odense, Denmark

Index

www.ingramcontent.com/pod-product-compliance
Lightning Source LLC
Chambersburg PA
CBHW080458200326
41458CB00012B/4016